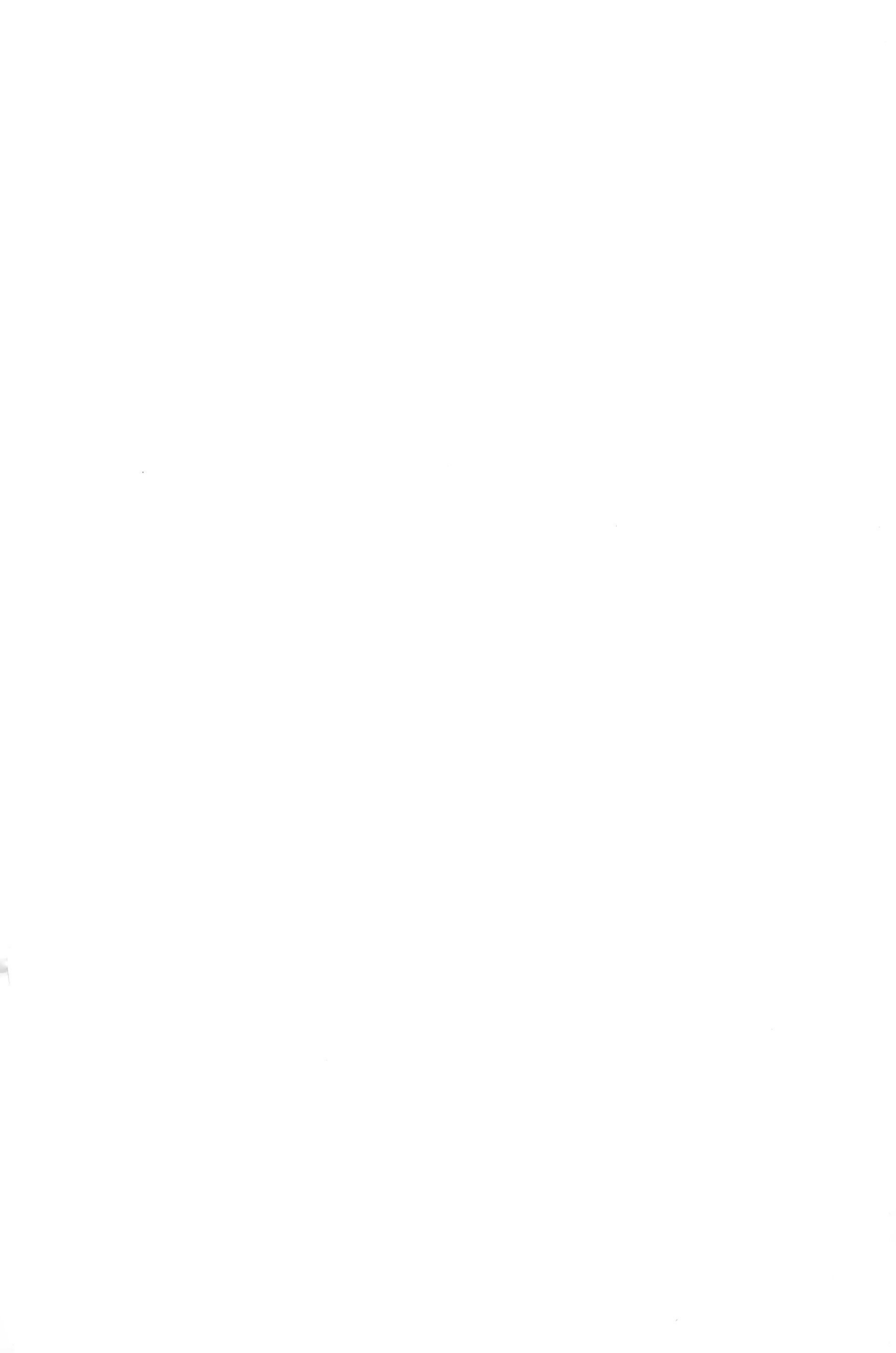

Photocatalytic Materials and Photocatalytic Reactions

Photocatalytic Materials and Photocatalytic Reactions

Guest Editor
Sugang Meng

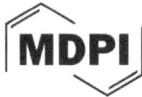

Basel • Beijing • Wuhan • Barcelona • Belgrade • Novi Sad • Cluj • Manchester

Guest Editor
Sugang Meng
College of Chemistry and
Materials Science
Huaibei Normal University
Huaibei
China

Editorial Office
MDPI AG
Grosspeteranlage 5
4052 Basel, Switzerland

This is a reprint of the Special Issue, published open access by the journal *Molecules* (ISSN 1420-3049), freely accessible at: https://www.mdpi.com/journal/molecules/special_issues/87U2U4T532.

For citation purposes, cite each article independently as indicated on the article page online and as indicated below:

Lastname, A.A.; Lastname, B.B. Article Title. *Journal Name* **Year**, *Volume Number*, Page Range.

ISBN 978-3-7258-3233-0 (Hbk)
ISBN 978-3-7258-3234-7 (PDF)
https://doi.org/10.3390/books978-3-7258-3234-7

© 2025 by the authors. Articles in this book are Open Access and distributed under the Creative Commons Attribution (CC BY) license. The book as a whole is distributed by MDPI under the terms and conditions of the Creative Commons Attribution-NonCommercial-NoDerivs (CC BY-NC-ND) license (https://creativecommons.org/licenses/by-nc-nd/4.0/).

Contents

About the Editor ix

Sugang Meng
Photocatalytic Materials and Photocatalytic Reactions
Reprinted from: *Molecules* 2025, 30, 269, https://doi.org/10.3390/molecules30020269 1

Jun Wang, Shuang Fu, Peng Hou, Jun Liu, Chao Li, Hongguang Zhang and Guowei Wang
Construction of TiO_2/CuPc Heterojunctions for the Efficient Photocatalytic Reduction of CO_2 with Water
Reprinted from: *Molecules* 2024, 29, 1899, https://doi.org/10.3390/molecules29081899 9

Zisheng Du, Kexin Gong, Zhiruo Yu, Yang Yang, Peixian Wang, Xiuzhen Zheng, et al.
Photoredox Coupling of CO_2 Reduction with Benzyl Alcohol Oxidation over Ternary Metal Chalcogenides ($Zn_mIn_2S_{3+m}$, m = 1–5) with Regulable Products Selectivity
Reprinted from: *Molecules* 2023, 28, 6553, https://doi.org/10.3390/molecules28186553 21

Iwona Pełech, Piotr Staciwa, Daniel Sibera, Konrad Sebastian Sobczuk, Wiktoria Majewska, Ewelina Kusiak-Nejman, et al.
The Influence of Heat Treatment on the Photoactivity of Amine-Modified Titanium Dioxide in the Reduction of Carbon Dioxide
Reprinted from: *Molecules* 2024, 29, 4348, https://doi.org/10.3390/molecules29184348 34

Baihua Long, Hongmei He, Yang Yu, Wenwen Cai, Quan Gu, Jing Yang and Sugang Meng
Bifunctional Hot Water Vapor Template-Mediated Synthesis of Nanostructured Polymeric Carbon Nitride for Efficient Hydrogen Evolution
Reprinted from: *Molecules* 2023, 28, 4862, https://doi.org/10.3390/molecules28124862 51

Ligang Ma, Wenjun Jiang, Chao Lin, Le Xu, Tianyu Zhu and Xiaoqian Ai
CdS Deposited In Situ on g-C_3N_4 via a Modified Chemical Bath Deposition Method to Improve Photocatalytic Hydrogen Production
Reprinted from: *Molecules* 2023, 28, 7846, https://doi.org/10.3390/molecules28237846 67

Minghao Zhang, Xiaoqun Wu, Xiaoyuan Liu, Huixin Li, Ying Wang and Debao Wang
Constructing In_2S_3/CdS/N-rGO Hybrid Nanosheets via One-Pot Pyrolysis for Boosting and Stabilizing Visible Light-Driven Hydrogen Evolution
Reprinted from: *Molecules* 2023, 28, 7878, https://doi.org/10.3390/molecules28237878 81

Keliang Wu, Yuhang Shang, Huazhen Li, Pengcheng Wu, Shuyi Li, Hongyong Ye, et al.
Synthesis and Hydrogen Production Performance of MoP/a-TiO_2/Co-$ZnIn_2S_4$ Flower-like Composite Photocatalysts
Reprinted from: *Molecules* 2023, 28, 4350, https://doi.org/10.3390/molecules28114350 94

Yonghui Wu, Zhipeng Wang, Yuqing Yan, Yu Wei, Jun Wang, Yunsheng Shen, et al.
Rational Photodeposition of Cobalt Phosphate on Flower-like $ZnIn_2S_4$ for Efficient Photocatalytic Hydrogen Evolution
Reprinted from: *Molecules* 2024, 29, 465, https://doi.org/10.3390/molecules29020465 110

Nicolás Sacco, Alexander Iguini, Ilaria Gamba, Fernanda Albana Marchesini and Gonzalo García
Pd:In-Doped TiO_2 as a Bifunctional Catalyst for the Photoelectrochemical Oxidation of Paracetamol and Simultaneous Green Hydrogen Production
Reprinted from: *Molecules* 2024, 29, 1073, https://doi.org/10.3390/molecules29051073 123

Shibing Chu and Qiuyu Gao
Unveiling the Low-Lying Spin States of [Fe$_3$S$_4$] Clusters via the Extended Broken-Symmetry Method
Reprinted from: *Molecules* **2024**, *29*, 2152, https://doi.org/10.3390/molecules29092152 . . . . . . **138**

Chuanfu Shan, Ziqian Su, Ziyi Liu, Ruizheng Xu, Jianfeng Wen, Guanghui Hu, et al.
One-Step Synthesis of Ag$_2$O/Fe$_3$O$_4$ Magnetic Photocatalyst for Efficient Organic Pollutant Removal via Wide-Spectral-Response Photocatalysis–Fenton Coupling
Reprinted from: *Molecules* **2023**, *28*, 4155, https://doi.org/10.3390/molecules28104155 . . . . . . **149**

Hongfei Shi, Haoshen Wang, Enji Zhang, Xiaoshu Qu, Jianping Li, Sisi Zhao, et al.
Boosted Photocatalytic Performance for Antibiotics Removal with Ag/PW$_{12}$/TiO$_2$ Composite: Degradation Pathways and Toxicity Assessment
Reprinted from: *Molecules* **2023**, *28*, 6831, https://doi.org/10.3390/molecules28196831 . . . . . . **166**

Yixiao Dan, Jialiang Xu, Jian Jian, Lingxi Meng, Pei Deng, Jiaqi Yan, et al.
In Situ Decoration of Bi$_2$S$_3$ Nanosheets on Zinc Oxide/Cellulose Acetate Composite Films for Photodegradation of Dyes under Visible Light Irradiation
Reprinted from: *Molecules* **2023**, *28*, 6882, https://doi.org/10.3390/molecules28196882 . . . . . . **187**

Muhammad Irfan, Noor Tahir, Muhammad Zahid, Saima Noreen, Muhammad Yaseen, Muhammad Shahbaz, et al.
The Fabrication of Halogen-Doped FeWO$_4$ Heterostructure Anchored over Graphene Oxide Nanosheets for the Sunlight-Driven Photocatalytic Degradation of Methylene Blue Dye
Reprinted from: *Molecules* **2023**, *28*, 7022, https://doi.org/10.3390/molecules28207022 . . . . . . **201**

Xuejiao Wang, Shuyuan Liu, Shu Lin, Kezhen Qi, Ya Yan and Yuhua Ma
Visible Light Motivated the Photocatalytic Degradation of P-Nitrophenol by Ca^{2+}-Doped AgInS$_2$
Reprinted from: *Molecules* **2024**, *29*, 361, https://doi.org/10.3390/molecules29020361 . . . . . . **220**

Jing Chen, Minghua Yang, Hongjiao Zhang, Yuxin Chen, Yujie Ji, Ruohan Yu and Zhenguo Liu
Boosting the Activation of Molecular Oxygen and the Degradation of Rhodamine B in Polar-Functional-Group-Modified g-C$_3$N$_4$
Reprinted from: *Molecules* **2024**, *29*, 3836, https://doi.org/10.3390/molecules29163836 . . . . . . **236**

Maria-Anna Gatou, Natalia Bovali, Nefeli Lagopati and Evangelia A. Pavlatou
MgO Nanoparticles as a Promising Photocatalyst towards Rhodamine B and Rhodamine 6G Degradation
Reprinted from: *Molecules* **2024**, *29*, 4299, https://doi.org/10.3390/molecules29184299 . . . . . . **250**

Chunmei Tian, Huijuan Yu, Ruiqi Zhai, Jing Zhang, Cuiping Gao, Kezhen Qi, et al.
Visible Light Photoactivity of g-C$_3$N$_4$/MoS$_2$ Nanocomposites for Water Remediation of Hexavalent Chromium
Reprinted from: *Molecules* **2024**, *29*, 637, https://doi.org/10.3390/molecules29030637 . . . . . . **278**

Ran Ding, Liang Li, Ya-Ting Yu, Bing Zhang and Pei-Long Wang
Photoredox-Catalyzed Synthesis of 3-Sulfonylated Pyrrolin-2-ones via a Regioselective Tandem Sulfonylation Cyclization of 1,5-Dienes
Reprinted from: *Molecules* **2023**, *28*, 5473, https://doi.org/10.3390/molecules28145473 . . . . . . **293**

Xin He, Yanan Wu, Jia Luo, Xianglin Dai, Jun Song and Yong Tang
First-Principles Study on Janus-Structured Sc$_2$CX$_2$/Sc$_2$CY$_2$ (X, Y = F, Cl, Br) Heterostructures for Solar Energy Conversion
Reprinted from: *Molecules* **2024**, *29*, 2898, https://doi.org/10.3390/molecules29122898 . . . . . . **307**

Meng-Yao Dai, Xu-Cai Zhao, Bo-Cheng Lei, Yi-Neng Huang, Li-Li Zhang, Hai Guo and Hua-Gui Wang
First Principle Study on the Z-Type Characteristic Modulation of GaN/g-C$_3$N$_4$ Heterojunction
Reprinted from: *Molecules* **2024**, *29*, 5355, https://doi.org/10.3390/molecules29225355 . . . . . . **323**

Angie V. Lasso-Escobar, Elkin Darío C. Castrillon, Jorge Acosta, Sandra Navarro, Estefanía Correa-Penagos, John Rojas and Yenny P. Ávila-Torres
Modulation of Electronic Availability in g-C$_3$N$_4$ Using Nickel (II), Manganese (II), and Copper (II) to Enhance the Disinfection and Photocatalytic Properties
Reprinted from: *Molecules* **2024**, *29*, 3775, https://doi.org/10.3390/molecules29163775 . . . . . . **337**

Fatemeh Abshari, Moritz Paulsen, Salih Veziroglu, Alexander Vahl and Martina Gerken
Mimicking Axon Growth and Pruning by Photocatalytic Growth and Chemical Dissolution of Gold on Titanium Dioxide Patterns
Reprinted from: *Molecules* **2025**, *30*, 99, https://doi.org/10.3390/molecules30010099 . . . . **356**

About the Editor

Sugang Meng

Sugang Meng is currently a full professor and leading researcher at Huaibei Normal University. He received his PhD degree from the Fuzhou University in 2013, under the supervision of Prof. Xianzhi Fu. From 2020 to 2021, he was a visiting scholar in Prof. Yi Xie's group at the University of Science and Technology of China. He has been honored with several awards within the Anhui Province, China, including TOYP (2022), Outstanding Young Postgraduate Tutor (2022), and the Natural Science and Technology Award (2019). He is currently an Editorial Member of the *Chinese Journal of Rare Metals*, a Young Scientist Committee Member of *Advanced Powder Materials*, a Guest Editor of *ChemSusChem, ChemNanoMat, ChemPhotoChem, ChemPhysChem, Molecules, Microstructures and Chemical Synthesis*, and an Editorial Board Member of *Colloid and Surface Science, Frontiers in Catalysis*, and *Modern Chemical Research*. He has successfully completed a project for the National Natural Science Foundation of China (NSFC), as well as 12 other projects. He has published >100 papers in various SCI journals. His current research is focused on the design and synthesis of low-dimensional nanostructured materials for photocatalysis and photo/thermalcatalysis.

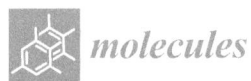

Editorial

Photocatalytic Materials and Photocatalytic Reactions

Sugang Meng [1,2]

[1] Key Laboratory of Green and Precise Synthetic Chemistry and Applications, Ministry of Education, College of Chemistry and Materials Science, Huaibei Normal University, Huaibei 235000, China; mengsugang@126.com

[2] Anhui Provincial Key Laboratory of Synthetic Chemistry and Applications, College of Chemistry and Materials Science, Huaibei Normal University, Huaibei 235000, China

1. Introduction

This Special Issue, titled "Photocatalytic Materials and Photocatalytic Reactions", focuses on designing advanced photocatalysts, understanding their structure-dependent properties, and seeking to exploit them in the fields of energy conversion, pollutant degradation, artificial photosynthesis, organic synthesis, etc. As early as 1912, in the age of coal, Giacomo Ciamician [1] proposed the theory that photochemistry could be a potential and promising strategy to realize the harmonious development of human society and nature. However, the pioneering work on photosynthesis was a study on photo-electrochemically water splitting, published in 1972 by Fujishima and Honda [2]. Throughout the next few years, photocatalysis was mainly studied in regard to the degradation of toxic compounds. In recent decades, photocatalysis has attracted extensive and ongoing attention, because it exhibits great potential for applications in artificial photosynthesis, including H_2 production and CO_2 reduction, organic synthesis, pollutant degradation, N_2 fixation, precious metal recovery, H_2O_2 photosynthesis, life science and medical research, space exploration, and other related fields (Figure 1) [3–9]. Meanwhile, photocatalysts have evolved from inorganic substances to new nanomaterials such as graphitic carbon nitride (g-C_3N_4), polymers, piezoelectric materials, ferroelectric materials, metal–organic frameworks (MOFs), covalent organic frameworks (COFs), single-atom catalysts (SACs), high-entropy alloys (HEAs), supramolecules, superlattices, topological insulators, localized surface plasmon resonance (LSPR), and diverse composite materials/heterojunctions, among other things (Figure 2) [6–16].

Our search results indicated a recent boom in photocatalysis research (Figure 3). About 243,000 studies on this topic have been published in the last 25 years. A total of 146 research areas and 212 countries/regions are involved. Photocatalysis is notable because it is driven by inexhaustible solar energy under mild reaction conditions. The design of advanced photocatalytic materials with good performance and the exploration of green photocatalytic reactions with carbon neutrality are significant for sustainability.

This Special Issue contains 23 original research articles related to photocatalytic materials, including metal oxides, metal sulfides, metal nitrides, metallo-organic compounds, g-C_3N_4, clusters, LSPR, and heterojunction/composite materials. Their applications included H_2 production, CO_2 reduction, organic synthesis, environmental remediation, disinfection, toxicity, and dual-function photoredox reactions.

Received: 30 December 2024
Revised: 6 January 2025
Accepted: 9 January 2025
Published: 11 January 2025

Citation: Meng, S. Photocatalytic Materials and Photocatalytic Reactions. *Molecules* **2025**, *30*, 269. https://doi.org/10.3390/molecules30020269

Copyright: © 2025 by the author. Licensee MDPI, Basel, Switzerland. This article is an open access article distributed under the terms and conditions of the Creative Commons Attribution (CC BY) license (https://creativecommons.org/licenses/by/4.0/).

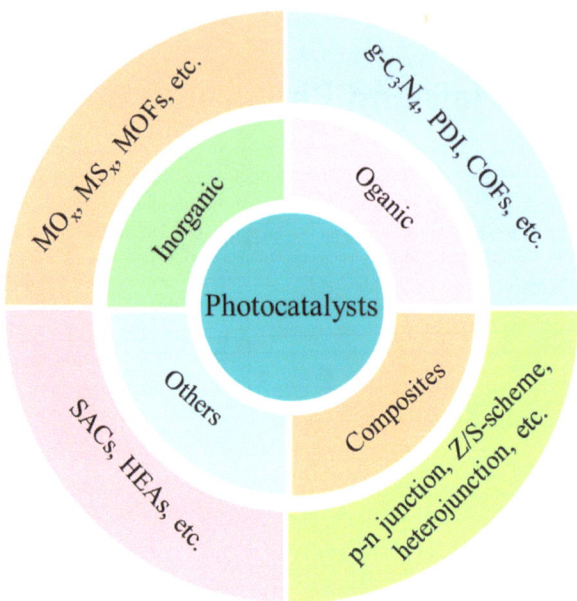

Figure 1. The types of materials explored for use as potential photocatalysts.

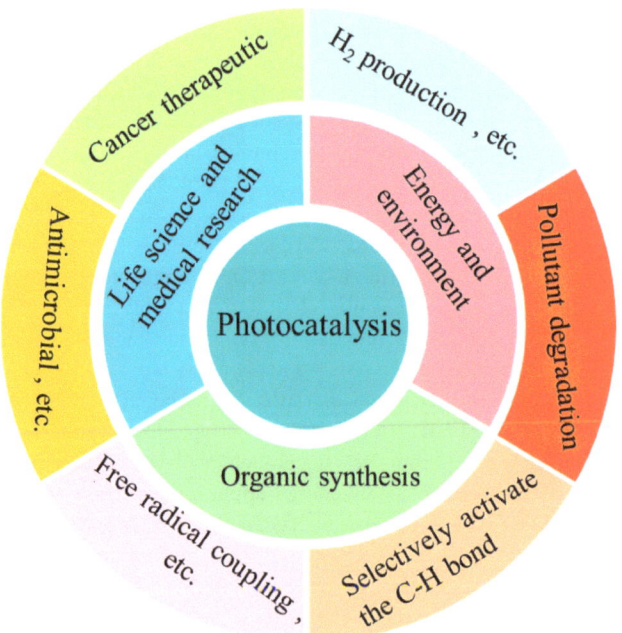

Figure 2. Various photocatalytic reactions.

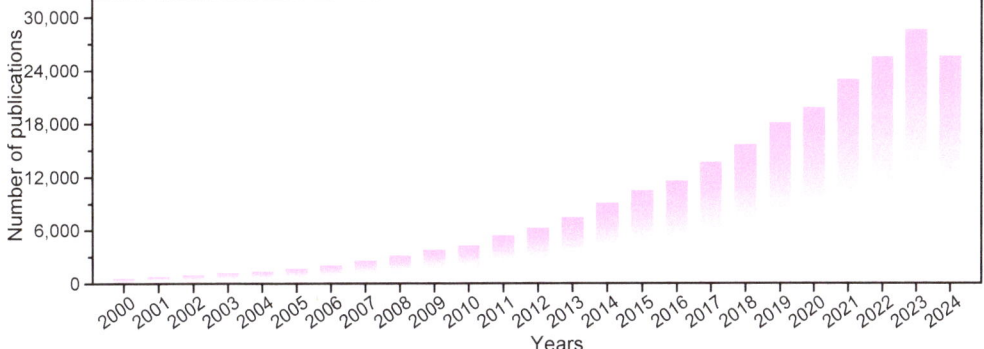

Figure 3. The number of annual journal publications that covered "photocatalysts*" as a subject prior to 9 December 2024, as recorded in the Web of Science database.

2. An Overview of the Published Articles

In the Special Issue's first contribution, Li et al. synthesized a new magnetic nanocomposite, Ag_2O/Fe_3O_4, to achieve the photocatalytic degradation of methyl orange (MO) under visible light irradiation. They observed that 99.5% of MO could be degraded by the Ag_2O/Fe_3O_4 (10%) photocatalyst within 15 min. In addition, the designed Ag_2O/Fe_3O_4 photocatalyst also exhibited broad applicability and stability. Their work demonstrated successful photocatalysis–Fenton coupling and overcame the challenges involved in a difficult catalyst recovery process and regarding low photocatalytic efficiency.

Next, in the study by Wang et al. (Contribution 2), a multicomponent composite $MoP/a\text{-}TiO_2/Co\text{-}ZnIn_2S_4$ was prepared through multiple hydrothermal processes. The effects of Co dopants, i.e., amorphous TiO_2 and MoP, increased visible light absorption, improving the separation of photoexcited charge carriers via heterojunction and hydrogen production sites, respectively. Thus, the high efficiency of photocatalytic H_2 production was realized on $MoP/a\text{-}TiO_2/Co\text{-}ZnIn_2S_4$. Compared to the pristine $ZnIn_2S_4$, the H_2 production of $MoP/a\text{-}TiO_2/Co\text{-}ZnIn_2S_4$ was enhanced by about three times.

Furthermore, in the research work by Meng et al. (Contribution 3), nanostructured polymeric carbon nitride ($g\text{-}C_3N_4$, PCN) was synthesized using a one-step thermal polymerization process with the assistance of hot water vapor. Vapor has a dual function used to prepare nanostructured PCN: besides being a green etching reagent, it can act as a gas bubble template. Moreover, reaction times, temperatures, mechanisms were also studied in the precursors of PCN. The H_2 production of nanostructured PCN increased by about four times in contrast to bulk PCN. This study offers a new and versatile strategy for fabricating nanostructured $g\text{-}C_3N_4$ with high photocatalytic performance.

Wang et al. (Contribution 4) outlined a visible light-induced regioselective cascade and the sulfonylation–cyclization of a cascade of 1,5-dienes under mild conditions. An array of 3-sulfonylated pyrrolin-2-one derivatives was constructed through lower catalyst loading and achieved good to excellent yields at room temperature. Importantly, this protocol can be used in large-scale synthesis.

Meanwhile, in the research paper by Meng et al. (Contribution 5), a series of $Zn_mIn_2S_{3+m}$ photocatalysts (m = 1, 2, 3, 4 and 5) was prepared and applied in dual-function photoredox reactions: the selective oxidation of alcohols and the reduction of CO_2 in one reaction system. In $Zn_5In_2S_8$, $Zn_4In_2S_7$, $Zn_3In_2S_6$, $Zn_2In_2S_5$, and $ZnIn_2S_4$, structures and properties was studied using experiments and theoretical calculation. The morphology, light absorption, and band structures were tuned by changing the Zn/In molar ratio. Moreover, the selectivity of gas products (H_2 and CO) and liquid products (hydrobenzoin and benzaldehyde) could also be regulated.

In the research work by Chen et al. (Contribution 6), Ag/PW12/TiO_2 composed of TiO_2, polyoxometalates (POMs) [$H_3PW_{12}O_{40}$] (PW12), and Ag nanoparticles was fabricated through successive electrospinning and photoreduction processes. Ag/PW12/TiO_2 exhibited high degradation efficiencies for methyl orange (MO, 99.29%), enrofloxacin (ENR, 93.65%), and tetracycline (TC, 78.19%). Moreover, for TC degradation and TC concentration, the Ag/PW12/TiO_2 dosage, the pH of the TC solution, and the intermediates and toxicities of the products were also investigated in detail.

Furthermore, in the study by Zhou et al. (Contribution 7), the Bi_2S_3-ZnO/CA film was fabricated by assembling Bi_2S_3, ZnO, and cellulose acetate (CA). In the Bi_2S_3-ZnO/CA film, the addition of Bi_2S_3 improved cavity density and uniformity. On the other hand, the addition of ZnO enabled the formation of heterojunctions with Bi_2S_3 to promote the separation and migration of photogenerated electron–hole pairs, thus improving the photocatalytic activity and stability of Bi_2S_3. This is evidenced by the fact that the RhB (rhodamine B) degradation efficiencies of ZnO/CA, 4Bi2S3/CA, and 4Bi_2S_3-ZnO/CA were about 26.51%, 50.26%, and 90.2%, respectively.

Shahid et al. (Contribution 8) prepared a 2D I-$FeWO_4$/GO composite photocatalyst by combining halogen-doped $FeWO_4$ (I-$FeWO_4$) and graphene oxide (GO). In the designed I-$FeWO_4$/GO composite, GO acted as a supporter, halogen facilitated H_2O_2 production, and the interface of the I-$FeWO_4$/GO heterostructure promoted charge separation and migration. Thus, the I-$FeWO_4$ displayed good photocatalytic performance for the degradation of methylene blue (MB). Under sunlight irradiation for 120 min, 97.0% of MB could be degraded by the I-$FeWO_4$.

Furthermore, Ai et al. (Contribution 9) fabricated 2D heterojunction g-C_3N_4@CdS using a water bath method. Interestingly, tiny CdS nanorods were grown in situ in the gaps between the 2D g-C_3N_4 nanosheets. Due to the band-band transfer mechanism of the g-C_3N_4@CdS photocatalyst, the charge carriers could be separated efficiently, and thus excellent H_2 production with the assistance of visible light and lactic acid was observed. The H2 production rate of G-CdS-3 could reach up to 1611.4 $\mu mol \cdot g^{-1} \cdot h^{-1}$, which was about 10 times that of CdS and 76 times that of g-C_3N_4.

In the research work by Wang et al. (Contribution 10), a 2D–3D hybrid junction In_2S_3/CdS/N-rGO was synthesized using a one-step pyrolysis method. The rational 2D–3D In_2S_3/CdS/N-rGO hybrid junctions not only provided more active sites but also formed multiple tight interfaces, which facilitated charge separation and migration. Thus, a high H_2 evolution rate (10.9 $mmol \cdot g^{-1} \cdot h^{-1}$) could be obtained with the assistance of visible light and Na_2S/Na_2SO_3 aqueous solution.

To remove high levels of toxic 4-nitrophenol (4-NP), Ma et al. (Contribution 11) designed the alkaline earth metal ion-doped photocatalyst Ca^{2+}-doped $AgInS_2$. The charge recombination and inactive production of superoxide radicals over $AgInS_2$ could be improved by doping Ca^{2+}. Thus, 63.2% of 4-NP was degraded under visible light for 120 min. In addition, capturing tests demonstrated that photoexcited holes and hydroxyl radicals were the main active species.

In the research work by Lu et al. (Contribution 12), cobalt phosphate (Co-Pi) was developed to modify $ZnIn_2S_4$ ($ZnIn_2S_4$/Co-Pi), aiming to suppress its charge recombination. Due to the transfer of photoexcited holes, $ZnIn_2S_4$/Co-Pi exhibited sustainable H_2 production with assistance of visible light and triethanolamine (TEOA). Specifically, 3593 $\mu mol \cdot g^{-1} \cdot h^{-1}$ of H_2 production was reached using $ZnIn_2S_4$/5%Co-Pi.

To remove hexavalent chromium, Guo et al. (Contribution 13) prepared a 2D g-C_3N_4/MoS_2 nanocomposite using an ultrasonic method. Due to the Z-scheme transfer mechanism, photoexcited charges could not only be separated efficiently at the g-C_3N_4/MoS_2 heterojunction but they also retained strong redox abilities. Thus, hexavalent chromium could be removed with high photocatalytic efficiency whenever it was exposed to UV light, visible light, or sunlight.

Furthermore, Garcia et al. (Contribution 14) fabricated a PdIn/TiO_2 hybrid photoelectrocatalyst for wastewater treatment with simultaneously clean energy production. In the reaction system, on the one hand, paracetamol was degraded by oxidation at the photoanode; on the other hand, hydrogen was produced through reduction at the photocathode. Thus, a dual-function redox reaction system was established.

To use sunlight for CO_2 reduction, Wang et al. (Contribution 15) designed TiO_2/CuPc heterojunctions by combining TiO_2 microspheres and copper phthalocyanines (CuPc). Benefiting from the heterojunction effect and the additional light-absorbing properties of TiO_2 and CuPc, a good reduction rate in 32.4 $\mu mol \cdot g^{-1} \cdot h^{-1}$ of CO_2 was achieved with TiO_2/CuPc at about 3.7 times that of the pristine TiO_2.

Unlike the experiments above, Gao et al. (Contribution 16) utilized the extended broken symmetry (EBS) method to investigate the low-lying spin states of the [Fe_3S_4] cluster, which is important for photosynthetic H_2O splitting. The results indicated that the EBS results matched well with the experimental data. The weaknesses of the BS method could be compensated for through the developed EBS method.

Meanwhile, Tang et al. (Contribution 17) investigated the Sc_2CX_2/Sc_2CY_2 (X, Y = F, Cl, Br) Janus heterojunction for photocatalysis and photovoltaics using first-principles calculations. The calculated results indicate that these Janus heterojunctions possess type-II band structures and direct Z-scheme transfer mechanisms, which thus facilitates their application in photocatalysis and photovoltaics.

In their research paper, P. Ávila-Torres et al. (Contribution 18) prepared metal-yielded coordination compounds Cu-g-C_3N_4, Ni-g-C_3N_4, and Mn-g-C_3N_4. The structural properties of disinfected E. coli bacteria were investigated. The results indicate that the textural property is a key characteristic.

Liu et al. (Contribution 19) studied hydroxyl groups on the g-C_3N_4 (HCN) for O_2 activation and pollutant degradation. The results show that hydroxyl groups can increase hydrophilicity and surface area, decrease interlayer distances, and promote the charge separation and transportation of the pristine g-C_3N_4, thus improving rhodamine B degradation.

Furthermore, A. Pavlatou et al. (Contribution 20) developed a new photocatalyst, namely magnesium oxide (MgO). MgO has a wide band gap and can produce hydroxyl radicals. It showed selectivity for rhodamine 6G and rhodamine B degradation under UV light. A total of 100% of rhodamine B could be degraded over MgO under UV light for 180 min.

In the research paper by Narkiewicz et al. (Contribution 21), triethylamine (TEA), diethylamine (DEA), and ethylenediamine (EDA) were used to modify TiO_2. The effect of amines and temperature on the photocatalytic reduction of CO_2 was investigated in detail. The results demonstrated that TEA-TiO_2 treated in the microwave reactor exhibited the highest activity.

Furthermore, in the research by Wang et al. (Contribution 22), the 2D GaN/g-C_3N_4 heterojunction was investigated using first-principle calculations. The calculated results indicate that the GaN/g-C_3N_4 heterojunction possesses type-II band structures, broad light absorption capabilities, and direct Z-scheme transfer mechanisms, and thus has potential applications in the field of photocatalysis.

In the final research paper, Gerken et al. (Contribution 23) investigated the interplay between photocatalytic growth and the chemical dissolution of gold structures on TiO_2/ITO patterns as a novel approach to mimic axonal dynamic connections. By optimizing gold growth and dissolution parameters, we demonstrated the potential for the precise control of the formation and removal of conductive pathways. This work bridges photocatalytic materials research and bio-inspired system development, offering new insights into the application of photodeposition and chemical etching in dynamic, adaptive systems.

3. Conclusions

In the face of increasingly severe environmental problems and resource challenges, green and sustainable development has become a global consensus and a guide for action. Photocatalysis is one of the most promising strategies for addressing the severe issues facing the environment and energy production and has attracted extensive and ongoing attention due to its inexhaustible, green, safe and economically viable characteristics. However, there are still many challenges involved in the practical application of photocatalysis, such as quantum efficiency, stability and reusability, selectivity, output-to-input ratio, and scaling-up. Fortunately, as a result of decades of hard work, photocatalysis has progressed to a new stage. Various and ingenious photocatalytic materials and photocatalytic reactions have been developed. Photocatalytic materials include but are not limited to nonmetallic LSPR materials, MOFs, COFs, SACs, SCCs, HEAs, heterojunctions, and composite materials. Photocatalytic reactions are involved in the fields of environmental, life science, medical research, space exploration, agriculture and food, energy, etc. However, designing advanced photocatalytic materials with good performance and exploring green photocatalytic reactions with carbon neutrality will require further progress.

Acknowledgments: The editors would like to express their great appreciation to all the authors, reviewers, and technical assistants who contributed to the Special Issue.

Conflicts of Interest: The author declares no conflicts of interest.

List of Contributions

1. Shan, C.; Su, Z.; Liu, Z.; Xu, R.; Wen, J.; Hu, G.; Tang, T.; Fang, Z.; Jiang, L.; Li, M. One-Step Synthesis of Ag_2O/Fe_3O_4 Magnetic Photocatalyst for Efficient Organic Pollutant Removal via Wide-Spectral-Response Photocatalysis–Fenton Coupling. *Molecules* **2023**, *28*, 4155.
2. Wu, K.; Shang, Y.; Li, H.; Wu, P.; Li, S.; Ye, H.; Jian, F.; Zhu, J.; Yang, D.; Li, B.; et al. Synthesis and Hydrogen Production Performance of $MoP/a-TiO_2/Co-ZnIn_2S_4$ Flower-like Composite Photocatalysts. *Molecules* **2023**, *28*, 4350.
3. Long, B.; He, H.; Yu, Y.; Cai, W.; Gu, Q.; Yang, J.; Meng, S. Bifunctional hot water vapor template-mediated synthesis of nanostructured polymeric carbon nitride for efficient hydrogen evolution. *Molecules* **2023**, *28*, 4862.
4. Ding, R.; Li, L.; Yu, Y.T.; Zhang, B.; Wang, P.L. Photoredox-Catalyzed Synthesis of 3-Sulfonylated Pyrrolin-2-ones via a Regioselective Tandem Sulfonylation Cyclization of 1, 5-Dienes. *Molecules* **2023**, *28*, 5473.
5. Du, Z.; Gong, K.; Yu, Z.; Yang, Y.; Wang, P.; Zheng, X.; Wang, Z.; Zhang, S.; Chen, S.; Meng, S. Photoredox Coupling of CO_2 Reduction with Benzyl Alcohol Oxidation over Ternary Metal Chalcogenides ($Zn_mIn_2S_{3+m}$, m = 1–5) with Regulable Products Selectivity. *Molecules* **2023**, *28*, 6553.
6. Shi, H.; Wang, H.; Zhang, E.; Qu, X.; Li, J.; Zhao, S.; Gao, S.; Chen, Z. Boosted photocatalytic performance for antibiotics removal with $Ag/PW_{12}/TiO_2$ composite: degradation pathways and toxicity assessment. *Molecules* **2023**, *28*, 6831.
7. Dan, Y.; Xu, J.; Jian, J.; Meng, L.; Deng, P.; Yan, J.; Yuan, Z.; Zhang, Y.; Zhou, H. In Situ Decoration of Bi_2S_3 Nanosheets on Zinc Oxide/Cellulose Acetate Composite Films for Photodegradation of Dyes under Visible Light Irradiation. *Molecules* **2023**, *28*, 6882.
8. Irfan, M.; Tahir, N.; Zahid, M.; Noreen, S.; Yaseen, M.; Shahbaz, M.; Mustafa, G.; Shakoor, R.A.; Shahid, I. The Fabrication of Halogen-Doped $FeWO_4$ Heterostructure Anchored over Graphene

8. Oxide Nanosheets for the Sunlight-Driven Photocatalytic Degradation of Methylene Blue Dye. *Molecules* **2023**, *28*, 7022.
9. Ma, L.; Jiang, W.; Lin, C.; Xu, L.; Zhu, T.; Ai, X. CdS Deposited In Situ on g-C_3N_4 via a Modified Chemical Bath Deposition Method to Improve Photocatalytic Hydrogen Production. *Molecules* **2023**, *28*, 7846.
10. Zhang, M.; Wu, X.; Liu, X.; Li, H.; Wang, Y.; Wang, D. Constructing In_2S_3/CdS/N-rGO Hybrid Nanosheets via One-Pot Pyrolysis for Boosting and Stabilizing Visible Light-Driven Hydrogen Evolution. *Molecules* **2023**, *28*, 7878.
11. Wang, X.; Liu, S.; Lin, S.; Qi, K.; Yan, Y.; Ma, Y. Visible Light Motivated the Photocatalytic Degradation of P-Nitrophenol by Ca^{2+}-Doped $AgInS_2$. *Molecules* **2024**, *29*, 361.
12. Wu, Y.; Wang, Z.; Yan, Y.; Wei, Y.; Wang, J.; Shen, Y.; Yang, K.; Weng, B.; Lu, K. Rational Photodeposition of Cobalt Phosphate on Flower-like $ZnIn_2S_4$ for Efficient Photocatalytic Hydrogen Evolution. *Molecules* **2024**, *29*, 465.
13. Tian, C.; Yu, H.; Zhai, R.; Zhang, J.; Gao, C.; Qi, K.; Zhang, Y.; Ma, Q.; Guo, M. Visible Light Photoactivity of g-C_3N_4/MoS_2 Nanocomposites for Water Remediation of Hexavalent Chromium. *Molecules* **2024**, *29*, 637.
14. Sacco, N.; Iguini, A.; Gamba, I.; Marchesini, F.A.; García, G. Pd: In-Doped TiO_2 as a Bifunctional Catalyst for the Photoelectrochemical Oxidation of Paracetamol and Simultaneous Green Hydrogen Production. *Molecules* **2024**, *29*, 1073.
15. Wang, J.; Fu, S.; Hou, P.; Liu, J.; Li, C.; Zhang, H.; Wang, G. Construction of TiO_2/CuPc Heterojunctions for the Efficient Photocatalytic Reduction of CO_2 with Water. *Molecules* **2024**, *29*, 1899.
16. Chu, S.; Gao, Q. Unveiling the Low-Lying Spin States of [Fe_3S_4] Clusters via the Extended Broken-Symmetry Method. *Molecules* **2024**, *29*, 2152.
17. He, X.; Wu, Y.; Luo, J.; Dai, X.; Song, J.; Tang, Y. First-Principles Study on Janus-Structured Sc_2CX_2/Sc_2CY_2 (X, Y= F, Cl, Br) Heterostructures for Solar Energy Conversion. *Molecules* **2024**, *29*, 2898.
18. Lasso-Escobar, A.V.; Castrillon, E.D.C.; Acosta, J.; Navarro, S.; Correa-Penagos, E.; Rojas, J.; Ávila-Torres, Y.P. Modulation of Electronic Availability in g-C_3N_4 Using Nickel (II), Manganese (II), and Copper (II) to Enhance the Disinfection and Photocatalytic Properties. *Molecules* **2024**, *29*, 3775.
19. Chen, J.; Yang, M.; Zhang, H.; Chen, Y.; Ji, Y.; Yu, R.; Liu, Z. Boosting the Activation of Molecular Oxygen and the Degradation of Rhodamine B in Polar-Functional-Group-Modified g-C_3N_4. *Molecules* **2024**, *29*, 3836.
20. Gatou, M.A.; Bovali, N.; Lagopati, N.; Pavlatou, E.A. MgO Nanoparticles as a Promising Photocatalyst towards Rhodamine B and Rhodamine 6G Degradation. *Molecules* **2024**, *29*, 4299.
21. Pełech, I.; Staciwa, P.; Sibera, D.; Sobczuk, K.S.; Majewska, W.; Kusiak-Nejman, E.; Morawski, A.T.; Wang, K.; Narkiewicz, U. The Influence of Heat Treatment on the Photoactivity of Amine-Modified Titanium Dioxide in the Reduction of Carbon Dioxide. *Molecules* **2024**, *29*, 4348.
22. Dai, M.Y.; Zhao, X.C.; Lei, B.C.; Huang, Y.N.; Zhang, L.L.; Guo, H.; Wang, H.G. First Principle Study on the Z-Type Characteristic Modulation of GaN/g-C_3N_4 Heterojunction. *Molecules* **2024**, *29*, 5355.
23. Abshari, F.; Paulsen, M.; Veziroglu, S.; Vahl, A.; Gerken, M. Mimicking Axon Growth and Pruning by Photocatalytic Growth and Chemical Dissolution of Gold on TiO_2 Patterns. *Molecules* **2024**, *30*, 99.

References

1. Ciamician, G. The photochemistry of the future. *Science* **1912**, *36*, 385. [CrossRef] [PubMed]
2. Fujishima, A.; Honda, K. Electrochemical photolysis of water at a semiconductor electrode. *Nature* **1972**, *238*, 37–38. [CrossRef]
3. Lei, J.; Zhou, N.; Sang, S.; Meng, S.; Low, J.; Li, Y. Unraveling the roles of atomically-dispersed Au in boosting photocatalytic CO_2 reduction and aryl alcohol oxidation. *Chin. J. Catal.* **2024**, *65*, 163–173. [CrossRef]
4. Che, Y.; Weng, B.; Li, K.; He, Z.; Chen, S.; Meng, S. Chemically bonded nonmetallic LSPR S-scheme hollow heterostructure for boosting photocatalytic performance. *Appl. Catal. B Environ. Energy* **2025**, *361*, 124656. [CrossRef]

5. Candish, L.; Collins, K.D.; Cook, G.C.; Douglas, J.J.; Gómez-Suárez, A.; Jolit, A.; Keess, S. Photocatalysis in the life science industry. *Chem. Rev.* **2021**, *122*, 2907–2980. [CrossRef] [PubMed]
6. Kumar, P.; Singh, G.; Guan, X.; Lee, J.; Bahadur, R.; Ramadass, K.; Kumar, P.; Kibria, M.G.; Vidyasagar, D.; Yi, J.; et al. Multifunctional carbon nitride nanoarchitectures for catalysis. *Chem. Soc. Rev.* **2023**, *52*, 7602–7664. [CrossRef] [PubMed]
7. Dhakshinamoorthy, A.; Li, Z.; Yang, S.; Garcia, H. Metal–organic framework heterojunctions for photocatalysis. *Chem. Soc. Rev.* **2024**, *53*, 3002–3035. [CrossRef] [PubMed]
8. Li, X.; Mitchell, S.; Fang, Y.; Li, J.; Perez-Ramirez, J.; Lu, J. Advances in heterogeneous single-cluster catalysis. *Nat. Rev. Chem.* **2023**, *7*, 754–767. [CrossRef]
9. Ham, R.; Nielsen, C.J.; Pullen, S.; Reek, J.N. Supramolecular coordination cages for artificial photosynthesis and synthetic photocatalysis. *Chem. Rev.* **2023**, *123*, 5225–5261. [CrossRef] [PubMed]
10. Sayed, M.; Yu, J.; Liu, G.; Jaroniec, M. Non-noble plasmonic metal-based photocatalysts. *Chem. Rev.* **2022**, *122*, 10484–10537. [CrossRef]
11. Zhang, H.; Gao, Y.; Meng, S.; Wang, Z.; Wang, P.; Wang, Z.; Chen, S.; Weng, B.; Zheng, Y.-M. Metal sulfide S-scheme homojunction for photocatalytic selective phenylcarbinol oxidation. *Adv. Sci.* **2024**, *11*, 2400099. [CrossRef] [PubMed]
12. Su, B.; Kong, Y.; Wang, S.; Zuo, S.; Lin, W.; Fang, Y.; Hou, Y.; Zhang, G.; Zhang, H.; Wang, X. Hydroxyl-Bonded Ru on Metallic TiN Surface Catalyzing CO_2 Reduction with H_2O by Infrared Light. *J. Am. Chem. Soc.* **2023**, *145*, 27415–27423. [CrossRef] [PubMed]
13. Meng, S.; Chen, C.; Gu, X.; Wu, H.; Meng, Q.; Zhang, J.; Chen, S.; Fu, X.; Liu, D.; Lei, W. Effcient photocatalytic H_2 evolution, CO_2 reduction and N_2 fxation coupled with organic synthesis by cocatalyst and vacancies engineering. *Appl. Catal. B Environ.* **2021**, *285*, 119789. [CrossRef]
14. Nishiyama, H.; Yamada, T.; Nakabayashi, M.; Maehara, Y.; Yamaguchi, M.; Kuromiya, Y.; Nagatsuma, Y.; Tokudome, H.; Akiyama, S.; Watanabe, T.; et al. Photocatalytic solar hydrogen production from water on a 100-m^2 scale. *Nature* **2021**, *598*, 304–307. [CrossRef] [PubMed]
15. Yang, J.; Li, L.; Xiao, C.; Xie, Y. Dual-Plasmon Resonance Coupling Promoting Directional Photosynthesis of Nitrate from Air. *Angew. Chem. Int. Ed.* **2023**, *62*, e202311911. [CrossRef] [PubMed]
16. Liu, D.; Xu, H.; Shen, J.; Wang, X.; Qu, C.; Lin, H.; Long, J.; Wang, Y.; Dai, W.; Fang, Y.; et al. Decoupling H_2 and O_2 Release in Particulate Photocatalytic Overall Water Splitting Using a Reversible O_2 Binder. *Angew. Chem. Int. Ed.* **2024**. [CrossRef]

Disclaimer/Publisher's Note: The statements, opinions and data contained in all publications are solely those of the individual author(s) and contributor(s) and not of MDPI and/or the editor(s). MDPI and/or the editor(s) disclaim responsibility for any injury to people or property resulting from any ideas, methods, instructions or products referred to in the content.

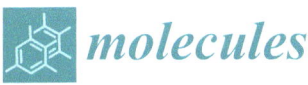

Article

Construction of TiO$_2$/CuPc Heterojunctions for the Efficient Photocatalytic Reduction of CO$_2$ with Water

Jun Wang [1], Shuang Fu [2], Peng Hou [2], Jun Liu [2], Chao Li [2], Hongguang Zhang [2,*] and Guowei Wang [3,*]

1. Academic Affairs Office, Qiqihar Medical University, Qiqihar 161006, China; 18845216002@163.com
2. College of Pharmacy, Qiqihar Medical University, Qiqihar 161006, China; fsjt1980@qmu.edu.cn (S.F.); houp@qmu.edu.cn (P.H.); liuj@qmu.edu.cn (J.L.); lichao@qmu.edu.cn (C.L.)
3. College of Pathology, Qiqihar Medical University, Qiqihar 161006, China
* Correspondence: zhanghg@qmu.edu.cn (H.Z.); wanggw@qmu.edu.cn (G.W.)

Abstract: Utilizing solar energy for photocatalytic CO$_2$ reduction is an attractive research field because of its convenience, safety, and practicality. The selection of an appropriate photocatalyst is the key to achieve efficient CO$_2$ reduction. Herein, we report the synthesis of TiO$_2$/CuPc heterojunctions by compositing CuPc with TiO$_2$ microspheres via a hydroxyl-induced self-assembly process. The experimental investigations demonstrated that the optimal TiO$_2$/0.5CuPc photocatalyst exhibited a significantly enhanced CO$_2$ photoreduction rate up to 32.4 $\mu mol \cdot g^{-1} \cdot h^{-1}$ under 300 W xenon lamp irradiation, which was 3.7 times that of the TiO$_2$ microspheres alone. The results of photoelectrochemical experiments indicated that the construction of the heterojunctions by introducing CuPc effectively promoted the separation and transport of photogenerated carriers, thus enhancing the catalytic effect of the photocatalyst.

Keywords: TiO$_2$/CuPc; heterojunction; photocatalysis; charge separation; CO$_2$ reduction

1. Introduction

The extensive exploitation of fossil fuels has dramatically increased the amount of carbon dioxide (CO$_2$) in the atmosphere, which has led to a global greenhouse effect that is worsening year by year and poses a serious threat to the survival of humankind [1,2]. Photocatalytic CO$_2$ reduction technology is an ideal way to mitigate the greenhouse effect due to its advantages, including mild operating conditions, low energy consumption, and the absence of secondary pollution [3–5]. The characteristics of the photocatalyst are generally considered to be among the most important factors determining the efficiency of photocatalytic CO$_2$ conversion. The development of an effective photocatalyst has therefore gained continuous attention.

Currently, various photocatalytic materials with enhanced CO$_2$ conversion effects have been developed [6–10]. Among them, titanium dioxide (TiO$_2$), a promising semiconductor material, has a wide range of applications in photocatalysis due to its unusual electronic and optical properties [11–14]. For this reason, it has received extensive research and attention. However, it still suffers a low CO$_2$ reduction efficiency, primarily due to the photogenerated electron-hole pairs being prone to recombination and the substantially wide bandgap (3.2 eV). So far, various strategies have been developed to enhance the photocatalytic performance of TiO$_2$ for CO$_2$ reduction, including the introduction of surface defects [15], the doping of heteroatoms [16], and the construction of heterojunctions [17]. Previous studies have successfully demonstrated that the construction of heterojunctions with narrow bandgap semiconductors is a reliable way to improve the photocatalytic activity of TiO$_2$ [18,19]. For example, Ejaz Hussain et al. synthesized Au@TiO$_2$/CdS hybrid catalysts through hydrothermal reactions and found that Au@TiO$_2$/CdS was the most active catalyst, producing 19.15 $mmol \cdot g^{-1} \cdot h^{-1}$ of hydrogen under sunlight [20]. Dai et al. successfully prepared TiO$_2$/CuS nanocomposites with cauliflower-like protrusions

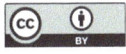

using a simple one-step hydrothermal method with the assistance of 3-mercaptopropionic acid (3-MPA) [21]. Their experimental results showed that the TiO_2/CuS nanocomposites exhibited a better photocatalytic performance compared to TiO_2 and CuS controls. Yin et al. synthesized visible-light-responsive $Ag_3PO_4/OH/TiO_2$ catalysts through the in situ growth of Ag_3PO_4 on the surface of TiO_2 with alkali treatment [22]. The introduction of Ag_3PO_4 effectively improved the light absorption ability of the photocatalysts, which enabled the catalysts to achieve a 90% degradation of RhB under visible light. Although the above approaches effectively improved the photocatalytic activity of TiO_2, it is still inefficient in photocatalytic CO_2 reduction because of its lack of catalytic sites.

Very recently, several studies have found that metal phthalocyanines (MPcs) can be used to construct efficient heterojunction photocatalysts with TiO_2 due to their suitable energy band structure and metal active center unit [23,24]. On the one hand, the porphyrin rings in metal phthalocyanines, analogous to chlorophylls, are widely used as photosensitizers to effectively improve the light absorption of photocatalysts. On the other hand, the central metal of metal phthalocyanines can provide efficient active sites for photocatalytic CO_2 reduction. For example, Altuğ Mert Sevim found that the photocatalytic degradation performance of a composite photocatalyst for 4-chlorophenol under visible-light irradiation was greatly enhanced through the introduction of metal phthalocyanine into TiO_2 [25]. It was also reported by Fei that $FePc/TiO_2$ catalysts demonstrated good photocatalytic activity for the degradation of organic contaminants [26]. Makoto Endo reported the synthesis of $ZnPc/TiO_2$ hybrid nanomaterials and evaluated their photocatalytic reduction of CO_2 [27]. It was found that modification of the TiO_2 with ZnPc could indeed improve its CO_2 photoconversion performance. The above examples successfully suggest that the construction of heterojunctions using metal phthalocyanines and TiO_2 for the efficient conversion of CO_2 is a reasonable design.

In this work, we successfully synthesized a series of TiO_2 microspheres loaded with different amounts of CuPc. The unique selective absorption for CuPc in the range of 500~800 nm can effectively solve the defect of poor visible-light utilization of TiO_2, resulting in heterojunctions with enhanced light absorption capabilities. It was found that the developed $TiO_2/0.5CuPc$ photocatalyst exhibited increased CO_2 reduction activity compared to pristine TiO_2. This enhancement of the photoactivity was attributed to the construction of heterojunctions, which promote the efficient separation of photogenerated charges, as demonstrated in the photoelectrochemical experiments. Moreover, the photocatalytic CO_2 conversion process was investigated through in situ diffuse reflectance infrared Fourier-transform spectroscopy (DRIFTS).

2. Results and Discussion

2.1. Catalyst Characterization

The crystal structure and composition of the as-synthesized samples were investigated using X-ray diffraction patterns (XRD). Typical XRD patterns depict the crystal structures of pure TiO_2, CuPc, and $TiO_2/0.5CuPc$ composites in Figure 1a. The TiO_2 sample exhibited seven characteristic diffraction peaks at 25.3°, 37.9°, 48.0°, 54.1°, 55.1°, 62.8°, and 68.7°, assigned to the (101), (004), (200), (105), (211), (204), and (116) crystal planes, respectively. These diffraction peaks could be indexed to the anatase TiO_2 crystal structure (JCPDS NO. 21-1272). In addition, it can be seen that the intensity of the characteristic diffraction peaks of TiO_2 was slightly reduced after the introduction of CuPc, which might be attributed to the fact that the characteristic peaks of TiO_2 were suppressed by the coated CuPc [28,29]. However, no significant new peaks attributed to CuPc appeared in the XRD spectrum of $TiO_2/0.5CuPc$ compared to that of TiO_2, indicating the low loading content of CuPc. The chemical structures of TiO_2 and $TiO_2/xCuPc$ were further analyzed using FTIR spectroscopy. As shown in Figure 1b, the broader absorption peak located in the range of 400–800 cm^{-1} can be attributed to the stretching vibration of Ti-O and Ti-O-Ti [30]. In contrast, the successful loading of CuPc onto TiO_2 can be identified by the characteristic peaks (1464, 1504, and 1728 cm^{-1}), which correspond to the phthalocyanine backbone and the central metal and ligand of CuPc [31]. As shown in Figure 1c, it was obvious that multiple peaks corresponding to the phthalocyanine backbone vibrations appeared in the TiO$_2$ samples after modification with CuPc. In addition, the intensity of the vibrational peak of the TiO$_2$ surface hydroxyl group located at 1640 cm^{-1} was significantly weaker after CuPc modification (the marked area), suggesting that CuPc interacted with the surface hydroxyl group (Figure 1b). The TEM images of the TiO$_2$ and TiO$_2$/0.5CuPc heterojunction are shown in Figure 1d,e. Obviously, the TiO$_2$ exhibited a spherical structure with a partially hollow core (Figure 1d). Many microspheres were clustered together and therefore exhibited poor dispersibility. It can be seen from Figure 1e that the CuPc modification did not affect the morphology of the TiO$_2$ microspheres and uniformly covered the surface of the TiO$_2$. In addition, as can be seen from Figure 1f, the color of the TiO$_2$ sample changed from light yellow to blue after loading with CuPc, indicating that the CuPc had been successfully loaded onto the surface of the TiO$_2$.

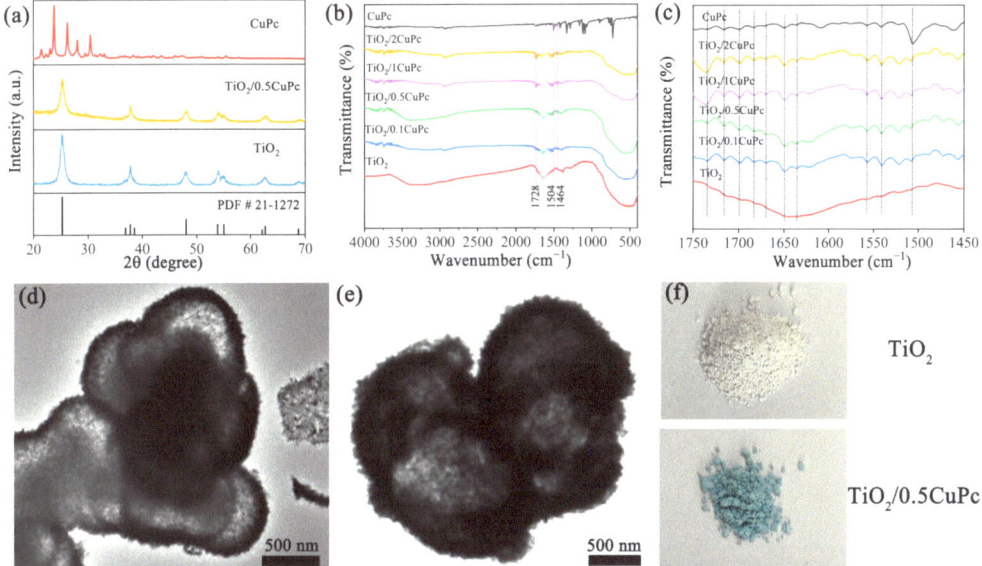

Figure 1. (**a**) XRD patterns of TiO$_2$, CuPc, and TiO$_2$/0.5CuPc. FTIR spectra at (**b**) 400–4000 cm^{-1} and (**c**) 1450–1750 cm^{-1} of TiO$_2$, CuPc, and TiO$_2$/xCuPc. TEM images of (**d**) TiO$_2$ and (**e**) TiO$_2$/0.5CuPc. (**f**) Photographs of TiO$_2$ and TiO$_2$/0.5CuPc.

Raman spectroscopy was utilized to further investigate the structures of TiO$_2$ and TiO$_2$/xCuPc. As expected, the Raman spectra prove that the TiO$_2$ microspheres exhibited an anatase phase (Figure 2a). The characteristic peaks at 146, 396, 516, and 637 cm^{-1} are assigned to the $E_{g(1)}$, B_{1g}, A_{1g}, and $E_{g(3)}$ lattice vibration modes of the anatase phase, respectively [32]. The Raman spectra of TiO$_2$/xCuPc show both TiO$_2$ and CuPc characteristic peaks, indicating that the TiO$_2$/xCuPc heterojunctions were successfully synthesized. It was observed that the intensity of the characteristic peaks of CuPc gradually increased with the increase in the amount of CuPc modification, while the intensity of the characteristic peaks of TiO$_2$ gradually decreased. In addition, the Raman vibration peak at 1523 cm^{-1} (the tensile of C-N-C bridge bonds in the CuPc) was shifted towards the long-wave-number direction after the formation of TiO$_2$/xCuPc heterojunctions, which may have been due to the occurrence of a self-assembly of CuPc on the TiO$_2$ surface (Figure 2b) [33,34].

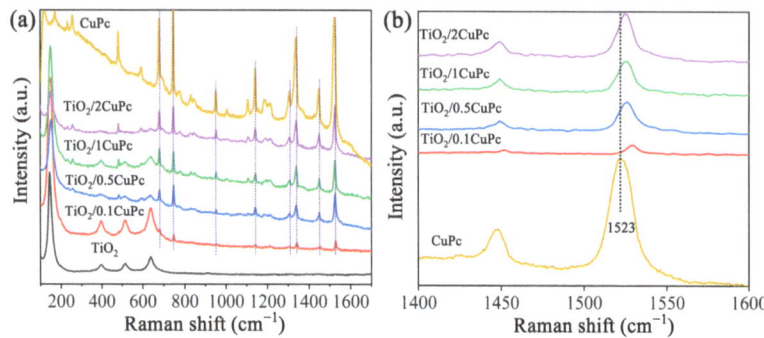

Figure 2. (a) Raman spectra and (b) partially magnified Raman spectra of TiO$_2$, CuPc, and TiO$_2$/xCuPc.

Figure 3 shows the UV-Vis DRS reflectance spectra of TiO$_2$, CuPc, and TiO$_2$/xCuPc. The absorption edge of the TiO$_2$ sample was observed at approximately 420 nm. However, the TiO$_2$/xCuPc heterojunctions exhibited strong light absorption in the visible region of 500~800 nm, which can be attributed to the resulting Q-band electron transition of CuPc from its highest occupied molecular orbital (HOMO) to its lowest unoccupied molecular orbital (LUMO) [35]. In addition, it can also be seen that the absorption intensity gradually increased as the amount of CuPc increased.

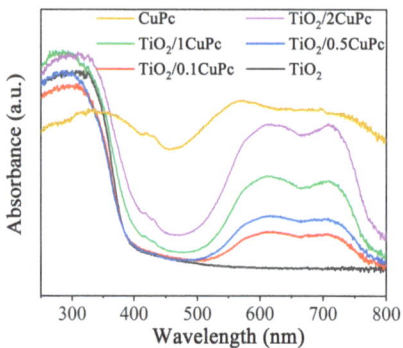

Figure 3. UV-vis DRS reflectance spectra of TiO$_2$, CuPc, and TiO$_2$/xCuPc.

The optical band gap of a catalyst can be calculated from its light absorption spectra according to the equation $\alpha h\nu = A(h\nu - E_g)^{n/2}$, where α, h, ν, A, and E_g represent the absorption coefficient, Planck constant, light frequency, proportionality, and band gap energy, respectively. For TiO$_2$ and CuPc, the values of n are 1 and 4, respectively. Based on the above equation, the calculated E_g values for TiO$_2$ and CuPc are 2.98 and 1.68 eV, respectively (Figure 4a,b). To further investigate the band structures of TiO$_2$ and CuPc, Mott–Schottky curves were obtained. A positive slope of the Mott–Schottky plot would indicate that TiO$_2$ is an n-type semiconductor, while a negative slope of the Mott–Schottky plot would indicate that CuPc is a p-type semiconductor. As shown in Figure 4c,d, the flat band potentials of TiO$_2$ and CuPc were determined to be -0.59 V and 0.92 V vs. Ag/AgCl, respectively. According to the formula E(RHE) = E(Ag/AgCl) + 0.197 + 0.059 pH, we could deduce that the conduction band potential (E_{CB}) of TiO$_2$ and the highest occupied molecular orbital (HOMO) energy level of CuPc were approximately 0.01 and 1.52 V vs. RHE, respectively. According to the empirical equation $E_g = E_{VB} - E_{CB}$, the valence band potential (E_{VB}) of TiO$_2$ and the lowest unoccupied molecular orbital (LUMO) energy level of CuPc were calculated to be 2.99 and -0.16 V vs. RHE, respectively. In addition, ultraviolet photoelectron spectroscopy (UPS) was also performed to determine the valence band energy (E_{VB}) of TiO$_2$ and CuPc (Figure 4e,f). The incident photon energy (hv) of the helium I source was 21.22 eV [36,37]. By subtracting the width of the peak from the excitation energy (21.22 eV), the valence band maximum of TiO$_2$ and the HOMO energy of CuPc were calculated to be 7.52 and 5.98 eV, respectively, on the absolute vacuum scale (AVS). According to the reference standard, 0 V for the reversible hydrogen electrode (RHE) is equal to 4.44 eV on the vacuum level. Therefore, the E_{VB} (versus RHE) value of TiO$_2$ and the HOMO energy of CuPc were calculated to be 3.08 and 1.54 V, respectively. That is, the conduction band energy (E_{CB}) of TiO$_2$ and the LUMO energy of CuPc were 0.10 and −0.14 V, respectively. These results are consistent with those found in the Mott–Schottky plot calculations.

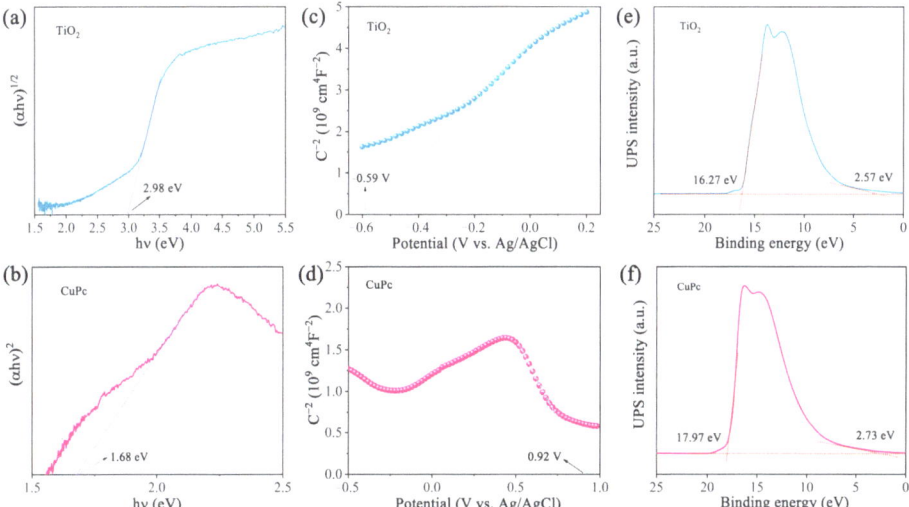

Figure 4. (**a**) Plot of $(\alpha h\nu)^{1/2}$ versus (hv) for the band gap energy of TiO$_2$ and (**b**) plot of $(\alpha h\nu)^2$ versus (hv) for the band gap energy of CuPc. Mott–Schottky plots of (**c**) TiO$_2$ and (**d**) CuPc. UPS spectra of (**e**) TiO$_2$ and (**f**) CuPc.

Photoelectrochemical experiments were applied to reveal the charge transfer kinetics of the heterojunctions. As shown in Figure 5a, the photocurrent density of TiO$_2$/0.5CuPc was higher than that of TiO$_2$, which indicates that the formation of a heterojunction can indeed effectively inhibit the recombination and further promote the separation of photogeneration carriers. The separation efficiency of photogeneration charges in the heterojunctions was further verified using the impedance spectroscopy spectra (EIS) (Figure 5b). It is obvious that the arc radius in the Nyquist plot of TiO$_2$/0.5CuPc is much smaller than that of the TiO$_2$ plot, suggesting that the charge transfer resistance in the heterojunction was reduced and facilitated rapid carrier separation and transfer. As shown in the inset of Figure 5b, the arc radius of TiO$_2$/0.5CuPc was similarly smaller than TiO$_2$ in the high-frequency region, suggesting better conductivity and proving the lower recombination rate of the carriers.

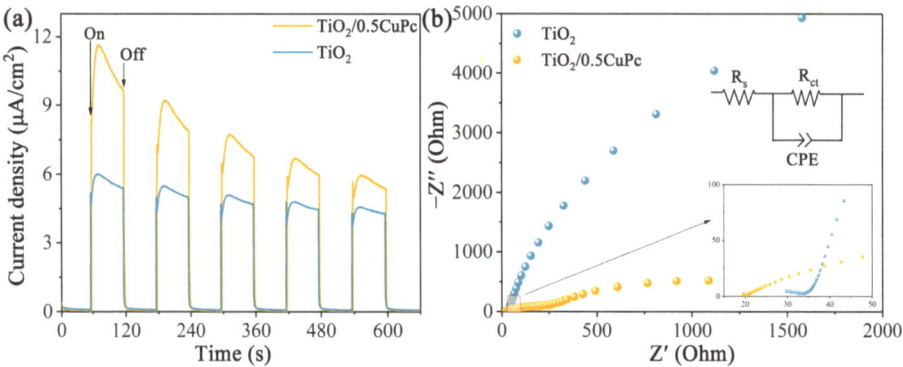

Figure 5. (**a**) Transient photocurrent responses and (**b**) EIS Nyquist plots of TiO_2 and $TiO_2/0.5CuPc$.

2.2. Photocatalytic Performance and Reaction Mechanism

The photocatalytic CO_2 reduction performance of the TiO_2 and $TiO_2/xCoPc$ was tested under 300 W Xe lamp illumination. As shown in Figure 6, the reduction products CH_4 and CO were detected. The sample of TiO_2 exhibited a low CO_2 reduction activity with a production rate of 8.7 $\mu mol \cdot g^{-1} \cdot h^{-1}$ for CO. However, integration with CuPc significantly enhanced the photocatalytic activity of TiO_2. It was noticed that the photocatalytic performance of the $TiO_2/xCoPc$ heterojunctions first increased and then decreased with the increase in CuPc loading. The higher the CuPc loading, the more severe the agglomeration of CuPc units at the TiO_2 surface, thus leading to a decrease in photocatalytic activity [38]. The maximum CO production performance rate of 32.4 $\mu mol \cdot g^{-1} \cdot h^{-1}$ was attained with the $TiO_2/0.5CoPc$ heterojunction, which was 3.7 times higher than that of the TiO_2 microspheres. In addition, the yield of CH_4 was almost negligible, which indicates that the $TiO_2/0.5CoPc$ heterojunction has high selectivity for CO_2 reduction to CO.

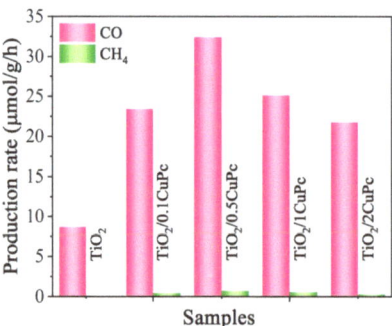

Figure 6. Photocatalytic activities for CO_2 reduction of the TiO_2 and $TiO_2/0.5CuPc$ heterojunction.

The mechanism of the CO_2 reduction process was investigated using electrochemical reduction measurements in different gas-bubbled systems. As shown in Figure 7a,b, it was obvious that the onset potential of $TiO_2/0.5CoPc$ heterojunction was lower than that of the TiO_2 microspheres in both N_2-saturated and CO_2-saturated electrolytes. Furthermore, the onset potential of the heterojunction in the CO_2-saturated electrolyte was lower than that in the N_2-saturated electrolyte, suggesting that the CuPc modification was more favorable for CO_2 activation [39].

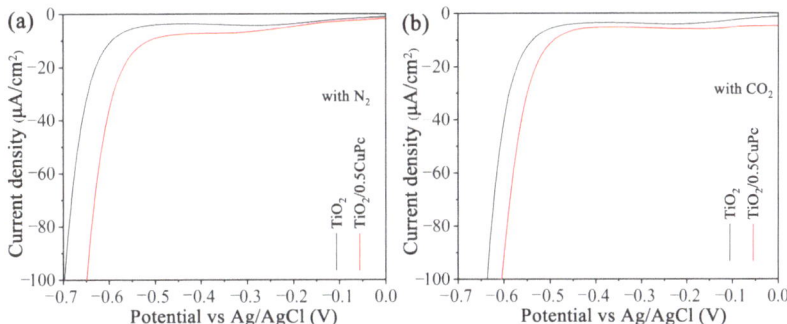

Figure 7. Electrochemical reduction curves of the TiO_2 and $TiO_2/0.5CuPc$ heterojunction in (**a**) a N_2-bubbled system and (**b**) a CO_2-bubbled system, respectively.

The intermediates in CO_2 conversion were explored using in situ diffuse reflectance infrared Fourier-transform spectroscopy (Figure 8). The absorption peaks located at 1338, 1386, and 1617 cm^{-1} are ascribed to bidentate carbonates (b-CO_3^{2-}), and the peaks at 1395, 1507, 1522, 1560, and 1576 cm^{-1} belong to monodentate carbonate (m-CO_3^{2-}) [40]. Bands at 1418, 1437, 1636, and 1652 cm^{-1} can also be observed, which can be assigned to the HCO_3^- groups. The absorption peak at 2077 cm^{-1} is attributable to CO. In addition, with the increase in irradiation time, it can be seen that a peak of the COO$^-$ radical at 1624 cm^{-1} and a peak of COOH* at 1733 cm^{-1} began to appear [41], and the peak intensity increased gradually. These results indicate that this photocatalytic reaction for the reduction of CO_2 was carried out efficiently. It is worth noting that the formation of the important intermediate COOH* is generally considered to be a rate-limiting step during the photocatalytic conversion of CO_2 to CO. It is obvious that the peak intensity of COOH* in the $TiO_2/0.5CoPc$ heterojunction was stronger compared to that of TiO_2 at the same light irradiation time, which indicates the better activity of the $TiO_2/0.5CoPc$ heterojunction for the photocatalytic conversion of CO_2.

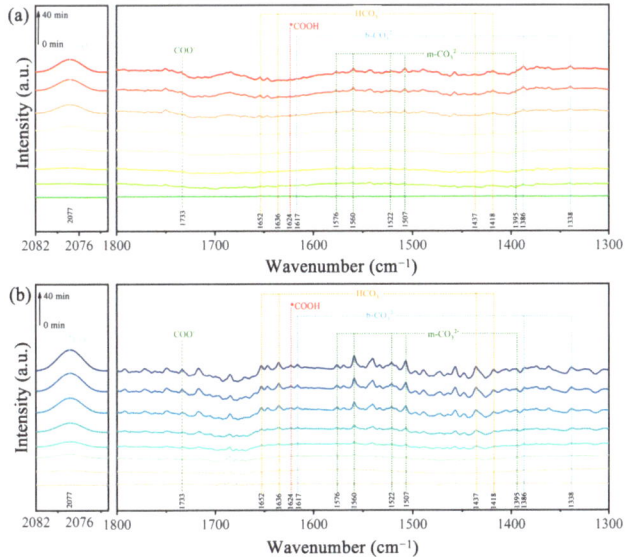

Figure 8. The in situ DRIFT spectra of (**a**) TiO_2 and (**b**) the $TiO_2/0.5CuPc$ heterojunction at different light irradiation intervals.

Based on the above discussions, a mechanism of charge transfer and separation to promote CO_2 conversion is proposed (Figure 9). First, the TiO_2 and CuPc absorbed enough light of different wavelengths for electron transition under the 300 W Xe lamp irradiation to generate photogenerated carriers (e^-/h^+ pairs). Because of the well-matched energy levels of TiO_2 and CuPc, the photogenerated electrons generated through the excitation of TiO_2 were transferred to the HOMO energy level of CuPc and recombined with the holes of CuPc. As a result, the remaining holes in the TiO_2 valence band could be used for the oxidation of H_2O to O_2, while the separated electrons in the LUMO energy level of CuPc were transferred to coordinated central metal ions for the CO_2 reduction reaction. Based on the in situ diffuse reflectance infrared Fourier-transform spectroscopy (DRIFTS) results, the possible CO_2 reduction pathways are as follows:

$$CO_2\ (g) \rightarrow CO_2{}^*$$
$$CO_2 + H^+ + e^- \rightarrow COOH^*$$
$$COOH^* + H^+ + e^- \rightarrow CO^* + H_2O$$
$$CO^* \rightarrow CO$$

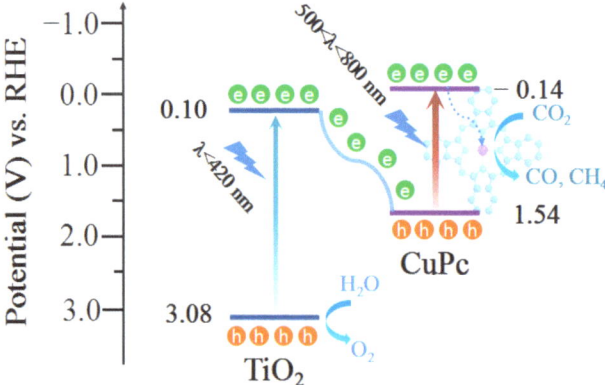

Figure 9. Schematic illustration of the proposed photocatalytic CO_2 reduction mechanism of the $TiO_2/0.5$CuPc heterojunction.

3. Materials and Methods

3.1. Materials

All of the chemical reagents were purchased from Aladdin Chemical Reagents Limited and were of analytical grade and used without further purification: titanium sulfate ($Ti(SO_4)_2$, 99%), ethylenediaminetetraacetic acid (EDTA, 99.5%), copper(II) phthalocyanine (CuPc, 97%), ethanol (C_2H_5OH, 99.99%), and sodium sulfate anhydrous (Na_2SO_4, 99%). Deionized water was used throughout.

3.2. Synthesis of TiO_2 Microspheres

The TiO_2 microspheres were synthesized through a simple hydrothermal method. At first, $Ti(SO_4)_2$ (0.2400 g, 1 mmol) and EDTA (1.4612 g, 5 mmol) were dissolved in 30 mL of deionized water under stirring. After that, the solution was transferred into an autoclave and was treated at 180 °C for 8 h in a temperature-controlled oven. The resulting product was filtered and washed with deionized water. Finally, the obtained solid was dried in an oven at 60 °C overnight.

3.3. Synthesis of TiO_2/CuPc Heterojunction

The TiO_2/CuPc heterojunctions were prepared using a hydroxyl-induced self-assembly process based on the reported method [35]. In a typical experiment, 40 mg of TiO_2 microspheres was dispersed in 25 mL of ethanol and sonicated for 30 min, noted as Solution A. Various amounts of CuPc powder were then dispersed in 25 mL of ethanol and sonicated for 30 min, noted as Solution B. Solution A and B were then mixed and sonicated for another 30 min. Afterwards, the above solution was evaporated in a water bath at 75 °C under magnetic stirring. After drying at 80 °C for 4 h in an oven, TiO_2/xCuPc heterojunctions (where x = 0.1, 0.5, 1, or 2) were obtained, with x representing the mass ratio percentage of CuPc to TiO_2. For example, weighing 40 mg of TiO_2 microspheres required the addition of 0.2 mg of CuPc, resulting in a mass percentage of CuPc to TiO_2 of 0.5%, noted as TiO_2/0.5CuPc. Similarly, if 0.04 mg, 0.4 mg, and 0.8 mg amounts of CuPc were added, respectively, we obtained TiO_2/0.1CuPc, TiO_2/1CuPc, and TiO_2/2CuPc.

3.4. Characterization

The morphology and structure of each samples were characterized by using transmission electron microscopy (JEOL, JEM-F200, Tokyo, Japan) with an acceleration voltage of 200 kV. X-ray powder diffraction analysis was recorded under ambient conditions with a Shimadzu XRD-6000 diffractor (Kyoto, Japan) with Cu K radiation (0.15405 nm) at 40 kV and 40 mA. Raman spectra of the samples were measured using a Renishaw inVia Reflex spectrometer system (λ = 532 nm) (London, UK). Fourier-transform infrared (FT-IR) spectra were recorded using a Thermo Scientific Nicolet iS50 (Waltham, MA, USA), with KBr as the diluent. UV-vis absorption spectra were recorded with a Shimadzu UV2700 spectrophotometer (Kyoto, Japan), using $BaSO_4$ as the reference. The electrochemical studies were detected on an H-type cell using an electrochemical workstation (IVIUM V13806, Amsterdam, The Netherlands). Ultraviolet photoelectron spectroscopy (UPS) measurements were performed on ESCALAB 250Xi (Waltham, MA, USA) with an unfiltered HeI (21.22 eV) gas discharge lamp and a total instrumental energy resolution of 100 meV. In situ diffuse reflectance infrared Fourier-transform spectroscopy (DRIFTS) measurements were performed by using the Nicolet iS50 Fourier-transform spectrometer (Waltham, MA, USA) equipped with an MCT diffuse reflectance accessory.

3.5. Photocatalytic CO_2 Reduction

Photocatalytic CO_2 reduction was conducted in a 100 mL quartz cell reactor equipped with a 300 W xenon lamp (PLSSXE300UV, PerfectLight, Beijing, China) as the light source. In detail, 10 mg of the photocatalyst and 10 mL of deionized water were added to the 100 mL quartz cell reactor. High-purity CO_2 gas (99.9%) was passed through the water and then into the reaction setup to reach an ambient pressure. The photocatalysts were allowed to equilibrate in the CO_2/H_2O system for 20 min under stirring, and were then irradiated with the 300 W xenon lamp. The amounts of CO and CH_4 that evolved were determined using a gas chromatograph (Techcomp GC-7900, Shanghai, China) equipped with both TCD and FID detectors. The production rates of CO and CH_4 were calculated according to the standard curve.

3.6. Photoelectrochemical Measurements

The film electrode was fabricated as follows: firstly, 10 mg of the sample, 0.1 mL of Nafion, and 0.9 mL of ethanol were mixed into a slurry thoroughly. Then, the slurry was coated onto the FTO glass electrode (1.0 cm × 1.0 cm). Lastly, the coated electrode was dried at 60 °C for 30 min. Photoelectrochemical (PEC) measurements were carried out using the IVIUM V13806 electrochemical workstation with a traditional three-electrode system. The as-prepared sample films were used as working electrodes in the sealed quartz cell. A platinum plate (99.9%) and a saturated KCl Ag/AgCl electrode were used as the counter electrode and reference electrode, respectively. A 0.2 mol·L^{-1} Na_2SO_4 solution was used as the electrolyte (pH = 6.8). PEC experiments were performed in a quartz cell using a 300 W xenon lamp as the illumination source. Mott–Schottky plots were implemented at frequencies of 1000 Hz. All of the experiments were performed at room temperature (about 25 ± 3 °C).

3.7. Electrochemical Reduction Measurements

Electrochemical reduction measurements were carried out in a traditional three-electrode system. The working electrode was a 0.3 cm diameter glassy carbon (GC) electrode, a saturated KCl Ag/AgCl electrode was used as the reference electrode, and a Pt sheet was used as the counter electrode. Five milligrams of each different sample mixed with 20 μL of a 5 wt % Nafion ionomer was dissolved in 0.18 mL of an aqueous ethanol solution. The catalyst ink was scanned with ultrasound for 30 min, and a suitable mass of the ink was uniformly dropped onto the clean GC electrode surface and dried in air. An IVIUM V13806 electrochemical workstation was employed to test the electrochemical activity and stability of the series of catalysts. High-purity N_2 or CO_2 (99.999%) were employed to bubble through the electrolyte to keep the gas saturated in the EC experiment. At the beginning, electrode potentials were cycled between two potential limits until perfectly overlapping; afterward, the I–V curves were obtained. For the electrolytes in the tests, 1 mol·L^{-1} Na_2SO_4 was used. The scan rate of the linear sweep voltammetry was 50 mV/s. All of the experiments were performed at room temperature (about 25 ± 3 °C).

3.8. In-Situ Diffuse Reflectance Infrared Fourier Transform Spectroscopy (DRIFTS)

In situ DRIFTS measurements were performed using a Nicolet iS50 Fourier-Transform Spectrometer equipped with an MCT diffuse reflectance accessory. Each spectrum was recorded at a resolution of 4 cm^{-1} by averaging 16 scans. The samples were compressed and stored in a custom-fabricated infrared reaction chamber sealed with a ZnSe window. Before measurement, each catalyst was purged with nitrogen at 170 °C for 3 h to remove any surface-adsorbed impurities. The samples were then cooled to room temperature and the background spectra were collected. Subsequently, a mixture of carbon dioxide and water vapor was introduced into the reaction chamber until the adsorption reached equilibrium. The samples were then swept with nitrogen to remove the unadsorbed gases. Subsequently, FT-IR spectra were collected at different irradiation intervals under 300 W xenon lamp irradiation.

4. Conclusions

In conclusion, this study successfully demonstrates the construction of TiO_2/CuPc heterojunctions that significantly enhance CO_2's photoreduction to CO. Benefiting from the complementary light-absorbing properties of CuPc and TiO_2, combined with the superior photogenerated charge separation efficiency, the developed TiO_2/0.5CuPc photocatalyst exhibited a better photocatalytic CO_2 reduction performance than that of pristine TiO_2. In addition, the presence of the metal Cu center in CuPc further acted as a catalytic site, enhancing the CO_2 reduction process. These findings not only highlight a facile strategy for enhancing TiO_2 photocatalyst activity but also pave the way for future advancements in photocatalytic technology for environmental remediation and the sustainable conversion of greenhouse gases into valuable resources.

Author Contributions: Conceptualization, H.Z. and G.W.; methodology, J.W. and S.F.; software, P.H. and C.L.; validation, J.L.; formal analysis, H.Z.; data curation, J.W.; writing—original draft preparation, G.W.; writing—review and editing, H.Z.; supervision, P.H.; project administration, H.Z. and G.W.; funding acquisition, H.Z. and G.W. All authors have read and agreed to the published version of the manuscript.

Funding: This work was financially supported by the Qiqihar city Science and Technology Programme of Joint Guidance Project (Grant No. LSFGG-2022034) and the Science and Technology Research Project of the Heilongjiang Provincial Department of Education (Grant No. 2020-KYYWF-0006).

Institutional Review Board Statement: Not applicable.

Informed Consent Statement: Not applicable.

Data Availability Statement: Data are contained within the article.

Conflicts of Interest: The authors declare no conflicts of interest.

References

1. Zhang, X.D.; Tang, Y.J.; Han, H.Y.; Chen, Z.L. Evolution Characteristics and Main Influencing Factors of Carbon Dioxide Emissions in Chinese Cities from 2005 to 2020. *Sustainability* **2023**, *15*, 14849. [CrossRef]
2. Chang, Y.F.; Huang, B.N. Factors Leading to Increased Carbon Dioxide Emissions of the Apec Countries: The Lmdi Decomposition Analysis. *Singap. Econ. Rev.* **2023**, *68*, 2195–2214. [CrossRef]
3. Liu, Y.Z.; Zhao, L.; Zeng, X.H.; Xiao, F.; Fang, W.; Du, X.; He, X.; Wang, D.H.; Li, W.X.; Chen, H. Efficient photocatalytic reduction of CO_2 by improving adsorption activation and carrier utilization rate through N-vacancy g-C_3N_4 hollow microtubule. *Mater. Today Energy* **2023**, *31*, 101211. [CrossRef]
4. Li, N.X.; Chen, Y.M.; Xu, Q.Q.; Mu, W.H. Photocatalytic reduction of CO_2 to CO using nickel(II)-bipyridine complexes with different substituent groups as catalysts. *J. CO2 Util.* **2023**, *68*, 102385. [CrossRef]
5. Wang, P.; Ba, X.H.; Zhang, X.W.; Gao, H.Y.; Han, M.Y.; Zhao, Z.Y.; Chen, X.; Wang, L.M.; Diao, X.M.; Wang, G. Direct Z-scheme heterojunction of PCN-222/$CsPbBr_3$ for boosting photocatalytic CO_2 reduction to HCOOH. *Chem. Eng. J.* **2023**, *457*, 141248. [CrossRef]
6. Ezugwu, C.I.; Ghosh, S.; Bera, S.; Faraldos, M.; Mosquera, M.E.G.; Rosal, R. Bimetallic metal-organic frameworks for efficient visible-light-driven photocatalytic CO_2 reduction and H_2 generation. *Sep. Purif. Technol.* **2023**, *308*, 122868. [CrossRef]
7. Jia, X.M.; Sun, H.Y.; Lin, H.L.; Cao, J.; Hu, C.; Chen, S.F. In-depth insight into the mechanism on photocatalytic selective CO_2 reduction coupled with tetracycline oxidation over $BiO_{1-x}Br$/g-C_3N_4. *Appl. Surf. Sci.* **2023**, *614*, 156017. [CrossRef]
8. Lu, S.W.; Liao, W.R.; Chen, W.H.; Yang, M.Q.; Zhu, S.Y.; Liang, S.J. Elemental sulfur supported on ultrathin titanic acid nanosheets for photocatalytic reduction of CO_2 to CH_4. *Appl. Surf. Sci.* **2023**, *614*, 156224. [CrossRef]
9. Tan, L.; Li, Y.R.; Lv, Q.; Gan, Y.Y.; Fang, Y.; Tang, Y.; Wu, L.Z.; Fang, Y.X. Development of soluble UiO-66 to improve photocatalytic CO_2 reduction. *Catal. Today* **2023**, *410*, 282–288. [CrossRef]
10. Zhao, L.; Zeng, X.H.; Wang, D.H.; Zhang, H.J.; Li, W.X.; Fang, W.; Huang, Z.H.; Chen, H. In-plane graphene incorporated borocarbonitride: Directional utilization of disorder charge via micro π-conjugated heterointerface for photocatalytic CO_2 reduction. *Carbon* **2023**, *203*, 847–855. [CrossRef]
11. Alkanad, K.; Hezam, A.; Al-Zaqri, N.; Bajiri, M.A.; Alnaggar, G.; Drmosh, Q.A.; Almukhlifi, H.A.; Krishnappagowda, L.N. One-Step Hydrothermal Synthesis of Anatase TiO_2 Nanotubes for Efficient Photocatalytic CO_2 Reduction. *ACS Omega* **2022**, *7*, 38686–38699. [CrossRef] [PubMed]
12. Bao, X.L.; Zhang, M.H.; Wang, Z.Y.; Dai, D.J.; Wang, P.; Cheng, H.F.; Liu, Y.Y.; Zheng, Z.K.; Dai, Y.; Huang, B.B. Molten-salt assisted synthesis of Cu clusters modified TiO_2 with oxygen vacancies for efficient photocatalytic reduction of CO_2 to CO. *Chem. Eng. J.* **2022**, *445*, 136718. [CrossRef]
13. Park, Y.H.; Kim, D.; Hiragond, C.B.; Lee, J.; Jung, J.W.; Cho, C.H.; In, I.; In, S.I. Phase-controlled 1T/2H-MoS_2 interaction with reduced TiO_2 for highly stable photocatalytic CO_2 reduction into CO. *J. CO2 Util.* **2023**, *67*, 102324. [CrossRef]
14. Gong, H.; Xing, Y.; Li, J.; Liu, S. Functionalized Linear Conjugated Polymer/TiO_2 Heterojunctions for Significantly Enhancing Photocatalytic H_2 Evolution. *Molecules* **2024**, *29*, 1103. [CrossRef] [PubMed]
15. Qian, X.Z.; Yang, W.Y.; Gao, S.; Xiao, J.; Basu, S.; Yoshimura, A.; Shi, Y.F.; Meunier, V.; Li, Q. Highly Selective, Defect-Induced Photocatalytic CO_2 Reduction to Acetaldehyde by the Nb-Doped TiO_2 Nanotube Array under Simulated Solar Illumination. *ACS Appl. Mater. Interfaces* **2020**, *12*, 55982–55993. [CrossRef]
16. Olowoyo, J.O.; Kumar, M.; Singhal, N.; Jain, S.L.; Babalola, J.O.; Vorontsov, A.V.; Kumar, U. Engineering and modeling the effect of Mg doping in TiO_2 for enhanced photocatalytic reduction of CO_2 to fuels. *Catal. Sci. Technol.* **2018**, *8*, 3686–3694. [CrossRef]
17. Yang, J.; Wang, J.; Zhao, W.J.; Wang, G.H.; Wang, K.; Wu, X.H.; Li, J.M. 0D/1D $Cu_{2-x}S/TiO_2$ S-scheme heterojunction with enhanced photocatalytic CO_2 reduction performance via surface plasmon resonance induced photothermal effects. *Appl. Surf. Sci.* **2023**, *613*, 156083. [CrossRef]
18. Feng, H.G.; Zhang, C.M.; Luo, M.H.; Hu, Y.C.; Dong, Z.B.; Xue, S.L.; Chu, P.K. A dual S-scheme $TiO_2@In_2Se_3@Ag_3PO_4$ heterojunction for efficient photocatalytic CO_2 reduction. *Nanoscale* **2022**, *14*, 16303–16313. [CrossRef] [PubMed]
19. Rehman, Z.U.; Bilal, M.; Hou, J.H.; Butt, F.K.; Ahmad, J.; Ali, S.; Hussain, A. Photocatalytic CO_2 Reduction Using TiO_2-Based Photocatalysts and TiO_2 Z-Scheme Heterojunction Composites: A Review. *Molecules* **2022**, *27*, 2069. [CrossRef] [PubMed]
20. Rafiq, K.; Sabir, M.; Abid, M.Z.; Jalil, M.; Nadeem, M.A.; Iqbal, S.; Rauf, A.; Hussain, E. Tuning of TiO_2/CdS Hybrid Semiconductor with Au Cocatalysts: State-of-the-Art Design for Sunlight-Driven H_2 Generation from Water Splitting. *Energy Fuels* **2024**, *38*, 4625–4636. [CrossRef]
21. Huang, S.; Qin, C.; Niu, L.; Wang, J.; Sun, J.; Dai, L. Strategies for preparing TiO_2/CuS nanocomposites with cauliflower-like protrusions for photocatalytic water purification. *New J. Chem.* **2022**, *46*, 10594–10602. [CrossRef]
22. Wang, X.; Yuan, S.; Geng, M.; Sun, M.; Zhang, J.; Zhou, A.; Yin, G. Combination of alkali treatment and Ag_3PO_4 loading effectively improves the photocatalytic activity of TiO_2 nanoflowers. *New J. Chem.* **2024**, *48*, 6789–6795. [CrossRef]
23. Keshipour, S.; Mohammad-Alizadeh, S. Nickel phthalocyanine@graphene oxide/TiO_2 as an efficient degradation catalyst of formic acid toward hydrogen production. *Sci. Rep.* **2021**, *11*, 16148. [CrossRef] [PubMed]
24. Li, Y.G.; Yang, M.R.; Tian, Z.M.; Luo, N.D.; Li, Y.; Zhang, H.H.; Zhou, A.N.; Xiong, S.X. Assembly of Copper Phthalocyanine on TiO_2 Nanorod Arrays as Co-catalyst for Enhanced Photoelectrochemical Water Splitting. *Front. Chem.* **2019**, *7*, 334. [CrossRef] [PubMed]

25. Sevim, A.M. Synthesis and characterization of Zn and Co monocarboxy-phthalocyanines and investigation of their photocatalytic efficiency as TiO$_2$ composites. *J. Organomet. Chem.* **2017**, *832*, 18–26. [CrossRef]
26. Fei, J.W.; Han, Z.B.; Deng, Y.; Wang, T.; Zhao, J.; Wang, C.H.; Zhao, X.M. Enhanced photocatalytic performance of iron phthalocyanine/TiO$_2$ heterostructure at joint fibrous interfaces. *Colloid Surf. A* **2021**, *625*, 126901. [CrossRef]
27. Endo, M.; Ochiai, T.; Nagata, M. Photoreduction of Carbon Dioxide By the Zinc Phthalocyanine Immobilized Titanium Dioxide. *ECS Meet. Abstr.* **2016**, *230*, 3654. [CrossRef]
28. Noor, S.; Waseem, M.; Rashid, U.; Anis-ur-Rehman, M.; Rehman, W.; Mahmood, K. Fabrication of NiO coated SiO$_2$ and SiO$_2$ coated NiO for the removal of Pb^{2+} ions. *Chin. Chem. Lett.* **2014**, *25*, 819–822. [CrossRef]
29. Li, J.Y.; Xu, R.K.; Deng, K.Y. Coatings of Fe/Al hydroxides inhibited acidification of kaolinite and an alfisol subsoil through electrical double-layer interaction and physical blocking. *Soil Sci.* **2014**, *179*, 495–502. [CrossRef]
30. Liccardo, L.; Bordin, M.; Sheverdyaeva, P.M.; Belli, M.; Moras, P.; Vomiero, A.; Moretti, E. Surface Defect Engineering in Colored TiO$_2$ Hollow Spheres Toward Efficient Photocatalysis. *Adv. Funct. Mater.* **2023**, *33*, 2212486. [CrossRef]
31. Zhang, M.Y.; Shao, C.L.; Guo, Z.C.; Zhang, Z.Y.; Mu, J.B.; Cao, T.P.; Liu, Y.C. Hierarchical Nanostructures of Copper(II) Phthalocyanine on Electrospun TiO$_2$ Nanofibers: Controllable Solvothermal-Fabrication and Enhanced Visible Photocatalytic Properties. *ACS Appl. Mater. Inter.* **2011**, *3*, 369–377. [CrossRef] [PubMed]
32. He, B.W.; Wang, Z.L.; Xiao, P.; Chen, T.; Yu, J.G.; Zhang, L.Y. Cooperative Coupling of H$_2$O Production and Organic Synthesis over a Floatable Polystyrene-Sphere-Supported TiO$_2$/Bi$_2$O$_3$ S-Scheme Photocatalyst. *Adv. Mater.* **2022**, *34*, 2203225. [CrossRef] [PubMed]
33. Tackley, D.R.; Dent, G.; Smith, W.E. IR and Raman assignments for zinc phthalocyanine from DFT calculations. *Phys. Chem. Chem. Phys.* **2000**, *2*, 3949–3955. [CrossRef]
34. Wu, H.; Bian, J.; Zhang, Z.; Zhao, Z.; Xu, S.; Li, Z.; Jiang, N.; Kozlova, E.; Hua, X.; Jing, L. Controllable synthesis of CuPc/N-rich doped (001) TiO$_2$ S-scheme nanosheet heterojunctions for efficiently wide-visible light-driven CO$_2$ reduction. *Appl. Surf. Sci.* **2023**, *623*, 157066. [CrossRef]
35. Sun, J.W.; Bian, J.; Li, J.D.; Zhang, Z.Q.; Li, Z.J.; Qu, Y.; Bai, L.L.; Yang, Z.D.; Jing, L.Q. Efficiently photocatalytic conversion of CO$_2$ on ultrathin metal phthalocyanine/g-C$_3$N$_4$ heterojunctions by promoting charge transfer and CO$_2$ activation. *Appl. Catal. B-Environ.* **2020**, *277*, 119199. [CrossRef]
36. Boruah, B.; Gupta, R.; Modak, J.M.; Madras, G. Novel insights into the properties of AgBiO$_3$ photocatalyst and its application in immobilized state for 4-nitrophenol degradation and bacteria inactivation. *J. Photochem. Photobiol. A Chem.* **2019**, *373*, 105–115. [CrossRef]
37. Ding, M.; Xiao, R.; Zhao, C.; Bukhvalov, D.; Chen, Z.; Xu, H.; Tang, H.; Xu, J.; Yang, X. Evidencing interfacial charge transfer in 2D CdS/2D MXene Schottky heterojunctions toward high-efficiency photocatalytic hydrogen production. *Solar Rrl* **2021**, *5*, 2000414. [CrossRef]
38. Prajapati, P.K.; Kumar, A.; Jain, S.L. First photocatalytic synthesis of cyclic carbonates from CO$_2$ and epoxides using CoPc/TiO$_2$ hybrid under mild conditions. *ACS Sustain. Chem. Eng.* **2018**, *6*, 7799–7809. [CrossRef]
39. Zhao, Z.L.; Bian, J.; Zhao, L.; Wu, H.J.; Xu, S.; Sun, L.; Li, Z.J.; Zhang, Z.Q.; Jing, L.Q. Construction of 2D Zn-MOF/BiVO$_4$ S-scheme heterojunction for efficient photocatalytic CO$_2$ conversion under visible light irradiation. *Chin. J. Catal.* **2022**, *43*, 1331–1340. [CrossRef]
40. Liu, H.; Chen, S.; Zhang, Y.; Li, R.; Zhang, J.; Peng, T. An effective Z-scheme hybrid photocatalyst based on zinc porphyrin derivative and anatase titanium dioxide microsphere for carbon dioxide reduction. *Mater. Today Sustain.* **2022**, *19*, 100164. [CrossRef]
41. Zhao, L.N.; Ji, B.A.; Zhang, X.F.; Bai, L.L.; Qu, Y.; Li, Z.J.; Jing, L.Q. Construction of Ultrathin S-Scheme Heterojunctions of Single Ni Atom Immobilized Ti-MOF and BiVO$_4$ for CO$_2$ Photoconversion of nearly 100% to CO by Pure Water. *Adv. Mater.* **2022**, *34*, 2205303. [CrossRef]

Disclaimer/Publisher's Note: The statements, opinions and data contained in all publications are solely those of the individual author(s) and contributor(s) and not of MDPI and/or the editor(s). MDPI and/or the editor(s) disclaim responsibility for any injury to people or property resulting from any ideas, methods, instructions or products referred to in the content.

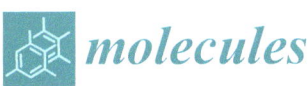

Article

Photoredox Coupling of CO$_2$ Reduction with Benzyl Alcohol Oxidation over Ternary Metal Chalcogenides (Zn$_m$In$_2$S$_{3+m}$, m = 1–5) with Regulable Products Selectivity

Zisheng Du [1], Kexin Gong [2], Zhiruo Yu [1], Yang Yang [1,2,3,*], Peixian Wang [4], Xiuzhen Zheng [1], Zhongliao Wang [1], Sujuan Zhang [1], Shifu Chen [1,2] and Sugang Meng [1,2,4,*]

[1] Key Laboratory of Green and Precise Synthetic Chemistry and Applications, Ministry of Education, College of Chemistry and Materials Science, Huaibei Normal University, Huaibei 235000, China
[2] Key Laboratory of Pollutant Sensitive Materials and Environmental Remediation, Key Laboratory of Clean Energy and Green Circulation, Huaibei Normal University, Huaibei 235000, China
[3] Shanghai Key Laboratory of Atmospheric Particle Pollution and Prevention (LAP3), Fudan University, Shanghai 200438, China
[4] State Key Laboratory Incubation Base for Green Processing of Chemical Engineering, School of Chemistry and Chemical Engineering, Shihezi 832003, China
* Correspondence: yangy@chnu.edu.cn (Y.Y.); mengsugang@126.com (S.M.); Tel.: +86-0561-3802235 (S.M.)

Abstract: Integrating photocatalytic CO$_2$ reduction with selective benzyl alcohol (BA) oxidation in one photoredox reaction system is a promising way for the simultaneous utilization of photogenerated electrons and holes. Herein, Zn$_m$In$_2$S$_{3+m}$ (m = 1–5) semiconductors (ZnIn$_2$S$_4$, Zn$_2$In$_2$S$_5$, Zn$_3$In$_2$S$_6$, Zn$_4$In$_2$S$_7$, and Zn$_5$In$_2$S$_8$) with various composition faults were synthesized via a simple hydrothermal method and used for effective selective dehydrocoupling of benzyl alcohol into high-value C–C coupling products and reduction of CO$_2$ into syngas under visible light. The absorption edge of Zn$_m$In$_2$S$_{3+m}$ samples shifted to shorter wavelengths as the atomic ratio of Zn/In was increased. The conduction band and valence band position can be adjusted by changing the Zn/In ratio, resulting in controllable photoredox ability for selective BA oxidation and CO$_2$ reduction. For example, the selectivity of benzaldehyde (BAD) product was reduced from 76% (ZnIn$_2$S$_4$, ZIS1) to 27% (Zn$_4$In$_2$S$_7$, ZIS4), while the selectivity of hydrobenzoin (HB) was increased from 22% to 56%. Additionally, the H$_2$ formation rate on ZIS1 (1.6 mmol/g/h) was 1.6 times higher than that of ZIS4 (1.0 mmol/g/h), and the CO formation rate on ZIS4 (0.32 mmol/g/h) was three times higher than that of ZIS1 (0.13 mmol/g/h), demonstrating that syngas with different H$_2$/CO ratios can be obtained by controlling the Zn/In ratio in Zn$_m$In$_2$S$_{3+m}$. This study provides new insights into unveiling the relationship of structure–property of Zn$_m$In$_2$S$_{3+m}$ layered crystals, which are valuable for implementation in a wide range of environment and energy applications.

Keywords: photocatalytic; CO$_2$ reduction; syngas; benzyl alcohol oxidation; ZnIn sulfide

Citation: Du, Z.; Gong, K.; Yu, Z.; Yang, Y.; Wang, P.; Zheng, X.; Wang, Z.; Zhang, S.; Chen, S.; Meng, S. Photoredox Coupling of CO$_2$ Reduction with Benzyl Alcohol Oxidation over Ternary Metal Chalcogenides (Zn$_m$In$_2$S$_{3+m}$, m = 1–5) with Regulable Products Selectivity. *Molecules* **2023**, *28*, 6553. https://doi.org/10.3390/molecules28186553

Academic Editor: Barbara Bonelli

Received: 17 July 2023
Revised: 6 September 2023
Accepted: 8 September 2023
Published: 10 September 2023

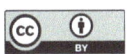

Copyright: © 2023 by the authors. Licensee MDPI, Basel, Switzerland. This article is an open access article distributed under the terms and conditions of the Creative Commons Attribution (CC BY) license (https:// creativecommons.org/licenses/by/ 4.0/).

1. Introduction

With the combustion of fossil fuels, a large amount of carbon dioxide (CO$_2$) is emitted into the air, leading to significant changes in both the environment and energy dynamics [1,2]. Solar-powered conversion of CO$_2$ into valuable fuels or feedstock has been recognized as a sustainable and environmentally friendly energy conversion technology to address these problems [3–8]. This approach is considered a win–win strategy as it can effectively reduce the greenhouse effect while also alleviating the pressure of energy scarcity. However, the conversion efficiencies of CO$_2$ are currently unsatisfactory due to the stable structure of CO$_2$. Additionally, typical photocatalytic systems are performed in water, which results in low evolution efficiency of O$_2$ due to the large overpotential [9]. Most CO$_2$ photoreduction studies focus on the reductive half-reaction, with less attention being paid to the oxidative half-reaction [10,11]. The use of sacrificial reagents such as isopropyl alcohol (IPA), triethanolamine (TEOA), sulfite, etc., to capture holes can accelerate the reaction rate but produces less value oxidation products [12–16]. Merging photocatalytic CO_2 reduction with organic synthesis into one system may be an ideal strategy [1,13]. Allowing the holes to react with organic substrates instead of H_2O or hole scavengers can facilitate the production of value-added chemicals and improve CO_2 reduction efficiency.

Among the organic substrates, benzyl alcohol (BA) is one of the most popular because it can be oxidized to value-added chemicals such as benzaldehyde (BAD) and C-C coupling products, including benzoin, deoxybenzoin, and hydrobenzoin (HB), which are widely used as versatile structural motifs in fine chemicals and pharmaceutical intermediates [17–19]. Metal sulfide semiconductors, known for their high redox ability, good visible-light responses, and rich variability in properties, have been widely used in photocatalytic fields, including CO_2 reduction, H_2 evolution, and BA oxidation, etc. [15,19–21]. Nevertheless, the majority of semiconductors demonstrate inadequate photocatalytic activities due to their limited light absorption properties and inefficient charge separation. To achieve the goal of industrial application, scientists have been actively researching catalyst modification techniques such as morphology control, defect engineering, heterojunction construction, and co-catalyst loading to overcome challenges related to slow electron transport behavior, high carrier recombination efficiency, and to effectively optimize the interface structure and behavior of catalysts, ultimately improving catalytic efficiency and selectivity. For example, Han et al. designed controllable Au–Pt@CdS hybrids for photoredox conversion of alcohol to valuable aldehyde and H_2 [22]. Qi et al. reported SiO_2-supported semiconductor CdS quantum dots, which exhibited high efficiency in dehydrogenative C–C coupling of BA into C–C coupled HB with high selectivity (95–100%) [17]. Kevin et al. prepared CdS QDs to achieve visible light-driven oxidation of BA with >90% selectivity for either BAD or C–C coupled products (including deoxybenzoin, benzil, and HB), by tuning the amount of Cd^0 deposited on the CdS QD surfaces in situ [23]. Intriguingly, ZnIn sulfide with a customized Zn/In ratio and controllable band structure has attracted significant attention [20]. The former work has demonstrated that the coproduction of C–C coupled products and hydrogen (H_2) can be controlled by altering the Zn/In ratio of $Zn_xIn_2S_{3+x}$ (x = 0.1, 0.2, 0.4, 0.6, and 0.8); however, the selectivity of specific C–C coupled product is very low [24]. The photocatalytic activities of $Zn_xIn_2S_{3+x}$ (x = 1–5) were explored for photocatalytic hydrogen production from water and CO_2 reduction [25]. Additionally, the $Zn_xIn_2S_{3+x}$ photocatalyst also showed high performances for lignin depolymerization to functionalized aromatics [26]. Previous studies have proven that doping, constructing heterojunction, or optimizing the atomic ratio of Zn and In can significantly enhance photocatalytic performance. However, the optimization of the atomic ratio offers a unique approach to improving photocatalytic performance. This is because by controlling the presence and distribution of composition faults, which disrupt the crystal structure's periodicity, the atomic ratio directly influences charge carrier dynamics and interfacial chemical reactions. Furthermore, the resulting anisotropic electrical conductivity from these composition faults promotes efficient charge separation and transfer, ultimately leading to improved photocatalytic activity. Unfortunately, not much attention has been given to the effects of composition faults of $Zn_xIn_2S_{3+x}$ layered crystals in the field of simultaneous photocatalytic CO_2 reduction and selective BA oxidation. This work aims to reveal the relationship between the structure and properties of $Zn_mIn_2S_{3+m}$ in CO_2 reduction and BA oxidation reactions in one system.

In this study, a series of ZnIn sulfides ($Zn_mIn_2S_{3+m}$ (m = 1–5, integer)) with various Zn/In ratios were synthesized via a simple hydrothermal method. $ZnIn_2S_4$, $Zn_2In_2S_5$, $Zn_3In_2S_6$, $Zn_4In_2S_7$, and $Zn_5In_2S_8$ were defined as ZIS1, ZIS2, ZIS3, ZIS4, and ZIS5, respectively. Their structure information and typical physicochemical properties were characterized by various characterization techniques, such as scanning electron microscopy (SEM), transmission electron microscopy (TEM), X-ray diffraction (XRD) spectra, UV-visible diffuse reflectance spectroscopy (UV–vis DRS), X-ray photoelectron spectroscopy (XPS), and so on. The relationship between structure and photogenerated charges were investigated by photocurrent, electrochemical impedance spectroscopy (EIS), and photoluminescence spectra, etc. Also, gas chromatography (GC) and high-performance liquid chromatography (HPLC) were employed to probe the products' composition, such as H_2, CO, BZ, BAD, HB, etc. Additionally, in situ diffuse reflectance infrared Fourier transform spectroscopy (DRIFTS) and density functional theory (DFT) calculation were carried out to explore the reaction mechanism on catalysts with different Zn/In ratios. The results showed that the band structure, H_2/CO ratio and selectivity of oxidation products of BA could be regulated by altering the Zn/In ratio. By conducting a thorough analysis of the photoproducts of H_2, CO, BZ, BAD, and HB, we aim to uncover important trends and insights that can contribute to the development of more efficient catalysts for these reactions.

2. Results and Discussion

2.1. Characterization of Catalysts

The XRD patterns of $Zn_mIn_2S_{3+m}$ (m = 1–5) composites showed similar patterns as shown in Figure 1. The peaks at 21.6, 26.8, 28.1, 47.0, 52.2, 55.9, and 76.8° can be assigned to (006), (102), (104), (112), (1012), (202), and (213) facets, respectively, which can be attributed to the hexagonal phase [26–28]. Oxides, binary sulfides, or organic compounds related to the reactants were not detected via the XRD analysis, indicating the prepared $Zn_mIn_2S_{3+m}$ (m = 1–5) samples were relatively pure, which was consistent with the reports [26,27]. It was reported that the chemical compositions of $Zn_mIn_2S_{3+m}$ are different, and the structure characteristics are similar, as a result, showing similar XRD patterns [25,28].

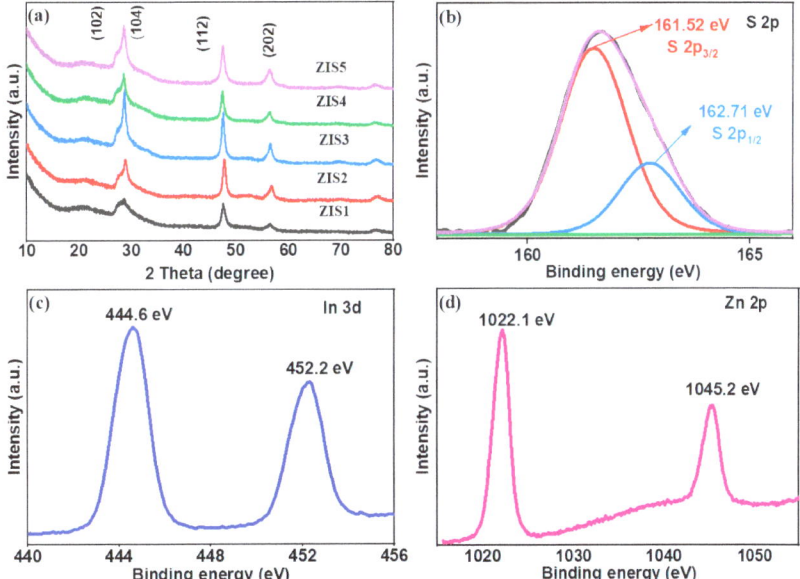

Figure 1. (a) XRD patterns of ZIS samples and high-resolution XPS spectra of (b) S 2p, (c) In 3d, (d) Zn 2p of ZIS4.

The X-ray photoelectron spectroscopy (XPS) was further employed to study the surface composition and chemical state of the ZIS4 sample. Figure 1b shows the high-resolution spectra of S 2p, in which the peak located at 161.7 eV can be attributed to S^{2-}. In Figure 1b, the deconvoluted S 2p XPS spectrum reveals distinct peaks at approximately 161.52 and 162.71 eV (with an energy difference of 1.19 eV), corresponding to S 2p3/2 and S 2p1/2, respectively [29,30]. The two characteristic peaks at approximately 444.6 and 452.2 eV correspond to In $3d_{5/2}$ and $3d_{1/2}$, respectively, demonstrating that the valence state of the indium was +3 [25,31]. The Zn 2p spectra of ZIS4 exhibit peaks around 1022.1 and

1045.2 eV, corresponding to the Zn $2p_{3/2}$ and $2p_{1/2}$ of Zn^{2+}, respectively [32]. The XRD and XPS results demonstrated that layer-structured $Zn_mIn_2S_{3+m}$ (m = 1–5) crystals were successfully synthesized.

Figure 2 displays the morphology and structure of prepared $Zn_mIn_2S_{3+m}$ photocatalysts. The scanning electron microscopy (SEM) images (Figure 2a,d,g) show clearly that the $ZnIn_2S_4$, $Zn_2In_2S_5$, and $Zn_3In_2S_6$ samples were composed of cross-linked nanosheets and the average diameter of the microspheres was about 1 µm. Interestingly, the shapes of microspheres for $Zn_4In_2S_7$ and $Zn_5In_2S_8$ were partially distorted (shown in Figure 2j,m).

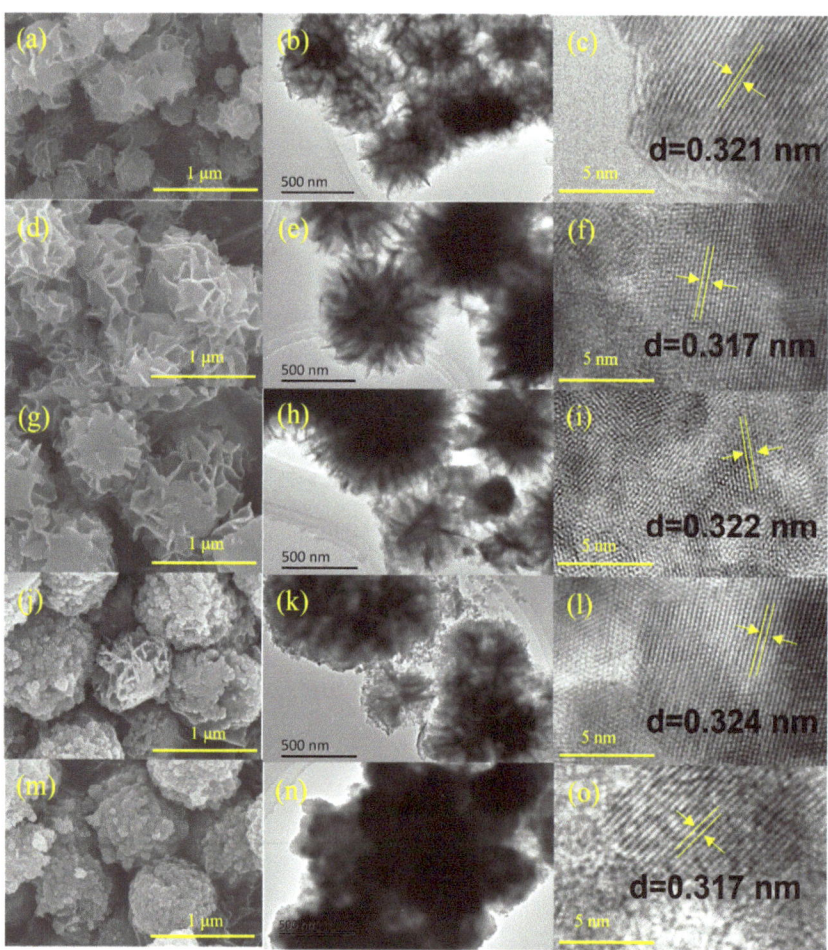

Figure 2. SEM, TEM, and HRTEM of ZIS1 (**a**–**c**), ZIS2 (**d**–**f**), ZIS3 (**g**–**i**), ZIS4 (**j**–**l**), and ZIS5 (**m**–**o**).

The transmission electron microscopy (TEM) images also display similar structures of $Zn_mIn_2S_{3+m}$ samples. With an increase of m, the sheets/petals that make up microspheres (Figure 2b) gradually become such small pieces (Figure 2n), which is consistent with SEM results. The high-resolution TEM (HRTEM) image of $Zn_mIn_2S_{3+m}$ catalysts are shown in Figure 2c,f,i,l,o. It is shown that the lattice fringes with an interplanar spacing of around 0.32 nm correspond to the (102) crystal plane of ZIS [25]. The XRD, XPS, SEM, as well as TEM results certified that all of the $Zn_mIn_2S_{3+m}$ (m = 1–5) layered crystals were successfully synthesized.

The BET-specific surface area and pore-size distribution of the prepared samples were measured by nitrogen adsorption-desorption analysis (shown in Figure 3). The estimated surface areas of the ZIS1, ZIS2, ZIS3, ZIS4, and ZIS5 samples were 42.5, 16.9, 13.9, 15.2, and 31.8 m^2/g, respectively. Additionally, the $Zn_mIn_2S_{3+m}$ samples also showed similar pore-size distributions, and the average pore diameters of ZIS1, ZIS2, ZIS3, ZIS4, and ZIS5 were about 52.3, 46.3, 47.3, 45.9, and 40.3 nm, respectively. A large pore size will facilitate effective transport pathways for product molecules and reactants [25]. The slightly decreased specific surface area may be caused by the distorted structure (SEM and TEM results).

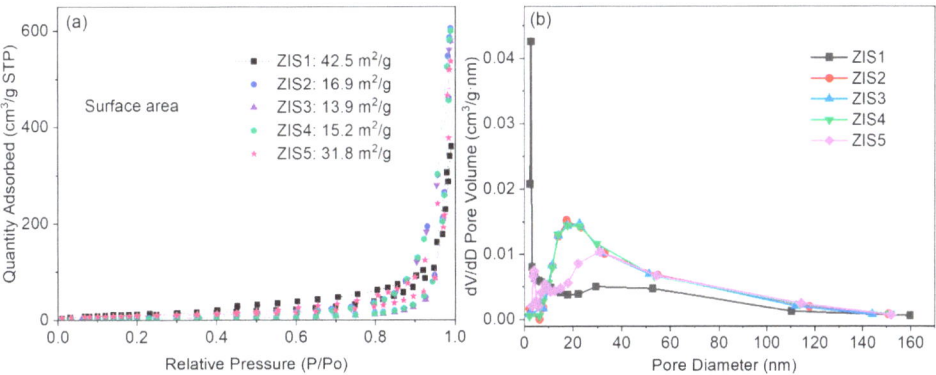

Figure 3. (**a**) Nitrogen adsorption-desorption isotherms and (**b**) pore-size distribution of ZIS samples.

The optical properties and energy band structure of $Zn_mIn_2S_{m+3}$ samples were studied using UV-vis diffuse reflectance spectroscopy (DRS) and Mott–Schottky measurements. As the value of m increased from 1 to 5, the absorption edges gradually shifted to shorter wavelengths (shown in Figure 4a), indicating an increase in band gap energy (Eg) of $Zn_mIn_2S_{m+3}$ samples with increasing Zn/In ratio. The Eg values of $Zn_mIn_2S_{m+3}$ were further calculated using the Kubelka–Munk function, $[F(R)h\nu]^{1/2}$, plotted against the energy of light (Figure 4b) [26]. It was observed that the Eg of $Zn_mIn_2S_{m+3}$ increased from 2.46 to 2.88 eV with an increasing molar ratio of Zn to In. Specifically, band gap energies of $ZnIn_2S_4$, $Zn_2In_2S_5$, $Zn_3In_2S_6$, $Zn_4In_2S_7$, and $Zn_5In_2S_8$ are approximately 2.46, 2.61, 2.73, 2.79, and 2.88 eV, respectively. The color of the five typical catalysts are shown in Figure S1, and it was evident clearly that the color gradually faded with the increase in Zn/In ratio. Further, density functional theory (DFT) calculations were conducted to estimate the trend of band gap with changing the Zn/In ratio in ZIS, and the corresponding data were displayed in Figure S2. The calculated Eg of ZIS1 and ZIS4 was 0.143 and 0.367 eV, respectively, demonstrating an increase in the Eg of $Zn_mIn_2S_{m+3}$ with increasing molar ratio of Zn to In.

The flat-band potential (E_{fb}) of the typical catalysts was further estimated by Mott–Schottky measurement. The Mott–Schottky curves indicated the samples exhibited n-type characteristics due to the positive slopes, and their flat-band potential was estimated to be −0.57, −0.59, −0.61, −0.65, −0.70 V vs. reversible hydrogen electrode (RHE), respectively (Figure 4c–g). The corresponding normal hydron electrode (NHE) potentials were calculated as −0.98, −1.00, −1.02, −1.06, −1.11 V vs. NHE. It has been reported that the conduction band minimum (CBM) of semiconductors is usually 0.1–0.2 V negative than the E_{fb} [33]. In this study, the CBMs of ZIS1, ZIS2, ZIS3, ZIS4, and ZIS5 were −1.08, −1.10, −1.12, −1.16, −1.21 V vs. NHE, respectively. According to Eg = E_{VB} − E_{CB}, the E_{VB} of ZIS1, ZIS2, ZIS3, ZIS4, and ZIS5 were 1.38, 1.51, 1.61, 1.63, and 1.67 V vs. NHE (shown in Figure 4h), respectively. These results and trends are consistent with previous reports [25,26].

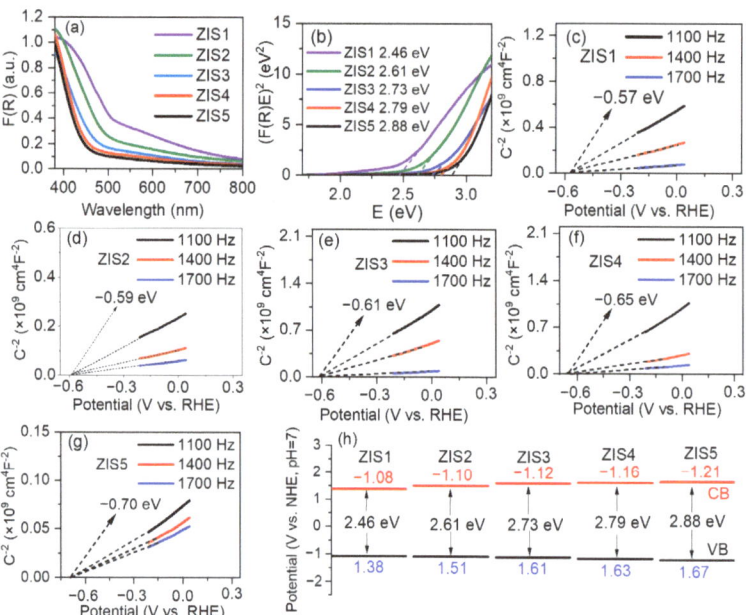

Figure 4. (**a**) UV-vis absorbance spectra, (**b**) Tauc plots, (**c**–**g**) Mott-Schottky plots, (**h**) energy band schematic diagram of typical catalysts.

The charge transfer behaviors are an important factor to explain the photocatalytic activity [19,34,35]. Photocurrent measurement was employed to assess the separation efficiency of photogenerated charge carries. As shown in Figure 5a, it is clear that the photocurrent increased sharply when the light was turned on and immediately returned to its initial negligible value when the light was switched off. ZIS4 exhibited the highest photocurrent, followed by ZIS1, ZIS3, ZIS2, and ZIS5 under light irradiation. Further, electrochemical impedance spectroscopy (EIS) was performed to study the charge transfer resistance of the typical photocatalysts [36,37]. From Figure 5b, it can be seen that ZIS1 has the smallest radii of the semicircles (nearly equal to ZIS5), implying that ZIS1 is beneficial for charge transfer. Photoluminescence (PL) spectra were also applied to investigate the transfer of photogenerated charge carriers [38,39]. In Figure 5c, ZIS4 exhibited the lowest PL intensity compared with other ZIS samples, meaning the ZIS4 had the lowest recommendation efficiency of electrons and holes; this was consistent with the photocurrent testing result. It can be inferred from the subsequent activity results that the product selectivity of both CO_2 reduction and BA oxidation was not directly related to the BET-specific surface area and charge separation efficiency, which can be affected by various facets, including active sites, defects, composition, morphology, etc. [25].

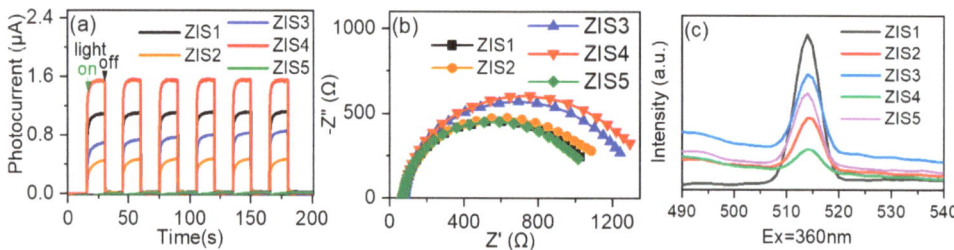

Figure 5. (**a**) Photocurrent density, (**b**) electrochemical impedance spectra (EIS), (**c**) steady-state photoluminescence spectra of typical catalysts.

2.2. Photoredox Reaction and Mechanism of CO_2 Reduction with Oxidation of BA

Subsequently, the photocatalytic CO_2 reduction reaction integrated with selective oxidation of benzyl alcohol (BA) under the irradiation of visible light ($\lambda > 420$ nm) was studied using $Zn_mIn_2S_{3+m}$ samples (Figure 6). Figure 6a shows that ZIS1 exhibited the highest H_2 formation rate of 1.6 mmol/g/h, followed by ZIS2, ZIS3, ZIS4, and ZIS5 at 1.5, 1.3, 1.0, and 0.7 mmol/g/h, respectively. While, the CO formation rate followed the order of ZIS5 (0.33 mmol/g/h) ≈ ZIS4 (0.32 mmol/g/h) > ZIS3 (0.17 mmol/g/h) > ZIS2 (0.15 mmol/g/h) > ZIS1 (0.13 mmol/g/h). This suggests that with increasing Zn content, the electrons preferentially react with CO_2 rather than H^+. The BET-specific surface area of the ZIS1 and ZIS4 samples was also measured using CO_2 adsorption–desorption analysis (shown in Figure S3). The surface areas of the ZIS1 and ZIS4 samples were determined to be 41.03 and 44.89 m^2/g, respectively, indicating that ZIS4 had a higher adsorption capacity of CO_2. DFT calculations were performed to understand the critical role of Zn/In ratio in the selective photoreduction of CO_2 to CO and H^+ to H_2 process over ZIS1 and ZIS4. The calculations revealed that the formation energy barrier of H^* on ZIS1 and ZIS4 is 0.89 and 0.92 eV, respectively (Figure 6b), confirming that H_2 formation is easier on ZIS1 than on ZIS4. Figure 6c shows that the formation energy barrier of $*CO_2$ and $*COOH$ on ZIS4 are lower than that of ZIS1, indicating that the CO_2 reduction process is more favorable on the ZIS4 catalyst. These calculated results align well with the experimental findings.

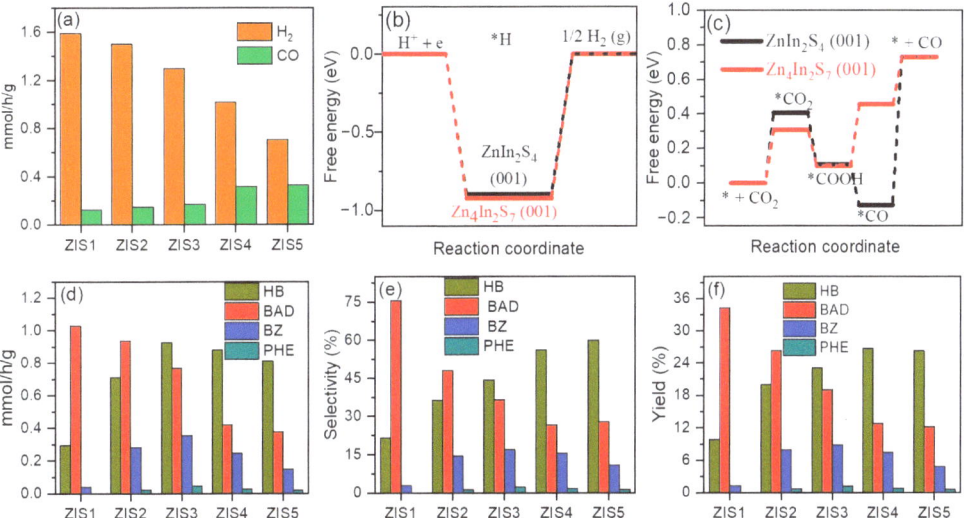

Figure 6. (**a**) Evolution rate of H_2 and CO over ZIS samples, free energy for generating (**b**) H_2 and (**c**) CO on ZIS1 and ZIS4 using DFT calculation, (**d**) generation rate, (**e**) selectivity, and (**f**) yield of products from BA oxidation over ZIS samples. "*" means the "active site".

Figure 6d displays that the formation rate of BAD was gradually decreased with increasing Zn/In ratio. On the other hand, the formation rates of the hydrogenation products, namely hydrogenation of benzyl alcohol (HB) and benzoin (BZ), increase with increasing Zn/In ratio and reach their highest values at ZIS3 (HB: 0.93 mmol/g/h and BZ: 0.35 mmol/g/h), after which they gradually decrease. Figure 6e shows that the selectivity of BAD was decreased from 76% (ZIS1) to 27% (ZIS4), while the selectivity of HB improved from 22% to 56% (ZIS4) and 60% (ZIS5). The yield of BAD also decreased from 34% (ZIS1) to 13% (ZIS4), while the yield of HB and BZ was increased from 10% and 1.2% to 27% and 8%, respectively (Figure 6f). These results demonstrated that both the H_2/CO ratio and oxidation products of BA can be adjusted by altering the Zn/In raion in ZIS. The standard curves for BAD, HB, BE, and PHE are presented in Figure S4, while the HPLC spectra illustrating the products generated from ZIS1 and ZIS4 are depicted in Figure S5.

Furthermore, a series of control experiments were conducted to confirm the importance of both the CO_2 atmosphere and BA substrate on the ZIS sample (shown in Figure S6). Without the addition of BA in the reaction system, the generation rates of H_2 and CO were found to be negligible compared to those obtained when BA was present. Substituting BA with TEOA resulted in an improvement in the generation rate of H_2, but a decrease in the generation rate of CO. When Ar was introduced into the cell instead of CO_2, no CO was detected, and the produced H_2 was also negligible. These findings suggest that CO is generated via CO_2 reduction. However, the yield of BAD was determined as 64.5%, with a selectivity of 100% for BAD, and no other C-C coupling products were detected. These results demonstrate that both a CO_2 atmosphere and a BA solution are essential for achieving a high generation rate of CO and C-C coupling products, such as HB and BZ.

To evaluate the stability of ZIS, ZIS4 was selected as the typical catalyst for testing. The catalytic stability of the ZIS4 sample was assessed through photocatalytic reusability analysis for three cycles, as shown in Figure 7. Figure 7a demonstrates that the H_2 evolution rates were 1.31, 1.28, and 1.05 mmol/g/h in the 1st, 2nd, and 3rd runs, respectively. The generation rate of CO was 0.30, 0.27, and 0.21 mmol/g/h in the 1st, 2nd, and 3rd runs, respectively. The corresponding liquid products are displayed in Figure 7b. The formation rate of HB and PHE did not significantly decrease, while the generation rate of BAD and BZ slightly decreased. Figure 7c,d reveals that even after three cycles, the selectivity and yield of liquid products remained close to those of the first cycle. Furthermore, XRD profiles and SEM images (Figures S7 and S8) of ZIS4 before and after long-time experiments confirmed the well-maintained crystalline phase and morphology. The preservation of the crystalline structure and negligible loss of gas and liquid generation rates over three runs indicate the durability of the ZIS4 sample, making it a promising candidate for potential applications in sustainable energy conversion.

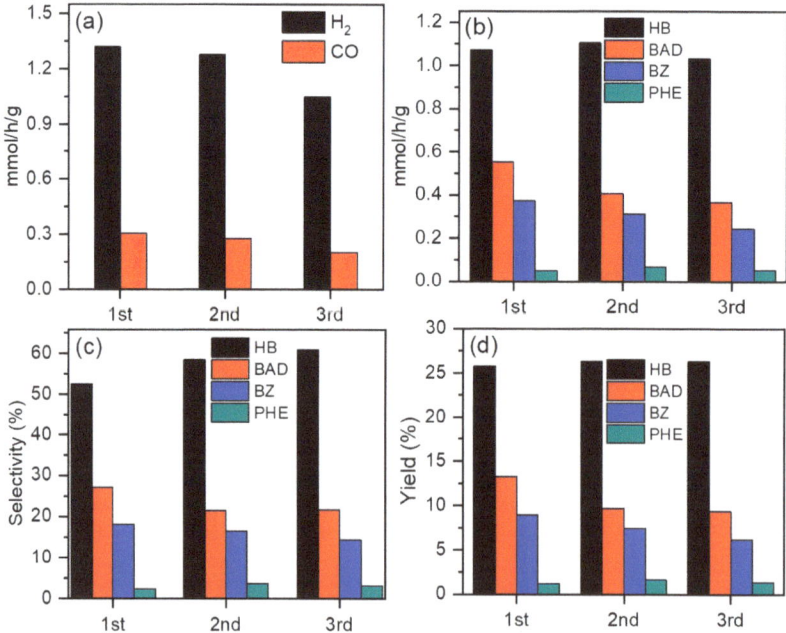

Figure 7. Photocatalytic CO_2 reduction and BA oxidation performances on the ZIS4 sample under visible-light irradiation over three cycles. (**a**) The generation rate of H_2 and CO, (**b**) generation rate, (**c**) selectivity, and (**d**) yield of products from BA oxidation.

Furthermore, the photocatalytic CO_2RR and BA oxidation catalyzed by the ZIS4 catalyst at room temperature were investigated using in situ diffuse reflectance infrared Fourier transform spectroscopy (DRIFTS). The corresponding data can be found in Figure 8. The reaction intermediates were determined by analyzing the observed peaks in the infrared spectra. The peaks at 1319 cm^{-1} were attributed to the presence of bidentate carbonate (b-CO_3^{2-}) [3]. Additionally, the peaks at 1540 cm^{-1} were assigned to the COOH* group, which serves as an important intermediate for CO formation [3]. The infrared spectra also revealed the reaction intermediates involved in the conversion of BA. The peak at 1207 cm^{-1} was assigned to the presence of the formyl group (HCO) in BAD, while the sharp peak at 1701 cm^{-1} was attributed to the vibration of the carbonyl (ν(CO)) stretch mode in BAD [40]. The stretching vibrations of C-H in BAD were found at 2853 cm^{-1}. The peaks in the range of 2900 to 3130 cm^{-1}, which gradually increased with reaction time, were assigned to HB, indicating the generation of more HB. The intense bands at 1452 and 1495 cm^{-1} were associated with aromatic δ(C-C) and ν(C–H) modes [40], which can be assigned to HB. Moreover, the peaks at 1583 cm^{-1} and 1601 cm^{-1} were attributed to the C=C skeleton vibration of mononuclear aromatic hydrocarbons, and the peak at 3062 cm^{-1} was assigned to C-H stretching vibration on the benzene ring of HB. These findings provide valuable information on the reaction mechanism and intermediates involved in the photocatalytic coupled system of CO_2 reduction and benzyl alcohol oxidation over the ZIS catalysts.

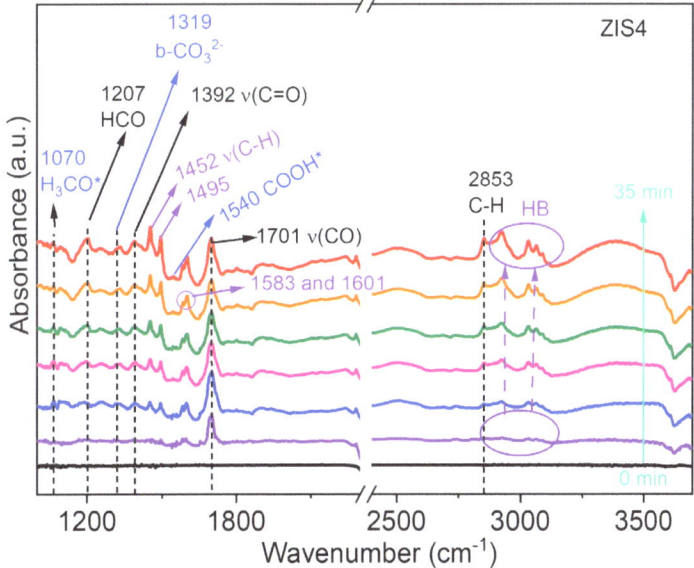

Figure 8. In situ DRIFTS spectra of the reaction intermediates in CO_2 photoreduction and BA oxidation over ZIS4 under light irradiation. "*" means the "active site".

3. Materials and Methods

3.1. Preparation of $Zn_mIn_2S_{3+m}$ Photocatalysts

$Zn_mIn_2S_{3+m}$ samples were synthesized by a simple hydrothermal method. For each preparation, 0.8 mmol $ZnSO_4\cdot 4H_2O$, 1.6 mmol $InCl_3\cdot 4H_2O$, 0.65 g CTAB, and 7 mmol thioacetamide (TAA) were dispersed into 70 mL deionized water. After stirring for 60 min, the above suspension was transferred into a 100 mL Teflon-lined autoclave (Anhui Kemi Machinery Technology Co., Ltd., Hefei, China) and heated at 160 °C for 12 h. After natural cooling to room temperature, the precipitate was washed with absolute ethanol and deionized water several times and dried at 60 °C in a vacuum oven. The as-obtained samples, $ZnIn_2S_4$, $Zn_2In_2S_5$, $Zn_3In_2S_6$, $Zn_4In_2S_7$, and $Zn_5In_2S_8$ were defined as ZIS1, ZIS2, ZIS3, ZIS4, and ZIS5, respectively.

3.2. Characterizations

The structures of samples were analyzed by powder X-ray diffraction (XRD) using a Bruker D8 advance X-ray diffractometer (Karlsruhe, Germany) with Cu Kα radiation (λ = 0.1540 nm) and a scanning speed of 3· min^{-1}. Fourier transform infrared spectroscopy (FT-IR) was measured on an iS50 (Waltham, MA, USA). The optical properties were characterized by UV-Vis diffuse reflectance spectroscopy (UV-Vis DRS) using a UV-Vis spectrophotometer (Shimadzu UV-3600, Kyoto, Japan). N_2 physisorption measurements were carried out at 77 K using a Micromeritics Tristar II 3020 surface area analyzer. Multipoint Brunauer-Emmett-Teller (BET) specific surface areas were then determined from the adsorption isotherms (Micromeritics ASAP 2460, Norcross, GA, USA). The X-ray photoelectron spectroscopy (XPS) was measured on a Thermo Fischer ESCALAB Xi$^+$ spectrometer with an Al Kα X-ray beam (Waltham, MA, USA). The binding energies were corrected regarding the C 1s peak of the surface adventitious carbon at 284.8 eV. Transmission electron microscopy (TEM) and high-resolution transmission electron microscopy (HRTEM) images were performed on a JEM-2100 with an accelerating voltage of 200 kV (Akishima-shi, Japan). The morphologies of the photocatalysts were carried out by scanning electron microscope (SEM, Regulus 8200, Tokyo, Japan).

3.3. Photoelectrochemical Measurements

Photoelectrochemical measurements: A 5 mg sample was dispersed in 400 µL of deionized water by sonication to obtain a uniform slurry. Then, 20 µL of slurry was deposited as a film on a 0.5 cm × 0.5 cm fluorine-doped tin oxide (FTO) conducting glass to obtain the working electrode. After drying at room temperature, the working electrode was obtained. Ag/AgCl was used as a reference electrode, and platinum wire as a counter electrode. The photocurrent test and flat band potential (M-S plots) were carried out in a three-electrode system in a 0.2 mol L^{-1} Na_2SO_4 solution. Electrochemical impedance spectra (EIS) are carried out in a mixture of 0.1 mol L^{-1} KCl and 0.1 mol L^{-1} $K_3[Fe(CN)_6]/K_4[Fe(CN)_6]$.

3.4. Photocatalytic Activity Testing

The coupling activity of photocatalytic CO_2 reduction and benzyl alcohol oxidation was tested in a visible high-temperature and high-pressure reactor. Typically, 5 mg photocatalyst and 5 mL acetonitrile containing 5 mM benzyl alcohol and 0.1 g K_2CO_3 were added into the reactor, which was then ultrasonicated to ensure even dispersion of the catalyst. The reactor was then vacuumed to remove air and finally was stirred in the dark for 30 min to achieve a dynamic dissolution equilibrium of CO_2 in an atmosphere of CO_2 gas. The Xe lamp (λ > 420 nm) was used to provide the light source for the reaction. Gas products were collected using a gas injection needle with a quantitative ring, and CO and other products were detected by a flame ionization detector (FID), while H_2 was detected by a thermal conductivity detector (TCD) gas chromatograph. The liquid products were collected, diluted with acetonitrile, and detected by high-performance liquid chromatography (HPLC).

3.5. DFT Calculations

The theoretical simulations were conducted via the Materials Studio (BIOVIA V2017, San Diego, CA, USA) equipped with the CASTEP mode. Also, we utilized the Perdew–Burke–Ernzerhof (PBE) form exchange-correlation functional within the generalized gradient approximation (GGA). The structures of the (001) plane of ZIS1 and ZIS4 were optimized. The formation energy barrier of H_2 and CO was conducted through the Vienna ab initio Simulation Package (VASP) with the projector augment wave method [41]. A generalized gradient approximation of the Perdew–Burke–Ernzerhof (PBE) functional was used as the exchange-correlation functional. The Brillouin zone was sampled with 2 × 2 × 1 K points for the surface calculation. The cutoff energy was set as 500 eV, and structure relaxation was performed until the convergence criteria of energy and force reached 1×10^{-5} eV and 0.02 eV Å^{-1}, respectively. A vacuum layer of 15 Å was constructed to eliminate interactions between periodic structures of the surface models. The van der Waals interaction was amended by the zero damping DFT-D3 method of Grimme [42]. The Gibbs free energy was calculated as $\Delta G = \Delta E + \Delta EZPE - T\Delta S$, where the ΔE, $\Delta EZPE$, and ΔS are electronic energy, zero-point energy, and entropy difference between products and reactants. The zero-point energies of isolated and absorbed intermediate products were calculated from the frequency analysis. The vibrational frequencies and entropies of molecules in the gas phase were obtained from the National Institute of Standards and Technology (NIST) database [43].

4. Conclusions

In summary, this study investigated the effects of composition faults in $Zn_mIn_2S_{3+m}$ on simultaneous photocatalytic CO_2 reduction and selective BA oxidation. By adjusting the element composition, the band gap energy (Eg) of $ZnmIn_2S_{m+3}$ could be controlled, resulting in adjustable redox ability. The CO_2 reduction activity and selectivity of BA oxidation products were found to be influenced by the Zn/In ratio in ZIS. Specifically, ZIS4 exhibited higher CO_2 adsorption capacity and lower CO_2 activation, while ZIS1 had a higher energy barrier for H_2 evolution. The presence of both a CO_2 atmosphere and a BA solution was crucial for achieving a high generation rate of CO and C-C coupling products. Moreover, the formation rate of BAD decreased with increasing Zn/In ratio, while the formation rates of hydrogenation products, HB and BZ, increased and reached their highest values at ZIS3. The selectivity of BAD decreased from ZIS1 to ZIS4, while the selectivity of HB increased. The yield of BAD decreased, while the yield of HB and BZ increased with increasing Zn/In ratio. These results highlight the potential of adjusting both the H_2/CO ratio and the oxidation products of BA by altering the Zn/In ratio in ZIS. Overall, this study provides valuable insights into the role of the Zn/In ratio in the simultaneous photocatalytic CO_2 reduction and selective BA oxidation process.

Supplementary Materials: The following supporting information can be downloaded at: https://www.mdpi.com/article/10.3390/molecules28186553/s1. Figure S1. Macro images of ZIS samples. Figure S2. The band gap of (a) ZIS1 and (b) ZIS4 by DFT calculation. Figure S3. CO2 adsorption-desorption isotherms of ZIS1 and ZIS4 samples. Figure S4. The HPLC spectra of (a) BAD, (c) HB, (e) BZ and (g) PHE; the corresponding standard curves of (b) BAD, (d) HB, (f) BZ and (h) PHE. Figure S5. The HPLC spectra of products generated from (a) ZIS1 and (b) ZIS4. Figure S6. Controlling experiments over ZIS4 sample. (a) generation rate of H2 and CO, (b) generation rate, (c) selectivity and (d) yield of products form BA oxidation.Figure S7. XRD patterns of ZIS4 before and after reaction. Figure S8. SEM image of ZIS4 after reaction.

Author Contributions: Conceptualization, S.C.; Methodology, K.G. and S.Z.; Software, Z.Y.; Validation, X.Z.; Formal analysis, Z.Y. and Z.W.; Investigation, Z.D., K.G., P.W., X.Z. and S.Z.; Data curation, Z.D.; Writing—original draft, Z.D. and Y.Y.; Writing—review & editing, S.M.; Supervision, Y.Y., S.C. and S.M.; Funding acquisition, Y.Y., S.C and S.M. All authors have read and agreed to the published version of the manuscript.

Funding: This work was supported by the National Natural Science Foundation of China (NSFC, 52002142 and 52272297); The Foundation of Anhui Province for Distinguished Young Scholars (2022AH020038); the Foundation of State Key Laboratory Incubation Base for Green Processing of Chemical Engineering (KF202201); The Foundation of Anhui Province for Outstanding Young Graduate-student Advisors (2022yjsds036); the Foundation of Educational Commission of Anhui Province (2022AH050373 and 2022AH010030); The Opening Project of Shanghai Key Laboratory of Atmospheric Particle Pollution and Prevention (LAP^3, grant no. FDLAP21005), and the Natural Science Foundation of Anhui Province (grant no. 2108085MB43).

Institutional Review Board Statement: Not applicable.

Informed Consent Statement: Not applicable.

Data Availability Statement: Not applicable.

Conflicts of Interest: The authors declared that there is no conflict of interest.

Sample Availability: Samples of the ZIS are available from the authors.

References

1. Yao, D.; Liang, K.; Chen, G.; Qu, Y.; Liu, J.; Chilivery, R.; Li, S.; Ji, M.; Li, Z.; Zhong, Z.; et al. Dual-functional reaction strategy boosts carbon dioxide reduction by coupling with selective benzyl alcohol oxidation on nano-Au/BiOCl photocatalysts. *J. Catal.* **2023**, *422*, 56–68. [CrossRef]
2. Ning, H.; Li, Y.; Zhang, C. Recent Progress in the Integration of CO_2 Capture and Utilization. *Molecules* **2023**, *28*, 4500. [CrossRef]
3. Zhou, M.; Wang, Z.; Mei, A.; Yang, Z.; Chen, W.; Ou, S.; Wang, S.; Chen, K.; Reiss, P.; Qi, K.; et al. Photocatalytic CO_2 reduction using La-Ni bimetallic sites within a covalent organic framework. *Nat. Commun.* **2023**, *14*, 2473. [PubMed]
4. Zhao, Y.; Waterhouse, G.I.N.; Chen, G.; Xiong, X.; Wu, L.-Z.; Tung, C.-H.; Zhang, T. Two-dimensional-related catalytic materials for solar-driven conversion of CO_x into valuable chemical feedstocks. *Chem. Soc. Rev.* **2019**, *48*, 1972–2010.
5. Lei, Q.; Yuan, H.; Du, J.; Ming, M.; Yang, S.; Chen, Y.; Lei, J.; Han, Z. Photocatalytic CO_2 reduction with aminoanthraquinone organic dyes. *Nat. Commun.* **2023**, *14*, 1087. [CrossRef] [PubMed]
6. Lv, J.; Xie, J.; Mohamed, A.G.A.; Zhang, X.; Feng, Y.; Jiao, L.; Zhou, E.; Yuan, D.; Wang, Y. Solar utilization beyond photosynthesis. *Nat. Rev. Chem.* **2023**, *7*, 91–105.
7. Chen, S.; Wei, J.; Ren, X.; Song, K.; Sun, J.; Bai, F.; Tian, S. Recent Progress in Porphyrin/g-C_3N_4 Composite Photocatalysts for Solar Energy Utilization and Conversion. *Molecules* **2023**, *28*, 4283. [CrossRef]
8. Chi, X.; Lan, Z.-A.; Chen, Q.; Zhang, X.; Chen, X.; Zhang, G.; Wang, X. Electronic Transmission Channels Promoting Charge Separation of Conjugated Polymers for Photocatalytic CO_2 Reduction with Controllable Selectivity. *Angew. Chem. Int. Ed.* **2023**, *62*, e202303785. [CrossRef]
9. Qi, M.-Y.; Lin, Q.; Tang, Z.-R.; Xu, Y.-J. Photoredox coupling of benzyl alcohol oxidation with CO_2 reduction over CdS/TiO_2 heterostructure under visible light irradiation. *Appl. Catal. B Environ.* **2022**, *307*, 121158.
10. Song, J.; Lu, Y.; Lin, Y.; Liu, Q.; Wang, X.; Su, W. A direct Z-scheme α-Fe_2O_3/$LaTiO_2N$ visible-light photocatalyst for enhanced CO_2 reduction activity. *Appl. Catal. B Environ.* **2021**, *292*, 120185. [CrossRef]
11. Wang, S.; Han, X.; Zhang, Y.; Tian, N.; Ma, T.; Huang, H. Inside-and-Out Semiconductor Engineering for CO_2 Photoreduction: From Recent Advances to New Trends. *Small Struct.* **2021**, *2*, 2000061.
12. Lu, K.-Q.; Li, Y.-H.; Zhang, F.; Qi, M.-Y.; Chen, X.; Tang, Z.-R.; Yamada, Y.M.A.; Anpo, M.; Conte, M.; Xu, Y.-J. Rationally designed transition metal hydroxide nanosheet arrays on graphene for artificial CO_2 reduction. *Nat. Commun.* **2020**, *11*, 5181. [CrossRef] [PubMed]
13. Han, C.; Li, Y.-H.; Li, J.-Y.; Qi, M.-Y.; Tang, Z.-R.; Xu, Y.-J. Cooperative Syngas Production and C−N Bond Formation in One Photoredox Cycle. *Angew. Chem. Int. Ed.* **2021**, *60*, 7962–7970. [CrossRef] [PubMed]
14. Meng, S.; Wu, H.; Cui, Y.; Zheng, X.; Wang, H.; Chen, S.; Wang, Y.; Fu, X. One-step synthesis of 2D/2D-3D NiS/$Zn_3In_2S_6$ hierarchical structure toward solar-to-chemical energy transformation of biomass-relevant alcohols. *Appl. Catal. B Environ.* **2020**, *266*, 118617. [CrossRef]
15. Feng, X.; Chen, H.; Yin, H.; Yuan, C.; Lv, H.; Fei, Q.; Zhang, Y.; Zhao, Q.; Zheng, M.; Zhang, Y. Facile Synthesis of P-Doped $ZnIn_2S_4$ with Enhanced Visible-Light-Driven Photocatalytic Hydrogen Production. *Molecules* **2023**, *28*, 4520. [CrossRef] [PubMed]
16. Pan, H.; Heagy, M.D. Bicarbonate reduction with semiconductor photocatalysts: Study of effect of positive hole scavengers. *MRS Commun.* **2018**, *8*, 1173–1177. [CrossRef]
17. Qi, M.-Y.; Li, Y.-H.; Anpo, M.; Tang, Z.-R.; Xu, Y.-J. Efficient Photoredox-Mediated C–C Coupling Organic Synthesis and Hydrogen Production over Engineered Semiconductor Quantum Dots. *ACS Catal.* **2020**, *10*, 14327–14335. [CrossRef]
18. Li, J.-Y.; Qi, M.-Y.; Xu, Y.-J. Efficient splitting of alcohols into hydrogen and C–C coupled products over ultrathin Ni-doped $ZnIn_2S_4$ nanosheet photocatalyst. *Chin. J. Catal.* **2022**, *43*, 1084–1091. [CrossRef]
19. Meng, S.; Chen, C.; Gu, X.; Wu, H.; Meng, Q.; Zhang, J.; Chen, S.; Fu, X.; Liu, D.; Lei, W. Efficient photocatalytic H_2 evolution, CO_2 reduction and N_2 fixation coupled with organic synthesis by cocatalyst and vacancies engineering. *Appl. Catal. B Environ.* **2021**, *285*, 119789. [CrossRef]
20. Wu, X.; Xie, S.; Zhang, H.; Zhang, Q.; Sels, B.F.; Wang, Y. Metal Sulfide Photocatalysts for Lignocellulose Valorization. *Adv. Mater.* **2021**, *33*, 2007129. [CrossRef]
21. Chava, R.K.; Kim, T.; Kim, Y.; Kang, M. Vanadium tetrasulfide as an earth-abundant and noble-metal-free cocatalyst for a solar-to-hydrogen conversion reaction. *J. Mater. Chem. C* **2023**, *11*, 1782–1790. [CrossRef]
22. Han, C.; Tang, Z.R.; Liu, J.; Jin, S.; Xu, Y.J. Efficient photoredox conversion of alcohol to aldehyde and H_2 by heterointerface engineering of bimetal-semiconductor hybrids. *Chem. Sci.* **2019**, *10*, 3514–3522. [CrossRef] [PubMed]
23. McClelland, K.P.; Weiss, E.A. Selective Photocatalytic Oxidation of Benzyl Alcohol to Benzaldehyde or C–C Coupled Products by Visible-Light-Absorbing Quantum Dots. *ACS Appl. Energy Mater.* **2018**, *2*, 92–96.
24. Luo, N.; Hou, T.; Liu, S.; Zeng, B.; Lu, J.; Zhang, J.; Li, H.; Wang, F. Photocatalytic Coproduction of Deoxybenzoin and H_2 through Tandem Redox Reactions. *ACS Catal.* **2019**, *10*, 762–769. [CrossRef]

25. Wu, Y.; Wang, H.; Tu, W.; Wu, S.; Chew, J.W. Effects of composition faults in ternary metal chalcogenides ($Zn_xIn_2S_{3+x}$, x = 1–5) layered crystals for visible-light-driven catalytic hydrogen generation and carbon dioxide reduction. *Appl. Catal. B Environ.* **2019**, *256*, 117810. [CrossRef]
26. Lin, J.; Wu, X.; Xie, S.; Chen, L.; Zhang, Q.; Deng, W.; Wang, Y. Visible-Light-Driven Cleavage of C-O Linkage for Lignin Valorization to Functionalized Aromatics. *ChemSusChem* **2019**, *12*, 5023–5031.
27. Shen, S.; Zhao, L.; Guo, L. $Zn_mIn_2S_{3+m}$ (m=1–5, integer): A new series of visible-light-driven photocatalysts for splitting water to hydrogen. *Int. J. Hydrogen Energy* **2010**, *35*, 10148–10154. [CrossRef]
28. Kalomiros, J.A.; Anagnostopoulos, A.N.; Spyridelis, J. Temperature dependence of the energy gap and some electrical properties of $Zn_2In_2S_5$ (II) single crystals. *Semicond. Sci. Technol.* **1989**, *4*, 536. [CrossRef]
29. Wu, L.; Li, M.; Zhou, B.; Xu, S.; Yuan, L.; Wei, J.; Wang, J.; Zou, S.; Xie, W.; Qiu, Y.; et al. Reversible Stacking of 2D $ZnIn_2S_4$ Atomic Layers for Enhanced Photocatalytic Hydrogen Evolution. *Small* **2023**, 2303821. [CrossRef]
30. Chava, R.K.; Son, N.; Kang, M. Band structure alignment transitioning strategy for the fabrication of efficient photocatalysts for solar fuel generation and environmental remediation applications. *J. Colloid Interface Sci.* **2022**, *627*, 247–260. [CrossRef]
31. Zhang, G.; Yang, J.; Huang, Z.; Pan, G.; Xie, B.; Ni, Z.; Xia, S. Construction dual vacancies to regulate the energy band structure of $ZnIn_2S_4$ for enhanced visible light-driven photodegradation of 4-NP. *J. Hazard. Mater.* **2023**, *441*, 129916. [CrossRef]
32. Liu, W.; Wang, Y.; Huang, H.; Wang, J.; He, G.; Feng, J.; Yu, T.; Li, Z.; Zou, Z. Spatial Decoupling of Redox Chemistry for Efficient and Highly Selective Amine Photoconversion to Imines. *J. Am. Chem. Soc.* **2023**, *145*, 7181–7189. [CrossRef] [PubMed]
33. Gu, X.; Chen, T.; Lei, J.; Yang, Y.; Zheng, X.; Zhang, S.; Zhu, Q.; Fu, X.; Meng, S.; Chen, S. Self-assembly synthesis of S-scheme g-C_3N_4/$Bi_8(CrO_4)O_{11}$ for photocatalytic degradation of norfloxacin and bisphenol A. *Chin. J. Catal.* **2022**, *43*, 2569–2580.
34. Zhang, M.; Zhang, Y.; Ye, L.; Yu, Z.; Liu, R.; Qiao, Y.; Sun, L.; Cui, J.; Lu, X. In situ fabrication $Ti_3C_2F_x$ MXene/$CdIn_2S_4$ Schottky junction for photocatalytic oxidation of HMF to DFF under visible light. *Appl. Catal. B Environ.* **2023**, *330*, 122635. [CrossRef]
35. Luo, Z.; Ye, X.; Zhang, S.; Xue, S.; Yang, C.; Hou, Y.; Xing, W.; Yu, R.; Sun, J.; Yu, Z.; et al. Unveiling the charge transfer dynamics steered by built-in electric fields in BiOBr photocatalysts. *Nat. Commun.* **2022**, *13*, 2230. [PubMed]
36. Meng, S.; Ye, X.; Zhang, J.; Fu, X.; Chen, S. Effective use of photogenerated electrons and holes in a system: Photocatalytic selective oxidation of aromatic alcohols to aldehydes and hydrogen production. *J. Catal.* **2018**, *367*, 159–170.
37. Zhao, S.; Luo, Y.; Li, C.; Ren, K.; Zhu, Y.; Dou, W. High-performance photothermal catalytic CO_2 reduction to CH_4 and CO by ABO_3 (A = La, Ce; B = Ni, Co, Fe) perovskite nanomaterials. *Ceram. Int.* **2023**, *49*, 20907–20919.
38. Yang, M.-Q.; Xu, Y.-J.; Lu, W.; Zeng, K.; Zhu, H.; Xu, Q.-H.; Ho, G.W. Self-surface charge exfoliation and electrostatically coordinated 2D hetero-layered hybrids. *Nat. Commun.* **2017**, *8*, 14224.
39. Shang, W.; Liu, W.; Cai, X.; Hu, J.; Guo, J.; Xin, C.; Li, Y.; Zhang, N.; Wang, N.; Hao, C.; et al. Insights into atomically dispersed reactive centers on g-C_3N_4 photocatalysts for water splitting. *Adv. Powder Mater.* **2023**, *2*, 100094.
40. Wang, Q.; Chen, L.; Guan, S.; Zhang, X.; Wang, B.; Cao, X.; Yu, Z.; He, Y.; Evans, D.G.; Feng, J.; et al. Ultrathin and Vacancy-Rich CoAl-Layered Double Hydroxide/Graphite Oxide Catalysts: Promotional Effect of Cobalt Vacancies and Oxygen Vacancies in Alcohol Oxidation. *ACS Catal.* **2018**, *8*, 3104–3115. [CrossRef]
41. Kresse, G.; Joubert, D. From ultrasoft pseudopotentials to the projector augmented-wave method. *Phys. Rev. B* **1999**, *59*, 1758. [CrossRef]
42. Grimme, S.; Ehrlich, S.; Goerigk, L. Effect of the damping function in dispersion corrected density functional theory. *J. Comput. Chem.* **2011**, *32*, 1456–1465. [CrossRef] [PubMed]
43. Nørskov, J.K.; Rossmeisl, J.; Logadottir, A.; Lindqvist, L.; Kitchin, J.R.; Bligaard, T.; Jonsson, H. Origin of the overpotential for oxygen reduction at a fuel-cell cathode. *J. Phys. Chem. B* **2004**, *108*, 17886–17892. [CrossRef]

Disclaimer/Publisher's Note: The statements, opinions and data contained in all publications are solely those of the individual author(s) and contributor(s) and not of MDPI and/or the editor(s). MDPI and/or the editor(s) disclaim responsibility for any injury to people or property resulting from any ideas, methods, instructions or products referred to in the content.

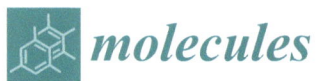

Article

The Influence of Heat Treatment on the Photoactivity of Amine-Modified Titanium Dioxide in the Reduction of Carbon Dioxide

Iwona Pełech [1,*], Piotr Staciwa [1], Daniel Sibera [1,2], Konrad Sebastian Sobczuk [1], Wiktoria Majewska [1], Ewelina Kusiak-Nejman [1], Antoni W. Morawski [1], Kaiying Wang [3] and Urszula Narkiewicz [1]

[1] Department of Inorganic Chemical Technology and Environment Engineering, Faculty of Chemical Technology and Engineering, West Pomeranian University of Technology in Szczecin, Pułaskiego 10, 70-322 Szczecin, Poland; piotr.staciwa@zut.edu.pl (P.S.); daniel.sibera@zut.edu.pl (D.S.); sk43128@zut.edu.pl (K.S.S.); ewelina.kusiak@zut.edu.pl (E.K.-N.); antoni.morawski@zut.edu.pl (A.W.M.); urszula.narkiewicz@zut.edu.pl (U.N.)

[2] Department of Construction and Road Engineering, Faculty of Civil and Environmental Engineering, West Pomeranian University of Technology in Szczecin, Piastów 50a, 70-311 Szczecin, Poland

[3] Department of Microsystems, University of South-Eastern Norway, 3184 Horten, Norway; kaiying.wang@usn.no

* Correspondence: iwona.pelech@zut.edu.pl

Citation: Pełech, I.; Staciwa, P.; Sibera, D.; Sobczuk, K.S.; Majewska, W.; Kusiak-Nejman, E.; Morawski, A.W.; Wang, K.; Narkiewicz, U. The Influence of Heat Treatment on the Photoactivity of Amine-Modified Titanium Dioxide in the Reduction of Carbon Dioxide. *Molecules* 2024, 29, 4348. https://doi.org/10.3390/molecules29184348

Academic Editor: Sugang Meng

Received: 1 August 2024
Revised: 9 September 2024
Accepted: 11 September 2024
Published: 13 September 2024

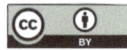

Copyright: © 2024 by the authors. Licensee MDPI, Basel, Switzerland. This article is an open access article distributed under the terms and conditions of the Creative Commons Attribution (CC BY) license (https://creativecommons.org/licenses/by/4.0/).

Abstract: Modification of titanium dioxide using ethylenediamine (EDA), diethylamine (DEA), and triethylamine (TEA) has been studied. As the reference material, titanium dioxide prepared by the sol–gel method using titanium(IV) isopropoxide as a precursor was applied. The preparation procedure involved heat treatment in the microwave reactor or in the high-temperature furnace. The obtained samples have been characterized in detail. The phase composition was determined through the X-ray diffraction method, and the average crystallite size was calculated based on it. Values for specific surface areas and the total pore volumes were calculated based on the isotherms obtained through the low-temperature nitrogen adsorption method. The bang gap energy was estimated based on Tauc's plots. The influence of the type and content of amine, as well as heat treatment on the photocatalytic activity of modified titanium dioxide in the photocatalytic reduction of carbon dioxide, was determined and discussed. It was clear that, regardless of the amount and content of amine introduced, the higher photoactivity characterized the samples prepared in the microwave reactor. The highest amounts of hydrogen, carbon monoxide, and methane have been achieved using triethylamine-modified titanium dioxide.

Keywords: titanium dioxide; carbon dioxide; photocatalyst; amines; hydrogen evolution

1. Introduction

Air pollution is one of the most serious adverse effects of economic growth that affects everyday living. Burning fossil fuels leads to uncontrolled increases in greenhouse gas concentrations in the atmosphere. As a result, progressive global warming puts the global ecosystem out of order. Carbon dioxide emission, due to the tremendous amounts of this gas produced every year, is perceived to be one of the biggest concerns given climate change. Worldwide emission of this gas is constantly growing, i.e., in 2023, it reached 35.8 Gt [1], so the containment of CO_2 emissions for years to come will be a difficult task.

Taking this into consideration, the scientific community struggles to find means to counter this effect. In order to mitigate the CO_2 concentration in the atmosphere, several solutions have been proposed. Among others, carbon capture and storage [2], electrochemical conversion [3], catalytic conversion [4] and photocatalytic reduction [5] can be distinguished. The latter solution is especially attractive due to the possibility of the use of solar energy and the possibility of acquiring useful products from CO_2.

Photocatalytic CO_2 reduction is a green, photo-induced process. Through the application of irradiation, carbon dioxide molecules can be transferred into useful products such as carbon monoxide, methane or hydrogen. An important component of photocatalytic CO_2 reduction is a proper photocatalyst. In general, three steps can be distinguished in a photocatalytic process: (I) the generation of photogenerated carriers, (II) transferring the generated electrons and holes to the surface of the photocatalyst, (III) the catalytic reaction on the surface of the photocatalyst [6].

Research regarding the search for a proper semiconductor in order to enhance the effectiveness of photocatalytic CO_2 reductions is in the pipeline. A suitable material must meet several requirements, i.e., a relatively narrow bandgap and a low recombination rate of charges strongly affect the photocatalysis efficiency. Finally, the photocatalyst should be cost-effective and stable during reaction [7]. There are several semiconductors that can be stated as promising photocatalysts, i.e., ZnO [8], Fe_2O_3 [9], Cu_2O [10] or TiO_2 [11]. However, none of the existing semiconductors meet the requirements for large-scale CCU (carbon capture and utilization) application, and further improvement of the efficiency of these materials is strongly advised.

Among existing photocatalysts, titanium dioxide is a very promising material because of its low cost, non-toxicity and availability. Moreover, many publications attest to the ease of its modification. It was proven that, through modification with Ag [12], Cu [13], I [14], Co [15], and N [16], titanium dioxide can become a highly efficient CO_2-reducing photocatalyst.

In the available papers, it is reported that amines, as titania modifiers, increase their adsorptive properties towards CO_2. Chen et al. [17] reported the increase in photocatalytic reduction of CO_2 using amine-modified brookite TiO_2 nanorods coupled with CuxS. Song et al. [18] prepared TiO_2 nanotubes modified by three kinds of amines (ethylenediamine, polyetherimide and tetraethylenepentamine). TEPA-modified TiO_2 nanotubes showed the highest CO_2 adsorption capacity. Ota et al. [19] developed a synthesis method of new amorphous titanium dioxide nanoparticles with a diameter of 3 nm, a high surface area and a large amount of OH groups. Amorphous TiO_2 nanoparticles were successfully modified with ethylenediamine and showed a higher CO_2 adsorption capacity than conventional TiO_2 and mesoporous SiO_2. Jiang et al. [20] developed a new low-cost, highly selective and stable sorbent-based pre-combustion CO_2 capture. Experimental results have shown that the selectivity of TiO_2 for separation of CO_2 from CO_2/CH_4 mixture can be significantly improved via amine modification. Ma et al. [21] modified TiO_2 using different amines, including diethylenetriamine (DETA), triethylenetetramine (TETA), and tetraethylenepentamine (TEPA), for CO_2 capture. Experimental results revealed that CO_2 uptake capacities of the titania composite sorbents increase with amine loading but decrease with the size of impregnated amines. The same conclusion, that the amine-modified materials exhibited enhanced CO_2 uptake compared to the initial titania, have been presented in our previous works [22,23].

As shown above, the amine modification of the photocatalyst has a positive effect on the enhancement of CO_2 adsorption. The influence of this type of modification on the photocatalytic activity of TiO_2 was reported. Mendonça et al. [24] used the activated carbon modified with ethylenediamine and impregnated with TiO_2 for improved photodegradation of sulfamethazine. Bao et al. [25] synthesized photocatalytically active N-doped TiO_2 nanoparticles by a one-pot hydrothermal method without calcination using structurally different amine sources as dopants under soft-chemistry conditions. TiO_2 modified with diethylamine was a suitable candidate due to its high visible-light absorption ability and having the highest efficiency in regard to the photodegradation of reactive brilliant red dye. Liao et al. [26] stated that amine functionalization of TiO_2 nanoparticles substantially increases the affinity of CO_2 on TiO_2 surfaces for more effective CO_2 activation. It also greatly enhances the photocatalytic rate of CO_2 reduction into CH_4 and CO. Karawek et al. [27] prepared a sandwich-type composite consisting of two 2-dimensional nanostructures (2D–2D) using the heterostructure of titanium dioxide nanosheets (TNS) and graphene oxide (GO). Alkanolamine MEA, DEA, and TEA were tested to promote the photoactivity of TNS in photoreducing CO_2. The TEA−TNS performed better than DEA−TNS and MEA−TNS due to increased CO_2 loading and faster CO_2 desorption rates. The best results came from the TEA-[Cu-TNS/GO] composite, in which the TEA was grafted onto the Cu-TNS/GO, attracting CO_2 for the photoreduction, and the copper ions enhanced the charge separation characteristics of the TNS. Jin et al. [28] demonstrated that surface modifications with primary amines on TiO_2 increase the activity in Co or methane production, regardless of metalcocatalysts.

In the present work, amines with different boiling points, and featured different numbers of nitrogen and carbon atoms were used to modify TiO_2: ethylenediamine (EDA, $C_2H_8N_2$, 116.9 °C), diethylamine (DEA, $C_4H_{11}N$, 55.5 °C), and triethylamine (TEA, $C_6H_{15}N$, 89.8 °C). Two different methods were used for modification—a microwave oven operating under pressure and a thermal oven for high-temperature processing—to determine how these conditions affect the photoactivity of the samples.

2. Results and Discussion

The phase composition of the obtained materials was studied using the X-ray diffraction method. In Figure 1, the diffraction patterns of the EDA-modified titania heated in the microwave reactor (Figure 1a) and high-temperature furnace (Figure 1b) are presented. All the visible reflexes were assigned to the anatase phase (ICDD 01-073-1764), and no other phases were identified in the samples. Exactly the same results were obtained for DEA-modified titania (Figure 2) and TEA-modified titania (Figure 3).

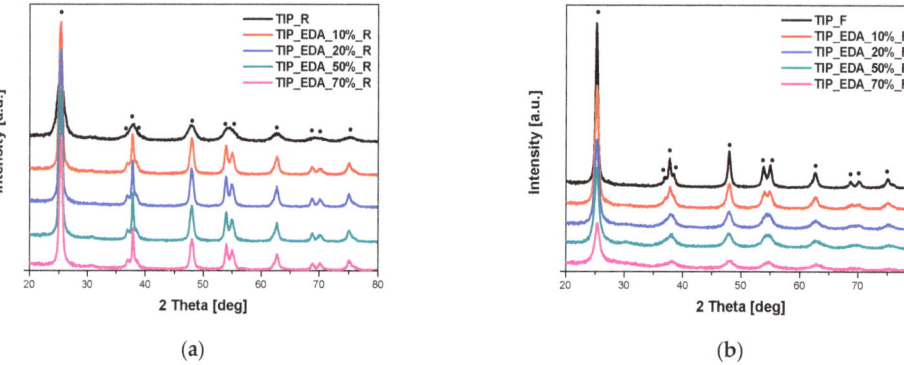

Figure 1. X-ray diffraction patterns of EDA-modified titania samples heated in the microwave reactor (**a**) and high-temperature furnace (**b**). Reflexes attributed to anatase are marked as •.

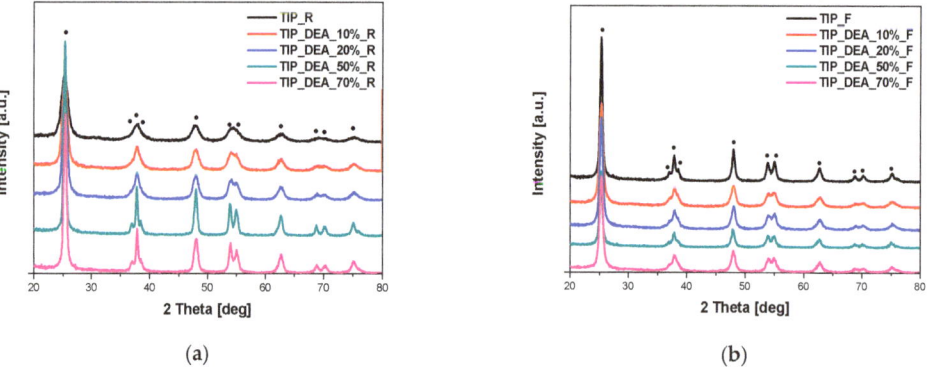

Figure 2. X-ray diffraction patterns of DEA-modified titania samples heated in the microwave reactor (**a**) and high-temperature furnace (**b**). Reflexes attributed to anatase are marked as •.

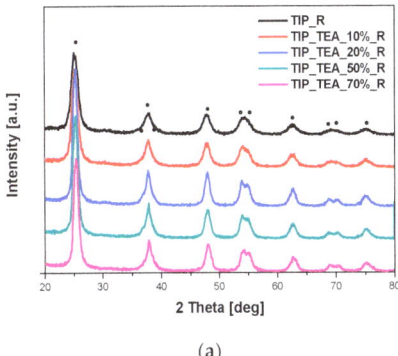
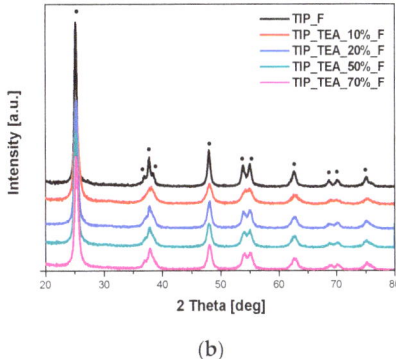

Figure 3. X-ray diffraction patterns of TEA-modified titania samples heated in the microwave reactor (**a**) and high-temperature furnace (**b**). Reflexes attributed to anatase are marked as •.

Based on the reflex located at the 2 theta angle of approximately 25° and assigned to the anatase phase, the average crystallite size was calculated. The obtained values are presented in Table 1. It was found that the average crystallite size for the reference sample obtained in the microwave reactor (TTIP_R) was smaller (14.3 nm) than for the same material obtained in the high-temperature furnace (TTIP_F, 21.9 nm); this was probably related to the difference in heating temperatures (400 °C in the tubular furnace and 250 °C in the microwave reactor). Microwave heating is an in situ energy conversion mode and radically differs from traditional heating processes. According to the available literature [29–32], microwave heating has significant advantages over conventional heating procedures and can heat materials to high temperatures with ultra-fast heating rates in a short time with high energy efficiency. Using this method, low values of the anatase average crystallite size can be achieved, as was mentioned above and in [33,34]. Higher temperatures in the case of traditional heat treatment result in the formation of larger particles [35,36].

The materials modified with DEA and TEA and prepared in the microwave reactor had lower values of average crystallite size than the appropriate reference sample. For both DEA- and TEA-modified titania, the average crystallite size was very similar, and no significant differences were noted. All the calculated values ranged from ~7 nm to ~10 nm. In the case of ethylenediamine, the amine content does not have a significant impact on the average crystallite size as well, which ranged from 15.4 nm for TTIP_EDA_10%_R to 16.9 nm for TTIP_EDA_70%_R. Higher values of the average crystallite size were achieved for the materials modified with EDA in comparison with TTIP_R, and especially with the samples modified using DEA and TEA. A similar dependence was noticed at [37], where the authors calculated the crystallite size by the Sherrer's formula and found that the crystallite sizes of the deposits in the case of 3-methoxypropylamine and dimethylamine, compared to ethanolamine, were approximately 17% and 24% less, respectively. Sun et al. [38] stated that, in low-pH conditions, the quantity of hydroxyl groups in hydrolysis is small, which prevents the crystallization of the samples and the growth of the TiO_2 crystallites. With increasing pH, more hydroxyl groups are available for the hydrolysis, which leads to better crystallization of TiO_2 and greater crystallite sizes [39,40]. Considering that EDA is the most basic amine among those used in studies, the above explanation may indicate why we obtained smaller crystallites of anatase using diethylamine and triethylamine.

All samples heated in the high-temperature furnace, regardless of the type of amine used for modification, were characterized by a lower average crystallite size than the reference sample, TTIP_F. For titania modified with EDA and heated in the tubular furnace, a slight decrease in the average crystallite size was noticed together with an increase in amine content in the sample. And so, for TTIP_EDA_10%_F, the average anatase crystallite size equalled 13.8 nm, whereas, for TTIP_EDA_70%_F, 9.0 nm was calculated. Similar to materials heated in the microwave reactor, the average crystallite size obtained for both DEA-

and TEA-modified titanium dioxide, was not significantly different. However, it should be noted that these differences, although small, were greater than in the case of samples heated in the microwave reactor. The values ranged from 12.7 nm (TTIP_DEA_10%_F) to 17.0 nm (TTIP_DEA_50%_F) and from 10.3 nm (TTIP_TEA_10%_F) to 14.5 nm (TTIP_TEA_20%_F).

Table 1. The average crystallite size calculated according to the Scherrer equation, textural properties of the amine-modified TiO_2 calculated based on low-temperature nitrogen adsorption isotherms and band gap energy estimated from Tauc's plots.

	Amine Content	Average Crystallite Size	S_{BET}	TPV	V_{micro}	V_{meso}	E_g
	[wt.%]	[nm]	[m²/g]	[cm³/g]	[cm³/g]	[cm³/g]	[eV]
		Microwave reactor					
TTIP_R	0	14.3	98	0.28	0.01	0.27	3.22
TTIP_EDA_10%_R	10	15.4	96	0.28	0.00	0.28	3.20
TTIP_EDA_20%_R	20	16.6	93	0.30	0.00	0.30	3.17
TTIP_EDA_50%_R	50	16.0	86	0.40	0.00	0.40	3.22
TTIP_EDA_70%_R	70	16.9	100	0.34	0.01	0.33	3.20
TTIP_DEA_10%_R	10	8.5	160	0.27	0.01	0.26	3.23
TTIP_DEA_20%_R	20	9.7	146	0.25	0.01	0.24	3.20
TTIP_DEA_50%_R	50	10.2	152	0.23	0.00	0.23	3.15
TTIP_DEA_70%_R	70	9.3	148	0.25	0.01	0.24	3.18
TTIP_TEA_10%_R	10	7.1	185	0.33	0.01	0.32	3.26
TTIP_TEA_20%_R	20	10.2	143	0.22	0.01	0.21	3.16
TTIP_TEA_50%_R	50	9.1	152	0.27	0.01	0.26	3.23
TTIP_TEA_70%_R	70	9.4	138	0.25	0.01	0.24	3.23
		High-temperature furnace					
TTIP_F	0	21.9	16	0.05	0.00	0.05	3.25
TTIP_EDA_10%_F	10	13.8	10	0.06	0.00	0.06	2.54
TTIP_EDA_20%_F	20	11.6	8	0.04	0.00	0.04	2.45
TTIP_EDA_50%_F	50	10.6	12	0.02	0.00	0.02	2.37
TTIP_EDA_70%_F	70	9.0	9	0.04	0.00	0.04	2.26
TTIP_DEA_10%_F	10	12.7	15	0.12	0.00	0.12	2.92
TTIP_DEA_20%_F	20	15.1	9	0.03	0.00	0.03	2.92
TTIP_DEA_50%_F	50	17.0	32	0.03	0.01	0.02	2.33
TTIP_DEA_70%_F	70	14.0	68	0.06	0.01	0.05	2.59
TTIP_TEA_10%_F	10	10.3	19	0.06	0.00	0.06	2.75
TTIP_TEA_20%_F	20	14.5	6	0.04	0.00	0.04	2.74
TTIP_TEA_50%_F	50	14.3	36	0.03	0.01	0.02	2.56
TTIP_TEA_70%_F	70	13.8	48	0.05	0.01	0.04	2.32

The obtained samples were also characterized using the low-temperature nitrogen adsorption method, and, based on the adsorption isotherms presented in Figures 4–6, different parameters have been calculated. The values of specific surface areas, the total pore volumes and the volumes of pores are presented in Table 1.

In Figure 4, the adsorption isotherms for EDA-modified titania prepared using a microwave reactor (Figure 5a) and high-temperature furnace (Figure 4b) are presented. For both the reference materials TTIP_R (Figure 4a) and TTIP_F (Figure 4b), the adsorption isotherms are of type II according to the IUPAC system, and their shape is characteristic of macroporous materials. For these samples, a H3 type of hysteresis loop is also observed [41,42], starting at a relative pressure of 0.45 p/p$_0$ and ending at a relative pressure of approximately 1 p/p$_0$, which indicates that the discussed materials are dominated by macropores not completely filled with pore condensate [41,42]. For the samples modified with EDA, regardless of the type of heat treatment, type II isotherms were obtained according to the IUPAC system, which is characteristic of macroporous materials. For the EDA-modified titania prepared using a microwave reactor, hysteresis loops of the H3 type were noticed, suggesting the presence of a pore network consisting of macropores [41,42]. On the contrary, in the case of EDA-modified titania prepared using a high-temperature furnace, hysteresis loops of the H4 type have been visible [41,42], and their presence indicates the existence of pores with the shape of narrow slits [41,42].

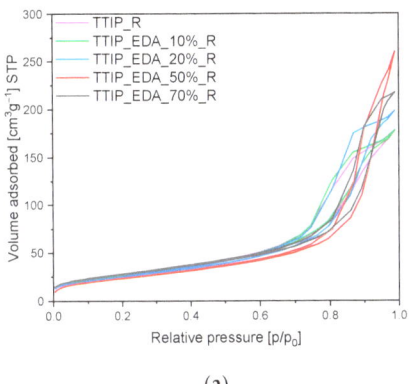
(a)

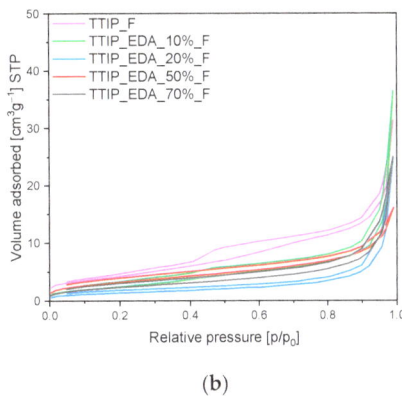
(b)

Figure 4. N_2 sorption isotherms of the EDA-modified titania dioxide prepared using (**a**) a microwave reactor and (**b**) a high-temperature furnace.

In Figure 5, the adsorption isotherms for diethylamine-modified titanium dioxide prepared using a microwave reactor (Figure 5a) and high-temperature furnace (Figure 5b) are shown. For DEA-modified titanium dioxide heated in the microwave reactor, similarly to the case of the reference material TTIP_R, the isotherms of type II were also obtained and the hysteresis loops of the H3 type were observed. For materials modified with an amine content of 10 wt.% and 20 wt.%, the hysteresis loop starts at a relative pressure of 0.5 p/p_0 and ends at a relative pressure of approximately 1 p/p_0. However, for the samples with an amine content of 50 wt.% and 70 wt.%, the hysteresis loop begins at a relative pressure of approximately 0.65 p/p_0 and ends at a relative pressure of approximately 1 p/p_0. This proves that, in samples with higher amine content (50 wt.% and 70 wt.%), the mesopores have a larger diameter than the mesopores in samples with lower amine content (10 wt.% and 20 wt.%); this was also true in the reference sample (TTIP_R).

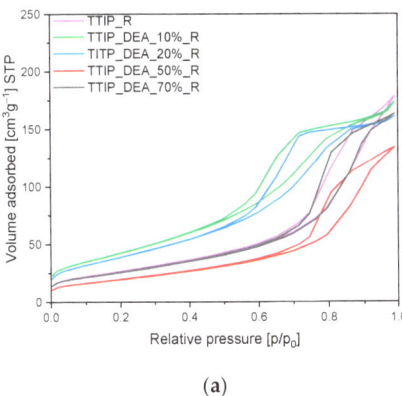
(a)

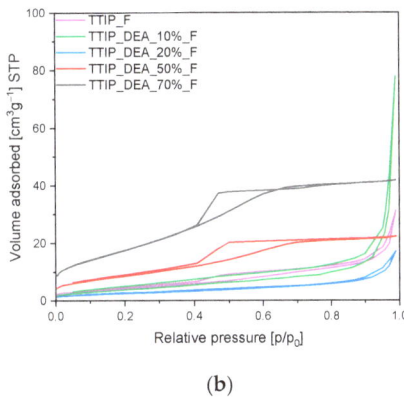
(b)

Figure 5. N_2 sorption isotherms of the diethylamine-modified titanium dioxide prepared using (**a**) microwave reactor and (**b**) high-temperature furnace.

In the case of the materials heated in the high-temperature furnace (Figure 5b), and exclusively in the case of materials with a higher content of amine (50 wt.% and 70 wt.%), type IVa isotherms were obtained according to the IUPAC system and hysteresis loops of the H2b type were observed. In contrast to this, for the samples modified with 10 wt.% and 20 wt.% of DEA obtained using a tubular furnace, type II isotherms were obtained, which are characteristic of macroporous materials. Hysteresis loops of the H4 type have also been observed [41,42], what indicates the presence of pores with the shape of narrow slits [41,42].

For triethylamine-modified titanium dioxide heated in the microwave reactor, the same as in the case of diethylamine-modified titanium dioxide, type II isotherms were obtained, and hysteresis loops of the H3 type were observed (Figure 6a). For the materials modified with an amine content of 10 wt.% and 20 wt.% hysteresis loop starts at a relative pressure of 0.4 p/p_0 and ends at a relative pressure of approximately 1 p/p_0. Whereas for samples with an amine content of 50 wt.% and 70 wt.%, H2b type isotherms were noticed with the hysteresis loops starting at a relative pressure of approximately 0.5 p/p_0 and ending at a relative pressure of approximately 1 p/p_0. It means that the samples with higher amine content (50 wt.% and 70 wt.%) possessed mesopores with larger diameters than the mesopores in samples with lower amine content (10 wt.% and 20 wt.%).

The same type of isotherm and hysteresis loop was noticed for the sample heated in the tubular furnace (Figure 6b), but only modified with amine content 50 wt.% and 70 wt.%. For the materials with lower amine content (10 wt.% and 20 wt.%) type II isotherms were obtained according to the IUPAC classification, which is characteristic of macroporous materials. Hysteresis loops of the H4 type have also been observed [41,42], which indicates the presence of pores in the shape of narrow slits [41,42].

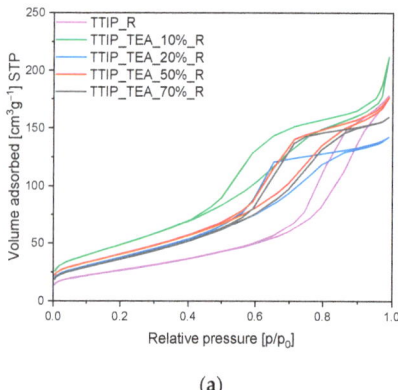
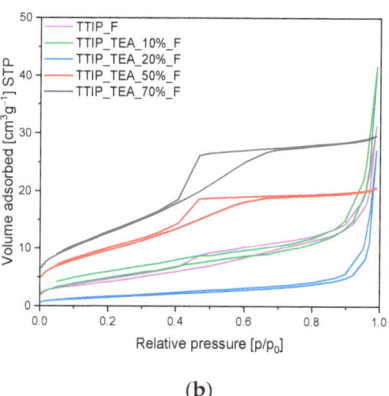

(a) (b)

Figure 6. N_2 sorption isotherms of the triethylamine-modified titanium dioxide prepared using (**a**) microwave reactor and (**b**) high-temperature furnace.

Based on the adsorption isotherms, the textural parameters of the tested materials were calculated and presented in Table 1. Generally, all the samples heated in the microwave reactor characterized higher values of surface area and total pore volume in comparison with the materials heated in the tubular furnace. The common feature of all the samples was that they did not have micropores.

In the case of ethylenediamine-modified titanium dioxide prepared using a microwave reactor, it was found that the content of amine in the samples had no influence on the values of specific surface areas, which ranged from 96 m^2/g for TTIP_EDA_10%_R to 100 m^2/g for TTIP_EDA_70%_R. Also, the values of S_{BET} did not differ significantly from the S_{BET} value of the reference sample (TTIP_R, 98 m^2/g). In the case of diethylamine- and triethylamine-modified titanium dioxide, higher values of surface area were achieved in comparison with the EDA-modified materials. The fact that the BET-specific surface areas increased might be due to the decrease in the crystallite size of titanium dioxide (Table 1). In both cases, there was no significant effect of DEA and TEA content on S_{BET} values. For diethylamine-modified titanium dioxide, the S_{BET} values equalled around 140 m^2/g, and for triethylamine-modified titanium dioxide, they were within the range of 140–150 m^2/g. Slightly higher values were recorded exclusively for the cases of samples modified with 10% of amine, namely TTIP_DEA_10_%_R and TTIP_TEA_10%_R, at 160 m^2/g and 185 m^2/g, respectively.

Ethylenediamine-modified titanium dioxide samples heated in the tubular furnace showed similar surface areas regardless of the amount of amine introduced. The values of S_{BET} ranged from 8 m^2/g for TTIP_EDA_20_%_F to 10 m^2/g for TTIP_EDA_50_%_R and were close to the values obtained for the reference material (16 m^2/g). In the case of diethylamine- and triethylamine-modified titanium dioxide, similar to the reference material, values of S_{BET} were noticed only for the materials with the addition of 10% and 20% of amine. For materials modified with 50% and 70% of diethylamine, S_{BET} equalled 32 m^2/g and 68 m^2/g, whereas for materials modified with 50% and 70% of triethylamine, the S_{BET} equalled 36 m^2/g and 48 m^2/g, respectively.

In general, all of the obtained materials were meso/macroporous. The total pore volume for the reference material obtained in a microwave reactor reached 0.28 cm^3/g. Regardless of the amine used and the content of amine, the data of the total pore volume for amine-modified materials were scattered and ranged from 0.21 cm^3/g for TTIP_DEA_50%_R to 0.40 cm^3/g for TTIP_EDA_50%. In the case of materials obtained using a tubular furnace, the values of the total pore volume were significantly lower and the total pore volume for the reference material TTIP_F equalled 0.05 cm^3/g. The values for the EDA, DEA and TEA-modified materials were similar.

Table 1 presents calculated band gap energy values for titania samples modified with selected amines. It can be clearly stated that, for all modified samples fabricated with the use of a microwave reactor, slight changes in band gap energy values, and thus insignificant red-shifts of the absorption edges, are observed. Additionally, the microwave treatment did not cause the colour change, and all samples stayed white or pale beige. The white colour and the slight batochromic shift of the adsorption edge for synthesized samples under the experimental conditions presented can indicate that the microwave-assisted pressure method is insufficient for carrying out the doping of TiO_2. However, all samples show high UV absorption due to the white colour, making them suitable for CO_2 photoreduction with simultaneous hydrogen formation (from photocatalytic water splitting) using an excitation source with a maximum wavelength below 380 nm.

When thermal annealing at 400 °C of the samples was applied, all samples showed red-shifts in the absorption edges concerning the reference sample (TTIP_F), a consequence of narrowing the band gaps, thus decreasing E_g values, which proves the occurrence of TiO_2 doping with nitrogen and/or carbon atoms. Regardless of the type of amine used, all samples showed high absorption of visible radiation due to their dark colour (from dark beige and grey to dark grey). Spadavecchia et al. [43] and Diker et al. [44] also stated that amines can be a source of nitrogen or carbon atoms, and the non-metal elements remaining after annealing in TiO_2 can act as dopants and shift the absorption edge into the visible part of the light. From Table 1, it can be seen that the band gap energy values decrease as the amines' theoretical concentration increases. For this preparation method, the dark colours of the synthesized samples are related to the boiling points of the amines used for modification (bp$_{DEA}$ = 55 °C and bp$_{TEA}$ = 89 °C). Even when the furnace is slowly heated to the required temperature (400 °C), DEA and TEA start boiling quickly and their vapours are removed with argon flow. This is also true for EDA, except that the boiling point for this amine is 117 °C, so the EDA evaporates more slowly, having a longer contact time with TiO_2.

All the tested materials were used as photocatalysts in the photocatalytic reduction of the carbon dioxide process. Hydrogen, methane and carbon monoxide were detected in the gas phase. Although hydrogen is not a direct product of CO_2 photoreduction, but rather a result of the water-splitting process, it is a valuable product and an essential component that is necessary for CO_2 conversion. The content of individual gasses was expressed in $\mu mol/g_{material}/dm^3$.

The hydrogen, carbon monoxide and methane contents in the gas phase during the 6 h process, obtained using ethylenediamine-, diethylamine-, and triethylamine-modified titanium dioxide heated in the microwave reactor, are presented in Figures 7a, 7b, 7c, respectively. Additionally, the hydrogen, carbon monoxide and methane contents in the gas phase for the reference material prepared with ammonia water (TTIP_R) have been marked in the same Figures. It is clearly visible that the photoactivity of the studied materials depended on the type of amine used for modification. The highest photoactivity in the photoreduction of carbon dioxide process showed TEA-modified titania, and the highest content of hydrogen (671 $\mu mol/g_{material}/dm^3$), carbon monoxide (388 $mol/g_{material}/dm^3$) and methane (136 $\mu mol/g_{material}/dm^3$) was obtained in the gas phase using this photocatalyst. A lower content of appropriate products in the gas phase was noticed for ethylenediamine- and diethylamine-modified titanium dioxide. For ethylenediamine-modified titanium dioxide, 243 $\mu mol/g_{material}/dm^3$ of hydrogen, 154 $\mu mol/g_{material}/dm^3$ of CO and 41 $\mu mol/g_{material}/dm^3$ of CH_4 was achieved, while, for diethylamine-modified titanium dioxide, 431 $\mu mol/g_{material}/dm^3$ of hydrogen, 297 $\mu mol/g_{material}/dm^3$ of CO and 68 $\mu mol/g_{material}/dm^3$ of CH_4 was obtained. Based on these results, the sample modified with triethylamine has been selected for further studies.

In Figure 8, the comparison between the content of hydrogen (Figure 8a), carbon monoxide (Figure 8b) and methane (Figure 8c) in the gas phase is shown and the values obtained using titanium dioxide modified with different contents of triethylamine prepared in the high-temperature furnace are presented. It is clear that higher photoactivity for hydrogen production was characterized for the samples with an amine content of 70% (183 $\mu mol/g_{material}/dm^3$). The remaining tested materials showed photoactivity at a similar level, what means that the hydrogen content in the gas phase for the sample modified with an amine content of 10% was practically the same as for the reference material. It should be noted that, in the case of carbon monoxide and methane, similar to what has been reported previously, the best results were achieved when titanium dioxide modified with an amine content of 70% was used. Generally, in the gas phase, the lowest values of the product were detected for methane. For the most photoactive material, triethylamine-modified titanium dioxide, 25 $\mu mol/g_{material}/dm^3$ of CH_4 was obtained.

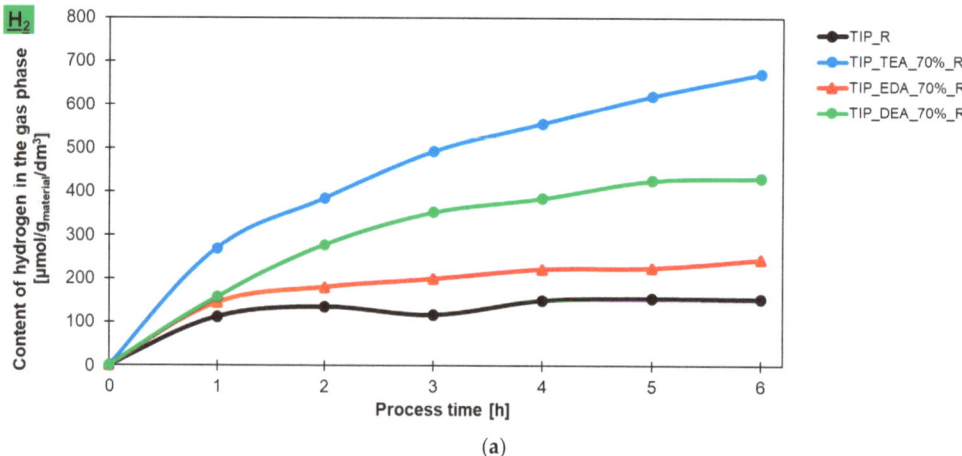

(a)

Figure 7. *Cont.*

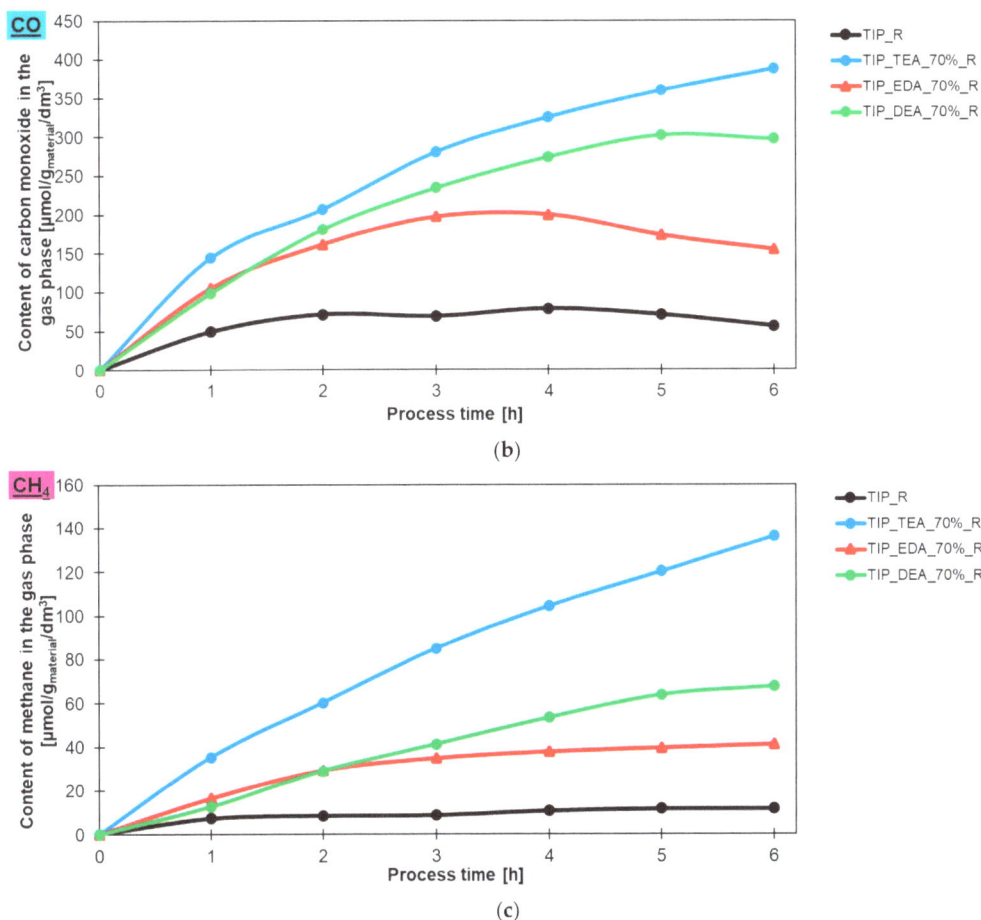

Figure 7. The content of hydrogen (**a**), carbon monoxide (**b**), and methane (**c**) in the gas phase obtained in the photocatalytic reduction of the carbon dioxide process using ethylenediamine-, diethylamine- and triethylamine-modified titanium dioxide heated in the microwave reactor.

Taking into account the results described above, the influence of amine content in triethylamine-modified materials prepared in the microwave reactor on the amount of hydrogen, carbon monoxide and methane (Figures 9a, 9b, 9c, respectively) produced in the photocatalytic reduction of carbon dioxide process has been checked. It was found that the highest content of hydrogen in the gas phase was detected for the sample modified with 70% of amine and the amount equalled 671 µmol/$g_{material}$/dm^3. Lower values were noticed for the sample modified with 50% and 10% of amine—231 µmol/$g_{material}$/dm^3 and 111 µmol/$g_{material}$/dm^3, respectively. It should also be noted that the sample TTIP_TEA_10%_R exhibited lower photoactivity than the reference material. In the case of carbon monoxide and methane production, a similar dependence was observed. What is important to note is that CO production decreased for the TTIP_TEA_10%_R and TTIP_TEA_50%_R in regard to what can be related to the occupation of active sites by products or unreacted CO_2, which prevents the reaction from proceeding further. Hydrogen production only increased in the sample modified with 70% of triethylamine (TTIP_TEA_70%_R), which suggests that saturation of the active sites in this photocatalyst occurs more slowly than for the other samples.

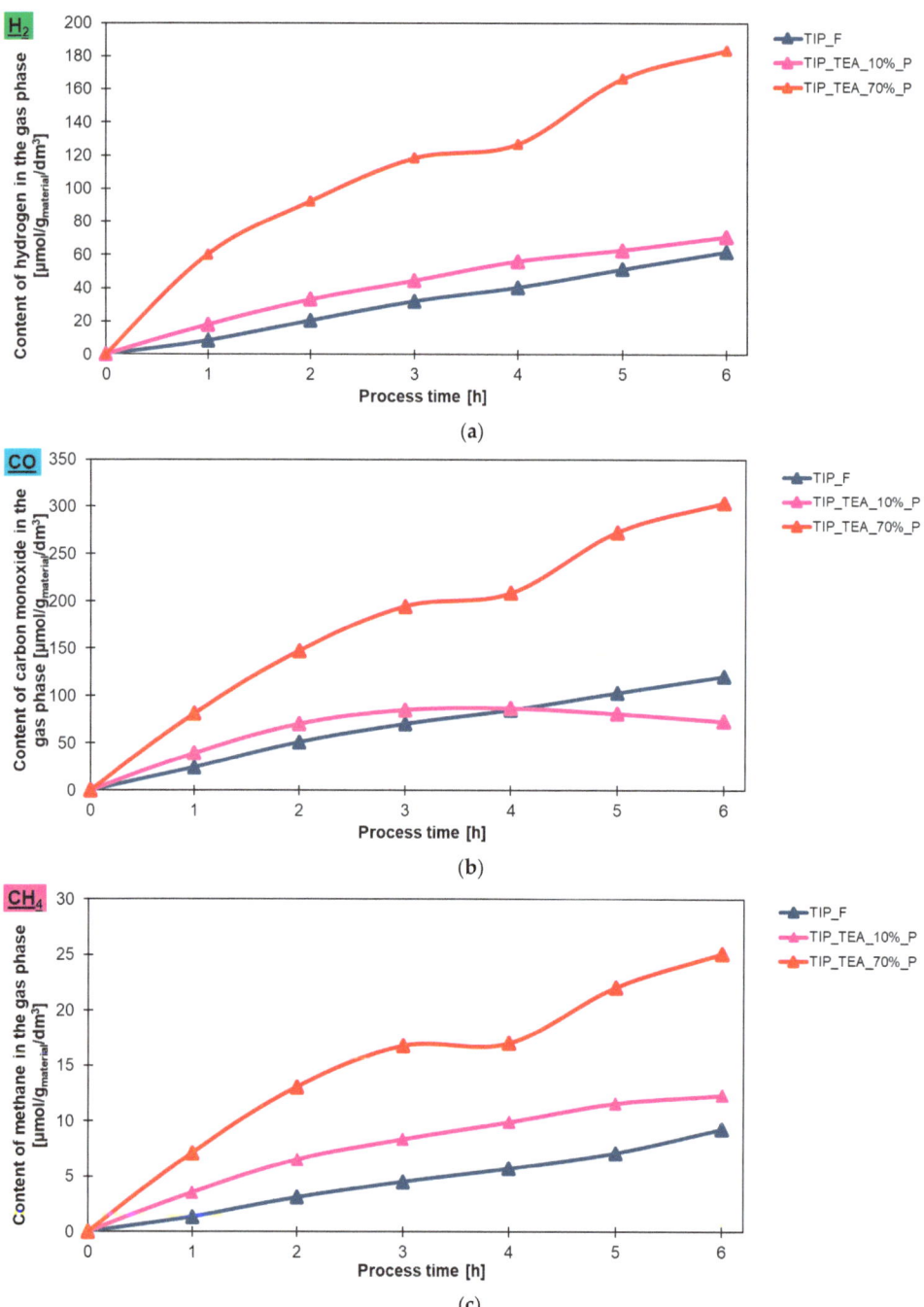

Figure 8. The content of (**a**) hydrogen, (**b**) carbon monoxide and (**c**) methane in the gas phase obtained in the photocatalytic reduction of carbon dioxide process using triethylamine-modified titanium dioxide heated in the microwave reactor and high-temperature furnace.

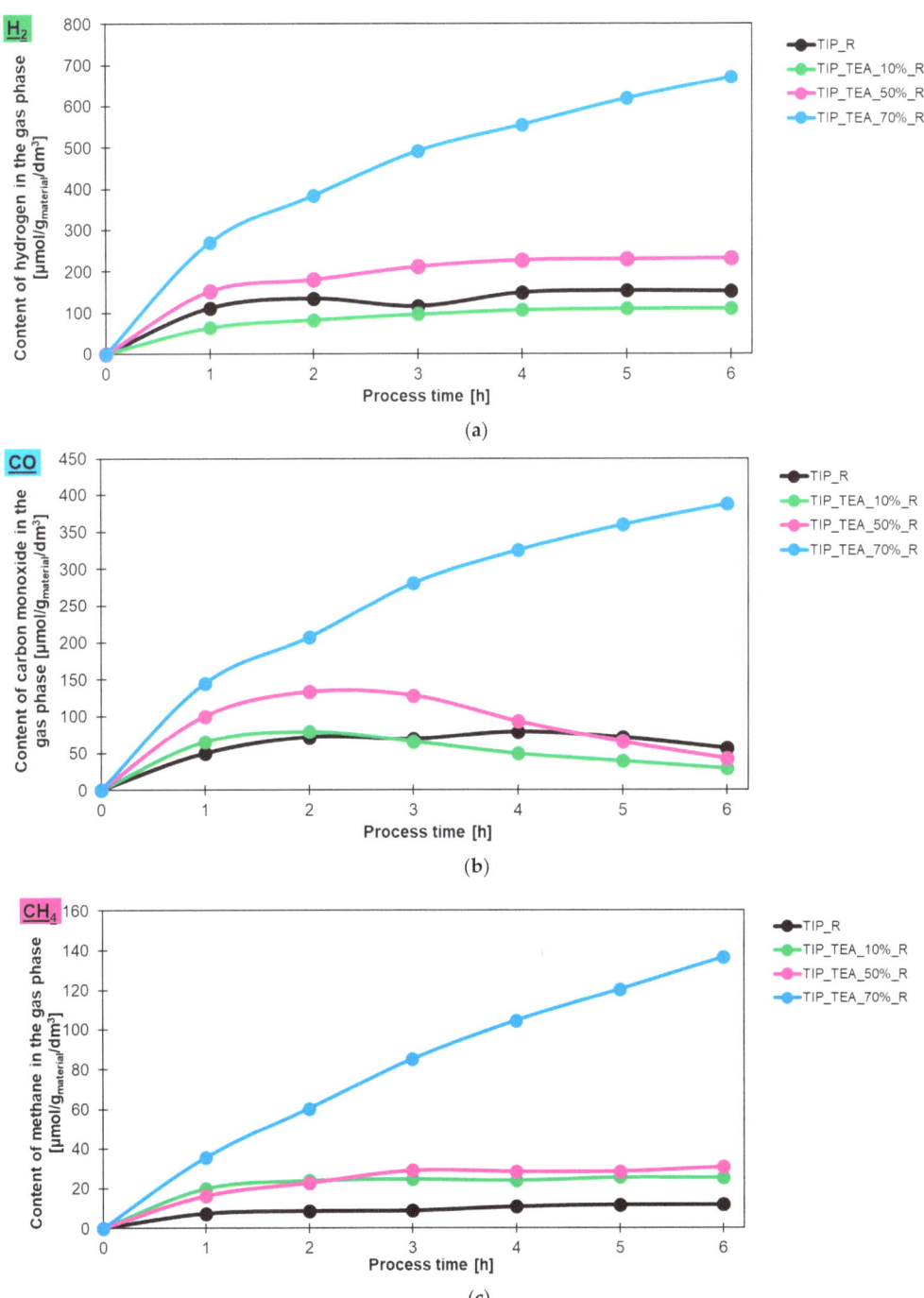

Figure 9. The content of (**a**) hydrogen, (**b**) carbon monoxide, (**c**) methane in the gas phase obtained in the photocatalytic reduction in the carbon dioxide process using triethylamine-modified titanium dioxide with different contents of amine and heated in the microwave reactor.

As is known from the available literature [45,46], photocatalytic activity depends on many factors, especially in regard to phase composition, particle size and the values of surface area. In our case, the average crystallite size and the BET-specific surface areas depended mainly on the heat treatment temperature, hence a lower content of products in the gas phase was noted for samples obtained in the high-temperature furnace. It was also visible that the use of ethylenediamine, instead of diethylamine and triethylamine, to modify titanium dioxide resulted in the formation of larger anatase crystallites for materials obtained under the same experimental conditions. This was probably due to the basicity of the individual amines and the amount of hydroxyl groups available for hydrolysis. More hydroxyl groups leads to better crystallization of TiO_2 and greater crystallite sizes, which was observed in the case of the samples modified using EDA. This is consistent with the literature data, which states that the crystallite size depends on many parameters, including temperature, process and precursors [47,48].

3. Experimental Part

3.1. Preparation of the Reference Material

To prepare the titanium dioxide, 50 mL of distilled water was added dropwise to the glass beaker containing 20 mL of titanium(IV) isopropoxide (TTIP) and 5 mL of ethyl alcohol. In order to change the pH, ammonia water (25% $NH_3 \cdot H_2O$) was dropped until the pH value was equal to 10. The whole mixture was continuously stirred for 24 h and then was left to age for 24 h. Then, the suspension was placed into a Teflon vessel and transferred to a microwave-assisted solvothermal reactor (ERTEC MAGNUM II, Wrocław, Poland). The process was conducted for 15 min under a pressure of 40 bar. Finally, the material was dried in a forced-air dryer at 80 °C, washed with distilled water, dried in a forced-air dryer at 80 °C and finally grounded in an agate mortar to a uniform consistency. The obtained sample was denoted as TTIP_R. Simultaneously, the sample was also taken without microwave treatment. The procedure was similar, with the exception that, after the ageing step, the material was dried in a forced-air dryer at 80 °C, grounded in an agate mortar and subjected to the heat treatment, which was performed in a high-temperature furnace (HST 12/400 Carbolite, Derbyshire, UK). For this purpose, the obtained powder was transferred into a quartz boat, placed in a high-temperature furnace and heated under an argon atmosphere at a temperature rising from 20 to 400 °C with a heating rate of 10 °C/min. When a temperature of 400 °C was reached, the heating process was continued for 1 h. Afterwards, the sample was cooled to room temperature under an argon atmosphere. The final product was washed with distilled water, dried in a forced-air dryer at 80 °C and finally grounded in an agate mortar to a uniform consistency. The obtained sample was denoted as TTIP_F.

3.2. Modification of Titanium Dioxide with Amines

To prepare amine-modified titanium dioxide, 50 mL of distilled water was added dropwise to the glass beaker containing 20 mL of titanium(IV) isopropoxide (TTIP) and 5 mL of ethyl alcohol. Then, the appropriate amine (ethylenediamine, diethylamine and triethylamine), in an amount of 10 wt.%, 20 wt.%, 50 wt.% and 70 wt.%, was added. The whole mixture was continuously stirred for 24 h, and was then left to age for 24 h. Then, the sample was placed into a Teflon vessel and transferred to a microwave reactor (ERTEC MAGNUM II). The process was conducted for 15 min under a pressure of 40 bar. Finally, the material was dried in a forced-air dryer at 80 °C, washed with distilled water, again dried in a forced-air dryer at 80 °C and finally grounded in an agate mortar to a uniform consistency. The obtained samples were denoted as TTIP_EDA_10%_R, TTIP_EDA_20%_R, TTIP_EDA_50%_R, TTIP_EDA_70%_R (ethylenediamine-modified titanium dioxide); TTIP_DEA_10%_R, TTIP_DEA_20%_R, TTIP_DEA_50%_R, TTIP_DEA_70%_R (diethylamine-modified titanium dioxide); and TTIP_TEA_10%_R, TTIP_TEA_20%_R, TTIP_TEA_50%_R, TTIP_TEA_70%_R (triethylamine-modified titanium dioxide).

Simultaneously, samples without microwave treatment were also made. The procedure was similar, with the exception that, after the ageing step, the material was dried in a forced-air dryer at 80 °C, grounded in an agate mortar and subjected to the heat treatment, which was performed in a high-temperature furnace (HST 12/400 Carbolite). For this purpose, the obtained powder was transferred into a quartz boat, placed in a high-temperature furnace and heated under an argon atmosphere, with the temperature rising from 20 to 400 °C at a heating rate of 10 °C/min. When a temperature of 400 °C was reached, the heating process was continued for 1 h. Afterwards, the sample was cooled to room temperature under an argon atmosphere. The final product was washed with distilled water, dried in a forced-air dryer at 80 °C and finally grounded in an agate mortar to a uniform consistency. The obtained samples were denoted as TTIP_EDA_10%_F, TTIP_EDA_20%_F, TTIP_EDA_50%_F, TTIP_EDA_70%_F (ethylenediamine-modified titanium dioxide); TTIP_DEA_10%_F, TTIP_DEA_20%_F, TTIP_DEA_50%_F, TTIP_DEA_70%_F (diethylamine-modified titanium dioxide); TTIP_TEA_10%_F, TTIP_TEA_20%_F and TTIP_TEA_50%_F, TTIP_TEA_70%_F (triethylamine-modified titanium dioxide).

3.3. Photocatalytic Reduction of Carbon Dioxide

The processes were conducted in a gas phase bottle-shaped reactor made of glass. The working volume of the reactor was 766 cm^3. A 150 W medium-pressure mercury lamp TQ150 Z3 (Heraeus, Hanau, Germany) was used in the photocatalytic tests. It was characterized by the wide range of both UV and visible light in the range of 250–600 nm, with the maximum at 365 nm. The lamp was placed in a quartz condenser. It was constantly cooled with water by a chiller equipped with a pump with a controlled temperature of 18 °C (Minichiller 280 OLÉ, Huber, Offenburg, Germany). The reactor was placed in a thermostatic chamber to maintain a stable temperature (20 °C) and exclude light sources. A measurement of 10 cm^3 of distilled water and glass fibre with the tested photocatalyst were placed in the reactor. The reactor was purified with pure CO_2 (Messer, Police, Poland) for 16 h to eliminate the air. During the whole process, the gas in the reactor was constantly mixed with the pump (flow rate of 1.6 dm^3/h). The process was performed at 20 °C and tested for 6 h. The gas samples for analysis were collected every 1 h. The gas phase composition was analyzed using an SRI 310C gas chromatograph (SRI Instruments, Torrance, CA, USA) equipped with a column with a molecular sieve with a mesh size of 5Å and a HID detector (Helium Ionization Detector). The carrier gas was helium. The analyses were performed under isothermal conditions at a temperature of 60 °C. The gas flow through the column was 60 cm^3/min, and the volume of the test gas was 1 cm^3. The content of the component in the gas phase was calculated in successive measurements based on the calibration curve.

3.4. Characterization Methods

The phase composition of the prepared samples was determined using the X-ray diffraction method Cu Kα radiation (λCu Kα = 0.1540 nm) on an Empyrean (Panalytical, Malvern, UK). The identification of the crystalline phases was performed using HighScore+ and the ICDD PDF-4+ 2015 database. The average crystallite size was calculated according to the following Scherrer equation based on obtained X-ray powder diffraction patterns:

$$D = (k \cdot \lambda)/(\beta \cdot \cos\theta)$$

where D—the average crystallite size in the direction perpendicular to the (hkl) reflection plane; k—a constant close to unity, dependent on the shape of the crystallite; λ—the X-ray wavelength; β—the peak broadening; θ—the XRD peak position.

To perform the low-temperature nitrogen adsorption/desorption studies, the equipment QUADRASORB evoTM gas sorption automatic system (Quantachrome Instruments, Anton Paar, Austria) was used together with a MasterPrep multi-zone flow/vacuum outgassing system under a vacuum of 1×10^{-5} mbar from Quantachrome Instruments (Boynton Beach, FL, USA). On the basis of the obtained adsorption/desorption isotherms, the specific surface area (S_{BET}) and pore volumes of the obtained materials were determined. Prior to analysis, 150 mg of the material was weighed and pre-dried at 90 °C in a laboratory dryer. The dried samples were transferred into measuring cells and degassed using Master-Prep (Ouantachrome Instruments, USA) at 100 °C for 12 h. The Brunauer–Emmett–Teller (BET) equation was used to determine the surface areas (S_{BET}), which were determined in the relative pressure range of 0.05–0.2. The total pore volume (V_{total}) was calculated from the volume of nitrogen held at the highest relative pressure ($p/p_0 = 0.99$). The volume of micropores (V_{micro} < 2 nm) with dimensions smaller than 2 nm was calculated as a result of integrating the pore volume distribution function using the DFT method; a mesopore volume (V_{meso}) with dimensions from 2 to 50 nm was calculated from the difference in the total pore volume (V_{total}) and the volume of micropores (V_{micro} < 2 nm).

The *band gap* of the reference and all amine-modified titania materials was determined from the optical *absorption* spectra by means of a Jasco V-650 spectrometer (JASCO International Co., Tokyo, Japan) equipped with a PIV-756 integrating sphere accessory spectrometer (JASCO International Co., Tokyo, Japan) for diffuse reflectance measurements. Barium sulphate ($BaSO_4$ pure p.a., Avantor Performance Materials Poland S.A., Gliwice, Poland) was used as a reference for determining the baseline. The Tauc plot was used to estimate the value of the semiconductor band gap energy.

4. Conclusions

Modification of titanium dioxide using ethylenediamine, diethylamine, and triethylamine heated in the microwave reactor or high-temperature furnace has been studied. Based on the X-ray diffraction method, it was found that, in all the tested materials, only the anatase phase was identified. The average crystallite size was higher for the raw material and materials modified with amines and heated in the high-temperature furnace instead of microwave reactor, due to the higher processing temperature. Regardless of the heating method, decrease of the average crystallite size after modification with amines in comparison with raw materials was noticed, apart from ethylenediamine-modified titanium dioxide heated in the microwave reactor, for which slightly higher values were noticed. Generally, all the samples heated in the microwave reactor were characterized with higher values of surface area, total pore volume and band gap energy in comparison with the materials heated in the tubular furnace. Modifying samples with amines utilizing microwave-assisted pressure treatment did not alter the E_g values, as can be indirectly evidenced by the white colour of the samples, making them capable of absorbing the UV radiation. On the other hand, thermal amine modification of titania at 400 °C using the high-temperature furnace leads to colour changes and the red-shift of the adsorption edge, which indicates the doping of TiO_2 with carbon and/or nitrogen. The main product detected in the gas phase was hydrogen, and the highest content was achieved using triethylamine-modified titanium dioxide with 70% of amine content and heated using microwaves.

Author Contributions: Conceptualization, I.P.; Methodology, I.P., P.S., D.S., K.S.S. and E.K.-N.; Validation, I.P.; Formal analysis, I.P., P.S., D.S. and E.K.-N.; Investigation, I.P., P.S., D.S., K.S.S., W.M. and E.K.-N.; Resources, I.P.; Data curation, I.P. and E.K.-N.; Writing—original draft, I.P., P.S., D.S. and E.K.-N.; Writing—review & editing, I.P., P.S., D.S., K.S.S., E.K.-N., A.W.M., K.W. and U.N.; Visualization, P.S., D.S., K.S.S. and E.K.-N.; Supervision, A.W.M., K.W. and U.N.; Project administration, I.P.; Funding acquisition, I.P. All authors have read and agreed to the published version of the manuscript.

Funding: The research was funded by the Initiative no FWD-Green-3, submitted within the call for proposals entitled "Synergistic metal/non-metal doping of titanium dioxide to produce hydrogen under UV and Vis light" financing within the framework of the Fund for Bilateral Relations, "FBR", the European Economic Area Financial Mechanism 2014–2021 and Norwegian Financial Mechanism 2014–2021 via Ministry of Development Funds and Regional Policy (Poland).

Institutional Review Board Statement: Not applicable.

Informed Consent Statement: Not applicable.

Data Availability Statement: No new data were created or analyzed in this study. Data sharing is not applicable to this article.

Conflicts of Interest: The authors declare no conflict of interest.

References

1. Zhu, L.; Deng, Z.; Davis, S.J.; Ciais, P. Global carbon emissions in 2023. *Nat. Rev. Earth Environ.* **2024**, *5*, 253–254. [CrossRef]
2. Raganati, F.; Miccio, F.; Ammendola, P. Adsorption of Carbon Dioxide for Post-combustion Capture: A Review. *Energy Fuels* **2021**, *35*, 12845–12868. [CrossRef]
3. Overa, S.; Ko, B.H.; Zhao, Y.; Jiao, F. Electrochemical Approaches for CO_2 Conversion to Chemicals: A Journey toward Practical Applications. *Acc. Chem. Res.* **2022**, *55*, 638–648. [CrossRef]
4. Garba, M.D.; Usman, M.; Khan, S.; Shehzad, F.; Galadima, A.; Ehsan, M.F.; Ghanem, A.S.; Humayun, M. CO_2 towards fuels: A review of catalytic conversion of carbon dioxide to hydrocarbons. *J. Environ. Chem. Eng.* **2021**, *9*, 104756. [CrossRef]
5. Lingampalli, S.R.; Ayyub, M.M.; Rao, C.N.R. Recent Progress in the Photocatalytic Reduction of Carbon Dioxide. *ACS Omega* **2017**, *2*, 2740–2748. [CrossRef] [PubMed]
6. Wang, R.; Wang, X.; Xiong, Y.; Hou, Y.; Wang, Y.; Ding, J.; Zhong, Q. Modulation of Trivalent/Tetravalent Metallic Elements in Ni-Based Layered Double Hydroxides for Photocatalytic CO_2 Reduction. *ACS Appl. Mater. Interfaces* **2022**, *14*, 35654–35662. [CrossRef] [PubMed]
7. Ahmad, I.; Zou, Y.; Yan, J.; Liu, Y.; Shukrullah, S.; Naz, M.Y.; Hussain, H.; Khan, W.Q.; Khalid, N.R. Semiconductor photocatalysts: A critical review highlighting the various strategies to boost the photocatalytic performances for diverse applications. *Adv. Colloid Interface Sci.* **2023**, *311*, 102830. [CrossRef] [PubMed]
8. Liu, X.; Ye, L.; Liu, S.; Ji, X. Photocatalytic Reduction of CO_2 by ZnO Micro/nanomaterials with Different Morphologies and Ratios of {0001} Facets. *Sci. Rep.* **2016**, *6*, 38474. [CrossRef]
9. Li, H.; Gao, Y.; Xiong, Z.; Liao, C.; Shih, K. Enhanced selective photocatalytic reduction of CO_2 to CH_4 over plasmonic Au modified g-C_3N_4 photocatalyst under UV–vis light irradiation. *Appl. Surf. Sci.* **2018**, *439*, 552–559. [CrossRef]
10. Wu, Y.A.; McNulty, I.; Liu, C.; Lau, K.C.; Liu, Q.; Paulikas, A.P.; Sun, C.J.; Cai, Z.; Guest, J.R.; Ren, Y.; et al. Facet-dependent active sites of a single Cu_2O particle photocatalyst for CO_2 reduction to methanol. *Nat. Energy* **2019**, *4*, 957–968. [CrossRef]
11. Rehman, Z.U.; Bilal, M.; Hou, J.; Butt, F.K.; Ahmad, J.; Ali, S.; Hussain, A. Photocatalytic CO_2 Reduction Using TiO_2-Based Photocatalysts and TiO_2 Z-Scheme Heterojunction Composites: A Review. *Molecules* **2022**, *27*, 2069. [CrossRef] [PubMed]
12. Zhang, Y.; Wang, X.; Dong, P.; Huang, Z.; Nie, X.; Zhang, X. TiO_2 Surfaces Self-Doped with Ag Nanoparticles Exhibit Efficient CO_2 Photoreduction under Visible Light. *RSC Adv.* **2018**, *8*, 15991–15998. [CrossRef]
13. Tseng, I.-H.; Wu, J.C.S.; Chou, H.-Y. Effects of sol–gel procedures on the photocatalysis of Cu/TiO_2 in CO_2 photoreduction. *J. Catal.* **2004**, *221*, 432–440. [CrossRef]
14. Zhang, Q.; Gao, T.; Andino, J.M.; Li, Y. Copper and iodine co-modified TiO_2 nanoparticles for improved activity of CO_2 photoreduction with water vapor. *Appl. Catal. B Environ.* **2012**, *123–124*, 257–264. [CrossRef]
15. Lan, D.; Pang, F.; Ge, J. Enhanced Charge Separation in NiO and Pd Co-Modified TiO_2 Photocatalysts for Efficient and Selective Photoreduction of CO_2. *ACS Appl. Energy Mater.* **2021**, *4*, 6324–6332. [CrossRef]
16. Michalkiewicz, B.; Majewska, J.; Kądziołka, G.; Bubacz, K.; Mozia, S.; Morawski, A.W. Reduction of CO_2 by adsorption and reaction on surface of TiO_2-nitrogen modified photocatalyst. *J. CO2 Util.* **2014**, *5*, 47–52. [CrossRef]
17. Chen, Z.; Zhu, X.; Xiong, J.; Wen, Z.; Cheng, G. A p–n Junction by Coupling Amine-Enriched Brookite–TiO2 Nanorods with CuxS Nanoparticles for Improved Photocatalytic CO_2 Reduction. *Materials* **2023**, *16*, 960. [CrossRef]
18. Song, F.; Zhao, Y.; Zhong, Q. Adsorption of carbon dioxide on amine-modified TiO_2 nanotubes. *J. Environ. Sci.* **2013**, *25*, 554–560. [CrossRef]
19. Ota, M.; Hirota, Y.; Uchida, Y.; Nishiyama, N. CO_2 Adsorption Property of Amine-Modified Amorphous TiO_2 Nanoparticles with a High Surface Area. *Colloids Interfaces* **2018**, *2*, 25. [CrossRef]
20. Jiang, G.; Huang, Q.; Kenarsari, S.D.; Hu, X.; Russell, A.G.; Fan, M.; Shen, X. A new mesoporous amine-TiO_2 based pre-combustion CO_2 capture technology. *Appl. Energy* **2015**, *147*, 214–223. [CrossRef]
21. Ma, L.; Bai, R.; Hu, G.; Chen, R.; Hu, X.; Dai, W.; Dacosta, H.; Fan, M. Capturing CO_2 with amine-impregnated titanium oxides. *Energy Fuels* **2013**, *27*, 5433–5439. [CrossRef]
22. Kapica-Kozar, J.; Piróg, E.; Kusiak-Nejman, E.; Wrobel, R.J.; Gesikiewicz-Puchalska, A.; Morawski, A.W.; Narkiewicz, U.; Michalkiewicz, B. Titanium dioxide modified with various amines used as sorbents of carbon dioxide. *New J. Chem.* **2017**, *41*, 1549–1557. [CrossRef]
23. Kapica-Kozar, J.; Michalkiewicz, B.; Wrobel, R.J.; Mozia, S.; Pirog, E.; Kusiak-Nejman, E.; Serafin, J.; Morawski, A.W.; Narkiewicz, U. Adsorption of carbon dioxide on TEPA-modified TiO_2/titanate composite nanorods. *New J. Chem.* **2017**, *41*, 7870–7885. [CrossRef]
24. Mendonça, T.A.P.; Nascimento, J.P.C.; Casagrande, G.A.; Vieira, N.C.S.; Gonçalves, M. Ethylenediamine-modified activated carbon photocatalyst with the highest TiO_2 attachment/dispersion for improved photodegradation of sulfamethazine. *Mater. Chem. Phys.* **2024**, *318*, 129203. [CrossRef]

25. Bao, N.; Niu, J.J.; Li, Y.; Wu, G.L.; Yu, X.H. Low-temperature hydrothermal synthesis of N-doped TiO$_2$ from small-molecule amine systems and their photocatalytic activity. *Environ. Technol.* **2012**, *34*, 2939–2949. [CrossRef] [PubMed]
26. Liao, Y.; Cao, S.-W.; Yuan, Y.; Gu, Q.; Zhang, Z.; Xue, C. Efficient CO$_2$ Capture and Photoreduction by Amine-Functionalized TiO$_2$. *Chem. Eur. J.* **2014**, *20*, 10220–10222. [CrossRef]
27. Karawek, A.; Kitjanukit, N.; Neamsung, W.; Kinkaew, C.; Phadungbut, P.; Seeharaj, P.; Kim-Lohsoontorn, P.; Srinives, S. Alkanolamine-Grafted and Copper-Doped Titanium Dioxide Nanosheets–Graphene Composite Heterostructure for CO$_2$ Photoreduction. *ACS Appl. Energy Mater.* **2023**, *6*, 10929–10942. [CrossRef]
28. Jin, L.; Shaaban, E.; Bamonte, S.; Cintron, D.; Shuster, S.; Zhang, L.; Li, G.; He, J. Surface Basicity of Metal@TiO$_2$ to Enhance Photocatalytic Efficiency for CO$_2$ Reduction. *ACS Appl. Mater. Interfaces* **2021**, *13*, 38595–38603. [CrossRef]
29. Wang, Z.; Shangguan, C.; Wang, Z.; Wang, T.; Wang, L.; Liu, M.; Sui, Y. Investigation on Crystallization and Magnetic Properties of (Nd, Pr, Ce)2Fe14B/α-Fe Nanocomposite Magnets by Microwave Annealing Treatment. *Materials* **2021**, *14*, 2739. [CrossRef]
30. Cichoň, S.; Macháč, P.; Fekete, L.; Lapčák, L. Direct microwave annealing of SiC substrate for rapid synthesis of quality epitaxial graphene. *Carbon* **2016**, *98*, 441–448. [CrossRef]
31. Mirzaei, A.; Neri, G. Microwave-assisted synthesis of metal oxide nanostructures for gas sensing application: A review. *Sens. Actuat. B Chem.* **2016**, *237*, 749–775. [CrossRef]
32. Kustov, L.; Vikanova, K. Synthesis of Metal Nanoparticles under Microwave Irradiation: Get Much with Less Energy. *Metals* **2023**, *13*, 1714. [CrossRef]
33. Andrade-Guel, M.; Díaz-Jiménez, L.; Cortés-Hernández, D.; Cabello-Alvarado, C.; Ávila-Orta, C.; Bartolo-Pérez, P.; Gamero-Melo, P. Microwave assisted sol–gel synthesis of titanium dioxide using hydrochloric and acetic acid as catalysts. *Boletín Soc. Española Cerámica Vidr.* **2019**, *58*, 171–177. [CrossRef]
34. Dufour, F.; Cassaignon, S.; Durupthy, O.; Colbeau-Justin, C.; Chanéac, C. Do TiO$_2$ Nanoparticles Really Taste Better When Cooked in a Microwave Oven? *Eur. J. Inorg. Chem.* **2012**, *2012*, 2707–2715. [CrossRef]
35. Chang, C.; Rad, S.; Gan, L.; Li, Z.; Dai, J.; Shahab, A. Review of the sol–gel method in preparing nano TiO$_2$ for advanced oxidation process. *Nanotechnol. Rev.* **2023**, *12*, 20230150. [CrossRef]
36. Hafizah, N.; Sopyan, I. Nanosized TiO$_2$ Photocatalyst Powder via Sol-Gel Method: Effect of Hydrolysis Degree on Powder Properties. *Int. J. Photoenergy* **2009**, *2009*, 962783. [CrossRef]
37. Lee, Y.-B.; Lee, J.-M.; Hur, D.-H.; Lee, J.-H.; Jeon, S.-H. Effects of Advanced Amines on Magnetite Deposition of Steam Generator Tubes in Secondary System. *Coatings* **2021**, *11*, 514. [CrossRef]
38. Sun, H.; Bai, Y.; Liu, H.; Jin, W.; Xu, N.; Chen, G.; Xu, B. Mechanism of nitrogen-concentration dependence on pH value: Experimental and theoretical studies on nitrogen-doped TiO$_2$. *J. Phys. Chem. C* **2008**, *112*, 13304–13309. [CrossRef]
39. Yu, J.; Su, Y.; Cheng, B.; Zhou, M. Effects of pH on the microstructures and photocatalytic activity of mesoporous nanocrystalline titania powders prepared via hydrothermal method. *J. Mol. Catal. A Chem.* **2006**, *258*, 104–112. [CrossRef]
40. Yin, S.; Aita, Y.; Komatsu, M.; Sato, T.J. One-Step Cohydrothermal Synthesis of Nitrogen-Doped Titanium Oxide Nanotubes with Enhanced Visible Light Photocatalytic Activity. *Eur. Ceram. Soc.* **2006**, *26*, 2735–2742. [CrossRef]
41. Sing, K.S.W. Reporting physisorption data for gas/solid systems with special reference to the determination of surface area and porosity (Provisional). *Pure Appl. Chem.* **1982**, *54*, 2201–2218. [CrossRef]
42. Thommes, M.; Kaneko, K.; Neimark, A.V.; Olivier, J.P.; Rodriguez-Reinoso, F.; Rouquerol, J.; Sing, K.S.W. Physisorption of gases, with special reference to the evaluation of surface area and pore size distribution (IUPAC Technical Report). *Pure Appl. Chem.* **2015**, *87*, 1051–1069. [CrossRef]
43. Spadavecchia, F.; Ardizzone, S.; Cappelletti, G.; Oliva, C.; Cappelli, S. Time effects on the stability of the induced defects in TiO$_2$ nanoparticles doped by different nitrogen sources. *J. Nanopart. Res.* **2012**, *14*, 1301. [CrossRef]
44. Diker, H.; Varlikli, C.; Mizrak, K.; Dana, A. Characterizations and photocatalytic activity comparisons of N-doped nc-TiO$_2$ depending on synthetic conditions and structural differences of amine sources. *Energy* **2011**, *36*, 1243–1254. [CrossRef]
45. Akpan, U.G.; Hameed, B.H. Parameters affecting the photocatalytic degradation of dyes using TiO$_2$-based photocatalysts: A review. *J. Hazard. Mater.* **2009**, *170*, 520–529. [CrossRef] [PubMed]
46. Hamidi, F.; Aslani, F. TiO$_2$-based Photocatalytic Cementitious Composites: Materials, Properties, Influential Parameters, and Assessment Techniques. *Nanomaterials* **2019**, *9*, 1444. [CrossRef]
47. Gao, L.; Zhang, Q. Effects of amorphous contents and particle size on the photocatalytic properties of TiO$_2$ nanoparticles. *Scr. Mater.* **2001**, *44*, 1195–1198. [CrossRef]
48. Jang, H.D.; Kim, S.K.; Kim, S.J. Effect of Particle Size and Phase Composition of Titanium Dioxide Nanoparticles on the Photocatalytic Properties. *J. Nanoparticle Res.* **2001**, *3*, 141–147. [CrossRef]

Disclaimer/Publisher's Note: The statements, opinions and data contained in all publications are solely those of the individual author(s) and contributor(s) and not of MDPI and/or the editor(s). MDPI and/or the editor(s) disclaim responsibility for any injury to people or property resulting from any ideas, methods, instructions or products referred to in the content.

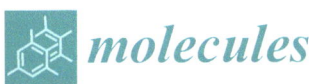

Article

Bifunctional Hot Water Vapor Template-Mediated Synthesis of Nanostructured Polymeric Carbon Nitride for Efficient Hydrogen Evolution

Baihua Long [1], Hongmei He [1], Yang Yu [1], Wenwen Cai [1], Quan Gu [2], Jing Yang [3,*] and Sugang Meng [4,*]

1. College of Material and Chemical Engineering, Pingxiang University, Pingxiang 337055, China
2. Key Laboratory of Applied Surface and Colloid Chemistry, Ministry of Education, School of Chemistry and Chemical Engineering, Shaanxi Normal University, Xi'an 710062, China
3. College of Health Science and Environmental Engineering, Shenzhen Technology University, Shenzhen 518118, China
4. Key Laboratory of Green and Precise Synthetic Chemistry and Applications, Ministry of Education, Huaibei Normal University, Huaibei 235000, China
* Correspondence: yangjingsztu@163.com (J.Y.); mengsugang@126.com (S.M.); Tel.: +86-18156139968 (S.M.)

Abstract: Regulating bulk polymeric carbon nitride (PCN) into nanostructured PCN has long been proven effective in enhancing its photocatalytic activity. However, simplifying the synthesis of nanostructured PCN remains a considerable challenge and has drawn widespread attention. This work reported the one-step green and sustainable synthesis of nanostructured PCN in the direct thermal polymerization of the guanidine thiocyanate precursor via the judicious introduction of hot water vapor's dual function as gas-bubble templates along with a green etching reagent. By optimizing the temperature of the water vapor and polymerization reaction time, the as-prepared nanostructured PCN exhibited a highly boosted visible-light-driven photocatalytic hydrogen evolution activity. The highest H_2 evolution rate achieved was 4.81 mmol·g^{-1}·h^{-1}, which is over four times larger than that of the bulk PCN (1.19 mmol·g^{-1}·h^{-1}) prepared only by thermal polymerization of the guanidine thiocyanate precursor without the assistance of bifunctional hot water vapor. The enhanced photocatalytic activity might be attributed to the enlarged BET specific surface area, increased active site quantity, and highly accelerated photo-excited charge-carrier transfer and separation. Moreover, the sustainability of this environmentally friendly hot water vapor dual-function mediated method was also shown to be versatile in preparing other nanostructured PCN photocatalysts derived from other precursors such as dicyandiamide and melamine. This work is expected to provide a novel pathway for exploring the rational design of nanostructured PCN for highly efficient solar energy conversion.

Keywords: carbon nitride; nanostructured; water vapor; H_2 evolution

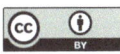

1. Introduction

The hydrogen evolution via photocatalytic water-splitting is potentially an efficient strategy to store clean energy and alleviate emerging energy issues in the future [1–4]. Polymeric carbon nitride (PCN) has long been proven to exhibit vast potential to achieve this magnificent goal [5–8]. Unfortunately, this stringent goal is greatly hindered by the low efficiency of bulk PCN due to inherent drawbacks, such as inferior separation and transfer for the photoexcited charge carriers, limited visible light absorption, extremely low specific surface area, and finite active sites [9–12]. In this regard, plenty of intelligent strategies have been developed to address the shortcomings mentioned above through the introduction of element doping or functional groups [13–16], modifications with defects or vacancies [17–19], regulating the nanostructure [20–23], adjusting morphology [24–27], or coupling with other semiconductors for heterojunctions and so forth [28–32]. Among these strategies, the nanostructure embedded in the PCN framework was demonstrated to be a simple and valid method for strikingly promoting the photocatalytic activity of PCN in many aspects [33]. In general, template methods such as hard-templating, soft-templating, and gas-templating were used to create the nanostructures, which resulted in a larger BET specific surface area, more active site quantity and improved the separation efficiency of photo-excited charged carriers.

Among these, the gas-templating method for nanostructure engineering was widely developed because it can circumvent not only the complexity of operations but also the use of extremely toxic chemical reagents that exist in the hard-templating and soft-templating methods. Additionally, this gas-templating method has the advantage of being simple, cost-effective, template-free, and suitable for large-scale synthesis. Normally, the gas-templating approach is primarily classified into two categories. The first is the self-induced gaseous templating method, which engineers the porous structure in PCN by using the self-generated gas as a template. For example, Tang et al. successfully obtained porous PCN with an extraordinary hydrogen evolution rate by direct thermal polymerization of urea at high temperatures in the air without using any additional chemical reagents. The porous structure is created by the emission of a large amount of ammonia gas and water vapor due to the existence of an oxygen element in the urea precursor, which is supposed to act as the gaseous template [34]. In another typical work, Chen et al. created nanoporous PCN with an increased BET specific surface area and pore volume via one-step polymerization of the single urea with self-supported gas, and the resulting nanostructured photocatalyst demonstrated a much higher hydrogen evolution rate [35]. The authors believe that the water vapor bubble served as a gaseous template in the proposed nanoporous PCN. Meanwhile, our groups also developed some simple sulfur-containing organic and inorganic compounds, such as trithiocyanuric acid, thiourea, guanidine thiocyanate, or ammonium thiocyanate, to serve as the unitary precursor for the one-pot production of nanoporous PCN at a high temperature [36–39]. The self-generated sulfur-containing gases produced at high temperatures are thought to be responsible for forming the nanostructure in PCN. However, the above synthesis method needed a high polymerization temperature to produce plenty of gas function as a gaseous template and also induced the destruction of the integrated PCN framework to some extent. The other method uses extra chemical reagents as dynamic gas-bubble templates. To date, specific types of chemical reagents, including NH_4Cl, $(NH_4)_2CO_3$, $NaHCO_3$, $(NH_4)_2SO_4$, $(NH_4)_2S_2O_8$ and sublimed sulfur, were intensely used as dynamic gas-bubble templates to promote the formation of nanostructured PCN [40–49]. During high-temperature calcining, the above chemical reagents can thermally decompose into a large number of gases as dynamic bubble templates, whose emissions induce the porous nanostructure in the PCN. Regrettably, the gases (NH_3, HCl, and SO_2) released by the above thermal decomposition of chemical reagents cannot be reused and are also sometimes detrimental to the environment, even though the method possesses the benefits of being low cost and easy to operate. Therefore, the exploration of green and pollution-free gas-bubble template methods to realize the synthesis of advanced nanostructured PCN is still of great urgency and interest.

Recently, the use of water vapor (completely green and abundant in the earth) for the pretreatment or preparation of the catalyst has been reported, and the as-prepared catalysts show astonishingly enhanced catalytic activity [17,50,51]. For instance, Huang et al. reported that an increase in the grain-boundary density in the Pd/Al_2O_3 catalyst is achieved by simple water vapor pretreatment and oxidation. The pretreatment catalyst showed a twelve-fold increase in methane oxidation compared to conventional pretreatments [50]. Yang et al. prepared the few-layered nanostructured PCN by using the bulk PCN and water vapor as the precursor and gas-bubble templates, respectively. The emissions of CO, H_2, and NO gas produced from the C/N-steam reforming reactions also played an important role in the formation of nanostructures in the PCN. Thus, the water vapor showed a dual function in their work, one was the dynamic gas-bubble template, and the other was a green initiator reagent for chemical etching [17]. However, their synthesis of nanostructured PCN required high-quality bulk PCN to serve as the precursor, which was relatively complex and time-consuming, although the method was demonstrated to be facile, green, and easy to scale up.

In this work, we proposed a one-step route for synthesizing nanostructured PCN to efficiently enhance its photocatalytic activity by judiciously introducing hot water vapor into the direct thermal polymerization of the guanidine thiocyanate precursor. The hot water vapor served a dual function as a dynamic gas-bubble template and an assisted chemical etching reagent in this synthesis. In particular, the supply of the water vapor is continuous throughout the whole synthesis procedure. We investigated the effect of the polymerization reaction time and the temperature of the water vapor on the morphology, structure, and optical/photoelectric properties of the as-prepared nanostructured PCN. Benefitting from the synchronous nanostructure and carbon vacancies embedded in the PCN, the optimized water-vapor treatment PCN was four times more effective than that of the bulk PCN treatment for photocatalytic hydrogen evolution. Moreover, this hot water vapor dual-function mediated method was also successfully extended to other PCN precursors (melamine and dicyandiamide) to obtain their corresponding derived nanostructured PCNs. The detailed synthesis processes were described, and comprehensive characterizations were conducted to elucidate the enhanced photocatalytic hydrogen evolution mechanism.

2. Results and Discussion

2.1. Morphology and Texture

The nanostructured photocatalysts were prepared via direct thermal polymerization and simultaneous chemical etching of the guanidine thiocyanate precursor with the assistance of N_2 flow, carrying the special temperature of the water vapor. We investigated the variability in water-vapor amounts in detail by accurately controlling the temperature of the water vapor and the reaction times during the polymerization process. Unfortunately, the guanidine thiocyanate precursor was burned off at water-vapor temperatures above 60 °C, and thus no photocatalysts were left in our present experimental conditions. The possible explanation is that the PCN or the intermediates of PCN formed during the polymerization process were completely etched by the excess water vapor. In addition, no photocatalysts were collected at the temperature of 60 °C water vapor for 4 h. The above synthesis results suggested that the selection of water vapor temperatures and reaction times is a key factor in providing an optimal amount of water vapor for preparing and modulating the nanostructured PCN.

The changes in the microstructure of the as-prepared photocatalysts were first characterized by SEM and TEM measurements. SEM observations revealed that CGS-CN displayed a compact, thick, and large aggregate morphology (Figure S1). The GS-CN-25 had a similar morphology to that of the CGS-CN due to the insufficient water vapor and short etching reaction time provided in this preparation system. In contrast, both GS-CN-60 and GS-CN-25-4h photocatalysts obtained upon increasing the temperature of the water vapor or prolonging the etching reaction time exhibited looser, thinner, and smaller aggregates. Excitingly, some nanosheets and pores were observed at the surface of the GS-CN-60 photocatalyst, and its contrast also illustrated its maximal BET specific surface area as evidenced by the BET analyses described below. The possible reason for this evolution is due to the significant contribution from the water vapor, which not only avoids the compact and large aggregates of CGS-CN but also its ability to etch the sheets to generate pores via the large number of gases (H_2, CO, CO_2, and NH_3) released during the simultaneous polymerization and etching procedure [51]. In other words, the released gases are able to explode many "tiny bombs" on the thick chunks of the CGS-CN, which leads to the generation of relatively loose, thin, small aggregates and even porous structural characteristics on the GS-CN-60.

TEM results further substantiated this visible evolution, displaying the bulk CGS-CN aggregates' gradual evolution into thin and semitransparent nanosheets along with certain surface pores on the GS-CN-60 photocatalyst by the hot water vapor dual-unction mediated method, as seen in Figure 1a,b. AFM topography and height profiles (Figure 1c–f) demonstrated that the GS-CN-60 existed as nanosheets with thicknesses ranging from 2 to 6 nm, while the average thickness of the bulk CGS-CN was around 20 nm. The unique morphological characteristics of the GS-CN-x photocatalysts directly affected their textural properties, as evidenced by the BET test.

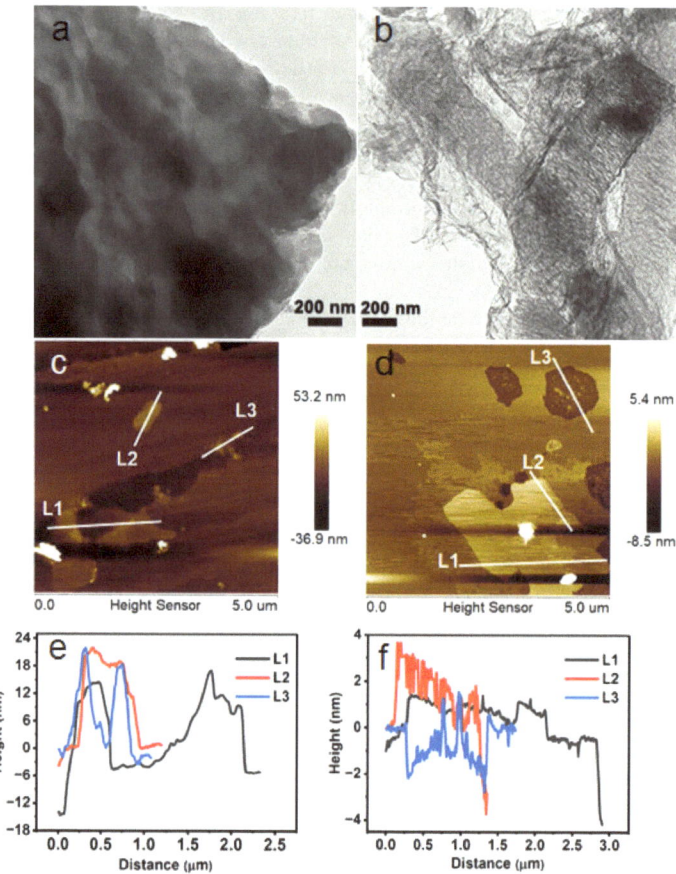

Figure 1. TEM images of: (**a**) bulk CGS-CN and (**b**) GS-CN-60. AFM images and corresponding height profile of: (**c**,**e**) bulk CGS-CN; and (**d**,**f**) GS-CN-60 ((**c**,**d**) corresponds to (**e**,**f**), respectively).

BET confirmed that the specific surface area gradually increased from CGS-CN, GS-CN-25, and GS-CN-25-4h to GS-CN-60, as shown in Figure 2. The GS-CN-60 had the largest surface area with 34.1 $m^2 \cdot g^{-1}$, which was about 1.7, 1.9, and 7.1 times higher than those of the GS-CN-25-4h, GS-CN-25, and bulk CGS-CN. Nevertheless, the surface area of GS-CN-25-4h (20.4 $m^2 g^{-1}$) only weakly increased compared to that of the GS-CN-25 (17.9 $m^2 g^{-1}$). These results reflected that the hot water vapor assisted by the dual function mediated strategy exerted the most significant impact on the surface area. Moreover, the adsorption–desorption isothermal curves for GS-CN-x photocatalysts all exhibited typical type IV with an H_3-type hysteresis loop and an enlarged pore volume (Figure 2), revealing that they possessed representative porous structural characteristics and were in line with the results of the SEM and TEM images. Consequently, the above results implied that the optimization of the nanostructured PCN with plentiful pores, high specific surface area, and expanded pore volume was successfully prepared by this hot water vapor dual-function mediated strategy by simply adjusting the relative amounts of water vapor, which promoted the guanidine thiocyanate precursor for suitable seed nucleation, growth, and synchronous etching during the polymerization processes.

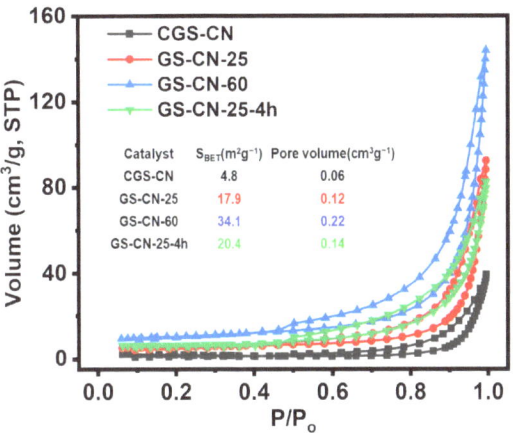

Figure 2. N$_2$ adsorption-desorption isotherms of bulk CGS-CN and GS-CN-x photocatalysts.

2.2. XRD and FTIR Analysis

Figure 3a represents the XRD patterns and diffraction peaks of all the photocatalysts. All tested photocatalysts exhibited two distinct diffraction peaks at around 13.3° and 27.2°, which are indexed to the (100) and (002) planes of hexagonal PCN. These reflections correspond to the in-plane structural heptazine units and interlamellar stacking distance, respectively. The results implied that the GS-CN-x could retain the primary heptazine structure of PCN after the water-vapor treatment reaction. Compared with bulk CGS-CN, the (100) diffraction peak intensity for GS-CN-25 showed no noticeable change, indicating that the in-planar layer size of GS-CN-25 had no significant influence (Figure S2). Nonetheless, the GS-CN-60 and GS-CN-25-4h photocatalysts exhibited a slightly weak diffraction peak at (100), attributed to the decrease in-planar layer size. Similarly, the relative intensity of the (002) diffraction peak for GS-CN-60 and GS-CN-25-4h also became weaker, which is attributed to the selective dismemberment of the PCN framework and the formation of the short-range ordered graphite molecular fragments upon increasing the temperature of the water vapor or prolonging the reaction time [52]. In addition, further observation indicated that the (002) peak position for GS-CN-x showed a progressive upshift compared to that of CGS-CN, highlighting the compacted interlayer stacking distance in the resulting water vapor treatment photocatalysts. The reason for this was that the undulated single layers in CGS-CN were planarized by the water-vapor treatment and thus resulted in a tight stack structure for these GS-CN-x photocatalysts [17].

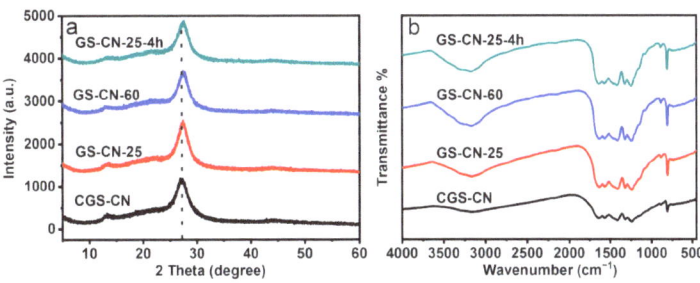

Figure 3. (**a**) XRD patterns of bulk CGS-CN and GS-CN-x photocatalysts; and (**b**) FT-IR spectra of bulk CGS-CN and GS-CN-x photocatalysts.

The FT-IR spectra presented in Figure 3b show that the GS-CN-x photocatalysts exhibited the same characteristic vibrational absorption peaks as that of CGS-CN. In any case, the identified peak positions at 810, 1200–1700, and 3000–3500 cm^{-1}, respectively, were assigned to the bending vibrations of heptazine units, stretching vibrations of aromatic C-N heterocycles, and stretching vibrations of the -NH$_x$ groups. Interestingly, the more vigorous intensity of these peaks in the region of 3100–3400 cm^{-1} for the GS-CN-x photocatalysts compared with that of the CGS-CN is indicative of more adsorbed H$_2$O on these GS-CN-x photocatalyst surfaces due to their sizeable open-up surface effects.

2.3. XPS and ESR Analysis

XPS further demonstrated the more subtle chemical structure and valence state of the photocatalysts. The XPS test confirmed the presence of carbon, nitrogen, and oxygen elements for all the photocatalysts, as illustrated in Figure 4a. The C 1s and N 1s high-resolution spectra of the GS-CN-x photocatalysts showed the same binding energies as that of the CGS-CN, indicating that the heptazine structure was hardly changed in the rigid water-vapor treatment conditions. The high-resolution C 1s spectrum revealed two labeled peaks with the binding energy centered at 288.0 and 284.6 eV (Figure 4b), which were assigned to sp^2-hybridized aromatic C atoms (N-C=N) in the heptazine rings and adventitious carbon, respectively. The high-resolution N 1s spectrum could be deconvoluted into four labeled peaks with the binding energy positioned at 398.5, 400.1, 401.2, and 404.0 eV, respectively (Figure 4c). The strongest N 1s peak at 398.5 eV corresponded to sp^2-hybridized aromatic N atoms (C=N-C) in the heptazine rings. The second strongest N 1s peak at 400.1 eV was indicative of tertiary N atoms from N-(C)$_3$ groups. The third N 1s peak at 401.2 eV was attributed to amino functional groups (C-N-H). The weakest N 1s peak at 404.0 eV was caused by π*-excitation. The analysis of the surface C/N atomic ratio results in Table S1 show that these GS-CN-x photocatalysts were deficient in carbon compared to CGS-CN. This result reflected the fact that the carbon vacancies were successfully incorporated into the GS-CN-x framework due to the preferential elimination of carbon atoms in the water-vapor treatment reaction. To distinguish the locations of carbon vacancies in the GS-CN-x framework, the summaries of C and N atomic contents were analyzed and quantified based on the peak area ratio (Figure S3). The atomic percentages of N-(C)$_3$ and C-N-H decreased, and that of C=N-C increased in N 1s XPS spectra for these GS-CN-x photocatalysts as compared with those of the bulk CGS-CN (Figure S3b), indicating that the elimination of the carbon atoms mainly occurred at the N-(C)$_3$ and C-N-H sites to generate carbon vacancies for these GS-CN-x photocatalysts. In addition, the increased atomic percentages of N-C=N in C 1s XPS spectra for GS-CN-x photocatalysts further cross-validate the above-mentioned deduction (Figure S3a). Nonetheless, the decreased atomic percentages of C-C/C=C for GS-CN-x photocatalysts could result from the part of graphitic carbon being removed from the surface by the reductive gas of H$_2$, which was generated through the water vapor etching reaction [51,53].

The direct evidence to confirm the formation of carbon vacancies in GS-CN-x can be further interpreted by EPR. As shown in Figure 4d, the Lorentzian line of bulk CGS-CN showed a feeble signal at g = 2.004. The EPR signal of PCN is stemmed from the unpaired electrons on sp^2-C atoms of aromatic C-N heterocycles, which leads to structural defects in the PCN framework. Moreover, the signal intensity increases gradually from CGS-CN, GS-CN-25, and GS-CN-25-4h to GS-CN-60. The increase of unpaired electrons on the sp^2-C atoms for GS-CN-x photocatalysts remarkably strengthened the intensity of the Lorentzian line, firmly showing that the concentration of carbon vacancies in the as-prepared GS-CN-x was increased and controllably tuned [54]. However, the bulk C/N atomic ratio in the EA analysis results (Table S2) suggested that the bulk C/N atomic ratio for these GS-CN-x photocatalysts was slightly decreased compared to the bulk CGS-CN, signifying that the carbon vacancies were more likely to be near the surface of the water-vapor-etched photocatalysts.

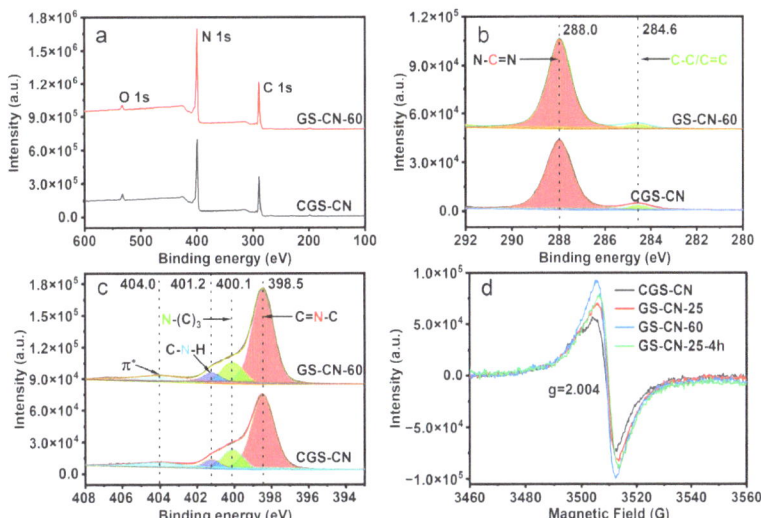

Figure 4. XPS patterns of bulk CGS-CN and GS-CN-x photocatalysts: (**a**) survey patterns; (**b**) high-resolution patterns of C1s; (**c**) high-resolution patterns of N1s; and (**d**) room-temperature EPR spectra of bulk CGS-CN and GS-CN-x photocatalysts.

2.4. UV-Visible and PL Analysis

The UV-vis absorption spectra of CGS-CN and GS-CN-x photocatalysts are shown in Figure 5a. The intrinsic absorption edge of the GS-CN-x showed a progressive blue shift compared to that of the bulk CGS-CN, which rendered the enlargement of the intrinsic bandgaps. It is noticeable that GS-CN-60 and GS-CN-25-4h photocatalysts show virtually identical absorption edges and intensities. Furthermore, no evident Urbach tail absorption in the visible-light region for the GS-CN-x was found, indicative of the absence of shallow trap states embedded in the bandgap of GS-CN-x generated by carbon vacancies [18,55]. This also indirectly demonstrated that the following enhancement of GS-CN-x photocatalytic activity was not directly correlated with their optical absorption. The corresponding bandgap energies of the photocatalysts were calculated based on the plots of $[F(R)h\nu]^{1/2}$ versus $h\nu$ (Figure 5b) and the bandgap energies of CGS-CN (2.56 eV), GS-CN-25 (2.68 eV), GS-CN-60 (2.73 eV), and GS-CN-25-4h (2.73 eV) were estimated. The broadened bandgap for the GS-CN-x catalysts was firmly demonstrated by a similar tendency in the gradual blue shift in the PL emission spectrum (Figure 5c). This hypochromic-shift phenomenon can be well explained as a consequence of the quantum size effect of the nanostructured materials. The values of the valence band were directly determined by XPS valence band spectroscopy (Figure 5d). The band edge of GS-CN-60 (1.97 eV) was revealed as a 0.21 eV negative shift compared to that of CGS-CN (2.18 eV). The conduction band values of CGS-CN and GS-CN-60 could be calculated as −0.38 eV and −0.76 eV, respectively, according to the Equation: $E_{CB} = E_{VB} - E_g$. The corresponding band alignments of CGS-CN and GS-CN-60 are schematically depicted in Figure S4, where the GS-CN-60 exhibited a more thermodynamically enhanced reduction power than that of the CGS-CN, indicative of the more powerful reduction ability of photoexcited electrons at GS-CN-60, which enabled the fast proton reduction in the following photocatalytic hydrogen evolution reaction.

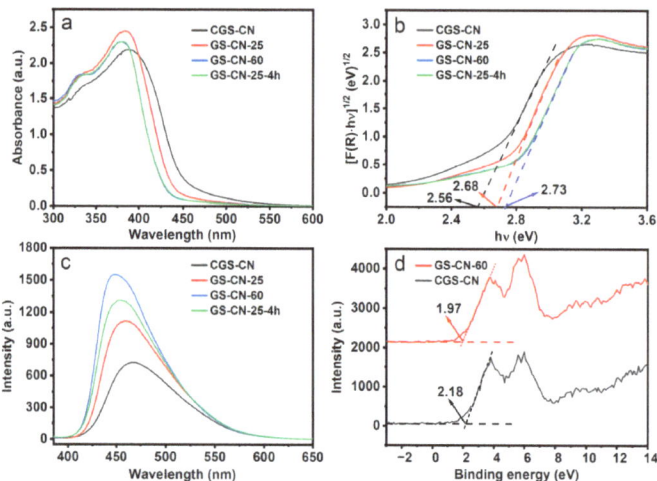

Figure 5. (**a**) UV-Vis diffuse reflectance spectra of bulk CGS-CN, GS-CN-x photocatalysts (noted: the nearly same absorption edge and intensity occurred in GS-CN-60 and GS-CN-25-4h); (**b**) The corresponding Kubelka–Munk transformed spectra of bulk CGS-CN and GS-CN-x photocatalysts; (**c**) FL emission spectra of bulk CGS-CN and GS-CN-x photocatalysts; and (**d**) XPS valence-band spectra of bulk CGS-CN and GS-CN-60 photocatalysts.

2.5. Time-Resolved PL and Photoelectrochemical Analysis

To better understand the recombination kinetics of photoexcited charge carriers, the time-resolved PL decay spectra of CGS-CN and GS-CN-x photocatalysts were recorded (Figure 6a). The fitted PL lifetime-decay curves, according to the two-exponential decay model, revealed that the average radiative lifetimes of CGS-CN, GS-CN-25, GS-CN-60, and GS-CN-25-4h were 6.68, 6.31, 5.42, and 5.47 ns, respectively. All the fitting decay parameters and the pertinent details are summarized in Table S3. The shortest lifetime of the singlet exciton in GS-CN-60 clearly implied that its depopulation of the excited states primarily occurred through non-radiative pathways, presumably through charge transfer of the electrons to some favorable carbon defect sites, and then promoted the rapid transfer and separation of charge carriers [56–59]. Concurrently, the change regularity of transient photocurrent responses of the photocatalysts can support the above explanation (Figure 6b). GS-CN-60 gave a higher photocurrent response than those of the other photocatalysts, indicative of its remarkably high charge-carrier separation efficiency. To further understand the dynamic behaviors of photo-generated charge carriers, electrochemical impedance spectroscopy (EIS) was conducted to investigate the properties of the electrode/electrolyte interface, and the result is illustrated in Figure 6c. The GS-CN-60 photocatalyst showed the smallest interfacial charge-transfer resistance due to the synergetic effect of the favorable porous and electronic structures, well in accordance with the photocurrent response. Owning a higher overall electronic conductivity, the photoexcited electron transfer kinetics from the bulk to the interface of GS-CN-60 was faster than that of the other photocatalysts, and therefore it is expected to guarantee high photocatalytic activity.

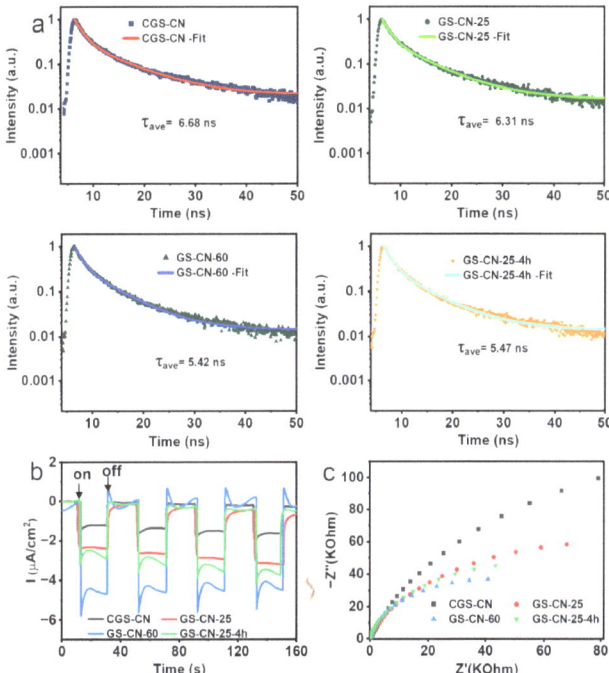

Figure 6. (**a**) Time-resolved PL decay spectra of bulk CGS-CN and GSCN-x photocatalysts kinetics monitored at their maximum emission wavelength (CGS-CN: 470 nm; GS-CN-25: 459 nm; GS-CN-60: 448 nm; GS-CN-25-4h: 453 nm) under 365 nm excitation; (**b**) transient photocurrent responses; and (**c**) EIS Nyquist plots of bulk CGS-CN and GS-CN-x photocatalysts.

2.6. Photocatalytic Activities

The photocatalytic activities of the as-prepared photocatalysts were examined by visible-light-induced photocatalytic H_2 evolution in coexistence with Pt catalyst and triethanolamine (TEOA) sacrificial electron donor. Initially, we investigated the influence of the concentration of TEOA on the rate of H_2 evolution by GS-CN-60 photocatalyst under visible light irradiation. As shown in Figure S5, the H_2 evolution rate reached a maximum at a concentration of 10 vol.% TEOA. Hereafter, we chose 10 vol.% TEOA as the sacrificial electron donor for the following experiment. The photocatalytic hydrogen evolution amounts versus irradiation time over the as-prepared photocatalysts were plotted in Figure 7a. The CGS-CN photocatalyst showed the lowest activity, with an H_2 evolution rate of 1.19 mmol·h^{-1}·g^{-1}. As expected, the photocatalytic H_2 generation activity was significantly enhanced for the GS-CN-x photocatalysts in comparison with that of CGS-CN, suggesting the positive contribution of the water vapor mediated strategy to the photocatalytic activity. The optimized H_2 evolution rate of 4.81 mmol·h^{-1}·g^{-1} was achieved for the GS-CN-60 photocatalyst, which was about four times higher than that of the bulk CGS-CN photocatalyst. This result clearly demonstrated the advantage of the hot water vapor treatment to create nanostructures in PCN. At the same time, the high activity was reproducible for the GS-CN-60 photocatalyst, as demonstrated by its excellent long-term stability over a period of 24 h. The generated amount of H_2 was about 13.2 mmol·g^{-1} in the first run and could retain the almost equivalent amount of H_2 in the subsequent five cycle runs, again revealing the robust stability of the GS-CN-60 for sustainable applications. Above all, the GS-CN-60 maintained a well-retained chemical structure even after five-cycle photocatalytic reactions, as demonstrated in the XRD and FT-IR spectroscopy results, which showed that there was no difference between the used photocatalyst and fresh photocatalyst (Figure S6). The wavelength-dependent apparent quantum yield curve of GSCN-60 matched well with its UV-Vis absorption spectrum, reflecting the light-induced nature of the reaction. Based on the above discussion, we are now in a position to try to understand the probable mechanisms behind the enhanced photocatalytic H_2 evolution activity of GSCN-60. In all, the exceptionally improved photocatalytic activity of GS-CN-60 was due to the synergistic action of high BET specific surface area in contrast to bulk CGS-CN, an enlarged bandgap, outstanding electron reduction ability, and an elevation of the mobility of photo-excited charge carriers. These results, taken together, definitely favored our proceeding with an investigation of the photocatalytic hydrogen evolution reaction.

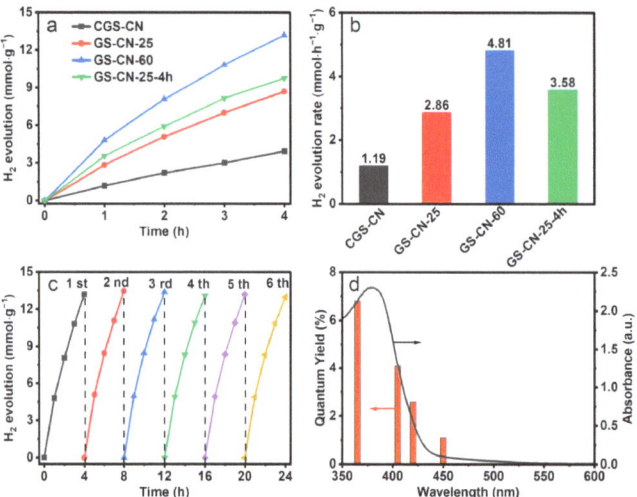

Figure 7. (**a**) Time-dependent evolution of H_2 produced on bulk CGS-CN and GS-CN-x photocatalysts; (**b**) H_2 evolution rate in the first hour on bulk CGS-CN and GS-CN-x photocatalysts; (**c**) recycling test of the GS-CN-60 photocatalyst; and (**d**) M of GS-CN-60 under different wavelengths of monochromatic light.

2.7. Photocatalytic Activities of the Other Prepared Nanostructured PCN

Last but not least, the generality of the effect of hot water vapor with a dual-function mediated strategy was not exclusive to the guanidine thiocyanate precursor. We also verified the effect of the hot water vapor treatment on the other precursors, such as dicyandiamide and melamine. The SEM and TEM results indicated that these water-vapor-treated CDCDA-CN-x and MA-CN-x photocatalysts also showed loose, thin, small aggregates compared with those of the corresponding bulk PCN (Figures S7 and S8), which was well reflected by the gradually increased BET specific surface area results (Table S4). The XRD, FTIR, UV-Visible absorption, and PL spectra of their bulk PCN and corresponding vapor treatment photocatalysts are shown for comparison (Figures S9–S11), indicating that DCDA-CN-x and MA-CN-x showed a similar variation trend with that of the GS-CN-x. These time-resolved PL, photocurrent-response, and EIS-Nyquist characterization results (Figure 8) revealed that these water-vapor-treatment photocatalysts exhibited greatly increased charge separation and electronic conductibility by virtue of their unique porous and electron structures. As expected, the DCDA-CN-x and MA-CN-x displayed obviously enhanced photocatalytic activity.

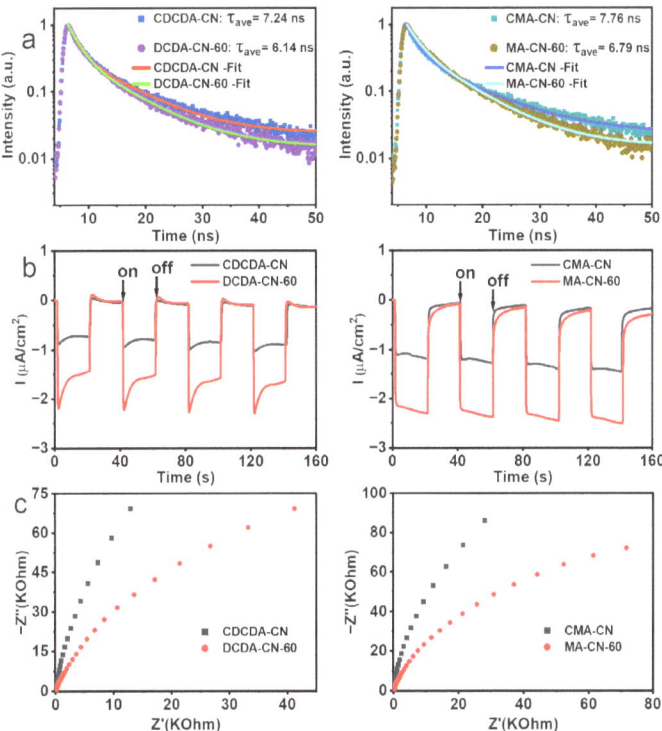

Figure 8. (**a**) Time-resolved PL decay spectra of CDCDA-CN, DCDA-CN-60, CMA-CN and MA-CN-60 photocatalysts kinetics monitored at their maximum emission wavelength (CDCDA-CN: 473 nm; DCDA-CN-60: 454 nm; CMA-CN: 473 nm; MA-CN-60: 445 nm) under 365 nm excitation; (**b**) Transient photocurrent responses; and (**c**) EIS Nyquist plots of CDCDA-CN, DCDA-CN-60, CMA-CN and MA-CN-60 photocatalysts.

The hydrogen-evolution rates of the DCDA-CN-60 and MA-CN-60 were 3.8 and 2.7 times higher than those of the bulk CDCDA-CN and CMA-CN, respectively (Figure 9). The difference in exfoliation behavior of PCN from the corresponding different precursors could well account for the different enhanced factors in the photocatalytic activity of H_2 evolution.

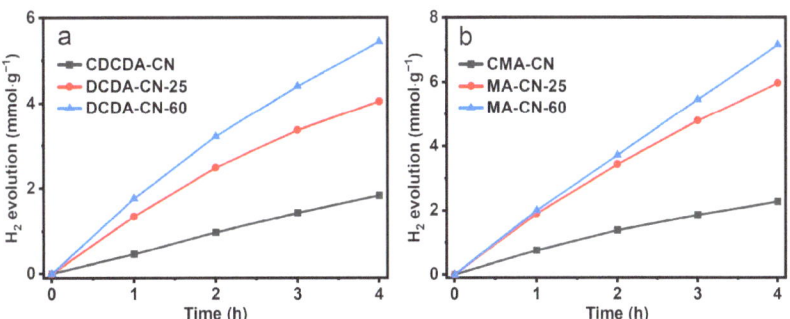

Figure 9. Photocatalytic H_2 evolution rates of: (**a**) CDCDA-CN and DCDA-CN-x; and (**b**) CMA-CN and MA-CN-x photocatalysts.

3. Materials and Methods

3.1. Materials

The guanidine thiocyanate, melamine, dicyandiamide, triethanolamine (TEOA), and $H_2PtCl_6 \cdot 6H_2O$ were of analytical grade and used as received without any further purification. Deionized water was used in all the experiments.

3.2. Preparation

2 g Guanidine thiocyanate was thoroughly ground into tiny powders with an agate mortar. After that, the powders were carefully transferred into a porcelain boat and subsequently heated to 550 °C at 5 °C·min^{-1} with nitrogen flow carrying a specific temperature of water vapor for 2 h in a tubular furnace. To avoid the hot water cooling during the transfer line between the gas-washing bottle and the entrance of the furnace, we twined the heat belt to keep the temperature of the transfer line at 100 °C. During the polymerization process, the hot water vapor, maintained at definite temperatures (25 °C, 60 °C, 80 °C, and 100 °C) via a hotplate magnetic stirrer, was carried into the tubular furnace at the assistance of nitrogen gas with a flow rate of 50 mL/min. Finally, the resulting photocatalysts labeled GS-CN-x (where x represents the temperature of water vapor) were obtained for further use. At the same time, the effect of increasing the water vapor etching reaction time to 4 h for preparing the nanostructure PCN was also explored. The final photocatalyst was denoted as GS-CN-x-y (where x represents the temperature of water vapor, and y represents the reaction time). The schematic diagram of this hot-water-vapor-assisted etching method for nanostructured PCN is illustrated in Scheme S1. In comparison, the preparation of bulk PCN as the control photocatalyst was the same as that of GS-CN-x, except for the absence of hot water vapor, which is denoted as CGS-CN for simplicity.

Similarly, we also used other precursors (melamine and dicyandiamide) to witness the same hot-water-vapor-treatment procedure to prepare their corresponding nanostructured PCN. The resulting photocatalysts were denoted as MA-CN-x (melamine as a precursor) and DCDA-CN-x (dicyandiamide as a precursor), where x still represents the temperature of the water vapor. In the meantime, their corresponding bulk PCN photocatalysts as control photocatalysts were also synthesized via calcining pure melamine and dicyandiamide in the absence of hot water vapor, which were denoted as CMA-CN and CDCDA-CN, respectively.

3.3. Characterization

The scanning emission microscope measurements were conducted using an FEI Nova Nano SEM 230 (Thermo Fisher Scientific, Waltham, MA, USA) Field Emission Scanning Electron Microscope. Transmission electron microscopy (TEM) images were obtained using an FEI Talos (Thermo Fisher Scientific, Waltham, MA, USA) field emission transmission electron microscope. X-ray photoelectron spectroscopy (XPS) data were collected on a Thermo ESCALAB 250 instrument (Thermo Fisher Scientific, Waltham, MA, USA) with a monochromatized Al Kα line source (200 W). The Fourier transform infrared (FT-IR) spectra were obtained on a Nicolet Nexus 670 FT-IR spectrometer (Thermo Nicolet Co., Madison, USA) in a range from 4000 to 400 cm^{-1}, and the photocatalysts were mixed with KBr at a concentration of ca. 1 wt%. Nitrogen adsorption–desorption experiments were performed at 77 K using Micromeritics Tristar II 3020 equipment (Micromeritics, Norcross, GA, USA). The specific surface area was calculated by the Brunauer-Emmet-Teller (BET) method. Elemental analysis (EA) was carried out on an elemental Analyzer (Elementar vario EL cube, Hanau, Germany). X-ray diffraction (XRD) measurements were performed on a Bruker D8 Advance diffractometer (Bruker, Billerica, MA, USA) with Cu Kα1 radiation (λ = 1.5406 Å). UV-Vis diffuse reflectance spectra (UV-Vis DRS) were collected on Lambda 650s Scan UV-Visible system (Perkin-Elmer, Waltham, MA, USA) using double beam optic, and Teflon was used as the reflectance standard. Electron paramagnetic resonance (EPR) spectra were tested by Bruker model A 300 spectrometer (Bruker, Billerica, MA, USA). The photoluminescence (PL) spectra were done at room temperature on a Hitachi F-7100 type of spectrophotometer (Hitachi Co., Tokyo, Japan). The time-resolved PL decay spectra were recorded at room temperature on an Edinburgh FI/FSTCSPC FLS-1000 spectrophotometer (Edinburgh, Livingston, UK). The electrochemical measurements were done on a CHI 760E electrochemical workstation (Chenhua Co., Ltd., Shanghai, China) in an electrolytic cell with standard three electrodes. The Ag/AgCl (3M KCl) was used as a reference electrode, and a Pt foil was used as a counter electrode. For the working electrode, the photocatalyst dispersion was dipped into the F-doped tin oxide (FTO) glass with a fixed area of 0.25 cm^2 and then dried at 120 °C for 2 h to improve adhesion for further use.

3.4. Photocatalytic H_2 Evolution Experiments

The photocatalytic reactions were performed in an 80 mL volume of Schlenk flask at 1 bar atmospheric pressure of Argon. Typically, 10 mg photocatalyst powder as a photosensitizer was ultrasonically dispersed in 10 vol.% TEOA aqueous solution (10 mL), which was used as the sacrificial electron donor. A 3 wt% Pt as the catalyst was loaded onto the surface of the photocatalyst by the photodeposition approach using $H_2PtCl_6 \cdot 6H_2O$. The reaction system was evacuated and then backfilled with the high-purity Argon gas (99.999%). This process was repeated three times to remove air completely, and at the last cycle, the Schlenk flask was backfilled with 1 bar of the high-purity Argon gas before irradiation under a 300 W Xe-lamp with UV cut-off filter ($\lambda > 420$ nm). The temperature of the reaction solution was kept at 25 °C by a flow of cooling water. After irradiation, 0.5 mL of the generated gas was extracted per hour and detected by gas chromatography (Fuli, GC-9790Plus, Wenling, China) equipped with a thermal conductive detector (TCD) using Argon as carrier gas. After four hours of terminating the reaction, the reaction system was repeated to evacuate and backfill the Argon gas for the next cycles of the hydrogen-evolution experiments to verify the stability of the photocatalyst.

The apparent quantum yield (*AQY*) for H_2 evolution was measured under a monochromatic light with a bandpass filter of 365, 405, 420, and 450 nm, respectively. The intensity of the light was 140, 127, 107, and 144 mW·cm^{-2} for the 365, 405, 420, and 450 nm monochromatic filters, respectively. The irradiation area was measured as 4.6 cm^2. According to the amount of hydrogen produced every hour in the photocatalytic reaction, the *AQY* was calculated by the Formula (1):

$$AQY = \frac{2 \times M \times N_A}{S \times P \times t \times \lambda/(h \times c)} \quad (1)$$

where *M* is the mole number of evolved H_2 (mol), N_A is Avogadro's constant (6.022 × 10^{23} mol^{-1}), *S* is the irradiated area (cm^2), *P* is the powder density of irradiation light (W·cm^{-2}), *t* is the irradiation time (s), λ is the wavelength of the monochromatic light (nm), *h* is the Planck constant (6.626 × 10^{-34} J·s), *c* is the velocity of light (3 × 10^8 m·s^{-1}).

4. Conclusions

In summary, nanostructured PCN can be successfully prepared by a green and sustainable water-vapor mediated method through one-pot simultaneous polymerization and chemical etching of the PCN precursors directly with hot water vapor. The nanostructured morphology with carbon vacancies can be created and is controllable by controlling the temperature of the water vapor and the reaction time in the synthesis process. Benefitting from the more exposed surface, increased photo-excited electrons reduction ability, and enhanced photo-excited charge carrier transfer and separation efficiency, the GSCN-60 realized substantially improved photocatalytic hydrogen evolution performance than that of the bulk CGS-CN. The present hot water vapor with a dual-function mediated approach could provide a novel pathway for the preparation of nanostructured PCN materials with high photocatalytic performance.

Supplementary Materials: The following supporting information can be downloaded at: https://www.mdpi.com/article/10.3390/molecules28124862/s1, Scheme S1: Proposed one-step synthesis of nanostructured PCN by introducing hot water vapor into the polymerization process of C/N precursors; Figure S1: SEM images of bulk CGS-CN and GS-CN-x photocatalysts; Figure S2: The high-magnification section of the XRD patterns for bulk CGS-CN and GS-CN-x photocatalysts; Figure S3: Summary of C atomic contents in the various photocatalysts determined by C1s spectra (a) and summary of N atomic contents in the various photocatalysts determined by N1s spectra (b); Figure S4: The energy band diagrams of bulk CGS-CN and GS-CN-60; Figure S5: H_2 evolution rate from different concentration of TEOA as a sacrificial electron donor by GS-CN-60 photocatalyst. Figure S6: XRD and FT-IR patterns of the GS-CN-60 for photocatalytic H_2 evolution before and after five cycling runs; Figure S7: SEM images of CDCDA-CN, DCDA-CN-60, CMA-CN, and MA-CN-60; Figure S8: TEM images of CDCDA-CN, DCDA-CN-60, CMA-CN, and MA-CN-60; Figure S9: XRD patterns of CDCDA-CN and DCDA-CN-x (a), CMA-CN and MA-CN-x (b); Figure S10: FTIR spectra of CDCDA-CN and DCDA-CN-x (a), CMA-CN and MA-CN-x (b); Figure S11: UV-Vis diffuse reflectance spectra (a), the corresponding Kubelka-Munk transformed spectra (b) and PL spectra of CDCDA-CN, DCDA-CN-x, CMA-CN and MA-CN-x (c); Table S1: Surface atomic ratio of all photocatalysts determined by XPS spectra; Table S2: The atom percentage of C, N, O and H atoms in the CGS-CN and GS-CN-60 photocatalysts determined by EA; Table S3: Lifetime and Relative Intensities of the fitting parameters of PL decay curves for CGS-CN and GS-CN-x photocatalysts; Table S4: BET specific surface areas (S_{BET}) of the photocatalysts.

Author Contributions: B.L.: Conceptualization, data curation, writing—original draft preparation, funding acquisition. H.H.: Investigation, data curation, validation. Y.Y. and W.C.: Investigation, data curation. Q.G.: Formal analysis, writing—review and editing. J.Y. and S.M.: Conceptualization, methodology, supervision, writing—review and editing, funding acquisition. All authors have read and agreed to the published version of the manuscript.

Funding: This work is thanks to financial support from the National Natural Science Foundation of China (51563020, 22101186), the Department of Education Project of Jiangxi Province (GJJ2202116), the Natural Science Foundation of Top Talent of SZTU (GDRC202114), the Foundation of Anhui Province for Distinguished Young Scholars (2022AH020038), and the Foundation of State Key Laboratory Incubation Base for Green Processing of Chemical Engineering (KF202201).

Institutional Review Board Statement: Not applicable.

Informed Consent Statement: Not applicable.

Data Availability Statement: Not applicable.

Conflicts of Interest: The authors declare no conflict of interest.

Sample Availability: Samples of the compounds are available from the authors.

References

1. Zhou, P.; Navid, I.A.; Ma, Y.; Xiao, Y.; Wang, P.; Ye, Z.; Zhou, B.; Sun, K.; Mi, Z. Solar-to-hydrogen efficiency of more than 9% in photocatalytic water splitting. *Nature* **2023**, *613*, 66–70. [CrossRef] [PubMed]
2. Nishiyama, H.; Yamada, T.; Nakabayashi, M.; Maehara, Y.; Yamaguchi, M.; Kuromiya, Y.; Nagatsuma, Y.; Tokudome, H.; Akiyama, S.; Watanabe, T.; et al. Photocatalytic solar hydrogen production from water on a 100-m² scale. *Nature* **2021**, *598*, 304–307. [CrossRef]
3. Meng, S.; Chen, C.; Gu, X.; Wu, H.; Meng, Q.; Zhang, J.; Chen, S.; Fu, X.; Liu, D.; Lei, W. Efficient photocatalytic H_2 evolution, CO_2 reduction and N_2 fixation coupled with organic synthesis by cocatalyst and vacancies engineering. *Appl. Catal. B* **2021**, *285*, 119789. [CrossRef]
4. Liu, J.; Liu, Y.; Liu, N.; Han, Y.; Zhang, X.; Huang, H.; Lifshitz, Y.; Lee, S.-T.; Zhong, J.; Kang, Z. Metal-free efficient photocatalyst for stable visible water splitting via a two-electron pathway. *Science* **2015**, *347*, 970–974. [CrossRef] [PubMed]
5. Wang, X.; Maeda, K.; Thomas, A.; Takanabe, K.; Xin, G.; Carlsson, J.M.; Domen, K.; Antonietti, M. A metal-free polymeric photocatalyst for hydrogen production from water under visible light. *Nat. Mater.* **2009**, *8*, 76–80. [CrossRef]
6. Liang, X.; Xue, S.; Yang, C.; Ye, X.; Wang, Y.; Chen, Q.; Lin, W.; Hou, Y.; Zhang, G.; Shalom, M.; et al. The Directional Crystallization Process of Poly (triazine imide) Single Crystals in Molten Salts. *Angew. Chem. Int. Ed.* **2023**, *62*, e202216434. [CrossRef]
7. Rahman, M.Z.; Mullins, C.B. Understanding Charge Transport in Carbon Nitride for Enhanced Photocatalytic Solar Fuel Production. *Acc. Chem. Res.* **2019**, *52*, 248–257. [CrossRef]
8. Ong, W.-J.; Tan, L.-L.; Ng, Y.H.; Yong, S.-T.; Chai, S.-P. Graphitic Carbon Nitride (g-C_3N_4)-Based Photocatalysts for Artificial Photosynthesis and Environmental Remediation: Are We a Step Closer to Achieving Sustainability? *Chem. Rev.* **2016**, *116*, 7159–7329. [CrossRef] [PubMed]

9. Lin, L.; Lin, Z.; Zhang, J.; Cai, X.; Lin, W.; Yu, Z.; Wang, X. Molecular-level insights on the reactive facet of carbon nitride single crystals photocatalysing overall water splitting. *Nat. Catal.* **2020**, *3*, 649–655. [CrossRef]
10. Wang, Q.; Li, Y.; Huang, F.; Song, S.; Ai, G.; Xin, X.; Zhao, B.; Zheng, Y.; Zhang, Z. Recent Advances in g-C_3N_4-Based Materials and Their Application in Energy and Environmental Sustainability. *Molecules* **2023**, *28*, 432. [CrossRef]
11. Aljuaid, A.; Almehmadi, M.; Alsaiari, A.A.; Allahyani, M.; Abdulaziz, O.; Alsharif, A.; Alsaiari, J.A.; Saih, M.; Alotaibi, R.T.; Khan, I. g-C_3N_4 Based Photocatalyst for the Efficient Photodegradation of Toxic Methyl Orange Dye: Recent Modifications and Future Perspectives. *Molecules* **2023**, *28*, 3199. [CrossRef]
12. Cao, D.; Wang, X.; Zhang, H.; Yang, D.; Yin, Z.; Liu, Z.; Lu, C.; Guo, F. Rational Design of Monolithic g-C_3N_4 with Floating Network Porous-like Sponge Monolithic Structure for Boosting Photocatalytic Degradation of Tetracycline under Simulated and Natural Sunlight Illumination. *Molecules* **2023**, *28*, 3989. [CrossRef] [PubMed]
13. Patnaik, S.; Sahoo, D.P.; Parida, K. Recent advances in anion doped g-C_3N_4 photocatalysts: A review. *Carbon* **2021**, *172*, 682–711. [CrossRef]
14. Kessler, F.K.; Zheng, Y.; Schwarz, D.; Merschjann, C.; Schnick, W.; Wang, X.; Bojdys, M.J. Functional carbon nitride materials-design strategies for electrochemical devices. *Nat. Rev. Mater.* **2017**, *2*, 17030. [CrossRef]
15. Xiao, X.; Gao, Y.; Zhang, L.; Zhang, J.; Zhang, Q.; Li, Q.; Bao, H.; Zhou, J.; Miao, S.; Chen, N.; et al. A Promoted Charge Separation/Transfer System from Cu Single Atoms and C_3N_4 Layers for Efficient Photocatalysis. *Adv. Mater.* **2020**, *32*, 2003082. [CrossRef]
16. Lin, J.; Tian, W.; Guan, Z.; Zhang, H.; Duan, X.; Wang, H.; Sun, H.; Fang, Y.; Huang, Y.; Wang, S. Functional Carbon Nitride Materials in Photo-Fenton-Like Catalysis for Environmental Remediation. *Adv. Funct. Mater.* **2022**, *32*, 2201743. [CrossRef]
17. Yang, P.; Ou, H.; Fang, Y.; Wang, X. A Facile Steam Reforming Strategy to Delaminate Layered Carbon Nitride Semiconductors for Photoredox Catalysis. *Angew. Chem. Int. Ed.* **2017**, *56*, 3992–3996. [CrossRef]
18. Yang, P.; Zhuzhang, H.; Wang, R.; Lin, W.; Wang, X. Carbon Vacancies in a Melon Polymeric Matrix Promote Photocatalytic Carbon Dioxide Conversion. *Angew. Chem. Int. Ed.* **2019**, *58*, 1134–1137. [CrossRef]
19. Niu, P.; Yin, L.-C.; Yang, Y.-Q.; Liu, G.; Cheng, H.-M. Increasing the Visible Light Absorption of Graphitic Carbon Nitride (Melon) Photocatalysts by Homogeneous Self-Modification with Nitrogen Vacancies. *Adv. Mater.* **2014**, *26*, 8046–8052. [CrossRef]
20. Talapaneni, S.N.; Singh, G.; Kim, I.Y.; Albahily, K.; Al-Muhtaseb, A.a.H.; Karakoti, A.S.; Tavakkoli, E.; Vinu, A. Nanostructured Carbon Nitrides for CO_2 Capture and Conversion. *Adv. Mater.* **2020**, *32*, 1904635. [CrossRef]
21. Tian, N.; Huang, H.; Du, X.; Dong, F.; Zhang, Y. Rational nanostructure design of graphitic carbon nitride for photocatalytic applications. *J. Mater. Chem. A* **2019**, *7*, 11584–11612. [CrossRef]
22. Chen, L.; Song, J. Tailored Graphitic Carbon Nitride Nanostructures: Synthesis, Modification, and Sensing Applications. *Adv. Funct. Mater.* **2017**, *27*, 1702695. [CrossRef]
23. Zheng, Y.; Lin, L.; Wang, X. Nanostructured Carbon Nitrides for Photocatalytic Water Splitting. In *Nanocarbons for Advanced Energy Conversion*, 1st ed.; Feng, X.L., Ed.; Wiley-VCH Verlag GmbH & Co. KGaA: Hoboken, NJ, USA, 2015; pp. 281–300.
24. Thomas, A.; Fischer, A.; Goettmann, F.; Antonietti, M.; Müller, J.-O.; Schlögl, R.; Carlsson, J.M. Graphitic carbon nitride materials: Variation of structure and morphology and their use as metal-free catalysts. *J. Mater. Chem.* **2008**, *18*, 4893–4908. [CrossRef]
25. Kröger, J.; Jiménez-Solano, A.; Savasci, G.; Lau, V.W.H.; Duppel, V.; Moudrakovski, I.; Küster, K.; Scholz, T.; Gouder, A.; Schreiber, M.-L.; et al. Morphology Control in 2D Carbon Nitrides: Impact of Particle Size on Optoelectronic Properties and Photocatalysis. *Adv. Funct. Mater.* **2021**, *31*, 2102468. [CrossRef]
26. Malik, R.; Tomer, V.K. State-of-the-art review of morphological advancements in graphitic carbon nitride (g-CN) for sustainable hydrogen production. *Renew. Sustain. Energy Rev.* **2021**, *135*, 110235. [CrossRef]
27. Long, B.; Zheng, Y.; Lin, L.; Alamry, K.A.; Asiri, A.M.; Wang, X. Cubic mesoporous carbon nitride polymers with large cage-type pores for visible light photocatalysis. *J. Mater. Chem. A* **2017**, *5*, 16179–16188. [CrossRef]
28. Zhang, J.; Liang, X.; Zhang, C.; Lin, L.; Xing, W.; Yu, Z.; Zhang, G.; Wang, X. Improved Charge Separation in Poly(heptazine-triazine) Imides with Semi-coherent Interfaces for Photocatalytic Hydrogen Evolution. *Angew. Chem. Int. Ed.* **2022**, *61*, e202210849.
29. Huang, D.; Yan, X.; Yan, M.; Zeng, G.; Zhou, C.; Wan, J.; Cheng, M.; Xue, W. Graphitic Carbon Nitride-Based Heterojunction Photoactive Nanocomposites: Applications and Mechanism Insight. *ACS Appl. Mater. Interfaces* **2018**, *10*, 21035–21055. [CrossRef]
30. Zhang, J.; Zhang, M.; Sun, R.-Q.; Wang, X. A Facile Band Alignment of Polymeric Carbon Nitride Semiconductors to Construct Isotype Heterojunctions. *Angew. Chem. Int. Ed.* **2012**, *51*, 10145–10149. [CrossRef]
31. Jiang, Z.; Wan, W.; Li, H.; Yuan, S.; Zhao, H.; Wong, P.K. A Hierarchical Z-Scheme α-Fe_2O_3/g-C_3N_4 Hybrid for Enhanced Photocatalytic CO_2 Reduction. *Adv. Mater.* **2018**, *30*, 1706108. [CrossRef]
32. Chen, S.; Wei, J.; Ren, X.; Song, K.; Sun, J.; Bai, F.; Tian, S. Recent Progress in Porphyrin/g-C_3N_4 Composite Photocatalysts for Solar Energy Utilization and Conversion. *Molecules* **2023**, *28*, 4283. [CrossRef]
33. Iqbal, W.; Yang, B.; Zhao, X.; Rauf, M.; Waqas, M.; Gong, Y.; Zhang, J.; Mao, Y. Controllable synthesis of graphitic carbon nitride nanomaterials for solar energy conversion and environmental remediation: The road travelled and the way forward. *Catal. Sci. Technol.* **2018**, *8*, 4576–4599. [CrossRef]
34. Martin, D.J.; Qiu, K.; Shevlin, S.A.; Handoko, A.D.; Chen, X.; Guo, Z.; Tang, J. Highly Efficient Photocatalytic H_2 Evolution from Water using Visible Light and Structure-Controlled Graphitic Carbon Nitride. *Angew. Chem. Int. Ed.* **2014**, *53*, 9240–9245. [CrossRef]

35. Zhang, Y.; Liu, J.; Wu, G.; Chen, W. Porous graphitic carbon nitride synthesized via direct polymerization of urea for efficient sunlight-driven photocatalytic hydrogen production. *Nanoscale* **2012**, *4*, 5300–5303. [CrossRef] [PubMed]
36. Zhang, J.; Sun, J.; Maeda, K.; Domen, K.; Liu, P.; Antonietti, M.; Fu, X.; Wang, X. Sulfur-mediated synthesis of carbon nitride: Band-gap engineering and improved functions for photocatalysis. *Energy Environ. Sci.* **2011**, *4*, 675–678. [CrossRef]
37. Zhang, G.; Zhang, J.; Zhang, M.; Wang, X. Polycondensation of thiourea into carbon nitride semiconductors as visible light photocatalysts. *J. Mater. Chem.* **2012**, *22*, 8083–8091. [CrossRef]
38. Long, B.; Lin, J.; Wang, X. Thermally-induced desulfurization and conversion of guanidine thiocyanate into graphitic carbon nitride catalysts for hydrogen photosynthesis. *J. Mater. Chem. A* **2014**, *2*, 2942–2951. [CrossRef]
39. Cui, Y.; Wang, Y.; Wang, H.; Cao, F.; Chen, F. Polycondensation of ammonium thiocyanate into novel porous g-C_3N_4 nanosheets as photocatalysts for enhanced hydrogen evolution under visible light irradiation. *Chin. J. Catal.* **2016**, *37*, 1899–1906. [CrossRef]
40. Madhurima, V.P.; Kumari, K.; Jain, P.K. A facile single-step approach to achieve in situ expanded g-C_3N_4 for improved photodegradation performance. *Polym. Adv. Technol.* **2023**, *34*, 578–586. [CrossRef]
41. Kamal Hussien, M.; Sabbah, A.; Qorbani, M.; Hammad Elsayed, M.; Raghunath, P.; Lin, T.-Y.; Quadir, S.; Wang, H.-Y.; Wu, H.-L.; Tzou, D.-L.M.; et al. Metal-free four-in-one modification of g-C_3N_4 for superior photocatalytic CO_2 reduction and H_2 evolution. *Chem. Eng. J.* **2022**, *430*, 132853. [CrossRef]
42. Khedr, T.M.; El-Sheikh, S.M.; Endo-Kimura, M.; Wang, K.; Ohtani, B.; Kowalska, E. Development of Sulfur-Doped Graphitic Carbon Nitride for Hydrogen Evolution under Visible-Light Irradiation. *Nanomaterials* **2023**, *13*, 62. [CrossRef]
43. Yu, S.; Li, C.; Wu, H.; Wang, Y.; Wang, L.; Dong, H.; Han, Z. Ultrathin Mesoporous Carbon Nitride Nanosheets Prepared Through a One-Pot Approach towards Enhanced Photocatalytic Activity. *Energy Technol.* **2020**, *8*, 2000719. [CrossRef]
44. Wang, C.; Zhang, G.; Zhang, H.; Li, Z.; Wen, Y. One-pot synthesis of porous g-C_3N_4 nanosheets with enhanced photocatalytic activity under visible light. *Diam. Relat. Mater.* **2021**, *116*, 108416. [CrossRef]
45. He, F.; Chen, G.; Yu, Y.; Zhou, Y.; Zheng, Y.; Hao, S. The sulfur-bubble template-mediated synthesis of uniform porous g-C_3N_4 with superior photocatalytic performance. *Chem. Commun.* **2015**, *51*, 425–427. [CrossRef]
46. Zhang, J.; Zhang, M.; Zhang, G.; Wang, X. Synthesis of Carbon Nitride Semiconductors in Sulfur Flux for Water Photoredox Catalysis. *ACS Catal.* **2012**, *2*, 940–948. [CrossRef]
47. Zhang, D.; Guo, Y.; Zhao, Z. Porous defect-modified graphitic carbon nitride via a facile one-step approach with significantly enhanced photocatalytic hydrogen evolution under visible light irradiation. *Appl. Catal. B* **2018**, *226*, 1–9. [CrossRef]
48. Wu, X.; Ma, H.; Zhong, W.; Fan, J.; Yu, H. Porous crystalline g-C_3N_4: Bifunctional $NaHCO_3$ template-mediated synthesis and improved photocatalytic H_2-evolution rate. *Appl. Catal. B* **2020**, *271*, 118899. [CrossRef]
49. Jiang, Y.; Sun, Z.; Tang, C.; Zhou, Y.; Zeng, L.; Huang, L. Enhancement of photocatalytic hydrogen evolution activity of porous oxygen doped g-C_3N_4 with nitrogen defects induced by changing electron transition. *Appl. Catal. B* **2019**, *240*, 30–38. [CrossRef]
50. Huang, W.; Johnston-Peck, A.C.; Wolter, T.; Yang, W.-C.D.; Xu, L.; Oh, J.; Reeves, B.A.; Zhou, C.; Holtz, M.E.; Herzing, A.A.; et al. Steam-created grain boundaries for methane C-H activation in palladium catalysts. *Science* **2021**, *373*, 1518–1523. [CrossRef]
51. Long, B.; Yan, G.; He, H.; Meng, S. Porous and Few-Layer Carbon Nitride Nanosheets via Surface Steam Etching for Enhanced Photodegradation Activity. *ACS Appl. Nano Mater.* **2022**, *5*, 7798–7810. [CrossRef]
52. Gao, S.; Wang, X.; Song, C.; Zhou, S.; Yang, F.; Kong, Y. Engineering carbon-defects on ultrathin g-C_3N_4 allows one-pot output and dramatically boosts photoredox catalytic activity. *Appl. Catal. B* **2021**, *295*, 120272. [CrossRef]
53. Tay, Q.; Kanhere, P.; Ng, C.F.; Chen, S.; Chakraborty, S.; Huan, A.C.H.; Sum, T.C.; Ahuja, R.; Chen, Z. Defect Engineered g-C_3N_4 for Efficient Visible Light Photocatalytic Hydrogen Production. *Chem. Mater.* **2015**, *27*, 4930–4933. [CrossRef]
54. Wang, X.; Meng, J.; Zhang, X.; Liu, Y.; Ren, M.; Yang, Y.; Guo, Y. Controllable Approach to Carbon-Deficient and Oxygen-Doped Graphitic Carbon Nitride: Robust Photocatalyst Against Recalcitrant Organic Pollutants and the Mechanism Insight. *Adv. Funct. Mater.* **2021**, *31*, 2010763. [CrossRef]
55. Wang, X.; Xia, Y.; Wang, H.; Jiao, X.; Chen, D. Etching-induced highly porous polymeric carbon nitride with enhanced photocatalytic hydrogen evolution. *Chem. Commun.* **2021**, *57*, 4138–4141. [CrossRef]
56. Guo, Y.; Li, J.; Yuan, Y.; Li, L.; Zhang, M.; Zhou, C.; Lin, Z. A Rapid Microwave-Assisted Thermolysis Route to Highly Crystalline Carbon Nitrides for Efficient Hydrogen Generation. *Angew. Chem. Int. Ed.* **2016**, *55*, 14693–14697. [CrossRef]
57. Shi, L.; Yang, L.; Zhou, W.; Liu, Y.; Yin, L.; Hai, X.; Song, H.; Ye, J. Photoassisted Construction of Holey Defective g-C_3N_4 Photocatalysts for Efficient Visible-Light-Driven H_2O_2 Production. *Small* **2018**, *14*, 1703142. [CrossRef] [PubMed]
58. Li, F.; Yue, X.; Zhang, D.; Fan, J.; Xiang, Q. Targeted regulation of exciton dissociation in graphitic carbon nitride by vacancy modification for efficient photocatalytic CO_2 reduction. *Appl. Catal. B* **2021**, *292*, 120179. [CrossRef]
59. Zhang, G.; Li, G.; Lan, Z.-A.; Lin, L.; Savateev, A.; Heil, T.; Zafeiratos, S.; Wang, X.; Antonietti, M. Optimizing Optical Absorption, Exciton Dissociation, and Charge Transfer of a Polymeric Carbon Nitride with Ultrahigh Solar Hydrogen Production Activity. *Angew. Chem. Int. Ed.* **2017**, *56*, 13445–13449. [CrossRef]

Disclaimer/Publisher's Note: The statements, opinions and data contained in all publications are solely those of the individual author(s) and contributor(s) and not of MDPI and/or the editor(s). MDPI and/or the editor(s) disclaim responsibility for any injury to people or property resulting from any ideas, methods, instructions or products referred to in the content.

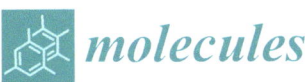

Article

CdS Deposited In Situ on g-C$_3$N$_4$ via a Modified Chemical Bath Deposition Method to Improve Photocatalytic Hydrogen Production

Ligang Ma [1], Wenjun Jiang [1], Chao Lin [1], Le Xu [2], Tianyu Zhu [1] and Xiaoqian Ai [2,*]

[1] School of Electronic Engineering, Nanjing Xiaozhuang University, Nanjing 211171, China; lgma@njxzc.edu.cn (L.M.)

[2] School of Physics and Information Engineering, Jiangsu Province Engineering Research Center of Basic Education Big Data Application, Jiangsu Second Normal University, Nanjing 210013, China

* Correspondence: aixiaoqian186@jssnu.edu.cn

Abstract: Ultra-thin two-dimensional materials are attracting widespread interest due to their excellent properties, and they are becoming ideal candidates for a variety of energy and environmental photocatalytic applications. Herein, CdS nanorods are successfully grown in situ between a monolayer of g-C$_3$N$_4$ using a chemical water bath method. Continuous ultrasound is introduced during the preparation process, which effectively prevents the accumulation of a g-C$_3$N$_4$ layer. The g-C$_3$N$_4$@CdS nanocomposite exhibits significantly enhanced photocatalytic activity for hydrogen production under visible-light irradiation, which is attributed to a well-matched band structure and an intimate van der Waals heterojunction interface. The mechanism of photocatalytic hydrogen production is discussed in detail. Moreover, our work can serve as a basis for the construction of other highly catalytically active two-dimensional heterostructures.

Keywords: monolayer g-C$_3$N$_4$; CdS; heterojunction; photocatalytic hydrogen production

Citation: Ma, L.; Jiang, W.; Lin, C.; Xu, L.; Zhu, T.; Ai, X. CdS Deposited In Situ on g-C$_3$N$_4$ via a Modified Chemical Bath Deposition Method to Improve Photocatalytic Hydrogen Production. *Molecules* **2023**, *28*, 7846. https://doi.org/10.3390/molecules28237846

Academic Editor: Sugang Meng

Received: 10 November 2023
Revised: 26 November 2023
Accepted: 28 November 2023
Published: 29 November 2023

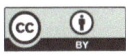

Copyright: © 2023 by the authors. Licensee MDPI, Basel, Switzerland. This article is an open access article distributed under the terms and conditions of the Creative Commons Attribution (CC BY) license (https://creativecommons.org/licenses/by/4.0/).

1. Introduction

With the rapid development of global industry, various problems, for example, climate warming, energy crisis, and environmental pollution, come along [1]. Using catalysts to harness inexhaustible solar energy is a green, sustainable, and promising method [2–5]. Under the irradiation of sunlight, a photocatalyst is excited to produce electron–hole pairs, and the electrons and holes undergo the reduction reaction and oxidation reaction, respectively, which can decompose organic pollutants into hydrocarbons [6–8], split water to produce hydrogen and oxygen [9], and reduce CO$_2$ to fuels such as CO and CH$_4$ [10]. In addition, excited electrons reduce nitrogen gas to ammonia, which is an important chemical feedstock and is widely used in agricultural waste [11]. In the photocatalytic reaction, the most critical choice is the photocatalyst, which determines the concentration of the electron–hole pairs produced under light irradiation.

In recent years, many semiconductor materials and nanocomposites have been developed in the field of photocatalysis, for example, CdS [12], ZnIn$_2$S$_4$ [13], PdS [14], and TiO$_2$ [15], among others [16]. Among the many semiconductors, graphite-like carbon nitride (g-C$_3$N$_4$) has become a research hotspot because of its suitable band structure and unique electric, optical, structural, and photochemical properties [17–20]. It is a non-metallic inorganic n-type semiconductor polymer composed of C and N elements, in which both C and N atoms are hybridized in the form of sp^2 and are connected to form a ring by the σ covalent bond, and, between the rings, they are connected by amino groups to form a π electron conjugated structure. Therefore, these unique structures of g-C$_3$N$_4$ can be applied to many fields. In 2009, Wang and his colleagues [21] first discovered that g-C$_3$N$_4$ produces hydrogen and oxygen under light irradiation, and this application for hydrogen evolution has attracted wide attention. Since then, a wide variety of g-C_3N_4-based photocatalysts have been designed to drive various reduction and oxidation reactions under light irradiation [17,22–25]. Here, the CdS materials have a suitable bandgap width of 2.4 eV and a good visible-light response, but there is serious photo-corrosion, which leads to a severe recombination of photogenerated carriers [6]. If CdS and g-C_3N_4 combine to form a heterojunction, there will inevitably be a photocatalytic performance of 1 plus 1 is greater than 2. Therefore, nanocomposites of g-C_3N_4 and CdS have been widely reported and studied [22,26,27]. The combination of excellent single-layer g-C_3N_4 and CdS will form a fast electron transport channel, and the separation efficiency of photogenerated electrons and holes can be greatly improved, thus showing an excellent rate of photohydrogen production. Jianjun Liu [28] systematically calculated the energy band structure and charge transfer of the heterojunction between g-C_3N_4 and CdS using the hybrid density functional approach. They suggested that the contact between CdS and monolayer g-C_3N_4 forms a van der Waals heterojunction, which will have an internal electric field that facilitates the separation of the electron–hole pair at the interface. Researchers [18,29] obtained a monolayer of g-C_3N_4 using ultrasound, and then they grew CdS using solvothermal, hydrothermal, and other methods. Although monolayer g-C_3N_4 obtained via ultrasound is easy to agglomerate to form bulk g-C_3N_4 in the process of the hydrothermal growth of other semiconductors, thus improving photocatalytic performance, there are still some limitations.

In this paper, CdS were grown in situ on monolayer g-C_3N_4, which is equivalent to a substrate. In order to better obtain monolayer g-C_3N_4, ultrasound was consistently maintained during the chemical bath deposited method, which is a method that has simple equipment and a low cost and allows for easy large-area preparation. Consequently, intimate contact interfaces between g-C_3N_4 and CdS were also obtained, which could accelerate the separation of photogenerated carriers. The experimental results show that the photocatalytic performance of the composites improved. The crystal structure, microstructure, and morphology of the composite were analyzed in detail. Moreover, photocatalytic mechanisms were also proposed, and they were demonstrated using characterization methods.

2. Results and Discussion

The crystal structures of the CdS, g-C_3N_4, and G-CdS nanocomposites were characterized using an X-ray diffractometer (XRD), as shown in Figure 1a. For pure g-C_3N_4, two diffraction peaks were found at 12.9° and 27.6°, which can be indexed as (100) and (002) diffraction planes for graphitic materials (JCPDS 87-1526) [21]. The (100) diffraction peaks and (002) diffraction peaks are associated with the in-plane repeated units and periodic graphitic stacking of the conjugated aromatic system [30,31], respectively, which indicates the existence of graphite-like layer structures. The obtained composite photocatalyst exhibited gradually appearing diffraction peaks at 25.1, 26.6, 44.1, and 52.1°, while the intensity of the diffraction peaks related to g-C_3N_4 gradually weakened with increasing concentrations of Cd and S. A comparison with the standard PDF card (65-3414) showed that these diffraction peaks are (100), (002), (110), and (112) of the CdS hexagonal wurtzite structure, respectively. The results of XRD indicate that the CdS of the hexagonal wurtzite structure was grown in situ on the g-C_3N_4 nanosheets through the CBD process, and the concentration of CdS gradually increased with the increase in Cd and S sources. The characteristic functional groups of the photocatalysts were analyzed using Fourier Transform Infrared (FTIR) spectroscopy. For g-C_3N_4, the spectrum reveals several notable features. The prominent absorption peak at 807 cm^{-1} can be attributed to the stretching vibration of heptazine ring units [32], as depicted in Figure 1b. Additionally, the broad band observed in the range of 1100–1700 cm^{-1} corresponds to the stretching vibration mode of the aromatic C-N heterocyclic skeleton, which is characteristic of the typical structure of g-C_3N_4. The spectrum for g-C_3N_4 also shows peaks in the range of 3000–3400 cm^{-1}, indicating the N-H bond stretching vibration of -NH_x [33], while the weak peak observed at 3437 cm^{-1} was attributed to the O-H stretching vibration, likely due to the presence of hydroxyl groups or the physical adsorption of H_2O molecules [34]. As for CdS, the spectrum exhibits distinct peaks at 3437 cm^{-1} and 1622 cm^{-1}, corresponding to the surface-adsorbed water molecules [35]. Additionally, the peaks at 1333 cm^{-1} and 1167 cm^{-1} are associated with the stretching vibration peak of Cd-S bonds. The peaks at 2924 cm^{-1} are attributable to the bending vibration of -CH$_2$ and -CH$_3$ groups [36,37]. Furthermore, in the G-CdS nanocomposites, both partial CdS vibration peaks and partial g-C$_3$N$_4$ vibration peaks were observed, indicating the successful combination of the two materials without impurities.

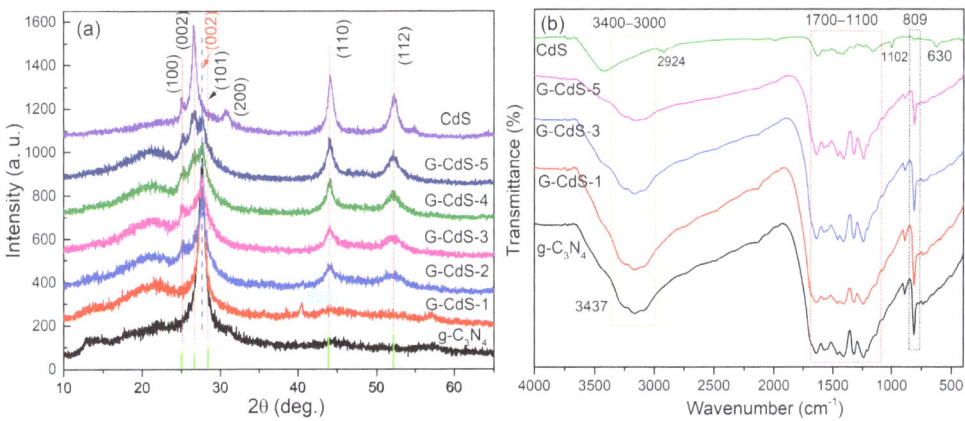

Figure 1. (**a**) XRD patterns and (**b**) FTIR patterns of CdS, g-C$_3$N$_4$, and G-CdS nanocomposites.

The microstructures and morphologies of the samples were characterized and analyzed using transmission electron microscopy (TEM), as shown in Figure 2. Both the amorphous and crystalline g-C$_3$N$_4$ exhibited an exceptionally thin nanosheet morphology. In contrast, the TEM morphology of pure CdS showed significant agglomeration (Figure 2b). Moreover, in the high-resolution TEM (HRTEM) images of the edge nanoparticles, lattice fringes with spacings of 0.351, 0.337, 0.2065, and 0.292 nm could be observed. The lattice fringes at 0.351 nm, 0.337 nm, and 0.2065 nm correspond to the hexagonal wurtzite structure of CdS, while the lattice fringe at 0.292 nm corresponds to the cubic structure of CdS. This indicates that CdS, in the absence of g-C$_3$N$_4$, consists of both hexagonal and cubic structures, which is consistent with the XRD results. For the G-CdS nanocomposites, many amorphous quantum dots with sizes around 8 nm emerged on the g-C$_3$N$_4$ nanosheet structures. This observation is consistent with the amorphous CdS results obtained from the XRD pattern. As the concentration of Cd and S further increased, nanorod-shaped nanowire structures with a length of approximately 50 nm and a width of around 4 nm emerged on the g-C$_3$N$_4$ nanosheet layer. Further confirmation through HRTEM revealed that these needle-shaped nanowire structures were composed of CdS material with a hexagonal wurtzite structure (the lattice fringes are marked in red in Figure 2). A clear and tight contact interface between g-C$_3$N$_4$ and CdS was achieved, which implies an intimate heterojunction between the two components, as indicated by the green dashed box in Figure 2g. Compared with Figure 2a, it can be seen that the thickness of the g-CN nanosheets is significantly thinner. This facilitated the effective transfer of charge carriers between the two semiconductors. This indicates that the CdS nanowire structures were grown in situ on g-C$_3$N$_4$ rather than being a mere physical mixture of the two materials. The high-resolution lattice stripe on the CdS nanorods was 0.333 nm, which means that the nanorods were preferentially grown in the (002) direction. For the G-CdS-5 nanocomposites, the nanorod-shaped CdS nanowire structures further grew in both length and width (Figure 2h). Therefore, according to the TEM morphology, it could be concluded that the concentrations of Cd and S sources influence the morphological evolution of CdS.

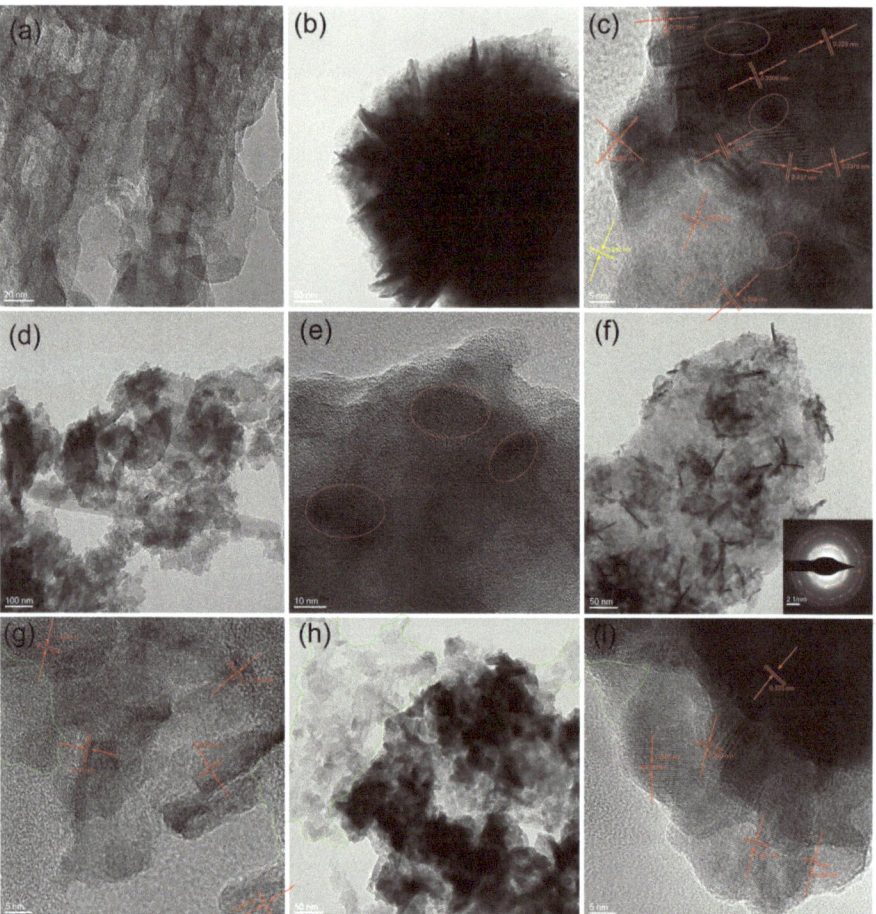

Figure 2. TEM images of (**a**) g-C$_3$N$_4$ without ultrasound, (**b**) CdS, (**d**) G-CdS-1, (**f**) G-CdS-3, and (**h**) G-CdS-5. HRTEM images (**c**) CdS, (**e**) G-CdS-1, (**g**) G-CdS-3, and (**i**) G-CdS-5. The red circled areas and green circled areas correspond to CdS and g-C$_3$N$_4$.

Moreover, elemental mapping techniques were utilized to investigate the elemental compositions of the G-CdS-3 nanocomposites. As depicted in Figure 3, it was observed that the G-CdS nanocomposites contained C, N, Cd, and S elements with no other impurities detected, which further confirms the successful synthesis of the composite samples. The results also show a uniform spatial distribution of C, N, Cd, and S elements, indicating the homogeneous distribution of the CdS nanowire structures on the surface of g-C$_3$N$_4$ or between the layers of g-C$_3$N$_4$.

The element compositions and chemical states in the samples were further investigated through X-ray photoelectron spectra (XPS). As shown in Figure 4a, in comparison to the CdS and g-C$_3$N$_4$ samples, the G-CdS nanocomposites contained Cd, S, C, N, and O elements, and the presence of a slight amount of O element may be attributed to the absorbed oxygen (such as H$_2$O and CO$_2$) on the surface of the sample, in good agreement with the elemental mapping results. All the high-resolution spectra were calibrated by setting the binding energy of the C-C peak to 284.8 eV. Figure 4b shows the C1s spectrum, which was fitted using Gaussian functions to analyze the types and quantities of functional groups present in the sample. In g-C$_3$N$_4$, the C1s core-level spectra consisted of four peaks located at 284.8, 286.3, 288.2, and 293.6 eV, which could be attributed to C=C, N≡C- groups [38],

N-C=N in typical s-triazine rings [39], and the carbon attached to uncondensed -NH$_2$ groups [40], respectively. The strength of the N-C=N bond gradually weakened, which was attributed to the increasing concentration of CdS. At the same time, the position of the bond energy also shifted, indicating that the coupling between g-C$_3$N$_4$ and CdS became stronger. Figure 4e shows that the N 1s spectrum has three peaks at 398.6 and 400.8 eV, which were attributed to the bi-coordinated N (C=N-C) and N-H bonds, respectively. These peaks also gradually weakened and shifted. With the increase in the CdS concentration, two distinct peaks with binding energies of 404.9 and 411.7 eV appeared, corresponding to the Cd 3d$_{5/2}$ and Cd 3d$_{3/2}$ states, respectively, of the Cd atoms in the Cd-S bonds [6,41,42]. At the same time, the S 2p peak gradually emerged, which could be deconvoluted into two doublets using Gaussian fitting, as displayed in Figure 4e. These two peaks were located at 161.3 (S 2p$_{3/2}$) and 162.3 (S 2p$_{1/2}$), which are characteristic of S species from CdS. It could clearly be seen that the two peaks moved towards a higher binding energy with the increase in the CdS concentration, which means that the crystallization quality and the coupling of the heterojunction further improved. These pieces of evidence, combined with the results of XRD, the FTIR spectra, and TEM, prove that there was a significant heterojunction between CdS and g-C$_3$N$_4$ in the G-CdS nanocomposites. This indicates that the G-CdS nanocomposite will exhibit excellent performance in terms of charge carrier transport. To determine the band structure, the valence band (VB) spectrum of XPS was measured to obtain the balance band potential ($E_{vb, XPS}$) using VB-XPS plots, as shown in Figure 4f. The intersection of the epitaxial linear part with the x-axis provides the $E_{VB, XPS}$ of CdS, and g-C$_3$N$_4$ with values of 0.4 and 1.23 eV, respectively. Then, the E_{VB} of the corresponding standard hydrogen electrode ($E_{VB, NHE}$) could be calculated as follows [43]: $E_{VB, NHE} = \phi + E_{VB, XPS} - 4.44$, where ϕ is the work function of the instrument (4.258 eV). Therefore, the $E_{VB, NHE}$ of CdS and g-C$_3$N$_4$ were calculated as 1.05 and 0.22 eV, respectively.

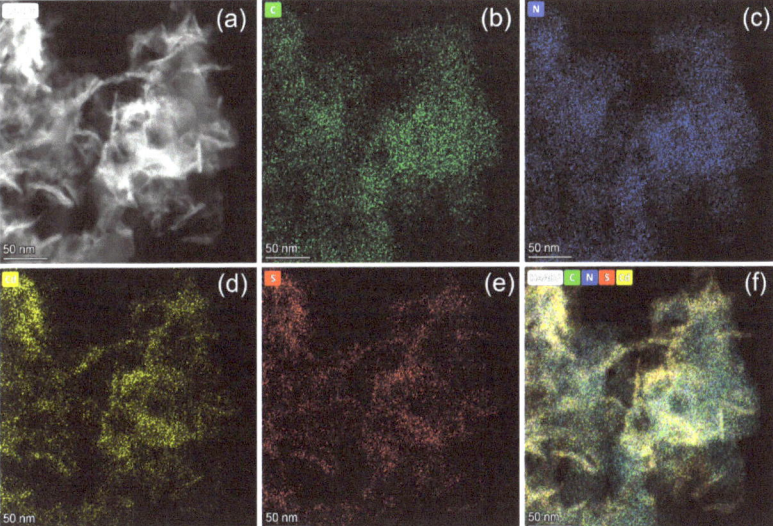

Figure 3. Element mapping of G-CdS-3 nanocomposites: (**a**) high-angle annular dark-field image, (**b**) C element, (**c**) N element, (**d**) Cd element, (**e**) S element, and (**f**) overlay diagram of element mapping.

The optical bandgap of a material determines the range of solar light absorption. Therefore, the optical properties were investigated using UV-vis diffuse reflectance spectra (Figure 5a). g-C$_3$N$_4$ and CdS exhibited sharp absorption band edges at 456 nm and 560 nm, respectively. Compared to g-C$_3$N$_4$, G-CdS exhibited a slight red shift in its diffuse reflectance spectrum, and the samples appeared darker in color, suggesting the formation of a composite structure of g-C$_3$N$_4$ and CdS in G-CdS. The redshift observed in the absorption spectra indicates a modification in the electronic band structure of g-C$_3$N$_4$, resulting from the formation of cyano group defects [38]. Consequently, the absorption edges of the G-CdS samples extend into the visible light region, enhancing the light absorption capability. According to the Tauc formula, the optical bandgap of the samples was calculated. The Tauc formula is as follows [6]: $\alpha h v = A(h v - E_g)^n$, where E_g, α, h, v, A, and n represent the optical bandgap, absorption coefficient, Planck's constant, incident light frequency, a constant, and n = 1/2 for CdS, respectively. The fitting results, as shown in Figure 5b, indicate that the intersection between the linear extrapolation and the x-axis represents the optical bandgap. The optical bandgaps of g-C$_3$N$_4$, G-CdS-1, G-CdS-2, G-CdS-3, G-CdS-4, G-CdS-5, and CdS were 2.86, 2.8, 2.49, 2.45, 2.4, 2.36, and 2.29 eV, respectively.

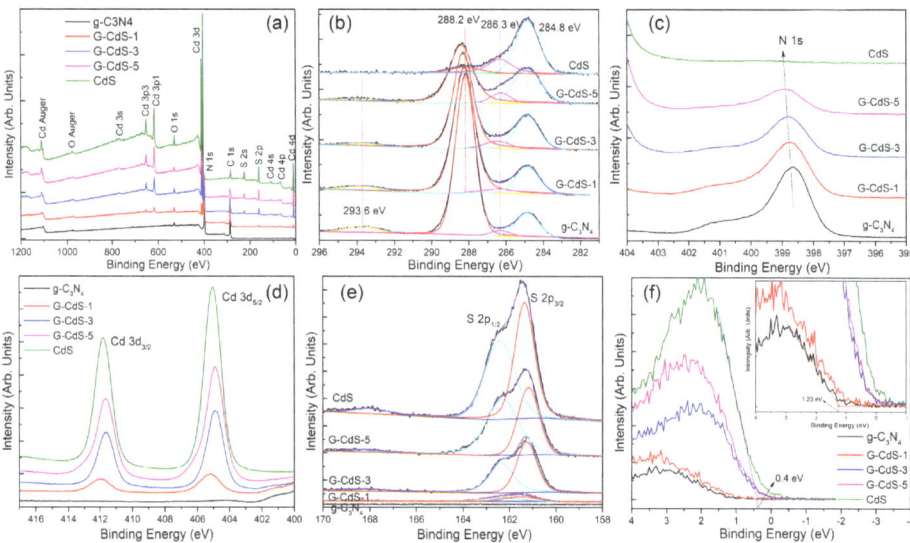

Figure 4. XPS spectra of g-C$_3$N$_4$, CdS, and G-CdS nanocomposites: (**a**) survey spectrum, (**b**) C 1s, (**c**) N 1s, (**d**) Cd 3d, (**e**) S 2p, and (**f**) valence-band spectra. (**b**,**e**) are the results of Gaussian fitting.

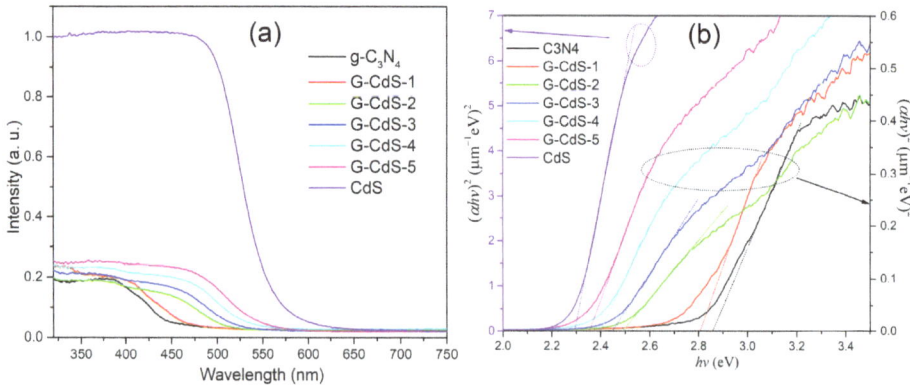

Figure 5. (**a**) UV-vis diffuse reflection spectra, and (**b**) the corresponding Tauc plots of $(\alpha h v)^2$ versus $h v$ for the g-C$_3$N$_4$, CdS, and G-CdS nanocomposites.

Figure 6 shows the photocatalytic hydrogen generation rate of the g-C_3N_4, CdS, and G-CdS nanocomposites. It can be seen from the figure that the hydrogen production of all the samples was linear with respect to the time of light irradiation. The g-C_3N_4 sample exhibited the lowest hydrogen production performance (20.98 µmol·g^{-1}·h^{-1}). Moreover, the hydrogen production performance gradually increased with the increase in CdS loading, and the hydrogen production performance of G-CdS-3 reached the maximum (1611.4 µmol·g^{-1}·h^{-1}), while the performance gradually decayed with the further increase in CdS loading. The hydrogen production of the G-CdS-3 was 76 times higher than that of g-C_3N_4 and 10 times higher than that of CdS. It is well known that the photogenerated electrons and holes produced by CdS under light irradiation are inherently strong recombination phenomena. Therefore, when CdS was grown in situ in the interlayer of g-C_3N_4, the aggregation of g-C_3N_4 decreased, and the specific surface area could be increased at an appropriate concentration, exposing more active sites, effectively increasing the photogenerated carrier separation rate and improving the photocatalytic performance of the nanocomposite. The photocatalytic hydrogen production properties of related g-C_3N_4@CdS nanocomposites were investigated, and a comparison of these properties is shown in Table 1. As shown in Table 1, the G-CdS nanocatalysts in this paper demonstrated excellent performance. Furthermore, by measuring the XRD patterns of the G-CdS-3 nanocomposites after the hydrogen production experiment, it was found that the diffraction patterns were basically unchanged compared with those of the fresh sample, as shown in Figure 7.

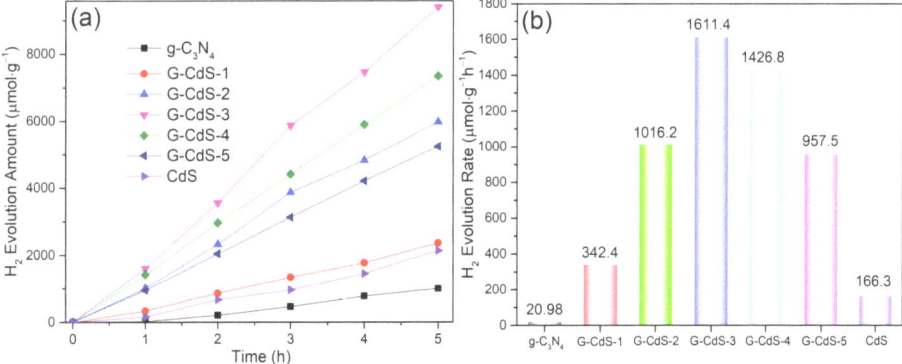

Figure 6. (**a**,**b**) Visible-light photocatalytic H_2 production rate of g-C_3N_4, CdS, and G-CdS nanocomposites.

Table 1. Comparison of H_2 evolution performance between G-CdS-3 and other reported photocatalysts.

Catalyst	Synthesis Method	Dosage (mg)	Type of Light Source	Sacrificial Reagent	H_2 Evolution Rate (µmol·g^{-1}·h^{-1})	Refs.
Pd-CdS/g-C_3N_4	hydrothermal method and borohydride reduction method	50	300 W Xe arc Lamp (λ > 400 nm)	0.5 M Na_2S and 0.5 M Na_2SO_3	293.0	[44]
CdS/g-C_3N_4	photodeposited method	10	300 W Xe arc Lamp (λ > 420 nm)	0.5 M Na_2S and 0.5 M Na_2SO_3	56.9	[45]
CdS/Au/g-C3N4	photodeposited method	100	Xenon Lamp (λ > 420 nm)	10 mL methanol	19.02	[46]
CdS/g-C3N4	hydrothermal synthesis	10	300 W Xe arc Lamp (λ > 400 nm)	20 mL triethanolamine	216.48	[47]
G-CdS	modified CBD method	50	300 W Xe arc Lamp (λ > 420 nm)	20% lactic acid aqueous solution	1611.4 µmol·g^{-1}·h^{-1}	This work

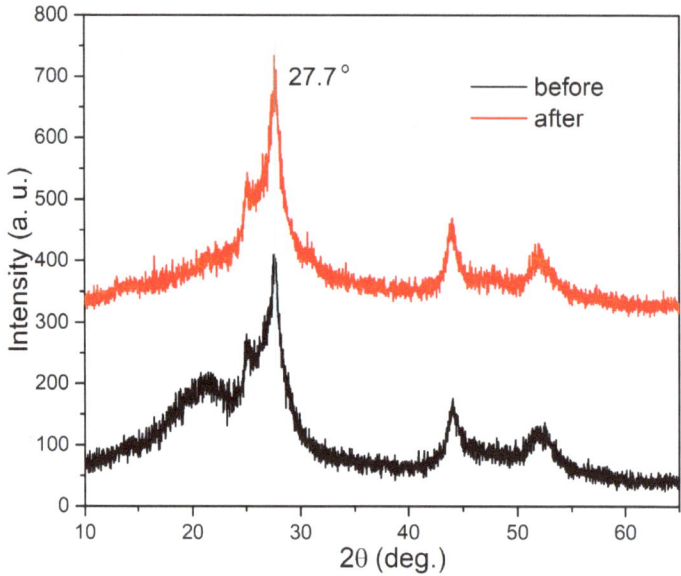

Figure 7. XRD patterns of G-CdS-3 before and after hydrogen production experiments.

By adding a certain amount of cadmium acetate and ammonia water into the ultrasonic g-C_3N_4 nanosheet aqueous solution, a cadmium complex, $[Cd(NH_3)_4]^{2+}$, was formed in the alkaline environment. Under the action of ultrasound, the $[Cd(NH_3)_4]^{2+}$ was uniformly attached to the g-C_3N_4 nanosheet. With the addition of thiourea, S^{2-} formed in the alkaline solution, where ammonium acetate acted as a buffer to control the release rate of S. In this way, Cd and S heteronucleated in the layer of g-C_3N_4 to form CdS. When the accumulation of Cd and S ions exceeded the solubility of CdS, CdS nanoparticles were deposited on g-C_3N_4. In the XRD pattern (Figure 1), the (002) diffraction peak of g-C_3N_4 could be significantly shifted to the lower diffraction angle, which means that the layer spacing of g-C_3N_4 becomes larger. With the progress of the reaction, CdS grew along the (002) crystal planes, and CdS nanorods were formed. The chemical equation of the reaction is as follows:

$$Cd + NH_3 \rightarrow [Cd(NH_3)_4]^{2+}$$

$$SC(NH_2)_2 + 3OH^- \rightarrow 2NH_3 + CO_3^{2-} + HS^-$$

$$HS^- + OH^- \rightarrow S^{2-} + H_2O$$

$$Cd^{2+} + S^{2-} \rightarrow CdS$$

Based on the results of XPS and the UV-vis absorption spectrum analysis, the band structures of the G-CdS nanocomposites are illustrated in Scheme 1. It can be seen that a Type II heterojunction formed between CdS and g-C_3N_4, which is consistent with the band structure calculated theoretically in the literature [28]. Under light irradiation, electron hole pairs were generated, and the well-matched Type II g-C_3N_4/CdS heterojunction could realize the positive synergistic effect of accelerating carrier separation and inhibiting CdS corrosion. In addition, during the preparation process, accompanied by ultrasound, g-C_3N_4 presented a monolayer or several layer structures, which had a van der Waals heterojunction with CdS. Therefore, the presence of an internal electric field in the heterojunction further promoted the separation of electron–hole pairs at the g-C_3N_4/CdS interface [28].

The separation of charge carriers in the G-CdS heterojunctions was also confirmed by photoluminescence and a photochemical test.

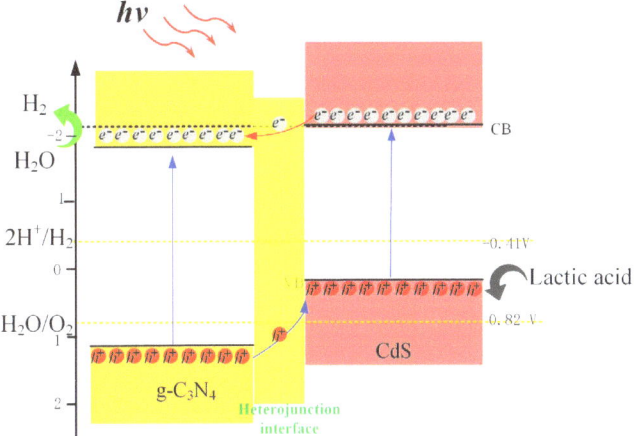

Scheme 1. Diagram of the band edge positions G-CdS nanocomposites.

In order to further investigate the luminescent properties of the composite related to the recombination of photogenerated charge carriers under light irradiation, the photoluminescence spectra were measured with an excitation wavelength of 370 nm, as shown in Figure 8. It can be observed in the figure that g-C_3N_4 and CdS exhibited strong photoluminescence peaks, while the intensity of the photoluminescence peak in the G-CdS-3 nanocomposites was the weakest. This suggests that the G-CdS-3 sample has a lower probability of photogenerated carrier recombination under light irradiation, indicating higher photocatalytic efficiency.

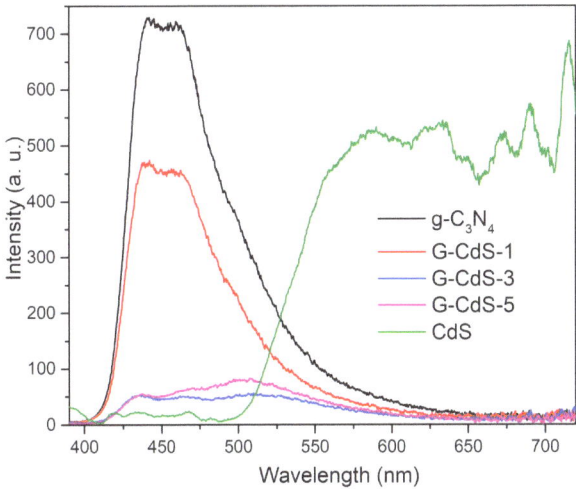

Figure 8. Photoluminescence emission spectra of CdS, g-C_3N_4, and G-CdS.

In addition, the interfacial charge transfer and separation capabilities of the g-C_3N_4, CdS, and G-CdS nanocomposites were also investigated in photoelectric chemistry experiments. As shown in Figure 9, the photoelectric response of the G-CdS nanocomposites was higher than that of g-C_3N_4 and CdS. Moreover, G-CdS-3 exhibited the best photocurrent density, which had high hydrogen production performance. Furthermore, electrochemical impedance spectroscopy (EIS) was employed to delineate the carrier transport and separation processes, as illustrated in Figure 10. Within EIS spectroscopy, the arc radius serves as a gauge for electron transfer capacity and efficiency in separating photogenerated carriers, and it expedites interfacial charge transfer [48]. Our experimental findings reveal the G-CdS-3 sample exhibits the smallest arc radius, underscoring its superior charge transfer and photogenerated electron–hole pair separation capabilities. This underscores an accelerated interface charge transfer rate within the sample.

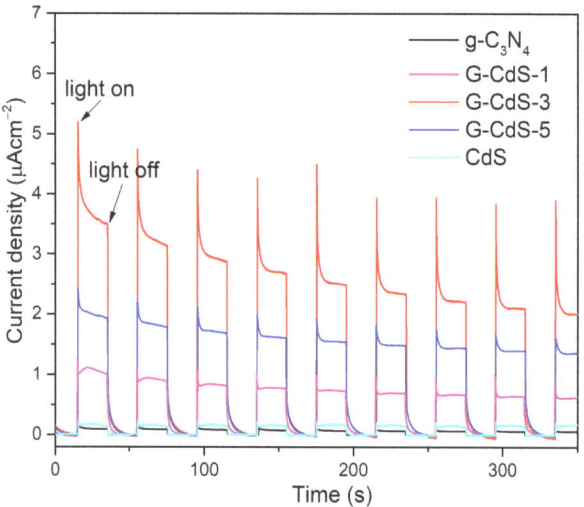

Figure 9. Photocurrent response curves of g-C_3N_4, CdS, and G-CdS nanocomposites.

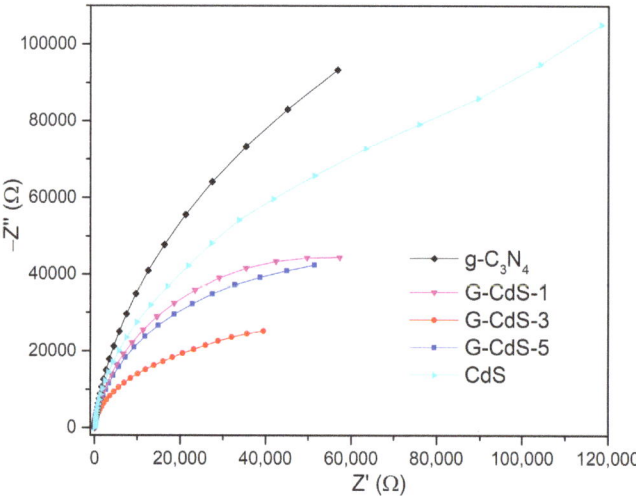

Figure 10. ESI Nyquist plots of g-CN, G-CdS, and CdS.

3. Experimental Section

3.1. Materials

Melamine (99%), cadmium acetate dihydrate ($Cd(CH_3COO)·H_2O$, 99.99%), ammonium acetate (CH_3COONH_4, 99%), ammonia solution ($NH_3·H_2O$, AR, 25–28%), and Thiourea (CH_4N_2S, 99%) were purchased from Aladdin Reagent Co., Ltd. (Shanghai,

China), and they were used directly without further purification. Deionized water with 18 MΩ cm was used in our experiment.

3.2. Synthesis of g-C_3N_4 Nanosheets

Firstly, 5g melamine powder was heated to 550 °C in an alumina crucible with a lid using a tube furnace at a heating rate of 5 °C/min and kept in the air for 2 h. The collected yellow bulk g-C_3N_4 was ground into a fine powder in an agate mortar. Secondly, g-C_3N_4 nanosheets were obtained via the thermal etching of bulk g-C_3N_4 at 500 °C in the air for 2 h. Finally, the g-C_3N_4 nanosheets were washed in deionized water and ethanol three to four times in sequence.

3.3. Synthesis of G-CdS Heterojunction

A schematic diagram of the deposition process of CdS on g-C_3N_4 is shown in Scheme 2. The g-C_3N_4@CdS (G-CdS) heterojunction was prepared using a modified chemical bath deposition (CBD) method [49] with ultrasonic microwave photocatalytic synthesis. In brief, 500 mg g-C_3N_4 and a certain amount of Cd(CH_3COO)·H_2O were mixed in 200 mL of deionized water for ultrasonic dispersion. Two hours later, 0.03 M CH_3COONH_4 was added, and NH_3·H_2O was added to adjust the pH to 11. The abovementioned mixed solution was heated to 60 °C for 30 min. Then, 0.004 M CH_4N_2S was added to the solution and heated to 90 °C for 30 min. When the reaction was over, the solution naturally cooled to room temperature. After the reaction, the solution was washed with deionized water and ethanol, and then it was filtered to obtain heterojunction materials. Finally, the obtained nanocomposites were dried at 60 °C for 12 h. The prepared samples were marked as G-CdS-1, G-CdS-2, G-CdS-3, G-CdS-4, and G-CdS-5, indicating the amount of Cd(CH_3COO)·H_2O as 0.002 M, 0.004 M, 0.006 M, 0.008 M, and 0.01 M, respectively. As a reference, the synthesis process of CdS is similar to that of G-CdS-3, except that g-C_3N_4 is not added.

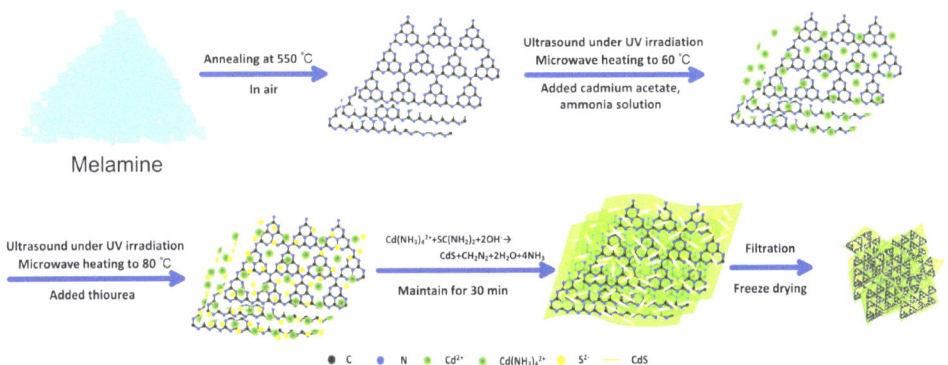

Scheme 2. Schematic diagram of the formation process of G-CdS heterostructure.

3.4. Characterization

The crystal structures of the g-C_3N_4, CdS, and G-CdS nanocomposites were characterized using an XRD with Cu Kα radiation, which operated at a voltage and current of 40 KV and 80 mA, respectively. The morphologies and microstructures of the nanocomposites were measured using TEM, Talos F200X G2, and HRTEM with an accelerated voltage of 200 KV, and super-X model energy dispersive spectroscopy was used to analyze the element distribution. For the TEM test, the ethanol solution containing 1 mg catalyst was dispersed evenly using ultrasound for 10 min, then dropped on the copper net, dried naturally, and measured. The characteristics of the functional groups in the synthetic materials were analyzed using FTIR, Thermo Scientific Nicolet iS20. The changes in the valence state and band structure of the elements in the nanocomposite were measured using XPS on a PHI 5000 Versaprobe III spectroscopy instrument with monochromatic Al

Kα radiation. Ultraviolet-visible diffuse reflectance spectra were obtained using a Hitachi UH4150 equipped with an integrating sphere. The steady-state photoluminescence was detected using a Hitachi F7000 spectrofluorometer with an excitation wavelength of 385 nm. The photocurrent performance and EIS spectroscopy were examined using a three-electrode electrochemical workstation (CHI660E, ChenHua Instrument Co., LTD, Shanghai, China). The reference electrode was Ag/AgCl, the counter electrode was a Pt plate, and the working electrode was an FTO glass with a catalyst. The electrolyte was a 0.5 M aqueous solution of Na_2SO_4.

3.5. Evaluation of Photocatalytic H_2 Production Activity

For the measurement of photocatalytic H_2 production, a reaction flask was filled with 50 mg photocatalyst, 20% lactic acid aqueous solution (10 mL) as a sacrificial agent, 100 mL of deionized water, and 3% wt Pt as a co-catalyst, using chloroplatinic acid as a Pt source. The mixed solution was ultrasonically dispersed for 30 min to obtain a uniformly dispersed suspension, which was then transferred to a quartz reactor connected to an online trace gas analysis system (Labsolar-6A, Perfectlight, Beijing, China). The system and the reactor were evacuated several times to ensure that the air was completely removed. The reactor was irradiated using a 300 W Xe arc lamp source, and the wavelength of the incident light was regulated by using a 420 nm long pass cut-off filter. The temperature of the reaction solution was maintained at 5 °C with a constant temperature water cooling system. The concentration of photocatalytic H_2 production after light irradiation was analyzed using an online gas chromatograph (GC9720PLUS, Fuli instruments, Zhejiang, China) with a thermal conductive detector. After the photocatalysis, the photocatalyst was centrifuged, washed several times, and then vacuum dried at 60 °C.

4. Conclusions

In summary, a van der Waals heterojunction was successfully fabricated by introducing a continuous ultrasonic step in the process of the chemical bath deposition method. Continuous ultrasound prevented g-C_3N_4 from agglomerating, and it remained in a monolayer or ultra-thin state. The microstructure, morphology, and optical properties of the G-CdS heterojunction were characterized using XRD, SEM, TEM, and UV absorption spectra. The results show that CdS of a hexagonal wurtzite structure grew preferentially on g-C_3N_4, showing a nanorod structure. Moreover, there was a clear and tight contact interface between g-C_3N_4 and CdS, as well as a tight heterojunction between the two components, which helped to efficiently transfer charge carriers between the two semiconductors. Photocatalytic H_2 production was also studied, and G-CdS-3 showed excellent photocatalytic performance; the catalytic mechanism was revealed using a Type II mechanism. PL and photocurrent spectra proved that a Type II heterojunction can accelerate carrier separation, reduce recombination, and improve photocatalytic H_2 production.

Author Contributions: Conceptualization, L.M. and X.A.; methodology, W.J. and C.L.; validation, L.M., W.J. and C.L.; formal analysis, L.M., T.Z. and X.A.; investigation, W.J., C.L. and L.X.; resources, L.M. and X.A.; data curation, L.M. and W.J.; writing—original draft preparation, L.M., W.J., C.L., L.X., T.Z. and X.A.; writing—review and editing, L.M., W.J., C.L., L.X., T.Z. and X.A.; supervision, L.M. and X.A.; project administration, L.M. and X.A.; funding acquisition, L.M. and X.A. All authors have read and agreed to the published version of the manuscript.

Funding: This work was jointly supported by the National Natural Science Foundation of China (No. 12204245) and the Natural Science Foundation of the Jiangsu Higher Education Institutions of China (Nos. 21KJB140018, 21KJD430006, and 22KJB510030).

Institutional Review Board Statement: Not applicable.

Informed Consent Statement: Not applicable.

Data Availability Statement: Data are contained within the article.

Conflicts of Interest: The authors declare no conflict of interest.

References

1. Dillon, M.E.; Wang, G.; Huey, R.B. Global metabolic impacts of recent climate warming. *Nature* **2010**, *467*, 704–706. [CrossRef] [PubMed]
2. Zhang, L.; Zhang, J.J.; Yu, H.G.; Yu, J.G. Emerging S-scheme photocatalyst. *Adv. Mater.* **2022**, *34*, 2107668. [CrossRef]
3. Lee, K.M.; Lai, C.W.; Ngai, K.S.; Juan, J.C. Recent developments of zinc oxide based photocatalyst in water treatment technology: A review. *Water Res.* **2016**, *88*, 428–448. [CrossRef] [PubMed]
4. Maeda, K.; Teramura, K.; Lu, D.; Takata, T.; Saito, N.; Inoue, Y.; Domen, K. Photocatalyst releasing hydrogen from water. *Nature* **2006**, *440*, 295. [CrossRef] [PubMed]
5. Zhao, Y.; Zhang, S.; Shi, R.; Waterhouse, I.; Tang, J.; Zhang, T. Two-dimensional photocatalyst design: A critical review of recent experimental and computational advances. *Mater. Today* **2020**, *34*, 78–91. [CrossRef]
6. Ma, L.; Ai, X.; Yang, X.; Cao, X.; Han, D.; Song, X.; Jiang, H.; Yang, W.; Yan, S.; Wu, X. Cd (II)-based metal-organic framework-derived CdS photocatalysts for enhancement of photocatalytic activity. *J. Mater. Sci.* **2021**, *56*, 8643–8657. [CrossRef]
7. Ma, L.; Ai, X.; Jiang, W.; Liu, P.; Chen, Y.; Lu, K.; Song, X.; Wu, X. Zn/Ce metal-organic framework-derived ZnO@CeO_2 nano-heterojunction for enhanced photocatalytic activity. *Colloid Interface Sci. Commun.* **2022**, *49*, 100636. [CrossRef]
8. Ma, L.; Ai, X.; Chen, Y.; Liu, P.; Lin, C.; Lu, K.; Jiang, W.; Wu, J.; Song, X. Improved photocatalytic activity via N-Type ZnO/p-Type NiO heterojunctions. *Nanomaterials* **2022**, *12*, 3665. [CrossRef]
9. Xiao, N.; Li, S.; Li, X.; Ge, L.; Gao, Y.; Li, N. The roles and mechanism of cocatalysts in photocatalytic water splitting to produce hydrogen. *Chin. J. Catal.* **2020**, *41*, 642–671. [CrossRef]
10. Modak, A.; Bhanja, P.; Dutta, S.; Chowdhury, B.; Bhaumik, A. Catalytic reduction of CO_2 into fuels and fine chemicals. *Green Chem.* **2020**, *22*, 4002–4033. [CrossRef]
11. Song, Y.; Johnson, D.; Peng, R.; Hensley, D.K.; Bonnesen, P.V.; Liang, L.; Huang, J.; Yang, F.; Zhang, F.; Qiao, R.; et al. A physical catalyst for the electrolysis of nitrogen to ammonia. *Sci. Adv.* **2018**, *4*, e1700336. [CrossRef] [PubMed]
12. Cheng, L.; Xiang, Q.; Liao, Y.; Zhang, H. CdS-based photocatalysts. *Energy Environ. Sci.* **2018**, *11*, 1362–1391. [CrossRef]
13. Wang, L.; Cheng, B.; Zhang, L.; Yu, J. In situ irradiated XPS investigation on S-scheme TiO_2@$ZnIn_2S_4$ photocatalyst for efficient photocatalytic CO_2 reduction. *Small* **2021**, *17*, 2103447. [CrossRef] [PubMed]
14. Li, X.-L.; Yang, G.; Li, S.; Xiao, N.; Li, N.; Gao, Y.; Lv, D.; Ge, L. Novel dual co-catalysts decorated Au@HCS@PdS hybrids with spatially separated charge carriers and enhanced photocatalytic hydrogen evolution activity. *Chem. Eng. J.* **2020**, *379*, 122350. [CrossRef]
15. Guo, Q.; Zhou, C.; Ma, Z.; Yang, X. Fundamentals of TiO_2 photocatalysis: Concepts, mechanisms, and challenges. *Adv. Mater.* **2019**, *31*, 1901997. [CrossRef]
16. Mamiyev, Z.; Balayeva, N.O. Metal sulfide photocatalysts for hydrogen generation: A review of recent advances. *Catalysts* **2022**, *12*, 1316. [CrossRef]
17. Fu, J.; Yu, J.; Jiang, C.; Cheng, B. g-C_3N_4-Based heterostructured photocatalysts. *Adv. Energy Mater.* **2018**, *8*, 1701503. [CrossRef]
18. Lu, M.; Pei, Z.; Weng, S.; Feng, W.; Fang, Z.; Zheng, Z.; Huang, M.; Liu, P. Constructing atomic layer g-C_3N_4-CdS nanoheterojunctions with efficiently enhanced visible light photocatalytic activity. *Phys. Chem. Chem. Phys.* **2014**, *16*, 21280–21288. [CrossRef]
19. Soheila, A.; Aziz, H. g-C_3N_4/carbon dot-based nanocomposites serve as efficacious photocatalysts for environmental purification and energy generation: A review. *J. Clean. Prod.* **2020**, *276*, 124319. [CrossRef]
20. Wen, J.; Xie, J.; Chen, X.; Li, X. A review on g-C_3N_4-based photocatalysts. *Appl. Surf. Sci.* **2017**, *391*, 72–123. [CrossRef]
21. Wang, X.; Maeda, K.; Thomas, A.; Takanabe, K.; Xin, G.; Carlsson, J.; Domen, K.; Antonietti, M. A metal-free polymeric photocatalyst for hydrogen production from water under visible light. *Nat. Mater.* **2009**, *8*, 76–80. [CrossRef] [PubMed]
22. Wang, Y.; Zhang, X.; Liu, Y.; Zhao, Y.; Xie, C.; Song, Y. Crystallinity and phase controlling of g-C_3N_4/CdS heterostructures towards high efficient photocatalytic H_2 generation. *Int. J. Hydrogen Energy* **2019**, *44*, 30151–30159. [CrossRef]
23. Ghosh, U.; Majumdar, A.; Pal, A. Photocatalytic CO_2 reduction over g-C_3N_4 based heterostructures: Recent progress and prospects. *J. Environ. Chem. Eng.* **2021**, *9*, 104631. [CrossRef]
24. Kadi, M.W.; Mohamed, R.; Ismail, A.; Bahnemann, D. Soft and hard templates assisted synthesis mesoporous CuO/g-C_3N_4 heterostructures for highly enhanced and accelerated Hg (II) photoreduction under visible light. *J. Colloid Interface Sci.* **2020**, *580*, 223–233. [CrossRef]
25. Zhu, Q.; Xu, Z.; Qiu, B.; Xing, M.; Zhang, J. Emerging cocatalysts on g-C_3N_4 for photocatalytic hydrogen evolution. *Small* **2021**, *17*, 2101070. [CrossRef]
26. Ran, Y.; Cui, Y.; Zhang, Y.; Fang, Y.; Zhang, W.; Yu, X.; Lan, H.; An, X. Assembly-synthesis of puff pastry-like g-C_3N_4/CdS heterostructure as S-junctions for efficient photocatalytic water splitting. *Chem. Eng. J.* **2022**, *431*, 133348. [CrossRef]
27. Zhao, Y.-F.; Sun, Y.; Yin, X.; Chen, R.; Yin, G.; Sun, M.; Liu, B. The 2D porous g-C_3N_4/CdS heterostructural nanocomposites with enhanced visible-light-driven photocatalytic activity. *J. Nanosci. Nanotechnol.* **2020**, *20*, 1098–1108. [CrossRef]
28. Liu, J. Origin of high photocatalytic efficiency in monolayer g-C_3N_4/CdS heterostructure: A hybrid DFT study. *J. Phys. Chem. C* **2015**, *119*, 28417–28423. [CrossRef]
29. Rong, X.; Qiu, F.; Zhao, H.; Yan, J.; Zhu, X.; Yang, D. Fabrication of single-layer graphitic carbon nitride and coupled systems for the photocatalytic degradation of dyes under visible-light irradiation. *Eur. J. Inorg. Chem.* **2015**, *2015*, 1359–1367. [CrossRef]
30. Zhao, D.; Wang, Y.; Dong, C.; Huang, Y.; Chen, J.; Xue, F.; Shen, S.; Guo, L. Boron-doped nitrogen-deficient carbon nitride-based Z-scheme heterostructures for photocatalytic overall water splitting. *Nat. Energy* **2021**, *6*, 388–397. [CrossRef]

31. Wang, Y.; Liu, X.; Liu, J.; Han, B.; Hu, X.; Yang, F.; Xu, Z.; Li, Y.; Jia, S.; Li, Z.; et al. Carbon quantum dot implanted graphite carbon nitride nanotubes: Excellent charge separation and enhanced photocatalytic hydrogen evolution. *Angew. Chem.* **2018**, *130*, 5867–5873. [CrossRef]
32. Tan, M.; Ma, Y.; Yu, C.; Luan, Q.; Li, J.; Liu, C.; Dong, W.; Su, Y.; Qiao, L.; Gao, L.; et al. Boosting photocatalytic hydrogen production via interfacial engineering on 2D ultrathin Z-scheme $ZnIn_2S_4$/g-C_3N_4 heterojunction. *Adv. Funct. Mater.* **2022**, *32*, 2111740. [CrossRef]
33. Qin, Y.; Li, H.; Lu, J.; Feng, Y.; Meng, F.; Ma, C.; Yan, Y.; Meng, M. Synergy between van der waals heterojunction and vacancy in $ZnIn_2S_4$/g-C_3N_4 2D/2D photocatalysts for enhanced photocatalytic hydrogen evolution. *Appl. Catal. B Environ.* **2020**, *277*, 119254. [CrossRef]
34. Gao, B.; Liu, L.; Liu, J.; Yang, F. Photocatalytic degradation of 2, 4, 6-tribromophenol over Fe-doped $ZnIn_2S_4$: Stable activity and enhanced debromination. *Appl. Catal. B Environ.* **2013**, *129*, 89–97. [CrossRef]
35. Devamani, R.H.P.; Kiruthika, R.; Mahadevi, P.; Sagithapriya, S. Synthesis and characterization of cadmium sulfide nanoparticles. *Int. J. Innov. Sci. Eng. Technol.* **2017**, *4*, 181–185.
36. Dastan, D.; Panahi, S.L.; Chaure, N.B. Characterization of titania thin films grown by dip-coating technique. *J. Mater. Sci. Mater. Electron.* **2016**, *27*, 12291–12296. [CrossRef]
37. Dastan, D.; Chaure, N.; Kartha, M. Surfactants assisted solvothermal derived titania nanoparticles: Synthesis and simulation. *J. Mater. Sci. Mater. Electron.* **2017**, *28*, 7784–7796. [CrossRef]
38. Wang, Z.; Wang, Z.; Zhu, X.; Ai, C.; Zeng, Y.; Shi, W.; Zhang, X.; Zhang, H.; Si, H.; Li, J.; et al. Photodepositing CdS on the active cyano groups decorated g-C_3N_4 in Z-scheme manner promotes visible-light-driven hydrogen evolution. *Small* **2021**, *17*, 2102699. [CrossRef]
39. Li, H.; An, M.; Zhao, Y.; Pi, S.; Li, C.; Sun, W.; Wang, H. Co nanoparticles encapsulated in N-doped carbon nanofibers as bifunctional catalysts for rechargeable Zn-air battery. *Appl. Surf. Sci.* **2019**, *478*, 560–566. [CrossRef]
40. Madhurima, V.; Kumari, K.; Jain, P. A facile single-step approach to achieve in situ expanded g-C_3N_4 for improved photodegradation performance. *Polym. Adv. Technol.* **2023**, *34*, 578–586. [CrossRef]
41. Ma, L.; Liu, W.; Cai, H.; Zhang, F.; Wu, X. Catalyst-and template-free low-temperature in situ growth of n-type CdS nanowire on p-type CdTe film and p-n heterojunction properties. *Sci. Rep.* **2016**, *6*, 38858. [CrossRef] [PubMed]
42. Jiang, N.; Xiu, Z.; Xie, Z.; Li, H.; Zhao, G.; Wang, W.; Wu, Y.; Hao, X. Reduced graphene oxide-CdS nanocomposites with enhanced visible-light photoactivity synthesized using ionic-liquid precursors. *New J. Chem.* **2014**, *38*, 4312–4320. [CrossRef]
43. Li, X.; Kang, B.; Dong, F.; Zhang, Z.; Luo, X.; Han, L.; Huang, J.; Feng, Z.; Chen, Z.; Xu, J.; et al. Enhanced photocatalytic degradation and H_2/H_2O_2 production performance of S-pCN/$WO_{2.72}$ S-scheme heterojunction with appropriate surface oxygen vacancies. *Nano Energy* **2021**, *81*, 105671. [CrossRef]
44. Güy, N. Directional transfer of photocarriers on CdS/g-C_3N_4 heterojunction modified with Pd as a cocatalyst for synergistically enhanced photocatalytic hydrogen production. *Appl. Surf. Sci.* **2020**, *522*, 146442. [CrossRef]
45. Jiang, W.; Zong, X.; An, L.; Hua, S.; Miao, X.; Luan, S.; Wen, Y.; Tao, F.; Sun, Z. Consciously constructing heterojunction or direct Z-scheme photocatalysts by regulating electron flow direction. *ACS Catal.* **2018**, *8*, 2209–2217. [CrossRef]
46. Ding, X.; Li, Y.; Zhao, J.; Zhu, Y.; Li, Y.; Deng, W.; Wang, C. Enhanced photocatalytic H_2 evolution over CdS/Au/g-C_3N_4 composite photocatalyst under visible-light irradiation. *APL Mater.* **2015**, *3*, 104410. [CrossRef]
47. Ji, C.; Du, C.; Steinkruger, J.; Zhou, C.; Yang, S. In-situ hydrothermal fabrication of CdS/g-C_3N_4 nanocomposites for enhanced photocatalytic water splitting. *Mater. Lett.* **2019**, *240*, 128–131. [CrossRef]
48. Wu, H.; Meng, S.; Zhang, J.; Zhang, X.; Wang, Y.; Chen, S.; Qi, G.; Fu, X. Construction of two-dimensionally relative p-n heterojunction for efficient photocatalytic redox reactions under visible light. *Appl. Surf. Sci.* **2020**, *505*, 144638. [CrossRef]
49. Ma, L.; Ai, X.; Wu, X. Effect of substrate and Zn doping on the structural, optical and electrical properties of CdS thin films prepared by CBD method. *J. Alloys Compd.* **2017**, *691*, 399–406. [CrossRef]

Disclaimer/Publisher's Note: The statements, opinions and data contained in all publications are solely those of the individual author(s) and contributor(s) and not of MDPI and/or the editor(s). MDPI and/or the editor(s) disclaim responsibility for any injury to people or property resulting from any ideas, methods, instructions or products referred to in the content.

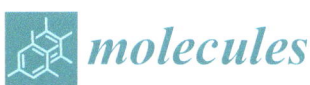

Article

Constructing In₂S₃/CdS/N-rGO Hybrid Nanosheets via One-Pot Pyrolysis for Boosting and Stabilizing Visible Light-Driven Hydrogen Evolution

Minghao Zhang, Xiaoqun Wu, Xiaoyuan Liu, Huixin Li, Ying Wang * and Debao Wang *

Key Lab of Inorganic Synthetic and Applied Chemistry, College of Chemistry and Molecular Engineering, Qingdao University of Science and Technology, Qingdao 266042, China
* Correspondence: y.wang@qust.edu.cn (Y.W.); dbwang@qust.edu.cn (D.W.)

Abstract: The construction of hybrid junctions remains challenging for the rational design of visible light-driven photocatalysts. Herein, In_2S_3/CdS/N-rGO hybrid nanosheets were successfully prepared via a one-step pyrolysis method using deep eutectic solvents as precursors. Benefiting from the surfactant-free pyrolysis method, the obtained ultrathin hybrid nanosheets assemble into stable three-dimensional self-standing superstructures. The tremella-like structure of hybrid In_2S_3/N-rGO exhibits excellent photocatalytic hydrogen production performance. The hydrogen evolution rate is 10.9 mmol·g^{-1}·h^{-1}, which is greatly superior to CdS/N-rGO (3.7 mmol·g^{-1}·h^{-1}) and In_2S_3/N-rGO (2.6 mmol·g^{-1}·h^{-1}). This work provides more opportunities for the rational design and fabrication of hybrid ultrathin nanosheets for broad catalytic applications in sustainable energy and the environment.

Keywords: In_2S_3/CdS/N-rGO; ultrathin nanosheets; photocatalysis; heterojunction; hydrogen evolution

1. Introduction

The photocatalytic decomposition of water to produce hydrogen has been identified as an effective and most promising strategy for dealing with environmental crises and energy scarcity [1]. Given the efficient use of solar energy, there have been many attempts in recent years to develop different photocatalysts for the decomposition of water under visible light [2]. Among which, chalcogenides and chalcogenide-based semiconductor materials have been widely investigated as photocatalysts for water splitting due to its inexpensive synthesis, low toxicity, large absorption coefficient, and narrow band gap energies [3]. The facile synthesis enables the rational design of chalcogenide catalysts with various shapes and structures and enriches the construction of hierarchical composites with other components to gain more interesting properties [4–10].

Cadmium sulfide (CdS) is widely used among many semiconducting metal sulfide materials due to its narrow band gap (2.4 eV), powerful reducibility, wide range of optical absorption wavelengths and a suitable energy band structure, which can effectively absorb visible light [7]. Nevertheless, CdS suffers from problems of stability in photocatalytic processes due to photocorrosion. There are still several issues with CdS that limit the rate of hydrogen production from pure CdS particles [11]. Up to now, numerous steps have been taken to address these problems [9,10,12], of which building heterojunctions with other semiconductors has been proven to be one of most the effective strategies [13–15]. For example, CdS/g-C₃N₄ nanoheterojunctions have been prepared using a hydrothermal method to improve its visible light photocatalytic performance for H₂ production [14]. Huang et al. reported the synthesis of CdS/ZnS nanocomposites for extraordinary photocatalytic H₂ generation via a type-II heterojunction [15]. Indium sulfide (In_2S_3) is an n-type semiconductor with a band gap of 2.0 to 2.4 eV, which has good stability as well as high photosensitivity [16]. Thanks to these advantages of both CdS and In_2S_3 semiconductors, more and more reports have focused on the synthesis of In_2S_3/CdS nanocomposites to form

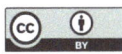

effective photocatalysts [17–21]. The suitable energy band structure between In_2S_3 and CdS benefits the construction of the In_2S_3/CdS heterojunction, which would accelerate the separation of photogenerated carriers and result in enhanced photocatalytic performance as compared to individual ones. For example, In_2S_3 nanoparticles have been deposited on CdS nanorod arrays for enhanced solar light-driven photoelectrochemical hydrogen evolution [22]. Yang et al. reported a Cu-doped In_2S_3/CdS heterojunction with a high spatial charge separation rate to boost photocatalytic hydrogen production [23].

However, sulfides have their inherent disadvantage of photocorrosion [24]. Thermodynamically, photocorrosion happens because of high oxidative h+ in the valence band which tends to oxidize lattice S^{2-} ions of CdS and In_2S_3 during the photocatalytic process. But the stability incensement could be achieved by adding a suitable sacrificial agent to scavenge the holes with competitive kinetics. For example, the photocatalytic activity and stability of sulfide photocatalysts can be efficiently improved by adding an S^{2-}/SO_3^{2-} mixture as an electron donor for hydrogen evolution from water.

On the other hand, graphene oxide has recently been introduced into semiconductor photocatalysts to further improve the efficiency of charge transfer and thereby improve photocatalytic activity and stability [25]. For example, Jia et al. reported the preparation of a N-doped graphene/CdS nanocomposite for water splitting under visible-light illumination, in which N-doped graphene could act as a protective layer to prevent photocorrosion of the CdS photocatalyst [26]. Liu et al. prepared a stacked nanostructure of GO–CdS@MoS_2 to diminish the shortage of serious photocorrosion and obtain a high photocatalytic H_2 evolution performance [27]. These sulfide/graphene composite preparation methods usually involve the pre-preparation of graphene and the release of poisonous substances. Thus, developing an environmentally friendly route is urgently needed to prepare sulfide/graphene composites.

Recently, deep eutectic solvents (DESs) have been accepted as novel media to apply to the fields of chemistry, materials, and catalysis because of the unique physicochemical properties including being environmentally friendly, its strong solvating ability, and its tunable compositions. More and more works have been reported exploring the potential of using DESs as reaction media for material synthesis, such as nanometals, zeolite-type materials, carbon materials, and metal–organic frameworks [28,29].

In this work, In and Cd-containing DES liquids were elaborately designed and applied to the synthesis of a hybrid In_2S_3/CdS/N-rGO photocatalyst via one-step pyrolysis, which is schematically shown in Figure 1. The unique liquid property of the DES precursor results in the in situ formation of tightly coupled interfaces in the hybrid. The in situ formed heterojunction with a spherical tremella-like structure could contribute to more active sites, highly efficient transfer and separation of photogenerated carriers, and the acquisition of strong redox stability. Under visible light, the hydrogen production rate of the In_2S_3/CdS/N-rGO photocatalyst achieved 10.9 mmol·g^{-1}·h^{-1}, which was 2.9 times that of a single component CdS and 4.2 times that of an In_2S_3 photocatalyst.

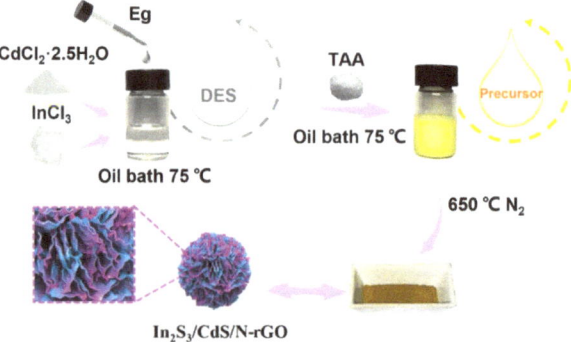

Figure 1. A schematic diagram for the preparation of the In2S3/CdS/N-rGO hybrid.

2. Results and Discussion

2.1. Formation of DES

The formation of deep eutectic solvents (DESs) of $CdCl_2 \cdot 2.5H_2O$, $InCl_3$, and ethylene glycol was first characterized. As shown in Figure 1, we collected FT-IR of $CdCl_2 \cdot 2.5H_2O$, $InCl_3$, ethylene glycol, and DESs. After DES formation, the chemical shift of –OH decreased because of hydrogen bond formation between Cl^- ions and the hydrogen atom in the DESs [30]. The absorption peak at 3429 cm^{-1} corresponds to the stretching of –OH in ethylene glycol. After DES formation with $CdCl_2 \cdot 2.5H_2O$ and $InCl_3$, the -OH was chelated by Cl^-. As a result, the –OH band moved to a lower wavenumber and significantly widened, which is evidence of hydrogen bond formation, enabling the components to be tightly coupled at the molecular level. At the same time, the oil bath temperature for the reaction to form a transparent and uniform liquid is about 75 °C. The melting point of the mixture was lower than the melting point of each component, which can also reveal the formation of DESs (the melting point of $InCl_3$ is 586 °C, and $CdCl_2 \cdot 2.5H_2O$ is 568 °C) [31]. The obtained DES liquids were used as precursors to synthesize the In_2S_3/CdS/N-rGO photocatalyst via a one-pot pyrolysis, as schematically shown in Figure 2.

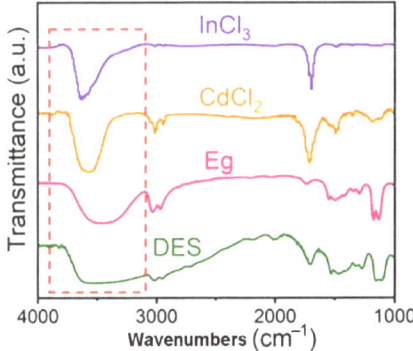

Figure 2. FT-IR spectra of $CdCl_2 \cdot 2.5H_2O$, $InCl_3$, ethylene glycol, and DES.

2.2. Material Characterization

The structure of the as-prepared photocatalysts was identified from the respective XRD patterns. As shown in Figure 3a, the XRD of the obtained In_2S_3/CdS/N-rGO photocatalyst shows significant characteristic diffraction peaks at 24.81°, 26.51°, 28.18°, 36.62°, 43.68°, 47.84°, 51.82°, and 66.77° corresponding to the (100), (002), (101), (102), (110), (103), (112), and (203) crystal faces of CdS (JCPDS, No. 41–1049). The diffraction peaks at 14.25°, 23.32°, 27.43°, 33.23°, 43.60°, and 47.70° are ascribed to the (103), (116), (109), (0012), (1015), and (2212) crystal faces of In_2S_3 (JCPDS, No. 25–0390). The narrow and sharp characteristic peaks indicate CdS and In_2S_3 samples have high crystallinity. In addition, In_2S_3 in the hybrid has a peak shift to a higher diffraction angle. It may come from the doping of smaller N or C atoms into In_2S_3 or from the formation of strong interface interactions between In_2S_3 and CdS and even the formation of a $CdIn_2S_4$ phase [20]. The XRD results support the presence of CdS and In_2S_3 substances. But there are no obvious diffraction peaks of graphene in the pattern, presumably due to the relatively weak intensity in comparison with the high crystallinity of In_2S_3 and CdS. The Raman spectrum was recorded to further identify the presence of graphene carbon. Figure 3b shows the Raman spectrum of the catalyst with two characteristic peaks around 1350 and 1580 cm^{-1}, confirming the presence of reduced graphene oxide carbon in the In_2S_3/CdS/N-rGO hybrid [25]. It is also evident that the Raman data are very noisy and the D band intensity is rather strong, which could be deduced from the lower content of rGO carbon in the hybrid, the doping of N atoms into rGO carbon, and the larger quantity of defects in rGO carbon because of the composition of In_2S_3/CdS in the in situ pyrolysis process.

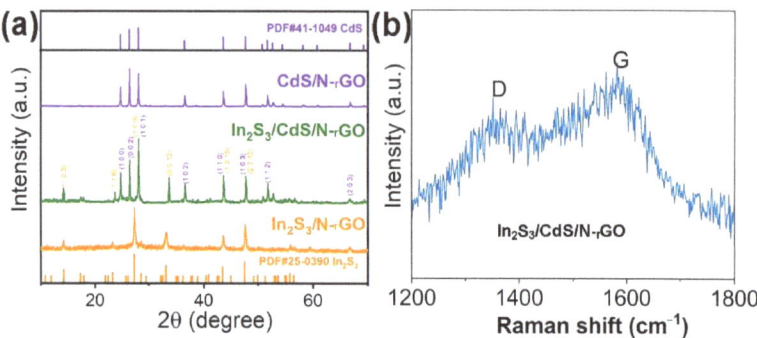

Figure 3. XRD patterns (**a**) and Raman spectrum (**b**) of the photocatalysts.

The morphology and surface microstructure of the $In_2S_3/CdS/N$-rGO photocatalyst were studied using SEM and TEM. As shown in Figure 4a, the $In_2S_3/CdS/N$-rGO photocatalyst has a layered shape of tremella, with a diameter of about 1–2 μm. The tremella shows staggered growth of ultrathin curved nanosheets. These nanosheets cluster together in different directions to form open cavities distributed across the entire surface of the microspheres (Figure 4b). This open cavity will produce rich voids and a large specific surface area and expose more active sites. It can also be seen from the TEM image in Figure 4c that the contrast between light and dark indicates the porous structure of the tremella microspheres composed of ultrathin nanosheets. The microstructure of the nanosheet was further characterized by the HRTEM image in Figure 4e. After zooming in (dotted red line regions), multiple layers of an almost transparent layer at the edge of the nanosheet can be identified, as marked by yellow lines. The lattice fringe of about 0.37 nm matches the distance between the layers of graphene oxide [30]. And Figure 4f shows two types of distinct lattice fringes, the 0.269 nm lattice matching (0012) the faces of In_2S_3 [32] and the 0.316 nm lattice for (101) the crystal surfaces of CdS [33]. Figure 4g shows a HAADF-STEM image of the hybrid, further confirming the tremella-like structure assembled by ultrathin nanosheet. The corresponding STEM-EDS elemental mappings in Figure 4h reveal a uniform distribution of Cd, In, S, C, O, and N elements in the $In_2S_3/CdS/N$-rGO hybrid. It can be concluded that the In_2S_3/CdS photocatalyst coated with a graphene oxide shell can be successfully prepared by the DES precursor-assisted one-pot pyrolysis method. The N-doped graphene oxide shell can inhibit the photocorrosion of metal sulfide to a certain extent and accelerate the electron transfer of charge at the interface, which would greatly improve the photocatalytic activity and stability.

Figure 5 shows XPS spectra of In 3d, Cd 3d, S 2p, C 1s, O 1s, and N 1s for different photocatalysts, respectively. The 443.4 eV and 451.0 eV peaks in Figure 5a match the In $3d_{5/2}$ and In $3d_{3/2}$ binding energy, indicating the presence of an In^{3+} state in the hybrid [34]. The characteristic peaks at 404.4 and 411.2 eV in Figure 5b correspond to the Cd $3d_{5/2}$ and Cd $3d_{3/2}$ binding energy of a Cd^{2+} valence state [35]. As shown in Figure 5c, the S 2p spectrum can be fitted into two peaks at 160.4 eV and 161.6 eV, attributed to the characteristic peaks of S $2p_{3/2}$ and S $2p_{1/2}$ of S^{2-} [36]. The C 1s spectrum of $In_2S_3/CdS/N$-rGO is shown in Figure 5d. The characteristic peak at 284.5 eV corresponds to sp^2 hybridization carbon and carbon atoms single- or double-bonded to the nitrogen atoms or oxygen [37]. The peaks at 285.6 and 288.7 eV correspond to the C–C/C=C and O–C=N/C-N functional groups [38]. The O 1s peak can be deconvoluted into four peaks at 530.9 eV, 532.1 eV, 533 eV, and 533.4 eV (Figure 5e), which come from surface-absorbed OH groups on In_2S_3/CdS as well as C=O, (CO*)OH, and C–O–C groups remained in rGO [39]. Figure 5f shows the $In_2S_3/CdS/N$-rGO photocatalyst and In_2S_3/N-rGO photocatalyst with respect to N 1s spectra, which can further prove the existence of N elements in In_2S_3/GO. $In_2S_3/CdS/N$-rGO shows three weak peaks. The three peaks are located at 400.5 eV, 400.13 eV, and 398.34 eV, which correspond to graphitic nitrogen, N of pyrroline, and pyridinic N [37,40].

These nitrogen-containing functional groups can confirm the existence of N-doped reduced graphene oxide. In addition, it is worth noting that compared to the binding energy of In 3d and N 1s in the composite photocatalyst $In_2S_3/CdS/N$-rGO, the elements in the In_2S_3/N-rGO photocatalyst move 0.3 eV in the direction of low binding energy, while the Cd 3d in the composite moves about 0.3 eV in the opposite direction. This indicates that a close coupling interface is formed between In_2S_3 and CdS, attributed to the homogenous contacting of components in the liquid DES precursor.

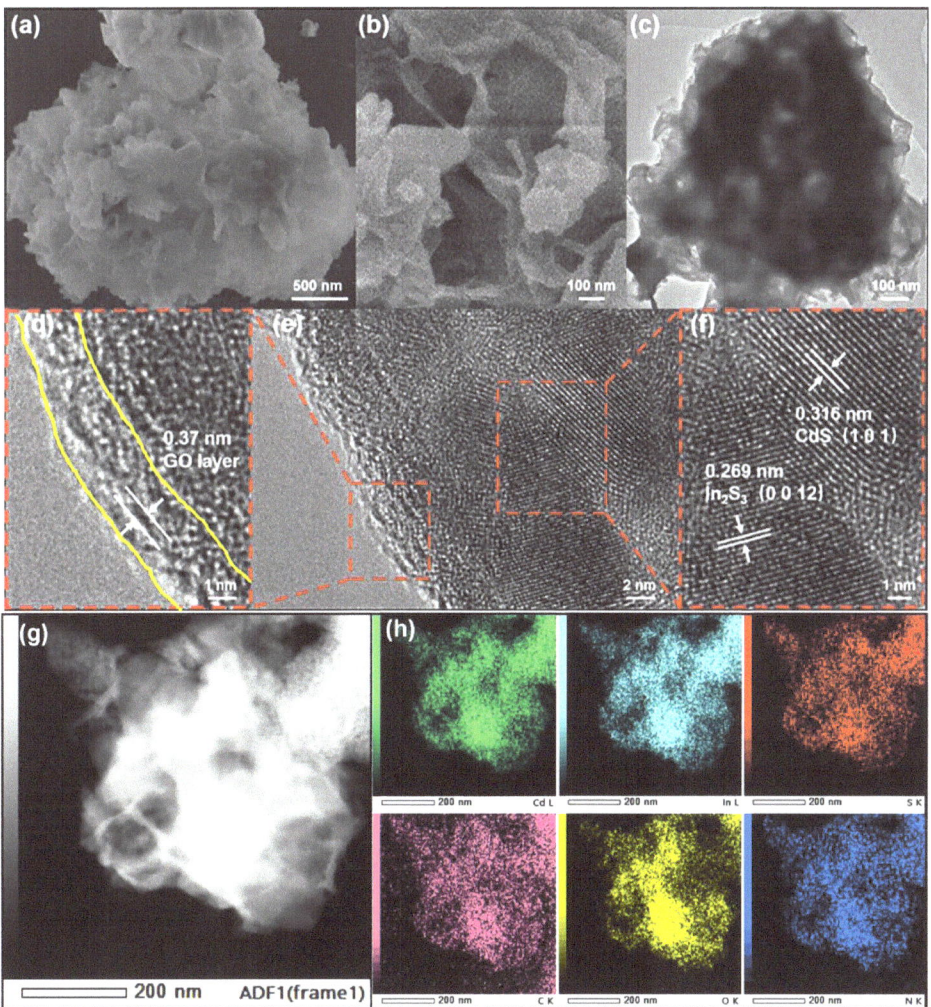

Figure 4. SEM (**a**,**b**), TEM (**c**), HRTEM (**d**–**f**), and HAADF-STEM image (**g**) and corresponding STEM-EDS elemental mappings (**h**) of $In_2S_3/CdS/N$-rGO photocatalyst.

In order to investigate the reason for improved photocatalytic hydrogen activity, a series of optical and electrochemical properties of the photocatalysts were measured to evaluate the charge transfer and separation ability. To investigate the optical absorption properties, UV-Vis diffuse reflectance spectroscopy (DRS) was carried out, as shown in Figure 6a. CdS/N-rGO exhibited a significant absorption edge at about 505 nm, suggesting good visible light absorption. Meanwhile, the absorption edge of the In_2S_3/N-rGO photocatalyst was close to 536 nm. After the In_2S_3/N-rGO was compounded with CdS/N-rGO, the absorption edges of In$_2$S$_3$/CdS/N-rGO (529 nm) fell well between those of CdS/N-rGO and In$_2$S$_3$/CdS/N-rGO, indicating that they can harvest more photon efficiency than CdS/N-rGO in the visible region via the compounding of In$_2$S$_3$/N-rGO. This result may be due to the narrow band gap and porous structure of In$_2$S$_3$ with a large specific surface area. It improves the utilization efficiency of sunlight and causes changes in the basic process of electron hole pair formation, improving photocatalytic performance.

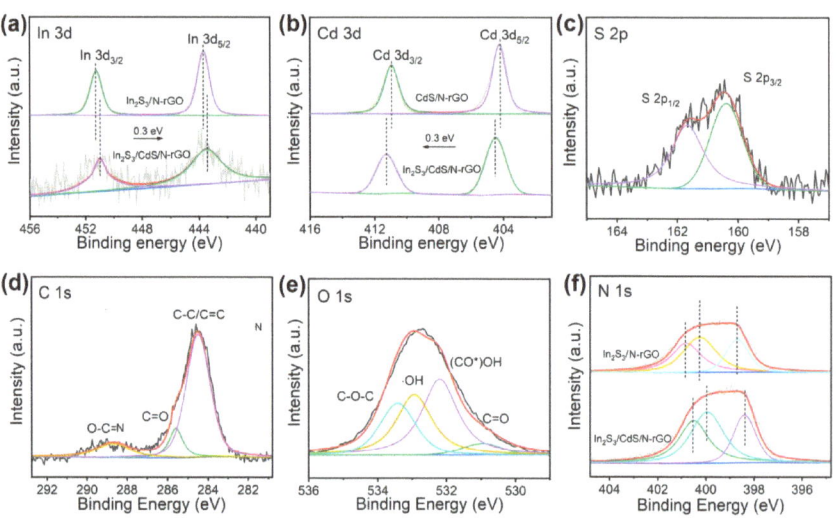

Figure 5. XPS spectra of (**a**) In 3d; (**b**) Cd 3d; (**c**) S 2p; (**d**) C 1s; (**e**) O 1s; and (**f**) N 1s of different photocatalysts.

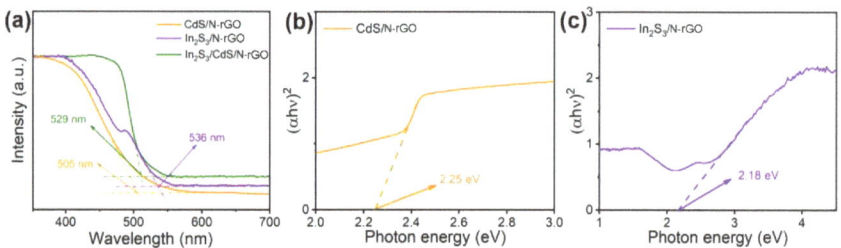

Figure 6. UV-Vis DRS spectra of different photocatalysts (**a**); corresponding Tauc plots for band gap estimation of (**b**) CdS/N-rGO and (**c**) In$_2$S$_3$/N-rGO.

The Tauc plots calculated by UV-Vis spectra through the Kubelka–Munk formula are shown in Figure 6b,c to estimate the band gaps of CdS/N-rGO and In$_2$S$_3$/N-rGO. The band gap energies (E_g) of the catalyst can be calculated by using the Tauc plot. According to previous reports, the band gap energies can be calculated by the equation $(\alpha h\nu) = K(h\nu - E_g)^{0.5}$ [41], where α is the absorption coefficient, ν is the optical frequency, K is a constant, and E_g is the band gap. By tangent to the X-axis, the band gaps of CdS/N-rGO and In$_2$S$_3$/N-rGO are estimated to be 2.25 eV and 2.18 eV, respectively.

2.3. Photocatalytic Hydrogen Evolution

The photocatalytic H$_2$ evolution activity of In$_2$S$_3$/CdS/N-rGO was investigated on an online photocatalytic system with a top light irradiation using 0.25 M Na$_2$S·9H$_2$O/0.35 M Na$_2$SO$_3$ as sacrificial reagents. As presented in Figure 7a, the photocatalytic hydrogen evolution performance of different photocatalysts were compared. A steady accumulation of H$_2$ is observed within 6 h. Figure 7b shows the corresponding hydrogen evolution rates. The $In_2S_3/CdS/N$-rGO photocatalyst has the highest value of 10.9 mmol·g^{-1}·h^{-1}, which is significantly improved compared to the catalytic performance of CdS/N-rGO and In_2S_3/N-rGO. The hydrogen evolution rate of the $In_2S_3/CdS/N$-rGO photocatalyst was 3.0 times and 4.2 times higher than that of CdS/N-rGO and In_2S_3/N-rGO photocatalysts, respectively. This performance is also higher than most of the non-noble metal CdS-based photocatalysts reported so far (Table 1).

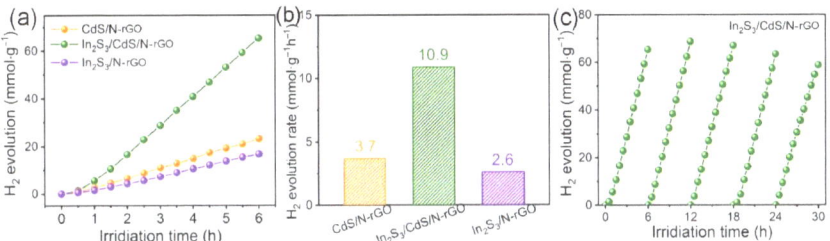

Figure 7. (a) Photocatalytic H_2 evolution and (b) H_2 evolution rates of different catalysts; (c) H_2 evolution cycling stability of $In_2S_3/CdS/N$-rGO.

Table 1. Comparison of the hydrogen evolution performance of the $In_2S_3/CdS/N$-rGO photocatalyst with other reported CdS-based photocatalysts.

Catalyst	Light Source	Scavengers	H_2 Evolution Rate (mmol·g^{-1}·h^{-1})	Ref.
$In_2S_3/CdS/N$-GO	$\lambda \geq 420$ nm	Na_2S and Na_2SO_3	10.9	This work
CdS-$Cu_{1.81}S$	$\lambda \geq 420$ nm	Na_2S and Na_2SO_3	2.714	[42]
CoS/CdS	$\lambda \geq 420$ nm	Na_2S and Na_2SO_3	0.143	[43]
CdS@Zn-C	$\lambda \geq 420$ nm	Na_2S and Na_2SO_3	6.6	[44]
$PbTiO_3$/CdS	$\lambda \geq 420$ nm	Na_2S and Na_2SO_3	0.849	[45]
Cd/CdS	$\lambda \geq 420$ nm	Na_2S and Na_2SO_3	1.753	[46]
Ti_3C_2@CdS	$\lambda \geq 420$ nm	methanol	0.088	[47]
CdS/NiO	$\lambda \geq 420$ nm	Na_2S and Na_2SO_3	1.77	[48]
CdS/np-rGO	$\lambda \geq 420$ nm	Na_2S and Na_2SO_3	2.171	[49]
Co@NC/CdS	$\lambda \geq 420$ nm	lactic acid	8.2	[50]
C/CdS	$\lambda \geq 420$ nm	Na_2S and triethanolamine	5.71	[51]

In addition, the stability of photocatalysts is also one of the important criteria for evaluating the performance of catalyst materials. As shown in Figure 7c, the $In_2S_3/CdS/N$-rGO photocatalyst was used in a 30-h cycle stability experiment for photocatalytic hydrogen evolution, with a total of five cycles and each for 6 h. The results indicate that the hydrogen production performance is only slightly lower than the initial value, demonstrating that the $In_2S_3/CdS/N$-rGO photocatalyst has good cycle stability while maintaining high performance.

2.4. Photoelectrochemical Properties

Generally, the photocatalytic performance greatly relates to the transfer and separation of photogenerated electron–hole pairs. PL intensity was applied to investigate the effectiveness of photoexcited electron–hole pair separation. As shown in Figure 8a, $In_2S_3/CdS/N$-rGO shows distinctly decreased PL intensity in comparison with CdS/N-rGO and In_2S_3/N-rGO. This implies that the recombination of photoinduced electron–hole pairs in $In_2S_3/CdS/N$-rGO was efficiently inhibited. In addition, transient photocurrent responses of the photocatalysts were measured by several on/off cycles under illumination (Figure 8b). After turning on the light, the I-t curve of the $In_2S_3/CdS/N$-rGO photocatalyst showed much higher photocurrent density than In_2S_3/N-rGO and CdS/N-rGO, indicating that the photoresponse sensitivity of photoexcited carriers could be indeed enhanced in the $In_2S_3/CdS/N$-rGO hybrid. This result is consistent with the PL results. In addition, EIS Nyquist plots are used to explore carrier dynamics, especially the charge transfer impedance at the semiconductor electrolyte interface. Figure 8c shows EIS Nyquist plots of different catalysts and the equivalent circuit model is shown in the inset. R_s is the solution resistance, R_{ct} represents the charge transfer resistance, and CPE is described as the constant phase element. By comparison, circle radii of In_2S_3/N-rGO and CdS/N-rGO are wider than that of $In_2S_3/CdS/N$-rGO, demonstrating that the internal hindrance of the $In_2S_3/CdS/N$-rGO heterojunction is less than that of the individual ingredient [35]. It is reasonable to conclude that forming an $In_2S_3/CdS/N$-rGO hybrid could greatly promote the directional migration and spatial separation of electron–hole charges from the above experiment results.

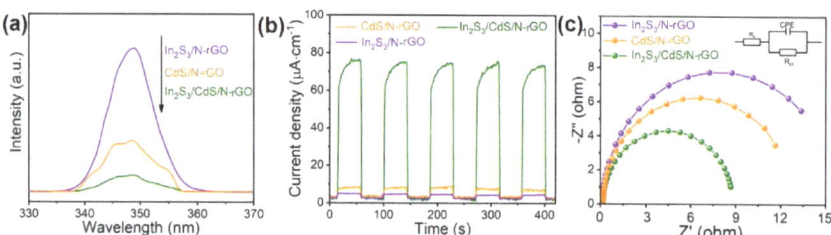

Figure 8. PL spectra (**a**); transient photocurrent responses curves (**b**); and EIS Nyquist plots (**c**) of different photocatalysts.

Figure 9 shows Mott–Schottky plots of CdS/N-rGO and In_2S_3/N-rGO measured at different frequencies. Both of them show positive slope values, indicating that they are all typical n-type semiconductors. The flat band potentials (E_{fb}) determined as the x-intercept in Mott–Schottky plots are −0.93 V for CdS/N-rGO and −1.32 V for In_2S_3/N-rGO versus Ag/AgCl. Based on the equation of E_{fb} (V vs. NHE) = E_{fb} (V vs. Ag/AgCl) + 0.61 [52], the normal hydrogen electrode (NHE) potentials were calculated to be E_{fb} (CdS) = −0.32 V and E_{fb} (In_2S_3/N-rGO) = −0.71 V from the flat band potentials.

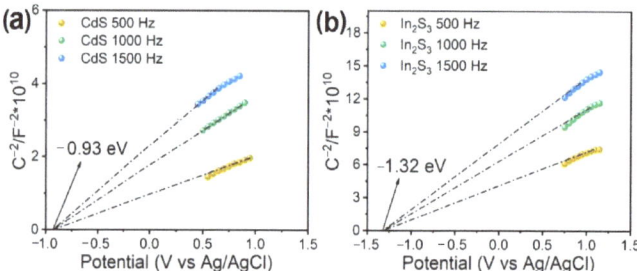

Figure 9. Mott–Schottky plots of (**a**) CdS/N-rGO and (**b**) In_2S_3/N-rGO.

2.5. Photocatalytic Hydrogen Evolution Mechanism

It is generally believed that coupling semiconductors with different valence band (VB) and conduction band (CB) energy potentials can promote effective interfacial charge transfer. Considering that an n-type semiconductor generally has a CB bottom of about 0.2 V higher than its E_{fb} value, the CB bottom is −0.12 V for CdS and −0.51 V for In_2S_3 when potential difference is set as 0.2 V. And the VB tops are determined to be 2.13 V (CdS) and 1.67 V (In_2S_3) by adding CB potential to the band gap value obtained from Figure 6b,c. According to the above experimental results, band structures of the obtained CdS/N-rGO and In_2S_3/N-rGO catalysts can be displayed in Figure 10. From the band alignment, In_2S_3 has a higher CB edge potential than CdS, while CdS has a deeper VB maximum. As a result, a type-II heterojunction can be formed with a staggered energy band alignment at the coupled interface between CdS and In_2S_3 which facilitates the charge separation and transfer process [53].

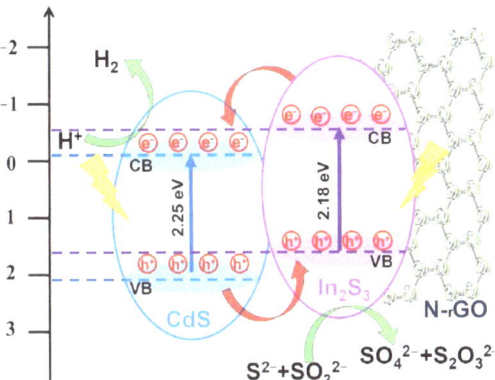

Figure 10. Photocatalytic hydrogen evolution mechanism of the In_2S_3/CdS/N-rGO photocatalyst.

According to the photochemical and photoelectrochemical experimental results discussed above, the combination of CdS and In_2S_3 in the type-II heterojunction could effectively accelerate the separation of photoexcited electrons and holes in space. Under visible light irradiation, photoinduced electrons in the CB of In_2S_3 would move to the CB of CdS, which would be captured by H^+ ions to produce H_2, whereas the holes transfer from the VB of CdS to the VB of In_2S_3, which would be captured by the sacrificial reagent. As a result, the accumulation of holes on the VB of CdS was prevented, inhibiting the photocorrosion of CdS and improving the stability of the photocatalyst. The elaborately designed DES liquid procedure enables the formation of the In_2S_3/CdS/N-rGO hybrid in one step, resulting in tightly coupled interfaces and an enhanced charge conductivity. In addition, the coupling of N-rGO plays significant roles in improving the photocatalytic performance. N-doping introduces electron-rich N into the graphene framework and enhances the electrical conductivity of rGO. N-doping forms additional defects and leads to a structural change in graphene carbon, which serve as active sites for the in situ growth of In_2S_3 and CdS, forming tightly coupled interfaces and enhancing the charge transfer of the hybrids [54]. Also, N-rGO can protect In_2S_3 and CdS from corrosion. Furthermore, the tremella-like structure provides more active sites for reactant species, such as hole scavengers, H^+, and H_2O, promoting reaction kinetics for enhanced photocatalytic activity [55]. In summary, the CdS/In_2S_3/N-rGO hybrid possesses a synergetic effect of visible light absorption enhancement, type-II heterojunction formation, and spherical tremella-like structure, which act together to achieve high photocatalytic performance.

3. Materials and Methods

3.1. Chemicals

Indium chloride ($InCl_3$, 98%) was purchased from Shanghai Macklin Biochemical Co., Ltd. Cadmium chloride ($CdCl_2 \cdot 2.5H_2O$), ethylene glycol, thioacetamide, sodium sulfide ($Na_2S \cdot 9H_2O$), anhydrous sodium sulfite, and absolute ethanol were purchased from Sinopharm Chemical Reagent Co., Ltd. All chemicals were used without further purification. Deionized water was used in all experiments.

3.2. Preparation of the Photocatalysts

The In_2S_3/CdS/N-rGO composite photocatalyst was prepared via the one-step pyrolysis method using DESs as precursors, as schematically shown in Figure 2. A total of 2.5 mmol of $InCl_3$, 2.5 mmol of $CdCl_2 \cdot 2.5H_2O$, and 17 mmol of ethylene glycol were firstly mixed into a glass bottle and heated in a 75 °C oil bath. The mixture converted to a transparent and homogeneous liquid after 30 min stirring. Then, 7.5 mmol of thiourea was added, and a uniform yellow liquid was formed after stirring for another 30 min. Finally, the liquid precursor was transferred to a covered porcelain boat. Then, the porcelain boat was placed in the center of the tube furnace and heated to 650 °C at a rate of 5 °C/min under N_2 atmosphere and kept for 4 h. After cooling to room temperature, the sample was washed, centrifuged three times with deionized water and ethanol, and dried to obtain the In_2S_3/CdS/N-rGO composite photocatalyst. Figure 1 schematically shows the synthesis procedure of the In_2S_3/CdS/N-rGO photocatalyst. CdS/N-rGO and In_2S_3/N-rGO photocatalysts were prepared via the same procedure, without the addition of $InCl_3$ for CdS/N-rGO and in the absence of $CdCl_2 \cdot 2.5H_2O$ for In_2S_3/N-rGO.

3.3. Materials Characterization

FT-IR spectra were recorded on Bruker Tensor 27 IR spectrometer and the sample was prepared by the KBr pellet method. Powder X-ray diffraction (XRD) characterizations were conducted on a D-MAX 2500/PC powder X-ray diffractometer. Scanning electron microscope (SEM) images were taken on a JSM-6700F microscope. TEM and high-resolution TEM (HRTEM) images were recorded on a JEM-F200 transmission electron microscope. XPS was conducted on a Thermo ESCALAB 250XI spectrometer. PL spectra were obtained by a Perkin Elmer LS-55. UV-Vis diffuse reflectance spectra (DRS) were conducted on a Lambda 750 s UV/VIS/NIR spectrophotometer.

3.4. Photocatalytic Reaction

The photocatalytic hydrogen production activity of the catalysts was evaluated on a CEL-SPH2N online photocatalytic hydrogen production system. A 300 W xenon lamp (Beijing Zhongjiao Jinyuan) equipped with 420 nm cut-off filter was applied to irradiation. By using a magnetic stirrer, 5 mg of the catalyst was dispersed in 100 mL of deionized water containing 0.25 M $Na_2S \cdot 9H_2O$/0.35 M Na_2SO_3 in a quartz reactor. The system was evacuated for 25 min to remove dissolved O_2 and CO_2 and the temperature was maintained at 7 °C. The hydrogen production was analyzed periodically using online gas chromatography (Agilent 7890 A) with intervals of 30 min. High purity nitrogen was used as a carrier gas.

3.5. Photoelectrochemical Properties

Electrochemical properties were carried out on a Moudulab XM electrochemical workstation in a 0.5 M Na_2SO_4 solution using a standard three-electrode system, the catalyst as working electrode, an Ag/AgCl electrode as a reference, and a Pt plate as a counter electrode. To prepare a working electrode, 12 mg of the catalyst, 50 μL Nafion, and 8 mg of carbon black were dispersed in 1 mL of ethanol, ultrasonically forming a homogeneous slurry. A total of 20 μL of slurry was dropped on a slide of FTO glass with an effective area of 1×1 cm^2. After being dried at 40 °C for 24 h, a working electrode was obtained. The transient photocurrent response (I-t) was performed without bias, illuminated by a 300 W xenon lamp (λ > 420 nm) switching on and off every 40 s.

4. Conclusions

In conclusion, a In_2S_3/CdS/N-rGO hybrid photocatalyst with a tremella-like structure was successfully prepared using a one-step pyrolysis method with DES liquids as precursors. The liquid DES precursor strategy has several advantages. (1) The homogeneous system enables sufficient contact between components. (2) The in situ growing and coupling of CdS/In_2S_3 and N-rGO were gained in one step, resulting in tightly coupled interfaces. (3) The tightly coupled N-rGO can effectively promote the rapid charge transfer and reduced electron hole recombination and can protect In_2S_3 and CdS from corrosion. (4) The tremella-like structure can provide more active sites. As a result, excellent photocatalytic hydrogen production performance was obtained. It can gain a high photocatalytic hydrogen production rate of 10.9 mmol·g^{-1}·h^{-1}. The liquid DES precursor strategy can be applied to prepare other transition metal sulfides/rGO hybrids, providing new candidates for highly efficient photocatalysts.

Author Contributions: Conceptualization, X.W. and Y.W.; methodology, M.Z. and X.W.; validation, M.Z., X.L. and H.L.; investigation, X.W.; writing—original draft preparation, X.W.; writing—review and editing, Y.W. and D.W.; supervision, Y.W. and D.W. All authors have read and agreed to the published version of the manuscript.

Funding: This work was supported by the National Natural Science Foundation of China (52072194, 51872152).

Institutional Review Board Statement: Not applicable.

Informed Consent Statement: Not applicable.

Data Availability Statement: The data presented in this study are available on request from the author.

Conflicts of Interest: The authors declare no conflict of interest.

References

1. Ravi, P.; Noh, J. Photocatalytic water splitting: How far away are we from being able to industrially produce solar hydrogen? *Molecules* **2022**, *27*, 7176. [CrossRef] [PubMed]
2. Huang, Z.M.; Ren, K.; Zheng, R.X.; Wang, L.M.; Wang, L. Ultrahigh carrier mobility in two-dimensional IV–VI semiconductors for photocatalytic water splitting. *Molecules* **2023**, *28*, 4126. [CrossRef] [PubMed]
3. Khan, M.M.; Rahman, A. Chalcogenides and chalcogenide-based heterostructures as photocatalysts for water splitting. *Catalysts* **2022**, *12*, 1338. [CrossRef]
4. Poudel, M.B.; Logeshwaran, N.; Kim, A.R.; Karthikeyan, S.C.; Vijayapradeep, S.; Yoo, D.J. Integrated core-shell assembly of Ni_3S_2 nanowires and CoMoP nanosheets as highly efficient bifunctional electrocatalysts for overall water splitting. *J. Alloys Compd.* **2023**, *960*, 170678. [CrossRef]
5. Poudel, M.B.; Logeshwaran, N.; Prabhakaran, S.; Kim, A.R.; Kim, D.H.; Yoo, D.J. Low-cost hydrogen production from alkaline/seawater over a single step synthesis of Mo_3Se_4-NiSe core-shell nanowire arrays. *Adv. Mater.* **2023**, e2305813. [CrossRef]
6. Lv, S.; Sun, Y.; Liu, D.; Song, C.; Wang, D. Construction of S-Scheme heterojunction $Ni_{11}(HPO_3)_8(OH)_6$/CdS photocatalysts with open framework surface for enhanced H_2 evolution activity. *J. Colloid Inter. Sci.* **2023**, *634*, 148–158. [CrossRef]
7. Ahmad, I.; Ben Ahmed, S.; Shabir, M.; Imran, M.; Hassan, A.M.; Alatawi, N.S. Review on CdS-derived photocatalysts for solar photocatalytic applications–advances and challenges. *J. Ind. Eng. Chem.* **2023**, in press. [CrossRef]
8. Lv, S.H.; Liu, D.Z.; Sun, Y.Y.; Li, M.X.; Zhou, Y.H.; Song, C.X.; Wang, D.B. Graphene oxide coupled high-index facets CdZnS with rich sulfur vacancies for synergistic boosting visible-light-catalytic hydrogen evolution in natural seawater: Experimental and DFT study. *J. Colloid Inter. Sci.* **2022**, *623*, 34–43. [CrossRef]
9. Tian, J.; Wen, X.; Hu, W.; Luo, L.; Wang, W.; Lin, K.; Zhan, H.; Ma, B. A highly efficient composite catalyst (Au/Ta_3N_5)/CdS for photocatalytic hydrogen production. *Catalysts* **2023**, *13*, 1103. [CrossRef]
10. Sun, Y.; Zhang, M.; Mou, X.; Song, C.; Wang, D. Construction of S-scheme $Mn0.1Cd0.9S/WO_3$ 1D/0D heterojunction assemblies for visible-light driven high-efficient H_2 evolution. *J. Alloys Compd.* **2022**, *927*, 167114. [CrossRef]
11. Ning, X.; Lu, G. Photocorrosion Inhibition of CdS-Based Catalysts for Photocatalytic Overall Water Splitting. *Nanoscale* **2020**, *12*, 1213–1223. [CrossRef] [PubMed]
12. Su, J.; Zhang, T.; Li, Y.; Chen, Y.; Liu, M. Photocatalytic Activities of Copper Doped Cadmium Sulfide Microspheres Prepared by a Facile Ultrasonic Spray-Pyrolysis Method. *Molecules* **2016**, *21*, 735. [CrossRef] [PubMed]
13. Nadikatla, S.K.; Chintada, V.B.; Gurugubelli, T.R.; Koutavarapu, R. Review of Recent Developments in the Fabrication of ZnO/CdS Heterostructure Photocatalysts for Degradation of Organic Pollutants and Hydrogen Production. *Molecules* **2023**, *28*, 4277. [CrossRef] [PubMed]
14. Niu, Y.; Shen, J.; Guo, W.; Zhu, X.; Guo, L.; Wang, Y.; Li, F. The Synergistic Effect in $CdS/g-C_3N_4$ Nanoheterojunctions Improves Visible Light Photocatalytic Performance for Hydrogen Evolution Reactions. *Molecules* **2023**, *28*, 6412. [CrossRef]
15. Huang, M.; Yu, M.; Si, R.; Zhao, X.; Chen, S.; Liu, K.; Pan, X. Tailoring Morphology in Hydrothermally Synthesized CdS/ZnS Nanocomposites for Extraordinary Photocatalytic H_2 Generation via Type-II Heterojunction. *Catalysts* **2023**, *13*, 1123. [CrossRef]
16. Mishra, S.R.; Gadore, V.; Ahmaruzzaman, M.D. Recent advances in In_2S_3-based photocatalysts for catalytic reduction of CO_2. *Chem. Phys. Impact* **2023**, *7*, 100324. [CrossRef]
17. Wei, L.; Zhang, J.; Ruan, M. Combined CdS/In_2S_3 Heterostructures with Cocatalyst for Boosting Carriers Separation and Photoelectrochemical Water Splitting. *Appl. Sur. Sci.* **2021**, *541*, 148431. [CrossRef]
18. Jiang, F.; Gunawan; Harada, T.; Kuang, Y.; Minegishi, T.; Domen, K.; Ikeda, S. $Pt/In_2S_3/CdS/Cu_2ZnSnS_4$ thin film as an efficient and stable photocathode for water reduction under sunlight radiation. *J. Am. Chem. Soc.* **2015**, *137*, 13691–13697. [CrossRef]
19. Sun, M.; Zhu, Y.; Yan, K.; Zhang, J. Dual-mode visible light-induced aptasensing platforms for bleomycin detection based on CdS-In2S3 heterojunction. *Biosens. Bioelectron.* **2019**, *145*, 111712. [CrossRef]
20. Hu, J.; Wu, J.; Zhang, S.; Chen, W.; Xiao, W.; Hou, H.; Lu, X.; Liu, C.; Zhang, Q. One-Pot Fabrication of 2D/2D $CdIn_2S_4/In_2S_3$ Heterojunction for Boosting Photocatalytic Cr(VI) Reduction. *Catalysts* **2023**, *13*, 826. [CrossRef]

21. Nawaz, M.; Akhtar, S.; Qureshi, F.; Almofty, S.A.; Nissapatron, V. Preparation of indium-cadmium sulfide nanoparticles with diverse morphologies: Photocatalytic and cytotoxicity study. *J. Mol. Struct.* **2022**, *1253*, 132288. [CrossRef]
22. Wu, J.; Wei, J.; Lv, B.; Wang, M.J.; Wang, X.L.; Wang, W.Z. Enhanced solar-light-driven photoelectrochemical water splitting performance of type II 1D/0D CdS/In$_2$S$_3$ nanorod arrays. *Chem. Phys. Lett.* **2023**, *830*, 140776. [CrossRef]
23. Yang, L.; Gao, T.; Yuan, S.; Dong, Y.; Chen, Y.; Wang, X.; Chen, C.; Tang, L.; Ohno, T. Spatial charge separated two-dimensional/two-dimensional Cu-In2S3/CdS heterojunction for boosting photocatalytic hydrogen production. *J. Colloid Inter. Sci.* **2023**, *652*, 1503–1511. [CrossRef] [PubMed]
24. Lee, B.R.; Jang, H.W. beta-In$_2$S$_3$ as water splitting photoanodes: Promise and challenges, electron. *Mater. Lett.* **2021**, *17*, 119–135.
25. Chang, D.W.; Baek, J.-B. Nitrogen-doped graphene for photocatalytic hydrogen generation. *Chem. Asian J.* **2016**, *11*, 1125–1137. [CrossRef]
26. Jia, L.; Wang, D.H.; Huang, Y.X.; Xu, A.W.; Yu, H.Q. Highly durable N-doped graphene/CdS nanocomposites with enhanced photocatalytic hydrogen evolution from water under visible light irradiation. *J. Phys. Chem. C* **2011**, *115*, 11466–11473. [CrossRef]
27. Liu, Q.; Wang, S.; Ren, Q.; Li, T.; Tu, G.; Zhong, S.; Zhao, Y.; Bai, S. Stacking design in photocatalysis: Synergizing cocatalyst roles and anti-corrosion functions of metallic MoS2 and graphene for remarkable hydrogen evolution over CdS. *J. Mater. Chem. A* **2021**, *9*, 1552–1562. [CrossRef]
28. Nam, N.N.; Do, H.D.K.; Trinh, K.T.L.; Lee, N.Y. Design Strategy and Application of Deep Eutectic Solvents for Green Synthesis of Nanomaterials. *Nanomaterials* **2023**, *13*, 1164. [CrossRef]
29. Zhang, C.; Fu, Y.; Gao, W.; Bai, T.; Cao, T.; Jin, J.; Xin, B. Deep Eutectic Solvent-Mediated Electrocatalysts for Water Splitting. *Molecules* **2022**, *27*, 8098. [CrossRef]
30. Zhang, D.; Mou, H.; Lu, F.; Song, C.; Wang, D. A Novel Strategy for 2D/2D NiS/Graphene Heterostructures as Efficient Bifunctional Electrocatalysts for Overall Water Splitting. *Appl. Catal. B Environ.* **2019**, *254*, 471–478. [CrossRef]
31. Isaifan, R.J.; Amhamed, A. Review on carbon dioxide absorption by choline chloride/urea deep eutectic solvents. *Adv. Chem.* **2018**, *2018*, 2675659a. [CrossRef]
32. Ma, D.; Wang, Z.; Shi, J.-W.; Zhu, M.; Yu, H.; Zou, Y.; Lv, Y.; Sun, G.; Mao, S.; Cheng, Y. Cu-In$_2$S$_3$ Nanorod Induced the Growth of Cu&In Co-Doped Multi-Arm CdS Hetero-Phase Junction to Promote Photocatalytic H$_2$ Evolution. *Chem. Eng. J.* **2020**, *399*, 125785. [CrossRef]
33. Shen, R.; Ren, D.; Ding, Y.; Guan, Y.; Ng, Y.H.; Zhang, P.; Li, X. Nanostructured CdS for Efficient Photocatalytic H$_2$ Evolution: A Review. *Sci. China Mater.* **2020**, *63*, 2153–2188. [CrossRef]
34. Park, J.; Lee, T.H.; Kim, C.; Lee, S.A.; Choi, M.J.; Kim, H.; Yang, J.W.; Lim, J.; Jang, W.H. Hydrothermally Obtained Type-II Heterojunction Nanostructures of In$_2$S$_3$/TiO$_2$ for Remarkably Enhanced Photoelectrochemical Water Splitting. *Appl. Catal. B Environ.* **2021**, *295*, 120276. [CrossRef]
35. He, B.; Bie, C.; Fei, X.; Cheng, B.; Yu, J.; Ho, W.; Al-Ghamdi, A.A.; Wangeh, S. Enhancement in the Photocatalytic H$_2$ Production Activity of CdS NrS by Ag$_2$S and NiS Dual Cocatalysts. *Appl. Catal. B Environ.* **2021**, *288*, 119994. [CrossRef]
36. She, H.; Sun, Y.; Li, S.; Huang, J.; Wang, L.; Zhu, G.; Wang, Q. Synthesis of Non-Noble Metal Nickel Doped Sulfide Solid Solution for Improved Photocatalytic Performance. *Appl. Catal. B Environ.* **2019**, *245*, 439–447. [CrossRef]
37. Marinoiu, A.; Raceanu, M.; Carcadea, E.; Varlam, M. Nitrogen-Doped Graphene Oxide as Efficient Metal-Free Electrocatalyst in PEM Fuel Cells. *Nanomaterials* **2023**, *13*, 1233. [CrossRef]
38. Wang, H.J.; Wan, Y.; Li, B.R.; Ye, J.; Gan, J.; Liu, J.; Liu, X.; Song, X.; Zhou, W.; Li, X.; et al. Rational design of Ce-doped CdS/N-rGO photocatalyst enhanced interfacial charges transfer for high effective degradation of tetracycline. *J. Mater. Sci. Technol.* **2024**, *173*, 137–148. [CrossRef]
39. Du, M.; Wang, Z.; Yang, C.; Deng, Y.; Wang, T.; Zhong, W.; Yin, W.; Jiao, Z.; Xia, W.; Jiang, B.; et al. N-doped reduced graphene oxide/Co$_{0.85}$Se microflowers with high mass loading as battery-type materials for quasi-solid-state hybrid supercapacitors. *J. Alloys Compd.* **2021**, *890*, 161801. [CrossRef]
40. He, Y.; Xu, G.; Wang, C.; Xu, L.; Zhang, K. Horsetail-Derived Si@N-Doped Carbon as Low-Cost and Long Cycle Life Anode for Li-Ion Half/Full Cells. *Electrochim. Acta* **2018**, *264*, 173–182. [CrossRef]
41. Xu, H.; Wang, Y.; Dong, X.; Zheng, N.; Ma, H.; Zhang, X. Fabrication of In$_2$O$_3$/In$_2$S$_3$ Microsphere Heterostructures for Efficient and Stable Photocatalytic Nitrogen Fixation. *Appl. Catal. B Environ.* **2019**, *257*, 117932. [CrossRef]
42. Liu, S.; Guo, X.; Wang, W.; Yang, Y.; Zhu, C.; Li, C.; Lin, W.; Tian, Q.; Liu, Y. CdS-Cu$_{1.81}$S Heteronanorods with Continuous Sublattice for Photocatalytic Hydrogen Production. *Appl. Catal. B Environ.* **2022**, *303*, 120909. [CrossRef]
43. Liu, S.; Ma, y.; Chi, D.; Sun, Y.; Chen, Q.; Zhang, J.; He, Z.; He, L.; Zhang, K.; Liu, B. Hollow Heterostructure CoS/CdS Photocatalysts with Enhanced Charge Transfer for Photocatalytic Hydrogen Production from Seawater. *Int. J. Hydrog. Energ.* **2022**, *47*, 9220–9229. [CrossRef]
44. Shi, Y.; Lei, X.; Xia, L.; Wu, Q.; Yao, W. Enhanced Photocatalytic Hydrogen Production Activity of CdS Coated with Zn-Anchored Carbon Layer. *Chem. Eng. J.* **2020**, *393*, 124751. [CrossRef]
45. Huang, X.; Lei, R.; Yuan, J.; Gao, F.; Jiang, C.; Feng, W.; Zhuang, J.; Liu, P. Insight into the Piezo-Photo Coupling Effect of PbTiO$_3$/CdS Composites for Piezo-Photocatalytic Hydrogen Production. *Appl. Catal. B Environ.* **2021**, *282*, 119586. [CrossRef]
46. Wang, Q.; Li, J.; Bai, Y.; Lian, J.; Huang, H.; Li, Z.; Lei, Z.; Shangguan, W. Photochemical Preparation of Cd/CdS Photocatalysts and Their Efficient Photocatalytic Hydrogen Production under Visible Light Irradiation. *Green. Chem.* **2014**, *16*, 2728–2735. [CrossRef]

47. Wang, Y.; Wang, X.; Ji, Y.; Bian, R.; Li, J.; Zhang, X.; Tian, J.; Yang, Q.; Shi, F. Ti$_3$C$_2$ Mxene Coupled with CdS Nanoflowers as 2D/3D Heterostructures for Enhanced Photocatalytic Hydrogen Production Activity. *Int. J. Hydrog. Energ.* **2022**, *47*, 22045–22053. [CrossRef]
48. Deng, C.; Ye, F.; Wang, T.; Ling, X.; Peng, L.; Yu, H.; Ding, K.; Hu, H.; Dong, Q.; Le, H.; et al. Developing Hierarchical CdS/NiO Hollow Heterogeneous Architectures for Boosting Photocatalytic Hydrogen Generation. *Nano Res.* **2022**, *15*, 2003–2012. [CrossRef]
49. Yuan, C.; Lv, H.; Zhang, Y.; Fei, Q.; Xiao, D.; Yin, H.; Lu, Z.; Zhang, Y. Three-Dimensional Nanoporous Heterojunction of CdS/np-rGO for Highly Efficient Photocatalytic Hydrogen Evolution under Visible Light. *Carbon* **2023**, *206*, 237–245. [CrossRef]
50. Li, X.; Gao, Y.; Li, N.; Ge, L. In-Situ Constructing Cobalt Incorporated Nitrogen-Doped Carbon/CdS Heterojunction with Efficient Interfacial Charge Transfer for Photocatalytic Hydrogen Evolution. *Int. J. Hydrogen Energy* **2022**, *47*, 27961–27972. [CrossRef]
51. Xu, M.; Kang, Y.; Jiang, L.; Jiang, L.; Tremblay, P.-L.; Zhang, T. The One-Step Hydrothermal Synthesis of CdS Nanorods Modified with Carbonized Leaves from Japanese Raisin Trees for Photocatalytic Hydrogen Evolution. *Int. J. Hydrogen Energy* **2022**, *47*, 15516–15527. [CrossRef]
52. Yu, G.; Gong, K.; Xing, C.; Hu, L.; Huang, H.; Gao, L.; Wang, D.; Li, X. Dual P-doped-site modified porous g-C$_3$N$_4$ achieves high dissociation and mobility efficiency for photocatalytic H$_2$O$_2$ production. *Chem. Eng. J.* **2023**, *461*, 142140. [CrossRef]
53. Zhu, Y.; Wan, T.; Wen, X.; Chu, D.; Jiang, Y. Tunable Type I and II heterojunction of CoOx nanoparticles confined in g-C3N4 nanotubes for photocatalytic hydrogen production. *Appl. Catal. B Environ.* **2019**, *244*, 814–822. [CrossRef]
54. Sahoo, S.; Shim, J.J. Nanostructured 3D zinc cobaltite/nitrogen-doped reduced graphene oxide composite electrode for supercapacitor applications. *J. Ind. Eng. Chem.* **2017**, *54*, 205–217. [CrossRef]
55. Yang, H.; Tang, J.; Luo, Y.; Zhan, X.; Liang, Z.; Jiang, L.; Hou, H.; Yang, W. MOFs-derived fusiform In$_2$O$_3$ mesoporous nanorods anchored with ultrafine CdZnS nanoparticles for boosting visible-light photocatalytic hydrogen evolution. *Small* **2021**, *17*, 2102307. [CrossRef]

Disclaimer/Publisher's Note: The statements, opinions and data contained in all publications are solely those of the individual author(s) and contributor(s) and not of MDPI and/or the editor(s). MDPI and/or the editor(s) disclaim responsibility for any injury to people or property resulting from any ideas, methods, instructions or products referred to in the content.

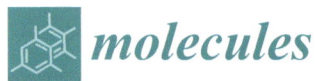

Article

Synthesis and Hydrogen Production Performance of MoP/a-TiO$_2$/Co-ZnIn$_2$S$_4$ Flower-like Composite Photocatalysts

Keliang Wu [1], Yuhang Shang [1], Huazhen Li [2], Pengcheng Wu [3], Shuyi Li [1], Hongyong Ye [1], Fanqiang Jian [1], Junfang Zhu [4], Dongmei Yang [4], Bingke Li [1,*] and Xiaofei Wang [5,*]

1. Henan Key Laboratory of Microbial Fermentation, School of Biology and Chemical Engineering, Nanyang Institute of Technology, Nanyang 473000, China; yehongyong2016@163.com (H.Y.)
2. Anhui Yansheng New Material Co., Ltd., Hefei 230039, China
3. School of Chemistry and Chemical Engineering, Shihezi University, Shihezi 832003, China
4. Department of Petroleum and Chemical, Bayingoleng Vocational and Technical College, Bazhou 841000, China
5. College of Materials and Chemical Engineering, West Anhui University, Lu'an 237012, China
* Correspondence: libingke86@nyist.edu.cn (B.L.); smilewxf@163.com (X.W.)

Abstract: Semiconductor photocatalysis is an effective strategy for solving the problems of increasing energy demand and environmental pollution. ZnIn$_2$S$_4$-based semiconductor photocatalyst materials have attracted much attention in the field of photocatalysis due to their suitable energy band structure, stable chemical properties, and good visible light responsiveness. In this study, ZnIn$_2$S$_4$ catalysts were modified by metal ion doping, the construction of heterojunctions, and co-catalyst loading to successfully prepare composite photocatalysts. The Co-ZnIn$_2$S$_4$ catalyst synthesized by Co doping and ultrasonic exfoliation exhibited a broader absorption band edge. Next, an a-TiO$_2$/Co-ZnIn$_2$S$_4$ composite photocatalyst was successfully prepared by coating partly amorphous TiO$_2$ on the surface of Co-ZnIn$_2$S$_4$, and the effect of varying the TiO$_2$ loading time on photocatalytic performance was investigated. Finally, MoP was loaded as a co-catalyst to increase the hydrogen production efficiency and reaction activity of the catalyst. The absorption edge of MoP/a-TiO$_2$/Co-ZnIn$_2$S$_4$ was widened from 480 nm to about 518 nm, and the specific surface area increased from 41.29 m^2/g to 53.25 m^2/g. The hydrogen production performance of this composite catalyst was investigated using a simulated light photocatalytic hydrogen production test system, and the rate of hydrogen production by MoP/a-TiO$_2$/Co-ZnIn$_2$S$_4$ was found to be 2.96 mmol·h^{-1}·g^{-1}, which was three times that of the pure ZnIn$_2$S$_4$ (0.98 mmol·h^{-1}·g^{-1}). After use in three cycles, the hydrogen production only decreased by 5%, indicating that it has good cycle stability.

Keywords: ZnIn$_2$S$_4$; Co doping; TiO$_2$; photocatalysis; hydrogen evolution

Citation: Wu, K.; Shang, Y.; Li, H.; Wu, P.; Li, S.; Ye, H.; Jian, F.; Zhu, J.; Yang, D.; Li, B.; et al. Synthesis and Hydrogen Production Performance of MoP/a-TiO$_2$/Co-ZnIn$_2$S$_4$ Flower-like Composite Photocatalysts. *Molecules* 2023, 28, 4350. https://doi.org/10.3390/molecules28114350

Academic Editor: Sugang Meng

Received: 3 April 2023
Revised: 12 May 2023
Accepted: 20 May 2023
Published: 25 May 2023

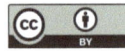

Copyright: © 2023 by the authors. Licensee MDPI, Basel, Switzerland. This article is an open access article distributed under the terms and conditions of the Creative Commons Attribution (CC BY) license (https://creativecommons.org/licenses/by/4.0/).

1. Introduction

The energy crisis is an ongoing global issue of increasing importance. Moreover, the rapid development of industrialization around the world has led to severe energy and environmental pressures [1]. Thus, there is an increased emphasis on research worldwide to successfully address the global energy crisis and to create new sustainable sources of energy [2]. The capture and conversion of solar energy by the photocatalytic splitting of water offers a promising strategy for converting inexhaustible solar energy into hydrogen (H$_2$) energy [3]. However, there are currently two main constraints that limit the large-scale application of hydrogen: (1) the large-scale green synthesis of hydrogen is a significant challenge; (2) the storage and transport of hydrogen is also difficult [4]. Hydrogen's shortcomings are partly explained by high infrastructure costs for production, storage, and distribution. These problems may result from their low energy density per volume, explosive characteristics, and ability to cause embrittlement in metals such as steel [5]. Many methods have been investigated for the production of hydrogen. The photocatalytic decomposition of water for hydrogen production is one of the simplest, most environmentally friendly and low-cost methods for producing hydrogen. Therefore, this method has attracted extensive research attention [6]. In particular, the production of hydrogen via the solar photolysis of water is gaining increasing attention due to its potential for solving the global energy crisis and mitigating environmental pollution problems [7,8]. Photogenerated charge carriers can be excited from photocatalysts under sunlight, and after the photogenerated electrons migrate to the surface of semiconductors, H^+ in water receives electrons that are reduced to H_2. The holes left behind are combined with sacrificial agents in the system and used to achieve continuous H_2 production.

In photocatalytic systems, the mobility of photogenerated carriers is an important factor affecting photocatalytic efficiency, with a fast migration rate and high separation efficiency positively contributing to the photocatalytic reaction [9]. The electrostatic potential of $ZnIn_2S_4$ with a hexagonal laminar structure is uniformly distributed within the plane, and the small potential of this material is well conducive to carrier migration [10]. Moreover, the positive charges are densely distributed in the indium sulfide tetrahedra and octahedra within the cell, while the negative charges are concentrated in the zinc indium tetrahedral [11]. Therefore, photogenerated electrons are easily transferred to the indium sulfide polyhedra, while the photogenerated holes more easily migrate to the zinc indium tetrahedra, which improves the separation efficiency of the photogenerated carriers [12]. Furthermore, the band gap of $ZnIn_2S_4$ is 2.3~2.5 eV and the energy band of $ZnIn_2S_4$ is narrow, which is also conducive to the generation of photogenerated carriers [13]. $ZnIn_2S_4$ is therefore an ideal photocatalytic material with broad application prospects.

In 2003, Lei et al. [14] synthesized $ZnIn_2S_4$ by a hydrothermal method and used this material as an effective visible-light-driven hydrogen precipitation photocatalyst for the first time. Guo's group [15] synthesized $ZnIn_2S_4$ microspheres by a hydrothermal/solvothermal process and explored their visible-light-driven photocatalytic hydrogen production performance. Their findings showed that these microsphere catalysts had a good potential for producing photocatalytic hydrogen from water when exposed to visible light [16].

However, pure $ZnIn_2S_4$ photocatalysts still suffer from low visible light utilization and low photocatalytic activity [17]. Moreover, the photocatalytic activity of $ZnIn_2S_4$ semiconductors is affected to some extent by their limited photogenerated electron and hole separation efficiency under visible light irradiation and low photogenerated carrier mobility [18]. Therefore, Yuan Wenhui et al. [19] prepared a series of Co-doped $ZnIn_2S_4$ photocatalysts using a solvothermal synthesis method. The successful incorporation of Co into the $ZnIn_2S_4$ lattice was confirmed by X-ray diffraction (XRD) and X-ray photoelectron spectroscopy (XPS). With increasing Co concentration, the absorption edge of the samples caused red-shift, but the Co also gradually disrupted the $ZnIn_2S_4$ morphology. Their photocatalytic results showed that Co^{2+} doping significantly improved the photocatalytic activity of $ZnIn_2S_4$. The optimum Co doping amount of 0.3 wt% for the $ZnIn_2S_4$ photocatalyst led to the highest photocatalytic activity [20]. Therefore, in this work, a doping amount of 0.3% was chosen to preserve the petal-like morphology and enhance the specific surface area of $ZnIn_2S_4$ while also improving its hydrogen production performance and utilization of sunlight [21,22].

TiO_2 has been widely investigated as a semiconductor photocatalyst material due to its many advantages, such as high stability and high photosensitivity. Therefore, TiO_2-based metal oxide photocatalysts are widely used in many practical applications [23]. However, TiO_2 particles easily agglomerate, have a low adsorption capacity for organic matter, and exhibit low solar energy utilization [24]. These factors limit the photocatalytic efficiency of TiO_2 and seriously affect its application in practical production [25]. The focus of photocatalytic research has therefore shifted from the improvement of traditional TiO_2 performance to the investigation of other catalysts with better performance in the visible light range. Amorphous TiO_2 is an important category of TiO_2 materials that exhibits the common "short-range order, long-range disorder" [26] structural feature seen in amorphous materials. Amorphous semiconductors have a large number of suspended bonds. Therefore, the energy band structures of amorphous materials exhibit a gap band between the valence band and the conduction band [27]. Amorphous TiO_2 with a lower band gap width can be obtained by modifying its electronic structure. This reduces the energy intensity required for electrons to transfer from the valence band to the conduction band [28]. Therefore, visible light irradiation can be used to activate these materials, improving their photocatalytic activity [29]. Zywitzki et al. reported amorphous titania-based photocatalysts synthesized using a facile, UV-light mediated method and evaluated as photocatalysts for hydrogen evolution from water/methanol mixtures. The resulting amorphous materials exhibited an overall higher hydrogen evolution rate (1.09 mmol·h^{-1}·g^{-1}) compared to a crystalline TiO_2 reference (P25 0.80 mmol·h^{-1}·g^{-1}) on a molar basis of the photocatalyst due to their highly porous structure and high surface area [30].

The photocatalytic activity of a photocatalyst is determined by its light absorption capacity as well as its electron–hole transfer and separation efficiency [31]. These factors are related to the catalyst surface properties, which play an important role in photocatalytic processes. For instance, the loading of co-catalysts on a photocatalyst surface to provide hydrogen production sites has been commonly reported in the literature [32]. Some common co-catalysts include alumina and potassium oxide. MoP is commonly used as an efficient catalyst for hydrodesulfurization (HDS) and hydrodenitrogenation (HDN) reactions [33]. Depending on the reversibility of hydrogen bonding to the catalyst, some catalysts used for HDS reactions are also useful for HER reactions because of the similar pathways and mechanisms of hydrogen production and hydrogenation as well as their low Tafel slope and low over potential. For example, Chen et al. [34] impregnated precursors on sponges to obtain MoP with a large specific surface area and enhanced photocatalytic activity. MoP cannot be directly used as a photocatalyst, but it can be used as an efficient hydrogen precipitation co-catalyst. Du et al. used MoP as a highly active co-catalyst on CdS nanorods for the first time, which significantly improved the photocatalytic activity of their CdS catalyst [35]. Thus, MoP is an efficient co-catalyst for hydrogen precipitation.

At present, the utilization of solar energy by metal oxide photocatalysts for hydrogen production has mainly focused on the UV wavelength range. Furthermore, most research is based on TiO_2 semiconductor photocatalytic materials. The majority of the wavelengths that make up solar energy, though, do not fall inside the visible spectrum. $ZnIn_2S_4$ shows promise as a visible-light-responsible ternary metal–sulfur compound photocatalyst, but its performance still needs to be improved. Therefore, in this work, $ZnIn_2S_4$ materials were prepared and modified (as shown in Figure 1): (1) Petal-shaped $ZnIn_2S_4$ catalysts were produced, their morphology was studied, and their photocatalytic performance was investigated. (2) Co-$ZnIn_2S_4$ was prepared by Co doping and ultrasonic exfoliation to broaden the absorption band edge and retain the petal-shaped morphology of the catalyst. (3) An a-TiO_2/Co-$ZnIn_2S_4$ composite photocatalyst was successfully prepared by coating amorphous TiO_2 on the Co-$ZnIn_2S_4$ surface, and the effect of loading different amounts of TiO_2 on the photocatalytic performance was investigated. At the same time, a TiO_2 and Co-$ZnIn_2S_4$ heterojunction was constructed, which led to the red-shift of the absorption band, enhanced light absorption properties, and a reduction in photogenerated electron–hole recombination. (4) Finally, MoP was loaded on the a-TiO_2/Co-$ZnIn_2S_4$ catalyst as a co-catalyst, which enhanced the light absorption intensity and provided reaction sites to promote the overall efficiency of catalytic hydrogen production. Therefore, MoP/a-TiO_2/Co-$ZnIn_2S_4$ flower-like composite photocatalysts with good photocatalytic hydrogen production activity and stability were prepared. This catalyst uses Co-$ZnIn_2S_4$ as the main body for photo generated electron excitation, and amorphous a-TiO_2 is combined with it to improve the efficiency of electron hole separation. Finally, MoP is used as a co-catalyst to provide hydrogen production sites, thus achieving efficient hydrogen production.

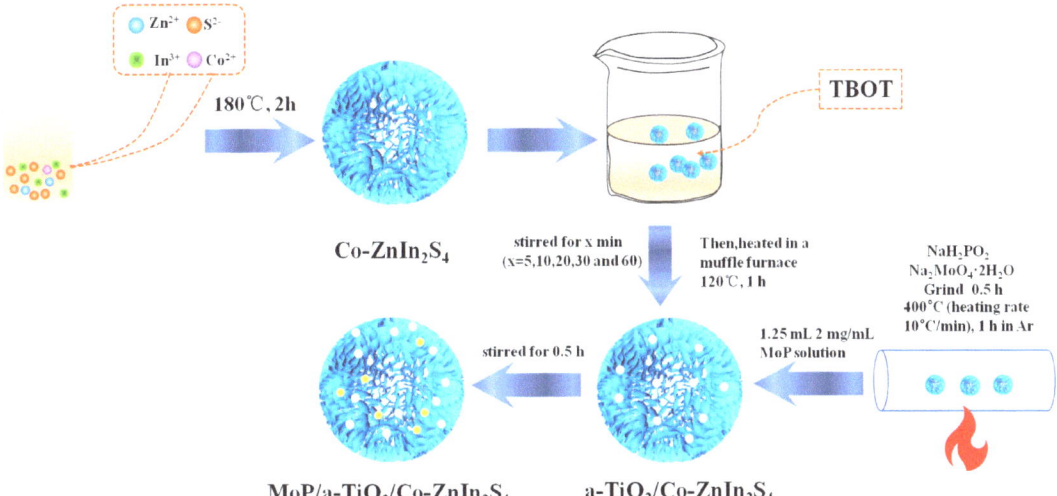

Figure 1. Steps for preparation of MoP/a-TiO$_2$/Co-ZnIn$_2$S$_4$ flower-like composite photocatalysts.

2. Results and Discussions

2.1. Structure, Morphology and Composition of Composite Photocatalysts

The synthesized ZnIn$_2$S$_4$ and loaded catalyst samples were characterized to investigate their morphology and microstructures, as shown by the SEM images in Figure 2. Figure 2a shows that the synthesized ZnIn$_2$S$_4$ was a petal-like microsphere consisting of a large number of nanoflakes, which are all made of ZnIn$_2$S$_4$ nanosheets. These nanoflakes were cross-linked to each other and formed many uniform slit-type pore structures between the petal layers. Figure 2b shows that Co doping did not change the flower-like structure of ZnIn$_2$S$_4$. No particles of Co aggregation were observed on the surface of the petals, so this demonstrated that Co was potentially doped into the lattice structure of ZnIn$_2$S$_4$. Figure 2c shows that the petals were loaded with a granular material, which indicated the successful loading of TiO$_2$. This was consistent with the catalyst morphology design. As shown in Figure 2d, the addition of MoP did not result in any obvious morphological changes. However, the MoP content was repeatedly low.

Element mapping (Figure 3 and Table 1) confirmed that MoP/TiO$_2$/Co-ZnIn$_2$S$_4$ contained S, Mo, In, Zn, Ti, O, P, and Co elements. All elements were evenly distributed without visible aggregation, further demonstrating the successful synthesis of the MoP/a-TiO$_2$/Co-ZnIn$_2$S$_4$ composite.

Table 1. Distribution of elements in the MoP/a-TiO$_2$/Co-ZnIn$_2$S$_4$ composite catalyst.

	In	S	Zn	Mo	P	Ti	O	Co
wt%	53.2	26.0	10.2	2.5	0.3	1.1	6.2	0.5

The morphological characteristics of the MoP/a-TiO$_2$/Co-ZnIn$_2$S$_4$ photocatalyst were further investigated by TEM, as shown in Figure 4. Figure 4a shows that the MoP/a-TiO$_2$/Co-ZnIn$_2$S$_4$ composite system had a nanoflower-like structure and intact, non-agglomerated microspheres. Figure 4b is a partial enlargement of Figure 4a, showing a more detailed view of the ZnIn$_2$S$_4$ nanosheets, which are very thin in the nanoflower. Some MoP/TiO$_2$ particles were visible on the nanosheets, which showed the successful loading of MoP and TiO$_2$ on the surface of ZnIn$_2$S$_4$. Figure 4c shows an electron diffraction pattern of the MoP/a-TiO$_2$/Co-ZnIn$_2$S$_4$ photocatalyst, demonstrating its good crystallinity. Lattice fringe spacings of 0.21, 0.32 and 0.35 nm were identified in Figure 4d, which respectively corresponded to MoP, ZnIn$_2$S$_4$, and TiO$_2$. This was consistent with the data in the relevant literature. Overall, this TEM analysis further demonstrated the successful preparation of MoP/a-TiO$_2$/Co-ZnIn$_2$S$_4$.

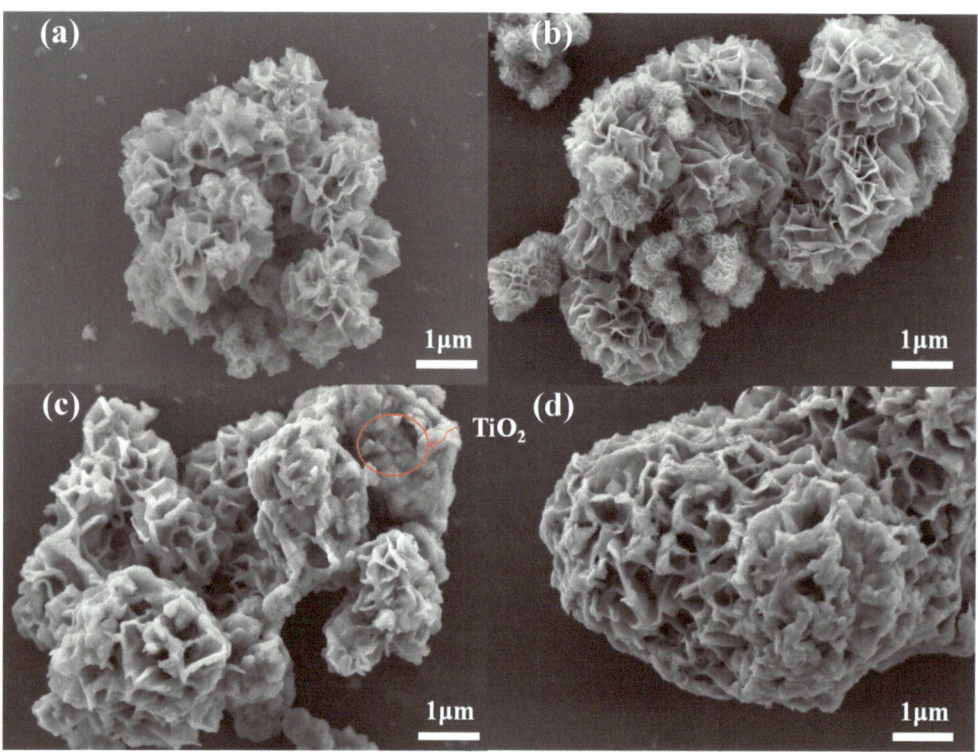

Figure 2. SEM micrographs of (**a**) ZnIn$_2$S$_4$, (**b**) Co-ZnIn$_2$S$_4$, (**c**) a-TiO$_2$/Co-ZnIn$_2$S$_4$, and (**d**) MoP/a-TiO$_2$/Co-ZnIn$_2$S$_4$.

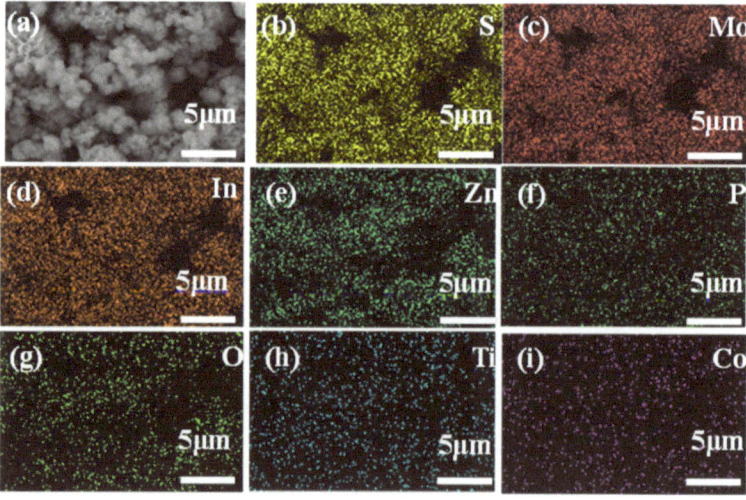

Figure 3. Elemental mapping of the MoP/a-TiO$_2$/Co-ZnIn$_2$S$_4$ composite catalyst. (**a**) scanning area, (**b**) S, (**c**) Mo, (**d**) In, (**e**) Zn, (**f**) P, (**g**) O, (**h**) Ti, (**i**) Co.

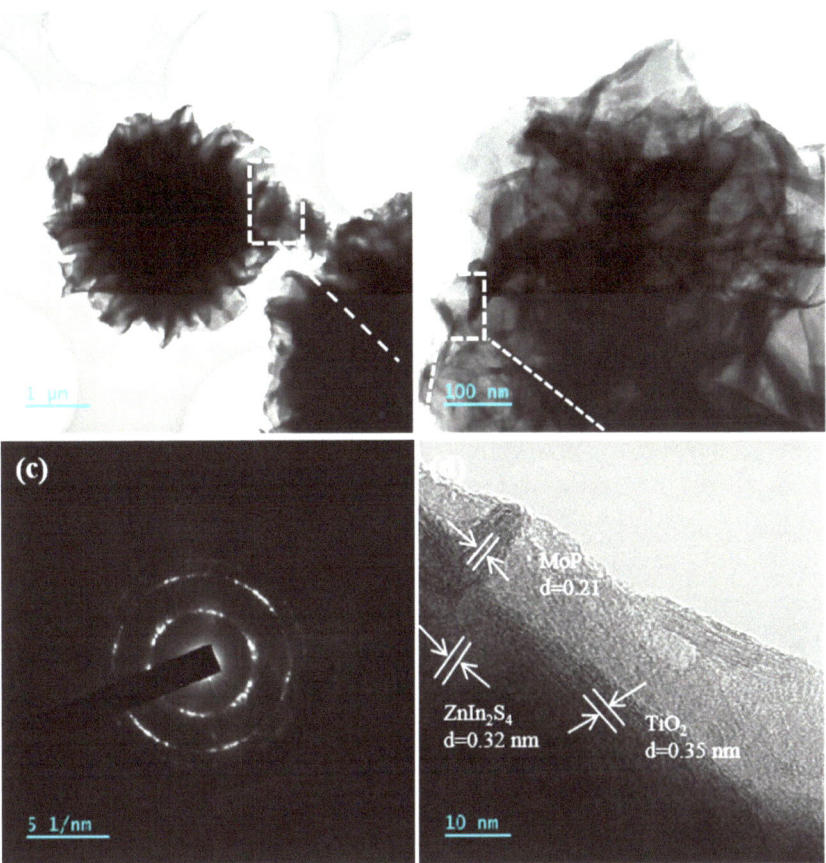

Figure 4. (**a**,**b**) TEM micrographs, (**c**) electron diffraction pattern, and (**d**) high-resolution TEM micrograph showing the lattice fringe spacing of MoP/a-TiO$_2$/Co-ZnIn$_2$S$_4$.

The catalyst samples were investigated by X-ray diffraction, as shown in Figure 5. Characteristic diffraction peaks were visible at 8.52°, 21.3°, 29.1°, and 49.3° for all four catalysts, and these peaks were consistent with standard cards JCPDS 49–1562 and JCPDS 48–1778. ZnIn$_2$S$_4$ is a direct bandgap semiconductor with a layered (according to card NO. 48–1778, a = b = c = 10.6, α = β = γ = 90°) and trigonal structure (ICSD-JCPDS card NO. 49–1562, a = b = 3.85, c = 24.68, α = 37.01°, β = 90°, γ = 120°), as shown in Figure 5. All polymorphs show certain photocatalytic performance under visible light, while the hexagonal ZnIn$_2$S$_4$ has better photocatalytic performance. The cubic ZnIn$_2$S$_4$ is a direct cubicspinel phase when the S atoms in the unit cell are ABC stacking [36]. The diffraction peak positions did not significantly shift upon modification, which indicated that the ZnIn$_2$S$_4$ was not significantly affected. The shape of the ZnIn$_2$S$_4$ peaks did not change after TiO$_2$ loading and no separate TiO$_2$ peaks were identified, indicating that partly amorphous TiO$_2$ was synthesized. The diffraction peaks also did not change after the addition of MoP, indicating the successful preparation of the composite MoP/a-TiO$_2$/Co-ZnIn$_2$S$_4$ catalyst.

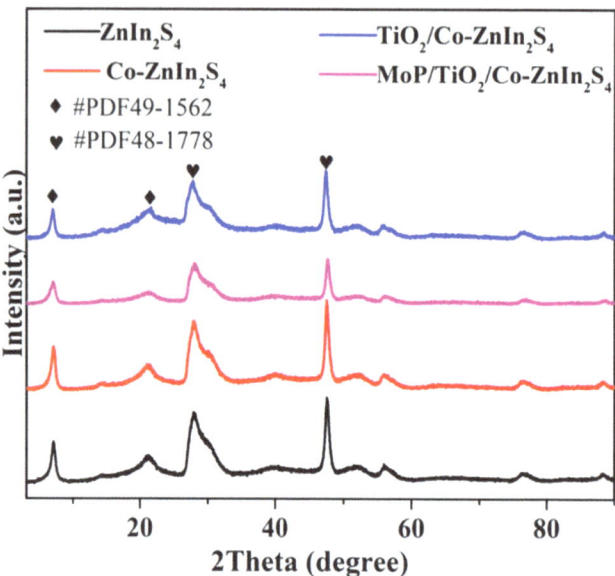

Figure 5. XRD patterns of the $ZnIn_2S_4$, $Co-ZnIn_2S_4$, $a-TiO_2/Co-ZnIn_2S_4$, and $MoP/a-TiO_2/Co-ZnIn_2S_4$, photocatalysts.

Figure 6a,b shows the N_2 adsorption–desorption isotherms and pore size distributions of $ZnIn_2S_4$, $Co-ZnIn_2S_4$, $a-TiO_2/Co-ZnIn_2S_4$ and $MoP/a-TiO_2/Co-ZnIn_2S_4$. All four isotherms were identified as type IV, and they contained H3 hysteresis loops. Moreover, the catalysts exhibited pore sizes ranging from 10 to 100 nm. As shown in Table 2, the specific surface area slightly changed after catalyst modification. Specifically, $MoP/a-TiO_2/Co-ZnIn_2S_4$ showed a slight increase in specific surface area compared with pure $ZnIn_2S_4$. The pore volume of $MoP/a-TiO_2/Co-ZnIn_2S_4$ was also slightly higher than that of pure $ZnIn_2S_4$. This was consistent with the SEM image shown in Figure 2c, in which some of the TiO_2 nanoparticles were supported on the $ZnIn_2S_4$ nanosheets. Therefore, the addition of TiO_2 and the MoP co-catalyst led to an increase in adsorption pore volume. Consequently, more adsorption and active sites were generated on the photocatalyst surface. Moreover, the modified catalysts exhibited lower pore sizes because TiO_2 was distributed between the $ZnIn_2S_4$ petals, which reduced the pore size.

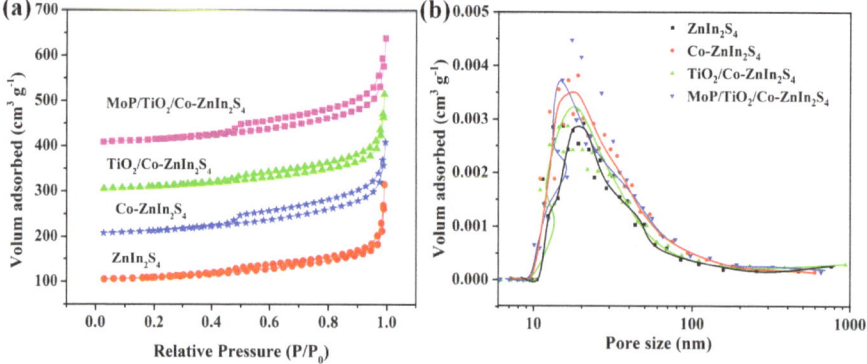

Figure 6. (**a**) N_2 adsorption–desorption isotherms and (**b**) pore size distributions of the $ZnIn_2S_4$, $Co-ZnIn_2S_4$, $a-TiO_2/Co-ZnIn_2S_4$, and $MoP/a-TiO_2/Co-ZnIn_2S_4$ photocatalysts.

Table 2. Specific surface area, pore volume, and average pore diameter of $ZnIn_2S_4$, $Co\text{-}ZnIn_2S_4$, $a\text{-}TiO_2/Co\text{-}ZnIn_2S_4$, and $MoP/a\text{-}TiO_2/Co\text{-}ZnIn_2S_4$.

Sample	Specific Surface Area (m²/g)	Pore Volume (cm³/g)	Average Pore Diameter (nm)
$ZnIn_2S_4$	41.293	0.3346	162.1
$Co\text{-}ZnIn_2S_4$	53.453	0.3242	121.3
$TiO_2/Co\text{-}ZnIn_2S_4$	46.669	0.3346	143.4
$MoP/a\text{-}TiO_2/Co\text{-}ZnIn_2S_4$	53.250	0.3703	139.1

The chemical state and chemical composition of the $MoP/a\text{-}TiO_2/Co\text{-}ZnIn_2S_4$ composite was analyzed by XPS. As shown in Figure 7, the XPS survey spectrum confirmed the presence of P, Mo, Ti, Zn, In and S elements in this composite photocatalyst. This was consistent with the EDS test results. The binding energy peaks at 445.1 eV, 225.9 eV, 139.8 eV and 161.9 eV were attributed to In3d, Mo3d, P2p and S 2p signals, respectively. This indicated the presence of MoP, TiO_2 and $ZnIn_2S_4$ in the $MoP/a\text{-}TiO_2/Co\text{-}ZnIn_2S_4$ composite photocatalyst. In the Ti 2p spectrum, the two main peaks near 458.7 eV and 464.5 eV were attributed to Ti $2p_{3/2}$ and Ti $2p_{1/2}$. These peaks were generated by the Ti^{4+} oxidation state of TiO_2. A single O1s peak near 530.0 eV was deconvoluted into three peaks. The peak at 530.0 eV was attributed to the presence of oxygen vacancies, and the peaks at 530.8 and 532.4 eV were caused by Ti–OH. This demonstrated that the synthesized TiO_2 was amorphous and that the presence of this TiO_2 increased the oxygen vacancy concentration of the catalyst. These results conclusively demonstrate that the $MoP/a\text{-}TiO_2/Co\text{-}ZnIn_2S_4$ composite photocatalyst was successfully prepared.

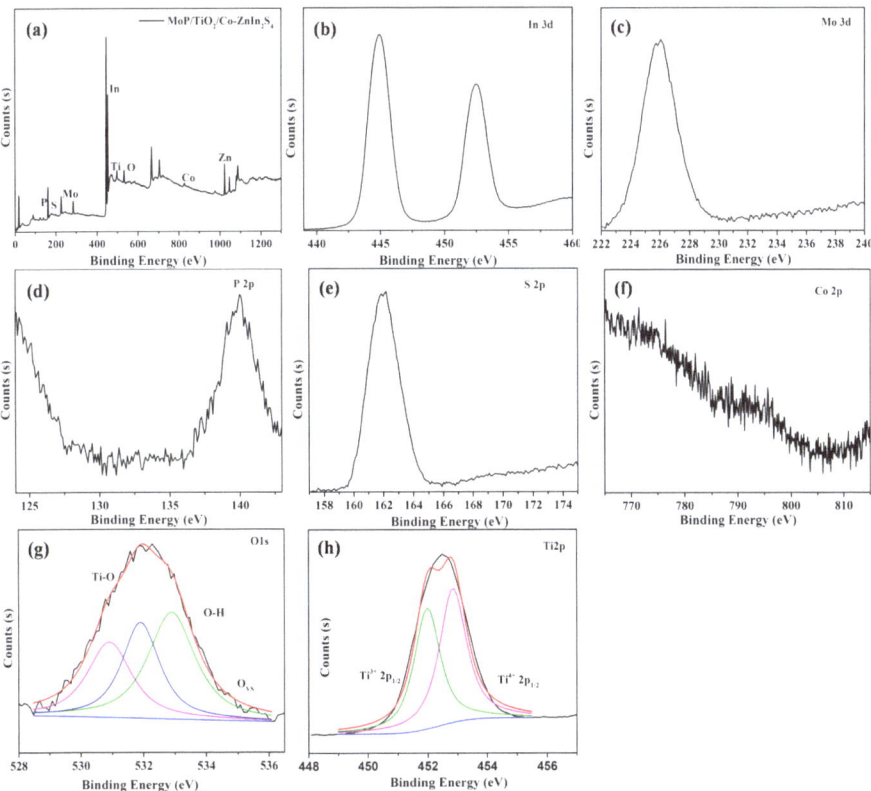

Figure 7. XPS spectra of the $MoP/a\text{-}TiO_2/Co\text{-}ZnIn_2S_4$ composite catalyst.

UV-vis diffuse reflectance spectra of TiO_2/Co-$ZnIn_2S_4$ were obtained using different TiO_2 loading times to explore the effect of TiO_2 on catalytic activity, as shown in Figure 8a. These spectra were denoted as X-TiO_2/Co-$ZnIn_2S_4$, where X represents the number of minutes. With increasing TiO_2 loading time, the light absorption intensity and range of this composite catalyst first increased and then decreased. In particular, at 20 min, the absorption side band of a-TiO_2/Co-$ZnIn_2S_4$ shifted to the right, and the highest absorption was achieved at this time. Therefore, 20-TiO_2/Co-$ZnIn_2S_4$ was selected as the basis for subsequent experiments. Figure 8b shows UV-vis diffuse reflectance spectra of $ZnIn_2S_4$, Co-$ZnIn_2S_4$, a-TiO_2/Co-$ZnIn_2S_4$ and MoP/a-TiO_2/Co-$ZnIn_2S_4$. The absorption edge of pure $ZnIn_2S_4$ synthesized in this study was 480 nm. As shown, the spectrum significantly changed after Co doping, reaching 500 nm. However, almost the same absorption was demonstrated after the addition of amorphous TiO_2. The absorption edge of MoP/a-TiO_2/Co-$ZnIn_2S_4$ was widened to about 518 nm, indicating that the MoP was photocatalyzed by the load. The band gap energies of $ZnIn_2S_4$, Co-$ZnIn_2S_4$, a-TiO_2/Co-$ZnIn_2S_4$ and MoP/a-TiO_2/Co-$ZnIn_2S_4$ were calculated using the curves shown in Figure 8b. As shown in Figure 8c, the band gap energy of MoP/a-TiO_2/Co-$ZnIn_2S_4$ was 2.7 eV. This analysis demonstrated the broader light absorption range and enhanced photocatalytic activity of the MoP/a-TiO_2/Co-$ZnIn_2S_4$ composite photocatalyst.

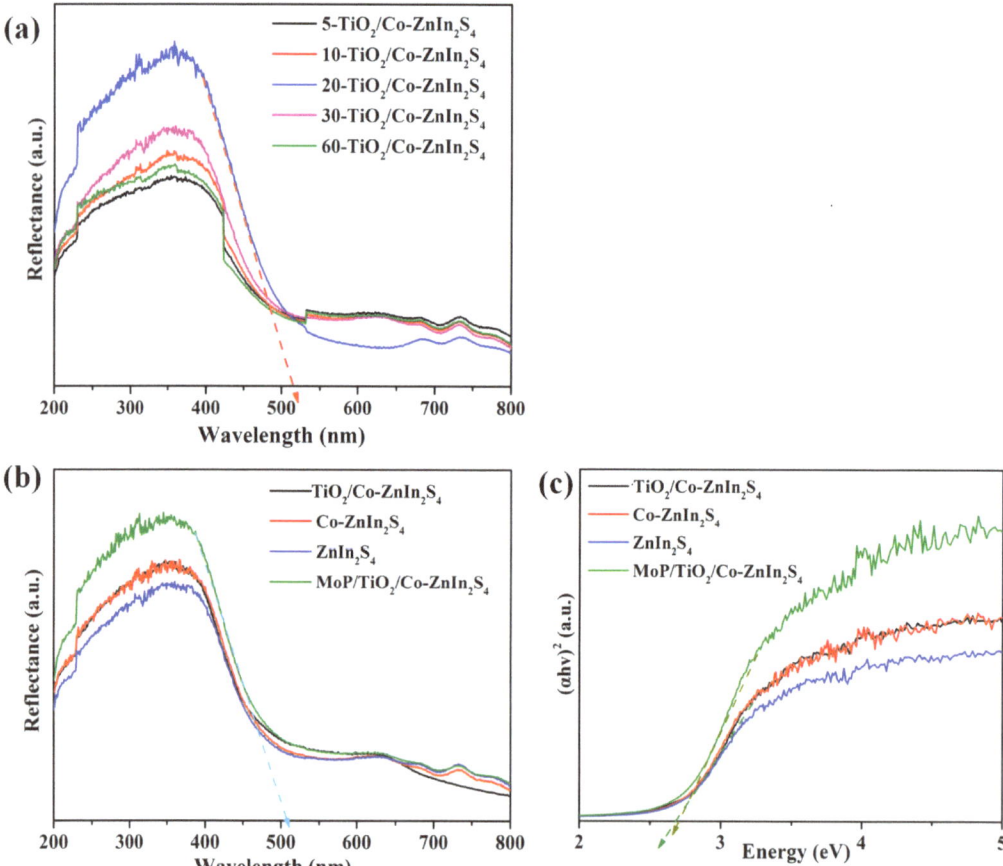

Figure 8. (**a**) UV-vis diffuse reflectance spectra of a-TiO_2/Co-$ZnIn_2S_4$ at different times; (**b**) UV-vis diffuse reflectance spectra and (**c**) bandgaps of $ZnIn_2S_4$, Co-$ZnIn_2S_4$, a-TiO_2/Co-$ZnIn_2S_4$, and MoP/a-TiO_2/Co-$ZnIn_2S_4$.

2.2. Photoelectrochemical Performance

The photoelectrical properties of the catalysts were characterized in order to study their photocatalytic activity. Figure 9a shows that the photocurrent starting positions of all the catalysts were significantly earlier than their dark current starting positions. In addition, compared with Co-ZnIn$_2$S$_4$, the initial positions of TiO$_2$/Co-ZnIn$_2$S$_4$ and MoP/a-TiO$_2$/Co-ZnIn$_2$S$_4$ were slightly shifted to the left. These results indicate that the composite catalyst had a lower activation energy and enhanced photocatalytic performance. Linear scan voltammetry curves of ZnIn$_2$S$_4$, Co-ZnIn$_2$S$_4$, a-TiO$_2$/Co-ZnIn$_2$S$_4$, and MoP/a-TiO$_2$/Co-ZnIn$_2$S$_4$ were obtained under both light and dark conditions, as shown in Figure 9b. This shows the photocurrent densities of ZnIn$_2$S$_4$, Co-ZnIn$_2$S$_4$, a-TiO$_2$/Co-ZnIn$_2$S$_4$ and MoP/a-TiO$_2$/Co-ZnIn$_2$S$_4$, which exhibited photocurrents of 1 µA/cm^2, 3 µA/cm^2, 4 µA/cm^2 and 4.5 µA/cm^2, respectively. This showed that Co doping significantly improved the performance of ZnIn$_2$S$_4$. Moreover, the separation efficiency of photogenerated electron–hole pairs was also significantly improved by the addition of TiO$_2$ supported on the ZnIn$_2$S$_4$ nanosheets. In addition, MoP/a-TiO$_2$/Co-ZnIn$_2$S$_4$ had a higher photocurrent density, therefore exhibiting more efficient carrier separation and transfer efficiency. The electrochemical impedance spectra shown in Figure 9c demonstrate that MoP/a-TiO$_2$/Co-ZnIn$_2$S$_4$ had lower high-frequency semicircles than Co-ZnIn$_2$S$_4$ or a-TiO$_2$/Co-ZnIn$_2$S$_4$ as well as lower resistance. This further indicated that MoP/a-TiO$_2$/Co-ZnIn$_2$S$_4$ had more efficient carrier separation and transfer efficiency. The line increase of curves Co-ZnIn$_2$S$_4$, a-TiO$_2$/Co-ZnIn$_2$S$_4$ and MoP/a-TiO$_2$/Co-ZnIn$_2$S$_4$ indicates that the charge transfer resistance decreases sequentially, which is also consistent with the higher carrier separation and transfer efficiency.

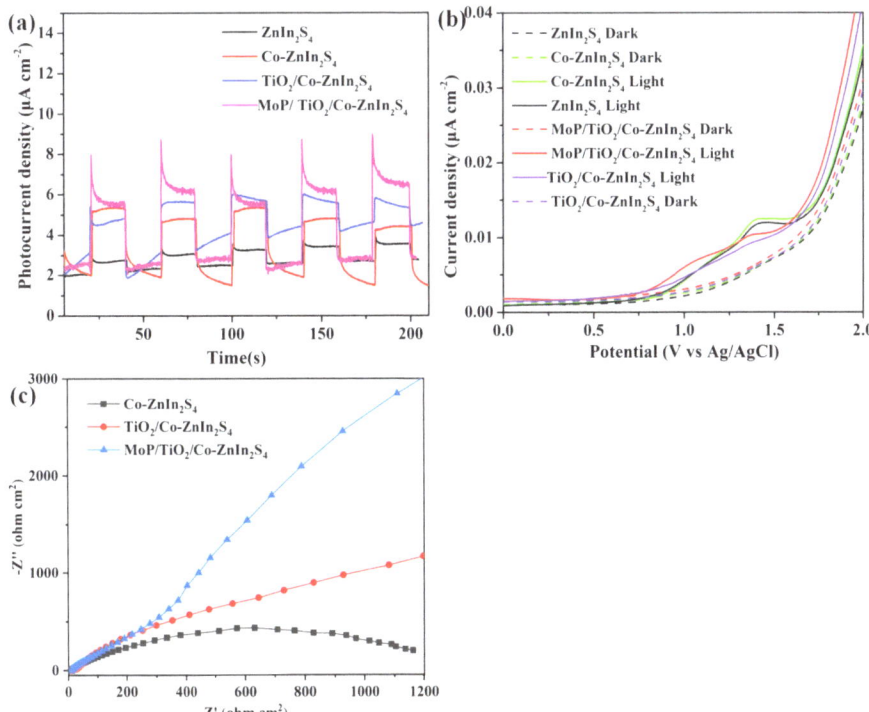

Figure 9. (**a**) Photocurrent response curves of Co-ZnIn$_2$S$_4$, a-TiO$_2$/Co-ZnIn$_2$S$_4$, and MoP/a-TiO$_2$/Co-ZnIn$_2$S$_4$; (**b**) linear scanning voltammograms and photocurrent response curves of ZnIn$_2$S$_4$, Co-ZnIn$_2$S$_4$, a-TiO$_2$/Co-ZnIn$_2$S$_4$, and MoP/a-TiO$_2$/Co-ZnIn$_2$S$_4$; (**c**) EIS curves of Co-ZnIn$_2$S$_4$, a-TiO$_2$/Co-ZnIn$_2$S$_4$, and MoP/a-TiO$_2$/Co-ZnIn$_2$S$_4$.

2.3. Photocatalytic Hydrogen Production Performance

The hydrogen production performance of the prepared catalysts was investigated, as shown in Figure 10. With increasing illumination time, hydrogen production increased for all four catalysts. As shown in Figure 10a, to explore the influence of the supported TiO_2 on catalytic activity, the photocatalytic hydrogen production performances of a-TiO_2/Co-$ZnIn_2S_4$ samples prepared by loading TiO_2 for different amounts of time were also investigated. The optimal hydrogen production rate of 3.88 mmol·g^{-1} was achieved by using 20-TiO_2/Co-$ZnIn_2S_4$, which was consistent with the UV-vis spectra shown in Figure 8a. The hydrogen production rates of $ZnIn_2S_4$, Co-$ZnIn_2S_4$, a-TiO_2/Co-$ZnIn_2S_4$, MoP/a-TiO_2/Co-$ZnIn_2S_4$ and P25 are shown in Figure 10b. As can be seen, Co doping, the addition of TiO_2, and the addition of MoP all led to enhanced hydrogen evolution. It also can be seen from Figure 10b that the hydrogen production using non-noble metal co-catalyst MoP (7.42 mmol·g^{-1}) is approximately twice as much as using Pt co-catalyst (3.88 mmol·g^{-1}). In addition, it can be observed from Figure 10b,c that the hydrogen production capacity and hydrogen production rate of Pt/P25 at 2.5 h is 6.43 mmol/g and 2.55 mmol·h^{-1}·g^{-1}, respectively. As shown in Figure 10c, the highest hydrogen production rate of 2.96 mmol·h^{-1}·g^{-1} was achieved by MoP/a-TiO_2/Co-$ZnIn_2S_4$; in contrast, the sample Pt/a-TiO_2/Co-$ZnIn_2S_4$ achieved 1.55 mmol·h^{-1}·g^{-1}. Each modification step (Co doping, addition of supported TiO_2, addition of MoP co-catalyst) further enhanced the hydrogen evolution rate compared with the unmodified $ZnIn_2S_4$. These results showed that the MoP/a-TiO_2/Co-$ZnIn_2S_4$ composite photocatalyst had excellent hydrogen production performance. It can be seen that the hydrogen production efficiency of the MoP/a-TiO_2/Co-$ZnIn_2S_4$ without Pt is still higher in comparison to that of P25 powder.

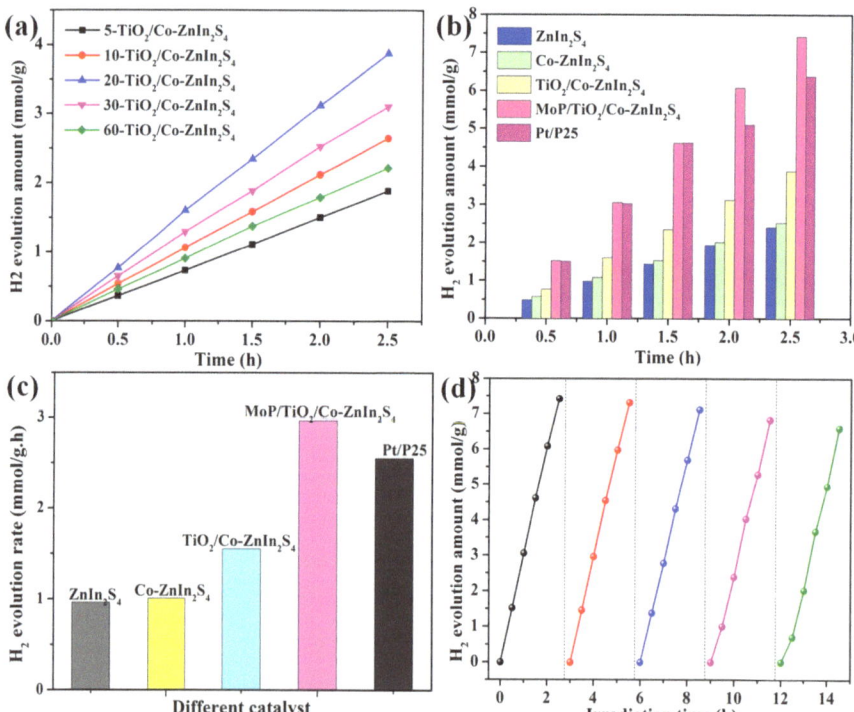

Figure 10. (**a**) Hydrogen production yields of a-TiO_2/Co-$ZnIn_2S_4$ samples prepared in different amounts of time for TiO_2 loading. (**b**) Hydrogen production yields of the prepared catalysts with increasing reaction time. (**c**) Hydrogen production rates of the prepared catalysts. (**d**) Hydrogen production of MoP/a-TiO_2/Co-$ZnIn_2S_4$ across 5 cycles.

Photocatalytic stability across multiple cycles is another important factor that influences the practical application of photocatalysts. Therefore, the MoP/a-TiO$_2$/Co-ZnIn$_2$S$_4$ composite catalyst was tested for cyclic hydrogen production. As shown in Figure 10d, after use in three cycles, the hydrogen production only decreased by 5%, indicating that it has good cycle stability. However, after 5 cycles, a slight decline in activity was observed (decline rate of 13.5%). This indicated a certain degree of catalytic stability. The degradation between cycles 3 and 4 (decline rate of 4.2%) was greater than that between cycles 1 and 2 (decline rate of 2.1%) due to the photocorrosion of ZnIn$_2$S$_4$.

2.4. Mechanism of Photocatalytic Hydrogen Evolution

According to the band gap structures and Fermi level of TiO$_2$ and ZnIn$_2$S$_4$, the possible transfer processes of photogenerated electron–hole pairs are proposed in Figure 11 [37]. The photogenerated electrons in the CB of ZnIn$_2$S$_4$ migrate to the CB of TiO$_2$ while the photoexcited holes in the VB of TiO$_2$ transfer to the VB of ZnIn$_2$S$_4$. The E$_{CB}$ of the photogenerated electrons is lower than the E$_0$ redox (H$^+$/H$_2$). The presumed process is, therefore, not feasible in this photocatalytic process. Another possible reaction mechanism is shown in Figure 11. In the photocatalytic reaction, the solid–solid contact interface between ZnIn$_2$S$_4$ and TiO$_2$ serves as the combination center of the photogenerated electrons in the CB of TiO$_2$ and the photogenerated holes in the VB of ZnIn$_2$S$_4$ [38]. The photogenerated electrons involved in the reaction have a stronger reduction ability than that of pure TiO$_2$, thus performing a better photocatalytic activity for HER. The photogenerated holes in the VB of TiO$_2$ oxidize water to O$_2$, while the photogenerated electrons in the CB of ZnIn$_2$S$_4$ simultaneously reduce H$^+$ to H$_2$. In summary, all of the above analyses show that the electron transfer process is identified as an S-scheme mechanism in this study.

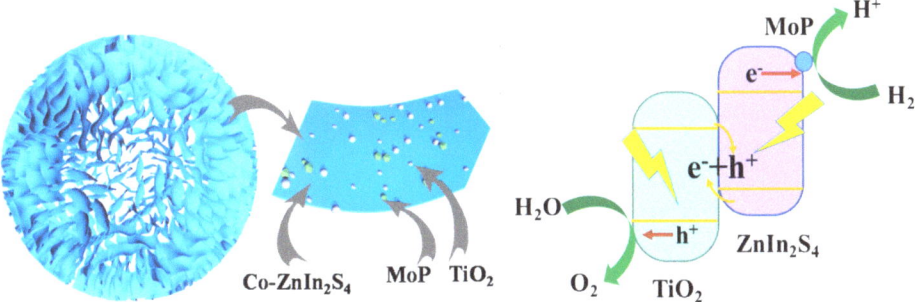

Figure 11. Composition diagram and photocatalytic reaction mechanism of MoP/a-TiO$_2$/Co-ZnIn$_2$S$_4$.

3. Experimental Section

3.1. Materials and Characterization

Zinc chloride (ZnCl$_2$, AR), indium chloride (InCl$_3$, AR), thioacetamide (TAA, AR), nickel chloride hexahydrate (NiCl$_2$·6H$_2$O, AR), tungsten chloride (WCl$_6$, AR), polyethylene glycol (HO(CH$_2$CH$_2$O)$_n$H, AR), melamine (C$_3$N$_3$(NH$_2$)$_3$, AR), and sodium citrate dehydrate (C$_6$H$_5$Na$_3$O$_7$·2H$_2$O, AR) were purchased from Shanghai Macklin Biochemical Co. (Shanghai, China) Triethanolamine (TEOA, AR) was purchased from Tianjin Beichen Founder Reagent Factory (Tianjin, China). Ethyl alcohol (CH$_3$CH$_2$OH, AR) was provided by Sinopharm Chemical Reagent Co., Ltd. (Shanghai, China). All materials were used as received.

Sample morphologies were analyzed using scanning electron microscopy (SEM, JSM-7900F, JEOL, Tokyo, Japan) coupled with energy-dispersive X-ray spectroscopy (OXFORD MAX-80, Oxford, UK). Transmission electron microscopy (TEM) was performed using a JSM-2100plus (JEOL, Tokyo, Japan). X-ray diffraction (XRD, Bruker (Billerica, MA, USA), D8 Advance) was used for crystal structure analysis. XRD patterns were obtained in the 2θ range of 20–90° with a scanning rate of 6°/min. Surface compositions were investigated by X-ray photoelectron spectroscopy (XPS) using an AMICUS ESCA3200 (Philadelphia,

PA, USA). The XPS spectra were corrected using the C1s peak at 284.8 eV. Ultraviolet-visible (UV-vis) diffuse reflectance spectra (DRS) were obtained in the 200–800 nm range by a UV-vis spectrophotometer (Shimadzu UV-2450, Kyoto, Japan). Photoluminescence (PL) spectra were collected using an Perkin-Elmer LS50B (Buckinghamshire, UK) with a 380 nm excitation wavelength at room temperature. BET surface areas and porosity were measured via nitrogen adsorption–desorption experiments using a Micromeritics ASAP 2020 (Micromeritics, Norcross, GA, USA).

3.2. Steps for Preparation of MoP/a-TiO$_2$/Co-ZnIn$_2$S$_4$ Flower-like Composite Photocatalysts

3.2.1. Preparation of Co-ZnIn$_2$S$_4$ Catalyst

A total of 0.136 g zinc chloride, 0.586 g indium chloride, and 0.301 g thioacetamide were weighed and added to 80 mL ethylene glycol. This mixture was stirred and centrifugally sonicated to dissolve the solid compounds. The solution was then transferred to a 100 mL hydrothermal kettle and heated in an oven at 180 °C for 2 h. After the reaction, the reaction solution was removed from the hydrothermal kettle and left to stand for 0.5 h. Next, centrifugation was used to obtain the solid product. The sample was then crushed with agate mortar to obtain ZnIn$_2$S$_4$. Doped Co-ZnIn$_2$S$_4$ was obtained by repeating this experimental procedure with the addition of 0.0069 g Co(NO$_3$)$_2$·6(H$_2$O).

3.2.2. Preparation of a-TiO$_2$/Co-ZnIn$_2$S$_4$ Catalyst

A total of 80 mg Co-ZnIn$_2$S$_4$ was added to 20 mL isopropanol. Then, 100 µL tetra-butyltitanate and 20 µL water were then added dropwise under stirring. Five samples were prepared and stirred for 5 min, 10 min, 20 min, 30 min and 60 min for the control test. These samples were centrifuged three times using isopropanol and then dried at 60 °C in an oven. The dried samples were ground and heated in a muffle furnace at 120 °C for 1 h to obtain a-TiO$_2$/Co-ZnIn$_2$S$_4$.

3.2.3. Preparation of MoP/a-TiO$_2$/Co-ZnIn$_2$S$_4$ Catalyst

A mixture of 1 g Na$_2$MoO$_4$·2H$_2$O and 10 g NaH$_2$PO$_2$ was ground in a mortar for 0.5 h until no crystal particles remained, and then transferred to a tubular furnace, under Ar protection at 400 °C (heating rate 10 °C/min), and calcined for 1 h to obtain MoP. A 2 mg/mL MoP solution was then prepared. Next, 0.5 g a-TiO$_2$/Co-ZnIn$_2$S$_4$ and 1.25 mL MoP solution were magnetically stirred for 0.5 h. MoP/a-TiO$_2$/Co-ZnIn$_2$S$_4$ was obtained by drying the resulting product in an oven at 60 °C followed by crushing with a mortar.

3.3. Photocatalysis and Photoelectrochemical Performance Measurements

3.3.1. Hydrogen Production Performance

Photocatalytic experiments were performed using an online photocatalytic hydrogen evolution system (Meiruichen, Beijing, China MC-SCO$_2$II-AG) at 5 °C using a 300 W Xe lamp equipped with a AM1.5G cutoff filter positioned 20 cm away from the reactor. A total of 10 mg of catalyst was dispersed in 100 mL of 0.1 M Na$_2$S and 0.1 M Na$_2$SO$_3$ solution and the mixture was stirred in vacuum for 30 min. We first ran tests in the dark for one hour to confirm no H$_2$ production. Hydrogen evolution, detected by an online gas chromatography (using FL9790, Fuli, Zhjiang, TCD with nitrogen as a carrier gas and 5 Å molecular sieve column) was observed only under light irradiation. At the end of the photocatalytic reaction, which lasted for 2.5 h, the reactor was refilled with 10 mL of Na$_2$S and Na$_2$SO$_3$ solutions and degassed. Then, 10 mg of P25 was dispersed in 100 mL of CH$_3$OH/H$_2$O solution, and 0.1 mL (1 mg/mL) of chloroplatinic acid was added.

3.3.2. Photoelectrochemical Performance

A CHI760E electrochemical workstation and a standard three-electrode system (platinum sheet, saturated silver chloride electrode, and the loaded FTO substrate) were used to analyze the catalysts. An aqueous 0.5 mol/L Na$_2$SO$_4$ solution was used as the electrolyte for transient photocurrent testing and electrochemical impedance spectroscopy (EIS) testing.

A xenon lamp light source system with an AM1.5G filter was used to simulate daylight for photocurrent testing.

Photocatalytic hydrogen production experiments were performed using a vacuum photocatalytic carbon dioxide reduction system with a xenon light source to simulate daylight. A working electrode for photochemical measurements was prepared using 7.5 mg of sample ($ZnIn_2S_4$, $Co-ZnIn_2S_4$, $a-TiO_2/Co-ZnIn_2S_4$ and $MoP/a-TiO_2/Co-ZnIn_2S_4$), which was sonicated for 30 min in a mixture containing 375 µL of ultrapure water, 125 of ethanol and 30 µL of naphthol. Then, 30 µL of the resulting suspension was used to drop-coat FTO glass, which was then heated for 30 min at 300 °C under Ar. A 1 cm × 1 cm glass substrate was then ultrasonicated first in acetone, then in ethanol and finally in water (15 min each step), after which it was dried by a flow of Ar. PEC measurements were conducted using a single compartment quartz cell with three electrodes. Data were recorded by the workstation equipment containing photoanode, saturated Ag/AgCl and 1 cm × 1 cm Pt piece as working, reference and counter electrodes, respectively. We used 0.2 M Na_2SO_4 with pH = 6.5 as electrolyte. PEC tests were conducted using a 150 W Xenon lamp equipped with a standard AM 1.5G filter. Quartz cell was positioned 10 cm away from the light source. The recorded potential was converted to reference hydrogen electrode (RHE) potentials using the following equation:

$$E_{RHE} = E_{Ag/AgCl} + pH * 0.059 + 0.195 \text{ V}$$

Linear sweep voltammetry (LSV) was conducted at 10 mV/s scan rate in the −0.4–1.2 V scan range relative to the Ag/AgCl electrode. EIS was performed under Xe lamp at 0 V with AC potential ranging from 100 K to 0.1 Hz.

4. Summary

In summary, a $MoP/a-TiO_2/Co-ZnIn_2S_4$ composite photocatalyst was successfully prepared by a facile hydrothermal method. The Co dopant in the flower-like $ZnIn_2S_4$ broadened the absorption band edge of the composite catalyst. Amorphous TiO_2 and $Co-ZnIn_2S_4$ were combined to form a heterojunction, which improved the photocarrier separation efficiency and the stability of the catalyst. More importantly, the introduction of amorphous TiO_2 created oxygen vacancies, which further improved the carrier density. Finally, the non-noble metal catalyst MoP nanoparticles were introduced into the system as co-catalysts, which became the hydrogen production sites and realized high-efficiency hydrogen production. The flower-like $MoP/a-TiO_2/Co-ZnIn_2S_4$ composite photocatalyst exhibited a hydrogen production rate of 2.96 mmol·h^{-1}·g^{-1}, which was 0.98 mmol·h^{-1}·g^{-1} of that of the pure $ZnIn_2S_4$. Therefore, this catalyst shows great promise for the green production of hydrogen. Moreover, this study also provides new insight into the design and underlying mechanism of direct Z-schemes for enhanced photocatalysis.

Author Contributions: Conceptualization, K.W.; Methodology, Y.S.; Formal analysis, H.Y. and D.Y.; Investigation, H.L., J.Z. and D.Y.; Data curation, S.L., F.J. and X.W.; Writing—original draft, P.W.; Writing—review & editing, K.W.; Visualization, X.W.; Funding acquisition, B.L. All authors have read and agreed to the published version of the manuscript.

Funding: The authors disclosed receipt of the following financial support for the research, authorship, and/or publication of this article: This work was supported by Anhui Yansheng New Material Co., Ltd. School-Enterprise Cooperation Project (202204610954), Cross projects of Nanyang Institute of Technology (330078), Doctoral research startup fund of Nanyang Institute of Technology (510140), Open subject of Henan Key Laboratory of microbial fermentation (HIMFT20210204) and School level project of Bayin College (bykyn-12).

Conflicts of Interest: We declare that we have no financial and personal relationships with other people or organizations that can inappropriately influence our work, there is no professional or other personal interest of any nature or kind in any product, service and/or company.

Sample Availability: Samples of the compounds are available from the authors.

References

1. Wang, Z.; Li, C.; Domen, K. Recent developments in heterogeneous photocatalysts for solar-driven overall water splitting. *Chem. Soc. Rev.* **2019**, *48*, 2109–2125. [CrossRef] [PubMed]
2. Paula, L.F.; Hofer, M.; Lacerda, V.P.; Bahnemann, D.W.; Patrocinio, A.O.T. Unraveling the photocatalytic properties of TiO_2/WO_3 mixed oxides. *Photochem. Photobiol.* **2019**, *18*, 2469–2483. [CrossRef] [PubMed]
3. Richards, B.S.; Hudry, D.; Busko, D.; Turshatov, A.; Howard, I.A. Photon Upconversion for Photovoltaics and Photocatalysis: A critical review. *Chem. Rev.* **2021**, *15*, 9165–9195. [CrossRef] [PubMed]
4. Hong, M.; Zhang, L.; Fang, H.; Feng, X.; Li, Z. Surface engineering of CdS quantum dots modified $SiO_2@C_3N_4$ nanospheres for effective photocatalytic hydrogen evolution. *Mater. Sci. Semicond. Process* **2021**, *136*, 106134–106142. [CrossRef]
5. Meng, S.; Chen, C.; Gu, X.; Wu, H.; Meng, Q.; Zhang, J.; Chen, S.; Fu, X.; Liu, D.; Lei, W. Efficient photocatalytic H_2 evolution, CO_2 reduction and N_2 fixation coupled with organic synthesis by cocatalyst and vacancies engineering. *Appl. Catal. B* **2021**, *285*, 119789. [CrossRef]
6. Yang, Z.; Wang, Y.; Liu, Y. Stability and charge separation of different $CH_3NH_3SnI_3/TiO_2$ interface: A first-principles study. *Appl. Surf. Sci.* **2018**, *441*, 394–400. [CrossRef]
7. Sun, M.; Wang, X.; Chen, Z.; Murugananthan, M.; Chen, Y.; Zhang, Y. Stabilized oxygen vacancies over heterojunction for highly efficient and exceptionally durable VOCs photocatalytic degradation. *Appl. Catal. B* **2020**, *273*, 119061–119072. [CrossRef]
8. Gu, X.; Chen, T.; Lei, J.; Yang, Y.; Zheng, X.; Zhang, S.; Zhu, Q.; Fu, X.; Meng, S.; Chen, S. Self-assembly synthesis of S-scheme g-C_3N_4/$Bi_8(CrO_4)O_{11}$ for photocatalytic degradation of norfloxacin and bisphenol A. *Chin. J. Catal.* **2022**, *43*, 2569–2580. [CrossRef]
9. Mao, S.; Zou, Y.; Sun, G.; Zeng, L.; Wang, Y.; Ma, D.; Guo, Y.; Cheng, Y.; Wang, C.; Shi, J.-W. Thio linkage between CdS quantum dots and UiO-66-type MOFs as an effective transfer bridge of charge carriers boosting visible-light-driven photocatalytic hydrogen production. *J. Colloid Interface Sci.* **2021**, *581*, 1–10. [CrossRef]
10. Zhao, W.; Li, J.; She, T.; Ma, S.; Cheng, Z.; Wang, G.; Zhao, P.; Wei, W.; Xia, D.; Leung, D.Y. Study on the Photocatalysis Mechanism of the Z-Scheme Cobalt Oxide Nanocubes/Carbon Nitride Nanosheets Heterojunction Photocatalyst with High Photocatalytic Performances. *J. Hazard. Mater.* **2021**, *402*, 123839–123845. [CrossRef]
11. Min, F.; Wei, Z.; Yu, Z.; Xiao, Y.; Guo, S.; Song, R.; Li, J. Construction of a hierarchical $ZnIn_2S_4$/g-C_3N_4 heterojunction for the enhanced photocatalytic degradation of tetracycline. *Dalton Trans.* **2022**, *51*, 535–547. [CrossRef]
12. Liang, Q.; Zhang, C.; Xu, S.; Zhou, M.; Zhou, Y.; Li, Z. In situ growth of CdS quantum dots on phosphorus-doped carbon nitride hollow tubes as active 0D/1D heterostructures for photocatalytic hydrogen evolution. *J. Colloid Interface Sci.* **2020**, *577*, 1–11. [CrossRef]
13. Min, F.; Wei, Z.; Yu, Z.; Xiao, Y.; Guo, S.; Song, R.; Li, J. Cubic quantum dot/hexagonal microsphere $ZnIn_2S_4$ heterophase junctions for exceptional visible-light-driven photocatalytic H_2 evolution. *J. Mater. Chem. A* **2017**, *5*, 8451–8460.
14. Lei, Z.B.; You, W.S.; Liu, M.Y.; Li, C. Preparation of $ZnIn_2S_4$ and the photocatalytic splitting water to produce hydrogen. In Proceedings of the Asia-Pacific Congress on Catalysis, Dailan, China, 13–15 March 2003; pp. 2142–2143.
15. Guo, X.; Liu, Y.; Yang, Y.; Mu, Z.; Wang, Y.; Zhang, S.; Wang, S.; Hu, Y.; Liu, Z. Effective visible-light excited charge separation in all-solid-state Ag bridged $BiVO_4$/$ZnIn_2S_4$ core-shell structure Z-scheme nanocomposites for boosting photocatalytic organics degradation. *J. Alloys Compd.* **2021**, *887*, 161389–161395. [CrossRef]
16. Chachvalvutikul, A.; Luangwanta, T.; Pattisson, S.; Hutchings, G.J.; Kaowphong, S. Enhanced photocatalytic degradation of organic pollutants and hydrogen production by a visible light–responsive Bi_2WO_6/$ZnIn_2S_4$ heterojunction. *Appl. Surf. Sci.* **2020**, *544*, 148885–148892. [CrossRef]
17. Tu, X.; Lu, J.; Li, M.; Su, Y.; Yin, G.; He, D. Hierarchically $ZnIn_2S_4$ nanosheet-constructed microwire arrays: Template-free synthesis and excellent photocatalytic performances. *Nanoscale* **2018**, *10*, 4735–4744. [CrossRef]
18. Si, M.; Zhang, J.; He, Y.; Yang, Z.; Yan, X.; Liu, M.; Zhuo, S.; Wang, S.; Min, X.; Gao, C.; et al. Synchronous and rapid preparation of lignin nanoparticles and carbon quantum dots from natural lignocellulose. *Green Chem.* **2018**, *20*, 3414–3419. [CrossRef]
19. Yuan, W.H.; Liu, X.C.; Li, L. Improving Photocatalytic Performance for Hydrogen Generation over Co-Doped $ZnIn_2S_4$ under Visible Light. *Acta Phys.-Chim. Sin.* **2013**, *29*, 151–156.
20. Jing, D.; Liu, M.; Guo, L. Enhanced Hydrogen Production from Water over Ni Doped $ZnIn_2S_4$ Microsphere Photocatalysts. *Catal. Lett.* **2010**, *140*, 167–171. [CrossRef]
21. Niu, B.; Cao, Y.L.; Xiao, J.F.; Lu, Z.; Xu, Z.M. Waste for Construction of Magnetic and Core–Shell Z-Scheme Photocatalysts: An Effective Approach to E-Waste Recycling. *Environ. Sci. Technol.* **2021**, *55*, 1279–1289. [CrossRef]
22. Xia, Y.; Li, Q.; Lv, K.; Tang, D.; Li, M. Superiority of graphene over carbon analogs for enhanced photocatalytic H_2-production activity of $ZnIn_2S_4$. *Appl. Catal. B* **2017**, *206*, 344–352. [CrossRef]
23. Xu, C.; Li, D.; Liu, X.; Ma, R.; Sakai, N.; Yang, Y.; Lin, S.; Yang, J.; Pan, H.; Huang, J.; et al. Direct Z-scheme construction of g-C_3N_4 quantum dots/TiO_2 nanoflakes for efficient photocatalysis. *Chem. Eng. J.* **2021**, *430*, 132861–132870. [CrossRef]
24. Tong, R.; Ng, K.W.; Wang, X.; Wang, S.; Wang, X.; Pan, H. Two-dimensional materials as novel co-catalysts for efficient solar-driven hydrogen production. *J. Mater. Chem. A* **2020**, *44*, 23202–23230. [CrossRef]
25. Nasir, M.S.; Yang, G.; Ayub, I.; Wang, S.; Yan, W. Tin diselenide a stable co-catalyst coupled with branched TiO_2 fiber and g-C_3N_4 quantum dots for photocatalytic hydrogen evolution. *Appl. Catal. B* **2020**, *270*, 118900–118909. [CrossRef]

26. Li, H.; Li, Y.; Wang, X.; Hou, B. 3D ZnIn$_2$S$_4$ nanosheets/TiO$_2$ nanotubes as photoanodes for photocathodic protection of Q235 CS with high efficiency undervisible light. *J. Alloys Compd.* **2019**, *771*, 892–899. [CrossRef]
27. Liu, J.; Liu, Z.; Piao, C.; Li, S.; Tang, J.; Fang, D.; Zhang, Z.; Wang, J. Construction of fixed Z-scheme Ag∣AgBr/Ag/TiO$_2$ photocatalyst composite film for malachite green degradation with simultaneous hydrogen production. *J. Power Sources* **2020**, *469*, 228430–228438. [CrossRef]
28. Li, W.; Wang, Z.; Kong, D.; Du, D.; Zhou, M.; Du, Y.; Yan, T.; You, J.; Kong, D. Visible-light-induced dendritic BiVO$_4$/TiO$_2$ composite photocatalysts for advanced oxidation process. *J. Alloys Compd.* **2016**, *688*, 703–711. [CrossRef]
29. Liu, Y.; Hong, Z.; Chen, Q.; Chen, H.; Chang, W.H.; Yang, Y.; Song, T.-B.; Yang, Y. Perovskite Solar Cells Employing Dopant-Free Organic Hole Transport Materials with Tunable Energy Levels. *Adv. Mater.* **2016**, *28*, 440–447. [CrossRef]
30. Zywitzki, D.; Jing, H.; Tüysüz, H.; Chan, C.K. High surface area, amorphous titania with reactive Ti^{3+} through a photo-assisted synthesis method for photocatalytic H$_2$ generation. *J. Mater. Chem. A* **2017**, *5*, 10957–10967. [CrossRef]
31. Yu, Z.Y.; Duan, Y.; Gao, M.R.; Lang, C.C.; Zheng, Y.R.; Yu, S.H. One-Dimensional Porous Carbon-Supported Ni/Mo$_2$C Dual Catalyst for Efficient Water Splitting. *Chem. Sci.* **2017**, *8*, 968–973. [CrossRef]
32. Xu, Y.; Li, N.; Wang, R.; Xu, L.; Liu, Z.; Jiao, T.; Liu, Z. Self-assembled FeP/MoP co-doped nanoporous carbon matrix for hydrogen evolution application. *Colloids Surf. A Physicochem. Eng. Asp.* **2022**, *636*, 128206–128212. [CrossRef]
33. Shen, Y.; Li, D.; Dang, Y.; Zhang, J.; Wang, W.; Ma, B. A ternary calabash model photocatalyst (Pd/MoP)/CdS for enhancing H$_2$ evolution under visible light irradiation. *Appl. Surf. Sci.* **2021**, *564*, 150432–150440. [CrossRef]
34. Zhang, L.; Fu, X.; Meng, S.; Jiang, X.; Wang, J.; Chen, S. Ultra-low content of Pt modified CdS nanorods: One-pot synthesis and high photocatalytic activity for H$_2$ production under visible light. *J. Mater. Chem. A* **2015**, *3*, 10360–10367. [CrossRef]
35. Du, C.; Shang, M.; Mao, J.; Song, W. Hierarchical MoP/Ni$_2$P heterostructures on nickel foam for efficient water splitting. *J. Mater. Chem. A* **2017**, *5*, 15940–15949. [CrossRef]
36. Yang, W.; Liu, B.; Fang, T.; Jennifer, W.A.; Christophe, L.; Li, Z.; Zhang, X.; Jiang, X. Layered crystalline ZnIn$_2$S$_4$ nanosheets: CVD synthesis and photo-electrochemical properties. *Nanoscale* **2016**, *8*, 18197–18203. [CrossRef]
37. Mora-Seró, I.; Bisquert, J. Fermi Level of Surface States in TiO$_2$ Nanoparticles. *Nano Lett.* **2003**, *3*, 945–949. [CrossRef]
38. Cao, S.; Yu, J.; Wageh, S.; Al-Ghamdi, A.A.; Mousavi, M.; Ghasemi, J.B.; Xu, F. H$_2$-production and electron-transfermechanism of a noble-metal-free WO$_3$@ZnIn$_2$S$_4$ S-scheme heterojunction photocatalyst. *J. Mater. Chem. A* **2022**, *10*, 17174–17184. [CrossRef]

Disclaimer/Publisher's Note: The statements, opinions and data contained in all publications are solely those of the individual author(s) and contributor(s) and not of MDPI and/or the editor(s). MDPI and/or the editor(s) disclaim responsibility for any injury to people or property resulting from any ideas, methods, instructions or products referred to in the content.

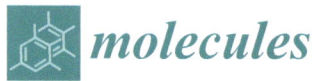

Article

Rational Photodeposition of Cobalt Phosphate on Flower-like ZnIn$_2$S$_4$ for Efficient Photocatalytic Hydrogen Evolution

Yonghui Wu [1], Zhipeng Wang [1], Yuqing Yan [1], Yu Wei [1], Jun Wang [1], Yunsheng Shen [1], Kai Yang [1], Bo Weng [2] and Kangqiang Lu [1,*]

[1] Jiangxi Provincial Key Laboratory of Functional Molecular Materials Chemistry, School of Chemistry and Chemical Engineering, Jiangxi University of Science and Technology, Ganzhou 341000, China
[2] cMACS, Department of Microbial and Molecular Systems, KU Leuven, 3001 Leuven, Belgium
* Correspondence: kqlu@jxust.edu.cn

Abstract: The high electrons and holes recombination rate of ZnIn$_2$S$_4$ significantly limits its photocatalytic performance. Herein, a simple in situ photodeposition strategy is adopted to introduce the cocatalyst cobalt phosphate (Co-Pi) on ZnIn$_2$S$_4$, aiming at facilitating the separation of electron–hole by promoting the transfer of photogenerated holes of ZnIn$_2$S$_4$. The study reveals that the composite catalyst has superior photocatalytic performance than blank ZnIn$_2$S$_4$. In particular, ZnIn$_2$S$_4$ loaded with 5% Co-Pi (ZnIn$_2$S$_4$/5%Co-Pi) has the best photocatalytic activity, and the H$_2$ production rate reaches 3593 μmol·g^{-1}·h^{-1}, approximately double that of ZnIn$_2$S$_4$ alone. Subsequent characterization data demonstrate that the introduction of the cocatalyst Co-Pi facilitates the transfer of ZnIn$_2$S$_4$ holes, thus improving the efficiency of photogenerated carrier separation. This investigation focuses on the rational utilization of high-content and rich cocatalysts on earth to design low-cost and efficient composite catalysts to achieve sustainable photocatalytic hydrogen evolution.

Keywords: photocatalytic H$_2$ evolution; indium zinc sulfide; cocatalyst; cobalt phosphate; photogenerated holes transfer

Citation: Wu, Y.; Wang, Z.; Yan, Y.; Wei, Y.; Wang, J.; Shen, Y.; Yang, K.; Weng, B.; Lu, K. Rational Photodeposition of Cobalt Phosphate on Flower-like ZnIn$_2$S$_4$ for Efficient Photocatalytic Hydrogen Evolution. *Molecules* **2024**, *29*, 465. https://doi.org/10.3390/molecules29020465

Academic Editor: Xiaomin Xu

Received: 29 December 2023
Revised: 12 January 2024
Accepted: 13 January 2024
Published: 17 January 2024

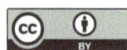

Copyright: © 2024 by the authors. Licensee MDPI, Basel, Switzerland. This article is an open access article distributed under the terms and conditions of the Creative Commons Attribution (CC BY) license (https:// creativecommons.org/licenses/by/ 4.0/).

1. Introduction

Rapid economic and social development depends on fossil fuels. However, due to the non-renewable nature of fossil fuels and the detrimental impact on the environment, it is imperative that we urgently seek sustainable energy sources capable of replacing them [1–5]. Hydrogen (H$_2$) energy, as a clean and renewable energy source, is one of the most promising alternative energy sources for fossil fuels [6–8]. Among various H$_2$ production methods, solar-driven water splitting for H$_2$ production is considered as a green and sustainable solar energy conversion technology, which can relieve the pressure of energy dilemma and environmental pollution [9–12]. Consequently, there is an urgent need to develop photocatalysts with high performance to promote the application of photocatalytic H$_2$ evolution technology [13]. Nowadays, due to their remarkable light absorption properties and special electronic structures, metal sulfides have become a hot topic in the field of solar energy conversion technology.

As a ternary sulfide, ZnIn$_2$S$_4$ has attracted global attention from researchers on account of its favorable layered structure, simple synthesis, good photostability and suitable electronic band structure [14,15]. In particular, the flower-like structure has a high surface area and improves the light absorption through multiple reflections, which plays an important role in enhancing the photocatalytic performance [16–18]. However, due to the high recombination rate of photogenerated electron–hole pairs, pure ZnIn$_2$S$_4$ exhibits low photocatalytic activity [19–22]. To address this problem, the rational introduction of cocatalyst is a viable approach to optimize the activity and stability of ZnIn$_2$S$_4$ [23]. Among the many cocatalysts, cobalt phosphate (Co-Pi) has demonstrated remarkable ability to transfer photogenerated holes from different light-collecting semiconductors in previous studies and has been reported to improve their overall performance [24]. Therefore, the rational introduction of the holes cocatalyst Co-Pi into $ZnIn_2S_4$ is expected to obtain a cost-effective and efficient composite photocatalyst to promote photocatalytic H_2 evolution. Moreover, in situ photodeposition is considered to be a promising method to enhance the photocatalytic activity of semiconductors, due to its advantages such as close contact, simple preparation and directional loading [25–27]. Consequently, rationally introducing Co-Pi into $ZnIn_2S_4$ by in situ photodeposition is expected to promote the migration of photogenerated holes of $ZnIn_2S_4$, thereby improving the photocatalytic performance of the composite photocatalyst.

Herein, we prepare the $ZnIn_2S_4$ nanoflower substrate material by the hydrothermal method, and the hybrid catalyst is constructed by in situ photodeposition of cobalt phosphate (Co-Pi) on $ZnIn_2S_4$ nanoflower. The $ZnIn_2S_4$/Co-Pi composite exhibits a significantly enhanced performance in the photocatalytic H_2 evolution compared to pure $ZnIn_2S_4$. Notably, the optimal $ZnIn_2S_4$/5%Co-Pi photocatalytic H_2 production rate is 3593 $\mu mol \cdot g^{-1} \cdot h^{-1}$, which surpasses most similar hybrid cocatalyst systems reported in the literature (Table 1). The photo/electrochemical tests and photoluminescence (PL) confirm that the photogenerated carrier separation efficiency of the composite catalyst is significantly improved. This work aims to provide insights for designing cost-effective and efficient mixed catalysts to enhance overall photocatalytic performance through rationally exploiting earth-abundant cocatalysts.

Table 1. Comparison of the hydrogen production properties of the $ZnIn_2S_4$-based catalysts.

Photocatalysts	Light Sources	Sacrificial Agents	H_2 ($\mu mol \cdot g^{-1} \cdot h^{-1}$)	Reference
$ZnIn_2S_4$-5%Co-Pi	300 W Xe lamp ($\lambda \geq 420$ nm)	TEOA	3593	this work
$ZnIn_2S_4$/$NiWO_4$	300 W Xe lamp ($\lambda \geq 420$ nm)	TEOA	1781	[28]
$ZnIn_2S_4$/BPQDs	300 W Xe lamp ($\lambda \geq 420$ nm)	TEOA	1207	[29]
J-$ZnIn_2S_4$/$CdIn_2S_4$	350 W Xe lamp ($\lambda \geq 420$ nm)	TEOA	1830	[30]
N-$ZnIn_2S_4$	350 W Xe lamp ($\lambda \geq 400$ nm)	Na_2S/Na_2SO_3	262.62	[31]
MoO_2/$ZnIn_2S_4$	300 W Xe lamp ($\lambda \geq 420$ nm)	TEOA	2722.5	[32]
ReS_2/$ZnIn_2S_4$	four 3 W 420 nm LED lamps	lactic acid (10 vol%)	2240	[33]
$ZnIn_2S_4$/$CoFe_2O_4$	300 W Xe lamp ($\lambda \geq 420$ nm)	Na_2S/Na_2SO_3	2260.5	[16]
$NiCo_2S_4$/$ZnIn_2S_4$	Xe lamp ($\lambda > 400$ nm)	-	770	[34]
$CoS_{1.097}$/$ZnIn_2S_4$	300 W Xe lamp (780 nm $\geq \lambda \geq$ 420 nm)	TEOA	2632.33	[35]

2. Results and Discussion

The preparation process diagram of the $ZnIn_2S_4$/Co-Pi (ZIS/Co-Pi) composite is shown in Figure 1a. Initially, $ZnIn_2S_4$ (ZIS) nanoflower is prepared by a one-step hydrothermal process. Subsequently, Co-Pi is introduced to ZIS nanoflower by in situ photodeposition to obtain ZIS/Co-Pi composites. Due to the best photocatalytic H_2 production performance of $ZnIn_2S_4$/5%Co-Pi (Z5CP), we mainly discuss this proportion of the composites in the subsequent characterization. According to Figure S1a,b, the color of ZIS nanoflower changes significantly before and after in situ photodeposition, with pure ZIS appearing as bright yellow, and Z5CP appearing as yellowish green. The morphology and microstructure of different samples are obtained by field emission scanning electron microscopy (FESEM). As depicted in Figure 1b, pure ZIS presents a spherical flower-like structure with a diameter of about 1 μm. The SEM image of Z5CP (Figure 1c) shows that Z5CP inherits the flower-like structure of ZIS. Notably, the flower-like structure can provide a number of active sites, and multiple layers of petals enable light to be reflected multiple times, which leads to enhanced light absorption [36,37]. In addition, the SEM image of Z5CP shows that the Co-Pi nanoparticles are highly dispersed, and no large Co-Pi particles were observed. As presented in Figure 1d, transmission electron microscopy (TEM) characterization further confirms the spherical flower-like structure of ZIS. Moreover, Figure 1e shows that the Co-Pi nanoparticles are attached to the ZIS nanoflower, proving the successful synthesis of Z5CP composites. As depicted in Figure 1f, the lattice distance of Z5CP is about 0.297 nm corresponding to the (104) crystal face of ZIS, and the Co-Pi synthesized by in situ photodeposition is amorphous. Furthermore, the EDS spectra (Figure S2) and the element mapping results (Figure 1g) confirm the existence of Zn, In, S, P, O, and Co elements in Z5CP. The spatial distribution of Zn, In, S, O, P, and Co elements in the elemental mapping images of Z5CP composite shows that Co-Pi grows uniformly on the surface of ZIS nanoflower.

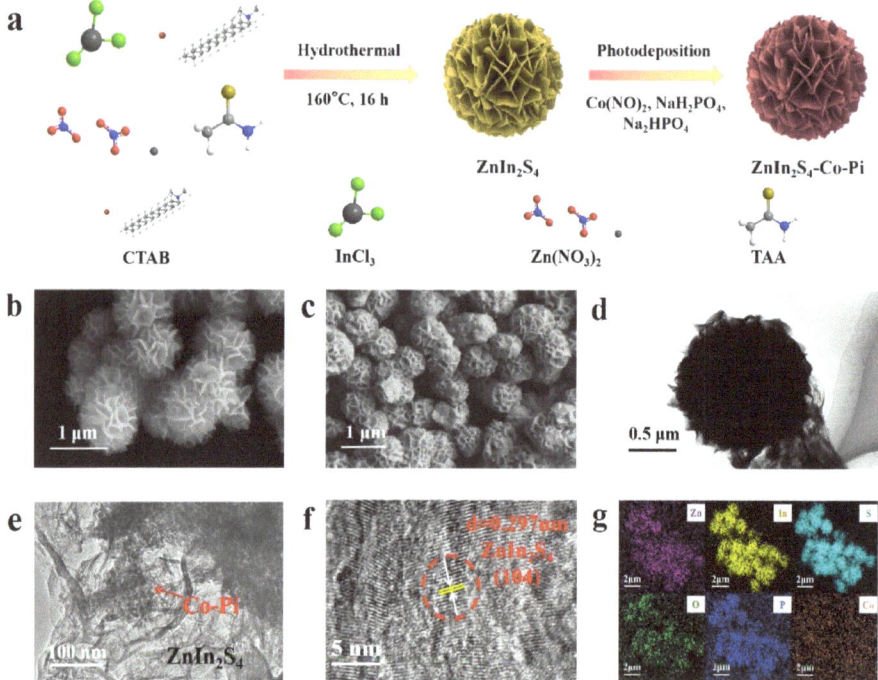

Figure 1. (**a**) Diagram illustrating the synthesis of ZIS/Co-Pi. (**b**,**c**) FESEM images of ZIS and Z5CP. (**d**–**f**) TEM images of Z5CP. (**g**) Mapping analysis results of Z5CP.

The phase structure and crystallinity are analyzed by the X-ray diffraction (XRD) map. Figure 2a displays the XRD spectra of both ZIS and Z5CP. For ZIS, the strong diffraction peaks at 27.5° and 47.2° belong to the (102) and (110) faces of hexagonal ZIS (JCPDS No.65-2023) [38]. For Z5CP composites, the XRD diffraction curve closely resembles that of ZIS except that there is a faint peak at 55.6° belonging to the (202) face of hexagonal ZIS, indicating that ZIS remains a stable crystal structure after coupling with Co-Pi [39]. However, in the Z5CP composite, the characteristic diffraction peak of Co-Pi is not observed due to the amorphous nature of in situ photodeposition of Co-Pi [40,41]. The optical characteristics of the photocatalysts are analyzed by UV-visible diffuse reflection spectroscopy (DRS). As depicted in Figure 2b, the pure ZIS displays a clear absorption edge around 520 nm, indicating a band gap of about 2.44 eV [42]. Compared with pure ZIS, the absorption intensity of Z5CP hybrid in the visible range (520~750 nm) increases with the strong absorption of Co-Pi, indicating that the introduction of Co-Pi can improve the visible light response of ZIS. Moreover, Figure 2b shows that there is no significant shift in absorption edge for the Z5CP composite, indicating that the Co-Pi cocatalyst only deposits on the ZIS surface and does not bind with the crystal lattice.

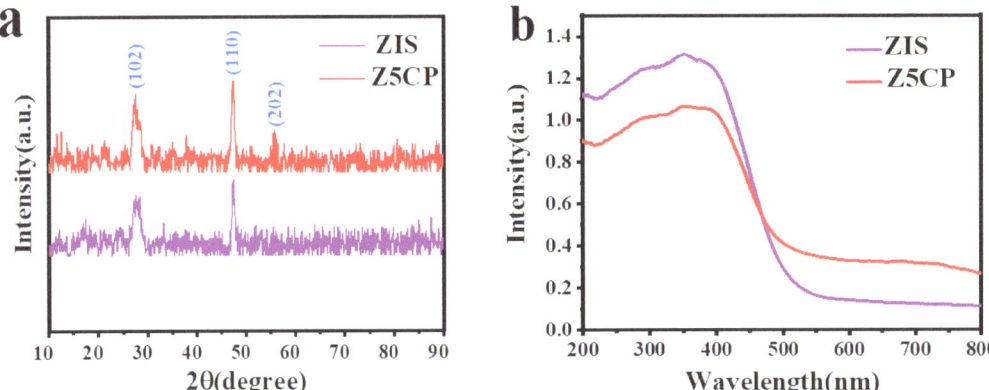

Figure 2. (**a**) X-ray diffraction (XRD) patterns and (**b**) UV–vis diffuse reflectance spectra (DRS) of ZIS and Z5CP.

The chemical composition and elemental states of Z5CP composite are further determined by X-ray photoelectron spectroscopy (XPS). As presented in Figure 3a, Zn, In, S, Co, and P elements exist in the hybrid products, which further demonstrates the successful photodeposition of Co-Pi on the surface of ZIS nanoflower. As shown in Figure 3b, the XPS spectrum of Zn 2p exhibits two distinct peaks at 1045 and 1022 eV, which correspond to the binding energies of Zn $2p_{1/2}$ and Zn $2p_{3/2}$ of Zn^{2+}, respectively. From the XPS spectrum of In 3d (Figure 3c), two peaks that center on binding energies 452.4 and 444.8 eV are respectively associated with In $3d_{3/2}$ and In $3d_{5/2}$, which indicate the +3 state of In. Moreover, as presented in Figure 3d, the peaks of 162.9 and 161.7 eV belong to S $2p_{1/2}$ and S $2p_{3/2}$, confirming the presence of S^{2-}. In the XPS spectrum of Co 2p (Figure 3e), the peak of Co $2p_{3/2}$ is at 781.3 eV (satellite peak at 784.3 eV), indicating the presence of Co^{2+} in the Z5CP composite [43–45]. In addition, the peak of P 2p (Figure 3f) at 133.5 eV indicates that P presents in the form of phosphate groups, which further proves the successful synthesis of Z5CP [46].

Photocatalytic H_2 production is performed with triethanolamine (TEOA) as the hole scavenger, and the photocatalytic properties of pure ZIS and different proportions of ZIS/Co-Pi composites under visible light are investigated. Figure 4a is a diagram of the photocatalytic activity of ZIS and composite with 1%, 5%, and 10% Co-Pi (hereinafter shown as Z1CP, Z5CP, and Z10CP, respectively). As shown in Figure 4a, due to the fast photogenerated electron–hole recombination rate, the pure ZIS is less active and the H_2 evolution rate is only 1832 $\mu mol \cdot g^{-1} \cdot h^{-1}$. After the introduction of Co-Pi cocatalyst, Z1CP, Z5CP, and Z10CP all show better H_2 evolution performance compared with blank ZIS. With the increase in Co-Pi content, the hydrogen yield increases gradually. However, when the Co-Pi content increases further, the H_2 evolution activity decreases, which may be due to the remarkable shielding effect of Co-Pi, thereby decreasing the photocatalytic active sites [47]. In particular, the Z5CP composite shows the highest H_2 evolution rate (3593 $\mu mol \cdot g^{-1} \cdot h^{-1}$), approximately two times higher than that of ZIS alone. This can be attributed to the fact that in situ photodeposition of Co-Pi promotes the transfer of photogenerated holes and reduces the recombination rate of photogenerated carriers. As shown in Table 1, the Z5CP composite prepared in this work has optimal photocatalytic H_2 production properties compared with the photocatalytic H_2 production activities of some representative ZIS-based composites reported in recent years. In addition, the stability of Z5CP is tested by the cyclic test. As depicted in Figure 4b, after five cycles, no apparent deactivation has been observed for Z5CP composite, indicating the excellent stability of Z5CP composite.

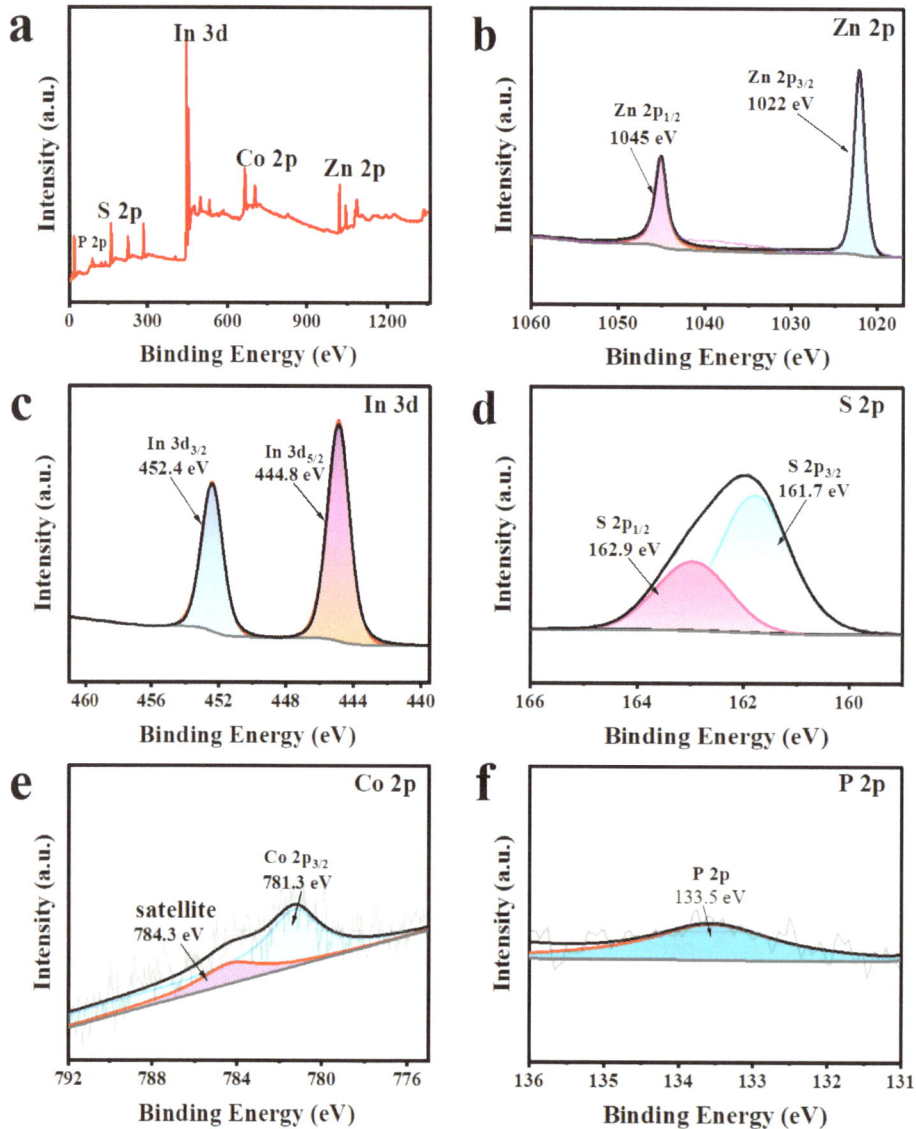

Figure 3. (**a**) XPS spectra of Z5CP, high-resolution spectra of (**b**) Zn 2p, (**c**) In 3d, (**d**) S 2p, (**e**) Co 2p, (**f**) P 2p.

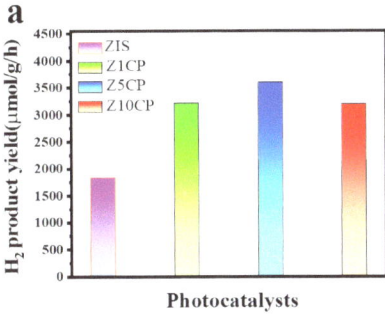
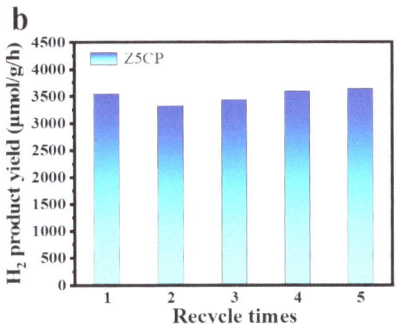

Figure 4. (**a**) Photocatalytic H_2 production over pure ZIS and Z5CP composites. (**b**) Stability plots of the photocatalytic H_2 production by Z5CP.

Photo/electrochemical tests are used to further characterize material reducing capacity and photogenerated carrier transfer efficiency. Linear sweep voltammetry (LSV) is first used to determine the H_2 evolution performance of ZIS and Z5CP samples. Figure 5a shows the polarization curve of ZIS and Z5CP composites. It can be seen that the overpotential of Z5CP is less than ZIS at the same current density, indicating that the H_2 evolution performance of Z5CP is better than that of ZIS [48]. The kinetics of photocatalysis in different samples can be compared by the Tafel slope. As shown in Figure S3, the Tafel slope of the Z5CP composite (0.21 V/decade) is smaller than that of ZIS (0.24 V/decade), indicating the better reduction effect and interfacial charge transfer efficiency of Z5CP, which is consistent with the photocatalytic H_2 production activity as well as other characterization results [49]. These results further demonstrate that Z5CP has faster reaction kinetics and excellent interface carrier separation efficiency. To study the charge separation and transfer of these ZIS/Co-Pi composites, instantaneous photocurrent (IT), electrochemical impedance spectroscopy (EIS) and steady-state photoluminescence (PL) spectra are measured on the ZIS and Z5CP samples [50]. As illustrated in Figure 5b, the optical current density of ZIS is small, indicating that the photogenerated carrier separation efficiency of ZIS is poor. However, it is found that after the introduction of Co-Pi, the optical current density of Z5CP is significantly improved compared with that of pure ZIS, indicating that Z5CP has better separation efficiency of electron (e^-) and hole (h^+) [51–55]. As shown in Figure 5c, the radius of curvature of Z5CP composite is smaller than ZIS, indicating that the charge transfer resistance of Z5CP is lower, which improves the separation and transfer rate of photogenerated carriers, thus enhancing the photocatalytic activity [56–60]. Furthermore, Figure 5d describes the steady−state photoluminescence (PL) spectra test of the sample. As shown in Figure 5d, the PL intensity of Z5CP is significantly lower than that of blank ZIS, indicating that the addition of cocatalyst Co-Pi effectively inhibits the recombination of photogenerated carriers [61–65]. Taken together, the results of these photo/electrochemical tests validate the improved separation and transfer of photogenerated charges in Z5CP, leading to the enhanced performance of photocatalytic H_2 evolution.

The information of chemical reaction area of the blank ZIS and the composite material Z5CP is obtained by the cyclic voltammetry test (CV). Figure 6a,b show the cyclic voltammetry (CV) curves of the blank ZIS and Z5CP composites, respectively. As illustrated in Figure 6c, the double-layer capacitance of Z5CP composite (3.99 $\mu F \cdot cm^{-2}$) is significantly larger than ZIS (1.83 $\mu F \cdot cm^{-2}$), which strongly proves that Z5CP has more active sites area than ZIS [45]. In addition, the flat charged position (E_{fb}) of the original ZIS is measured with Mott–Schottky (MS). Generally, the slope of the positive one indicates that the semiconductor is an intrinsic n-type semiconductor [51]. As can be seen from Figure 6d, ZIS belongs to the n-type semiconductor. Moreover, Figure S4 shows the detailed fitting parameters of MS. According to the x-intercept of the block, its E_{fb} is determined to be −0.52 V (vs. Ag/AgCl). In general, the conduction band position of n-type semiconductors is about 0.2 V more negative than that of E_{fb} [66–68]. Therefore, the conduction charge position (E_{CB}) of the ZIS is −0.72 V (vs. Ag/AgCl). From the formula $E_{NHE} = E_{Ag/AgCl} + 0.20$ V, the E_{CB} of ZIS is −0.52 V (vs. NHE). According to the band gap of ZIS (2.44 eV), the valence band potential (E_{VB}) of ZIS is 1.92 V (vs. NHE).

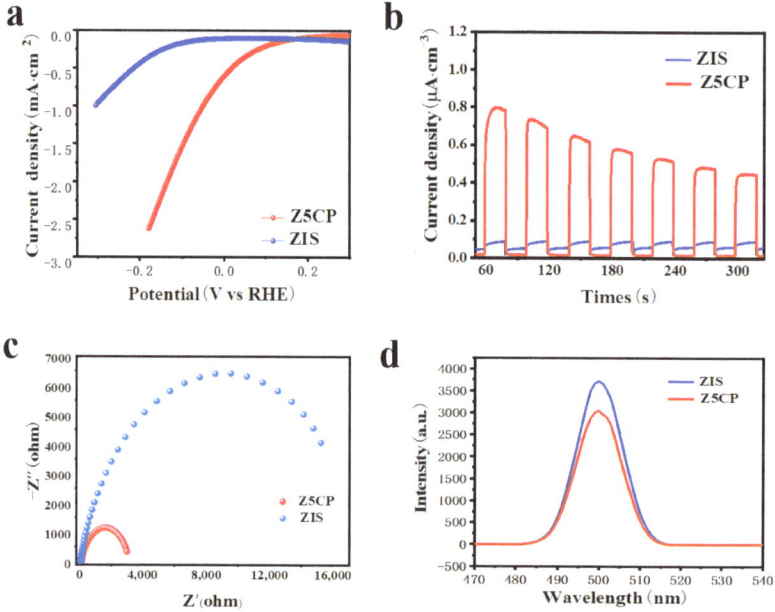

Figure 5. (**a**) Polarization curves. (**b**) Transient photocurrent spectra. (**c**) EIS Nyquist plots. (**d**) Steady−state photoluminescence (PL) emission spectra with an excitation wavelength of 500 nm.

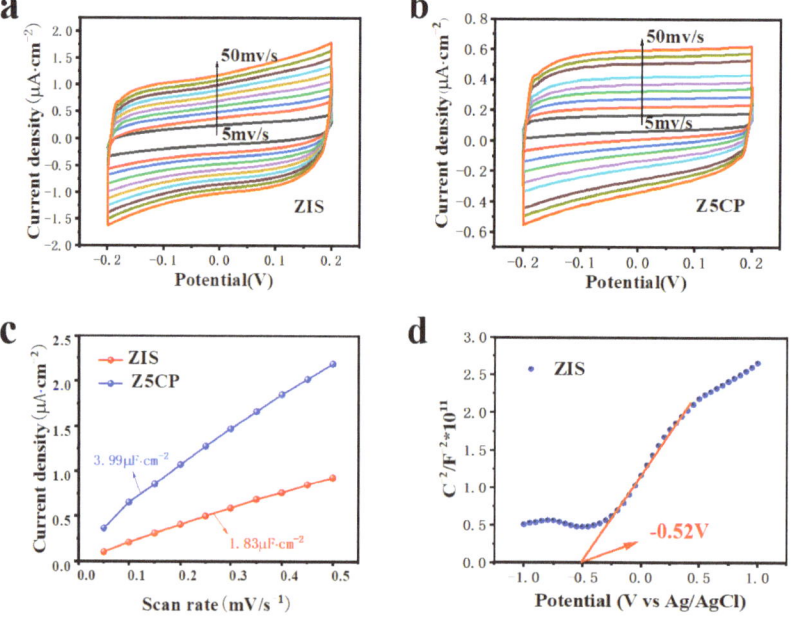

Figure 6. (**a**,**b**) Cyclic voltammetry curves of the ZIS and Z5CP. (**c**) Current density scan rate plot. (**d**) Mott−Schottky plots for ZIS.

Combined with the above experiments and characterization, we propose a viable mechanism for photocatalytic H_2 production of Z5CP under visible light. As shown in Figure 7, under visible light irradiation, Z5CP effectively absorbs the photon energy, and then the electrons on the valence band (VB) are excited and transition to the conduction band (CB), and the corresponding positive electric holes are generated on the valence band (VB). The electron (e^-) migrated to the semiconductor surface binds to the H^+ adsorbed in water to form H_2. However, ZIS has a high electrons and holes recombination rate; therefore, its photocatalytic activity is limited. Notably, Co-Pi has the excellent property of transferring photogenerated holes, and the holes of ZIS are transferred to Co-Pi and drive cycles to catalyze the $Co^{2+/3+} \to Co^{4+} \to Co^{2+/3+}$ reaction [24]. At the same time, ZIS rapidly exports holes to oxidize the sacrificial reagent of triethanolamine (TEOA); therefore, the resulting photogenerated hole (h^+) is effectively separated and consumed by it. Therefore, the photogenerated carrier separation efficiency of the composite photocatalyst Z5CP is improved, which allows more electrons to transfer to the catalyst surface to react with H^+ to produce more H_2. This is also the main factor for the significant improvement of the photocatalytic H_2 evolution performance of Z5CP composite.

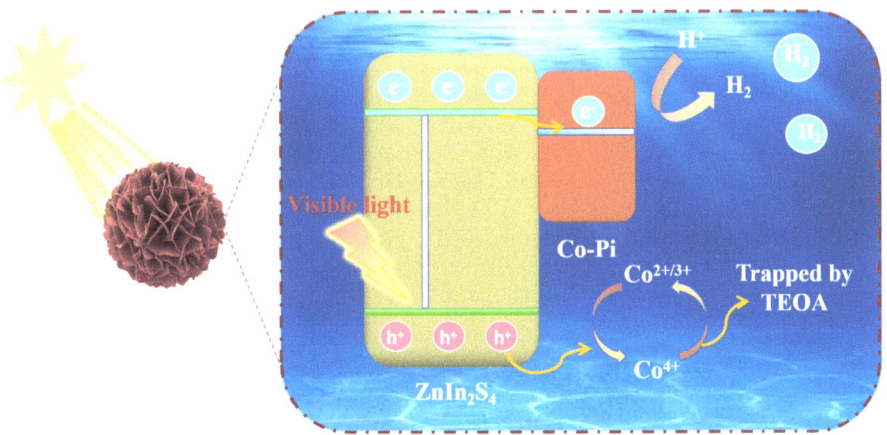

Figure 7. Mechanism diagram of Z5CP in the visible light-driven photocatalytic H_2 production reaction.

3. Experimental Section

3.1. Materials

Concentrated sulfuric acid (H_2SO_4), triethanolamine ($C_6H_{15}NO_3$, TEOA), anhydrous ethanol (C_2H_5OH), N,N-dimethylformamide (C_3H_7NO), disodium hydrogen phosphate dihydrate ($Na_2HPO_4 \cdot 2H_2O$), and sodium dihydrogen phosphate tetrahydrate ($NaH_2PO_4 \cdot 4H_2O$) are supplied by Xilong Scientific Co., Ltd. (Shantou, China). Cobalt nitrate hexahydrate ($Co(NO_3)_2 \cdot 6H_2O$), cetyltrimethylammonium bromide ($C_{19}H_{42}BrN$, CTAB), zinc nitrate hexahydrate ($Zn(NO_3)_2 \cdot 6H_2O$), indium chloride tetrahydrate ($InCl_3 \cdot 4H_2O$), and Nafion solution (5 wt%) ($C_9HF_{17}O_5S$) are supplied by Sinopharm Chemical Reagent Co., Ltd. (Shanghai, China).

3.2. Synthesis of $ZnIn_2S_4$ (ZIS)

Typically, $Zn(NO_3)_2 \cdot 6H_2O$ (304.2 mg), $InCl_3 \cdot 4H_2O$ (624.4 mg), and cetyltrimethylammonium bromide (CTAB) (230.6 mg) were added to a beaker containing 20 mL of deionized water and magnetically stirred for 30 min. Then, the thioacetamide (604.8 mg) was added to a beaker containing 10 mL deionized water and mixed to the above solution. Afterwards, the mixture was added to a Teflon liner and stirred for 30 min, and the liner was transferred to stainless steel autoclave heating in an oven at 433 K for 16 h. After cooling, the products were separated by filtration and washed several times with deionized water and ethanol. The resulting samples were dried under vacuum at 333 K for 12 h. Ultimately, a bright yellow solid was obtained.

3.3. Synthesis of $ZnIn_2S_4$/Co-Pi (ZIS/Co-Pi)

In a typical experiment, the prepared 200 mL (0.1 mol/L) NaH_2PO_4 and 200 mL (0.1 mol/L) Na_2HPO_4 solution were mixed and adjusted with pH to around 7. Subsequently, 80 mL of neutral buffer was measured, and the calculated amount of $Co(NO_3)_2 \cdot 6H_2O$ was added to make it evenly dispersed by ultrasound. Furthermore, 40 mg of $ZnIn_2S_4$ was weighed and introduced into the aforementioned system which was then sealed using a sealing ring with several ventilation holes. Then, the system was subjected to Ar gas flow under magnetic stirring for 30 min followed by irradiation from a xenon lamp while maintaining stirring for an additional duration of 60 min after sealing. After the photodeposition, the samples were filtered with deionized water, and the samples were obtained after vacuum drying at 333 K for 12 h. The loading amount of Co-Pi in ZIS/xCo-Pi was altered by changing the amount of $Co(NO_3)_2 \cdot 6H_2O$. In the experimental design, the loading ratios of deposited Co-Pi in $ZnIn_2S_4$ are 1%, 5%, and 10%, respectively.

3.4. Activity Evaluation of Photocatalytic H_2 Evolution

Photocatalytic H_2 production was performed in a 50 mL airtight quartz reactor. In the entire quartz reactor, 5 mg of the catalyst was dispersed into a solution containing 5 mL of deionized water and 1 mL of triethanolamine (TEOA). Before the reaction, high purity Ar was injected into the quartz reactor for 30 min to exhaust the residual air in the reactor. A 300 W xenon lamp ($\lambda > 420$ nm) was selected as the light source, and after 2 h of illumination, 1 mL of gas was extracted into the gas chromatograph (thermal conductivity detector TCD, Agilent Technologies GC 7820A, Santa Clara, CA, USA) to detect the hydrogen yield obtained after the reaction. In order to evaluate the stability of ZIS/Co-Pi composite, the photocatalyst was separated and centrifuged. The recovered photocatalyst is then subjected to a subsequent cycle under the same conditions.

3.5. Characterization Methods

The morphological characteristics were tested through scanning electron microscopy (SEM, FESEM ZEISS sigma 500, Oberkochen, Batenwerburg, Germany) and transmission electron microscopy (TEM, Jeol JEM-2100F instrument, Jeol, Akishima, Tokyo). The determination of crystal structures was determined by X-ray diffraction (XRD) with Cu Kα (λ = 0.15406 nm, Bruker D8 Advance, Billerica, MA, USA). The surface composition of the samples was determined by X-ray photoelectron spectrometer (XPS, Thermo Fisher, K-Alpha, Waltham, MA, USA). The UV-visible diffuse reflectance spectrometer (DRS, Shimadzu UV-2600, Kyoto, Japan) was used to test the optical response of the catalyst. Photoluminescence (PL) spectra were obtained using a spectrofluorometer (FLS 980, Edinburgh Instruments Ltd., Edinburgh, UK) with an excitation wavelength of 500 nm. Furthermore, all the electrochemical measurements of the photocurrent, the electrochemical impedance spectra (EIS), the Mott–Schottky (MS), cyclic voltammetry (CV), and linear sweep voltammetry (LSV) curves were carried out in the three-electrode cell, in which Ag/AgCl was used as a reference electrode, a Pt wire was used as a counter electrode, and an indium in oxide (ITO) conductive glass was used with the samples as a working electrode in 0.1 M Na_2SO_4 electrolyte (pH = 7.56), all measurements were carried out on CH instruments CHI-660E electrochemical workstation (Shanghai Chenhua CHI-660E, Shanghai, China).

4. Conclusions

In summary, we synthesize spherical $ZnIn_2S_4$ nanoflower substrate material by the hydrothermal method, and reasonably construct a novel photocatalyst of indium zinc sulfide/cobalt phosphate ($ZnIn_2S_4$/Co-Pi) hybrid photocatalyst by the in situ photodeposition method. In the presence of cocatalyst cobalt phosphate (Co-Pi), the hybrid photocatalyst shows outstanding photocatalytic hydrogen evolution performance. Through changing the photodeposition amount of Co-Pi, it is observed that the highest H_2 production rate of indium zinc sulfide ($ZnIn_2S_4$/5% Co-Pi) loaded with 5% cobalt phosphate (Co-Pi) is 3593 µmol·g^{-1}·h^{-1}, which is significantly higher than that of pure $ZnIn_2S_4$. The steady-state photoluminescence (PL) and electrochemical impedance spectroscopy (EIS) of the photocatalyst show that $ZnIn_2S_4$/Co-Pi composite has weaker PL intensity and lower charge transport resistance than blank $ZnIn_2S_4$, demonstrating that the hybrid photocatalyst has faster electron transfer and charge separation. Simultaneously, the larger double-layer capacitance and smaller overpotential of catalyst indicate that $ZnIn_2S_4$/Co-Pi composite has larger active area and better hydrogen evolution performance. This work makes reasonable use of the earth-abundant cocatalysts to design low-cost and efficient composite catalysts to promote the prospect of photocatalytic hydrogen evolution.

Supplementary Materials: The following supporting information can be downloaded at: https://www.mdpi.com/article/10.3390/molecules29020465/s1, Figure S1: Schematic representation of the samples for $ZnIn_2S_4$ (a) and $ZnIn_2S_4$-5%Co-Pi (b); Figure S2: EDS spectrum of $ZnIn_2S_4$-5%Co-Pi; Figure S3: Tafel slope plots for $ZnIn_2S_4$ and $ZnIn_2S_4$-5%Co-Pi; Figure S4: Mott-Schottky plots for $ZnIn_2S_4$.

Author Contributions: Conceptualization, Y.W. (Yonghui Wu) and K.L.; methodology, Z.W.; software, Y.W. (Yonghui Wu) and Z.W.; validation, Y.W. (Yu Wei), Y.Y. and J.W.; formal analysis, Y.S.; investigation, Y.Y.; resources, K.L. and B.W.; data curation, K.Y. (Kai Yang); writing—original draft preparation, Y.W. (Yonghui Wu); writing—review and editing, K.L.; visualization, Y.W. (Yonghui Wu); supervision, K.L.; project administration, K.Y. and B.W.; funding acquisition, K.L. All authors have read and agreed to the published version of the manuscript.

Funding: This work received financial support from Jiangxi Provincial Natural Science Foundation (20224BAB203018), Postdoctoral Research Projects of Jiangxi Province (2021RC11, 204302600031), Jiangxi Province "Double Thousand Plan" (jxsq2023102143), High Level Talent Research Launch Project of JXUST (205200100518), Jiangxi University of Science and Technology students' innovation and entrepreneurship training program (Preparation of graphene aerogel/semiconductor composite photocatalytic materials and their performance research, 202210407022), National Natural Science Foundation of China (21962006, 21902132), Jiangxi Provincial Academic and Technical Leaders Training Program-Young Talents (20204BCJL23037), Program of Qingjiang Excellent Young Talents, JXUST (JXUSTQJBJ2020005). The authors would like to thank Chen Weiwei from Shiyanjia Lab (www.shiyanjia.com) for the XPS analysis and Jiangxi Qianvi New Materials Co., Ltd. for SEM analysis.

Institutional Review Board Statement: Not applicable.

Informed Consent Statement: Not applicable.

Data Availability Statement: Data are contained within the article.

Conflicts of Interest: The authors declare no conflict of interest.

References

1. Gong, Y.-N.; Zhong, W.; Li, Y.; Qiu, Y.; Zheng, L.; Jiang, J.; Jiang, H.-L. Regulating Photocatalysis by Spin-State Manipulation of Cobalt in Covalent Organic Frameworks. *J. Am. Chem. Soc.* **2020**, *142*, 16723–16731. [CrossRef]
2. Su, B.; Zheng, M.; Lin, W.; Lu, X.F.; Luan, D.; Wang, S.; Lou, X.W. S-Scheme Co_9S_8@$Cd_{0.8}Zn_{0.2}$S-DETA Hierarchical Nanocages Bearing Organic CO_2 Activators for Photocatalytic Syngas Production. *Adv. Energy Mater.* **2023**, *13*, 2203290. [CrossRef]
3. Su, Q.; Zuo, C.; Liu, M.; Tai, X. A Review on Cu_2O-Based Composites in Photocatalysis: Synthesis, Modification, and Applications. *Molecules* **2023**, *28*, 5576. [CrossRef] [PubMed]
4. Paul, R.; Zhai, Q.; Roy, A.K.; Dai, L. Charge transfer of carbon nanomaterials for efficient metal-free electrocatalysis. *Interdiscip. Mater.* **2022**, *1*, 28–50. [CrossRef]
5. Yang, F.; Hu, P.; Yang, F.; Hua, X.-J.; Chen, B.; Gao, L.; Wang, K.-S. Photocatalytic applications and modification methods of two-dimensional nanomaterials: A review. *Tungsten* **2023**. [CrossRef]
6. Camara, F.; Gavaggio, T.; Dautreppe, B.; Chauvin, J.; Pécaut, J.; Aldakov, D.; Collomb, M.-N.; Fortage, J. Electrochemical Properties of a Rhodium(III) Mono-Terpyridyl Complex and Use as a Catalyst for Light-Driven Hydrogen Evolution in Water. *Molecules* **2022**, *27*, 6614. [CrossRef] [PubMed]
7. Wan, S.; Xu, J.; Cao, S.; Yu, J. Promoting intramolecular charge transfer of graphitic carbon nitride by donor–acceptor modulation for visible-light photocatalytic H_2 evolution. *Interdiscip. Mater.* **2022**, *1*, 294–308. [CrossRef]

8. Ma, M.-Y.; Yu, H.-Z.; Deng, L.-M.; Wang, L.-Q.; Liu, S.-Y.; Pan, H.; Ren, J.-W.; Maximov, M.Y.; Hu, F.; Peng, S.-J. Interfacial engineering of heterostructured carbon-supported molybdenum cobalt sulfides for efficient overall water splitting. *Tungsten* 2023, 5, 589–597. [CrossRef]
9. Wu, K.; Shang, Y.; Li, H.; Wu, P.; Li, S.; Ye, H.; Jian, F.; Zhu, J.; Yang, D.; Li, B.; et al. Synthesis and Hydrogen Production Performance of MoP/a-TiO$_2$/Co-ZnIn$_2$S$_4$ Flower-like Composite Photocatalysts. *Molecules* 2023, 28, 4350. [CrossRef]
10. Yoshimura, N.; Yoshida, M.; Kobayashi, A. Efficient Hydrogen Production by a Photoredox Cascade Catalyst Comprising Dual Photosensitizers and a Transparent Electron Mediator. *J. Am. Chem. Soc.* 2023, 145, 6035–6038. [CrossRef]
11. Lu, K.-Q.; Lin, X.; Tang, Z.-R.; Xu, Y.-J. Silicon nanowires@Co$_3$O$_4$ arrays film with Z-scheme band alignment for hydrogen evolution. *Catal. Today* 2019, 335, 294–299. [CrossRef]
12. Hu, N.; Cai, Y.; Li, L.; Wang, X.; Gao, J. Amino-Functionalized Titanium Based Metal-Organic Framework for Photocatalytic Hydrogen Production. *Molecules* 2022, 27, 4241. [CrossRef] [PubMed]
13. Liu, Z.-Y.; Lin, Y.-D.; Hao, Y.; Chen, H.-N.; Guo, Z.-W.; Li, X.-X.; Zheng, S.-T. Recent advances in polyoxoniobate-catalyzed reactions. *Tungsten* 2022, 4, 81–98. [CrossRef]
14. Liu, C.; Zhang, Q.; Zou, Z. Recent advances in designing ZnIn$_2$S$_4$-based heterostructured photocatalysts for hydrogen evolution. *J. Mater. Sci. Technol.* 2023, 139, 167–188. [CrossRef]
15. Zhang, Y.; Wu, Y.; Wan, L.; Ding, H.; Li, H.; Wang, X.; Zhang, W. Hollow core–shell Co$_9$S$_8$@ZnIn$_2$S$_4$/CdS nanoreactor for efficient photothermal effect and CO$_2$ photoreduction. *Appl. Catal. B* 2022, 311, 121255. [CrossRef]
16. Jiang, X.; Fan, D.; Yao, X.; Dong, Z.; Li, X.; Ma, S.; Liu, J.; Zhang, D.; Li, H.; Pu, X.; et al. Highly efficient flower-like ZnIn$_2$S$_4$/CoFe$_2$O$_4$ photocatalyst with p-n type heterojunction for enhanced hydrogen evolution under visible light irradiation. *J. Colloid Interface Sci.* 2023, 641, 26–35. [CrossRef]
17. Jiang, X.; Kong, D.; Luo, B.; Wang, M.; Zhang, D.; Pu, X. Preparation of magnetically retrievable flower-like AgBr/BiOBr/NiFe$_2$O$_4$ direct Z-scheme heterojunction photocatalyst with enhanced visible-light photoactivity. *Colloids Surf. A* 2022, 633, 127880. [CrossRef]
18. Shi, R.; Yang, P.; Song, X.; Wang, J.; Che, Q.; Zhang, A. ZnO flower: Self-assembly growth from nanosheets with exposed {1 1$^-$ 0 0} facet, white emission, and enhanced photocatalysis. *Appl. Surf. Sci.* 2016, 366, 506–513. [CrossRef]
19. Yuan, L.; Yang, M.-Q.; Xu, Y.-J. A low-temperature and one-step method for fabricating ZnIn$_2$S$_4$–GR nanocomposites with enhanced visible light photoactivity. *J. Mater. Chem. A* 2014, 2, 14401. [CrossRef]
20. Jin, P.; Wang, L.; Ma, X.; Lian, R.; Huang, J.; She, H.; Zhang, M.; Wang, Q. Construction of hierarchical ZnIn$_2$S$_4$@PCN-224 heterojunction for boosting photocatalytic performance in hydrogen production and degradation of tetracycline hydrochloride. *Appl. Catal. B* 2021, 284, 119762. [CrossRef]
21. Chen, J.; Wu, S.-J.; Cui, W.-J.; Guo, Y.-H.; Wang, T.-W.; Yao, Z.-W.; Shi, Y.; Zhao, H.; Liu, J.; Hu, Z.-Y.; et al. Nickel clusters accelerating hierarchical zinc indium sulfide nanoflowers for unprecedented visible-light hydrogen production. *J. Colloid Interface Sci.* 2022, 608, 504–512. [CrossRef]
22. Ding, Y.; Maitra, S.; Wang, C.; Halder, S.; Zheng, R.; Barakat, T.; Roy, S.; Chen, L.H.; Su, B.L. Vacancy defect engineering in semiconductors for solar light-driven environmental remediation and sustainable energy production. *Interdiscip. Mater.* 2022, 1, 213–255. [CrossRef]
23. Busser, G.W.; Mei, B.; Pougin, A.; Strunk, J.; Gutkowski, R.; Schuhmann, W.; Willinger, M.-G.; Schlögl, R.; Muhler, M. Photodeposition of Copper and Chromia on Gallium Oxide: The Role of Co-Catalysts in Photocatalytic Water Splitting. *ChemSusChem* 2014, 7, 1030–1034. [CrossRef] [PubMed]
24. Lu, K.-Q.; Qi, M.-Y.; Tang, Z.-R.; Xu, Y.-J. Earth-Abundant MoS$_2$ and Cobalt Phosphate Dual Cocatalysts on 1D CdS Nanowires for Boosting Photocatalytic Hydrogen Production. *Langmuir* 2019, 35, 11056–11065. [CrossRef] [PubMed]
25. Su, H.; Wang, W. Dynamically Monitoring the Photodeposition of Single Cocatalyst Nanoparticles on Semiconductors via Fluorescence Imaging. *Anal. Chem.* 2021, 93, 11915–11919. [CrossRef] [PubMed]
26. Zhao, H.; Mao, Q.; Jian, L.; Dong, Y.; Zhu, Y. Photodeposition of earth-abundant cocatalysts in photocatalytic water splitting: Methods, functions, and mechanisms. *Chin. J. Catal.* 2022, 43, 1774–1804. [CrossRef]
27. Wang, M.; Liu, Y.; Li, D.; Tang, J.; Huang, W. Isoelectric point-controlled preferential photodeposition of platinum on Cu$_2$O-TiO$_2$ composite surfaces. *Chin. Chem. Lett.* 2019, 30, 985–988. [CrossRef]
28. Zhang, M.; Tan, P.; Yang, L.; Zhai, H.; Liu, H.; Chen, J.; Ren, R.; Tan, X.; Pan, J. Sulfur vacancy and p-n junction synergistically boosting interfacial charge transfer and separation in ZnIn$_2$S$_4$/NiWO$_4$ heterostructure for enhanced photocatalytic hydrogen evolution. *J. Colloid Interface Sci.* 2023, 634, 817–826. [CrossRef]
29. Qu, Y.; Ren, J.; Sun, D.; Yu, Y. Synergetic control of specific orientation and self-distribution of photoelectrons in micro-nano ZnIn$_2$S$_4$/black phosphorus quantum dots (BPQDs) heterojunction to enhance photocatalytic hydrogen evolution. *J. Colloid Interface Sci.* 2023, 642, 204–215. [CrossRef]
30. Li, Y.; Li, S.; Meng, L.; Peng, S. Synthesis of oriented J type ZnIn$_2$S$_4$@CdIn$_2$S$_4$ heterojunction by controllable cation exchange for enhancing photocatalytic hydrogen evolution. *J. Colloid Interface Sci.* 2023, 650, 266–274. [CrossRef]
31. Chong, W.-K.; Ng, B.-J.; Kong, X.Y.; Tan, L.-L.; Putri, L.K.; Chai, S.-P. Non-metal doping induced dual p-n charge properties in a single ZnIn$_2$S$_4$ crystal structure provoking charge transfer behaviors and boosting photocatalytic hydrogen generation. *Appl. Catal. B* 2023, 325, 122372. [CrossRef]

32. Dong, W.; Zhou, S.-A.; Ma, Y.; Chi, D.-J.; Chen, R.; Long, H.-M.; Chun, T.-J.; Liu, S.-J.; Qian, F.-P.; Zhang, K. N-doped C-coated $MoO_2/ZnIn_2S_4$ heterojunction for efficient photocatalytic hydrogen production. *Rare Met.* **2023**, *42*, 1195–1204. [CrossRef]
33. Xu, J.; Zhong, W.; Chen, F.; Wang, X.; Yu, H. In situ cascade growth-induced strong coupling effect toward efficient photocatalytic hydrogen evolution of $ReS_2/ZnIn_2S_4$. *Appl. Catal. B* **2023**, *328*, 122493. [CrossRef]
34. Wu, K.; Jiang, R.; Zhao, Y.; Mao, L.; Gu, X.; Cai, X.; Zhu, M. Hierarchical $NiCo_2S_4/ZnIn_2S_4$ heterostructured prisms: High-efficient photocatalysts for hydrogen production under visible-light. *J. Colloid Interface Sci.* **2022**, *619*, 339–347. [CrossRef] [PubMed]
35. Feng, X.; Shang, H.; Zhou, J.; Ma, X.; Gao, X.; Wang, D.; Zhang, B.; Zhao, Y. Heterostructured core–shell $CoS_{1.097}@ZnIn_2S_4$ nanosheets for enhanced photocatalytic hydrogen evolution under visible light. *Chem. Eng. J.* **2023**, *457*, 141192. [CrossRef]
36. Li, Q.; Lu, Q.; Guo, E.; Wei, M.; Pang, Y. Hierarchical $Co_9S_8/ZnIn_2S_4$ Nanoflower Enables Enhanced Hydrogen Evolution Photocatalysis. *Energy Fuels* **2022**, *36*, 4541–4548. [CrossRef]
37. Zhao, F.; Zhang, M.; Yan, D.; Hu, X.; Fan, J.; Sun, T.; Liu, E. S-Scheme Co_9S_8 Nanoflower/Red Phosphorus Nanosheet Heterojunctions for Enhanced Photocatalytic H_2 Evolution. *ACS Appl. Nano Mater.* **2023**, *6*, 14478–14487. [CrossRef]
38. Liang, Q.; Gao, W.; Liu, C.; Xu, S.; Li, Z. A novel 2D/1D core-shell heterostructures coupling MOF-derived iron oxides with $ZnIn_2S_4$ for enhanced photocatalytic activity. *J. Hazard. Mater.* **2020**, *392*, 122500. [CrossRef]
39. Jiang, X.; Wang, Z.; Zhang, M.; Wang, M.; Wu, R.; Shi, X.; Luo, B.; Zhang, D.; Pu, X.; Li, H. A novel direct Z-scheme heterojunction $BiFeO_3/ZnFe_2O_4$ photocatalyst for enhanced photocatalyst degradation activity under visible light irradiation. *J. Alloys Compd.* **2022**, *912*, 165185. [CrossRef]
40. Ge, L.; Han, C.; Xiao, X.; Guo, L. In situ synthesis of cobalt–phosphate (Co–Pi) modified $g-C_3N_4$ photocatalysts with enhanced photocatalytic activities. *Appl. Catal. B* **2013**, *142–143*, 414–422. [CrossRef]
41. Xu, J.; Li, Q.; Sui, D.; Jiang, W.; Liu, F.; Gu, X.; Zhao, Y.; Ying, P.; Mao, L.; Cai, X.; et al. In Situ Photodeposition of Cobalt Phosphate (CoH_xPO_y) on $CdIn_2S_4$ Photocatalyst for Accelerated Hole Extraction and Improved Hydrogen Evolution. *Nanomaterials* **2023**, *13*, 420. [CrossRef] [PubMed]
42. Zhang, G.; Chen, D.; Li, N.; Xu, Q.; Li, H.; He, J.; Lu, J. Construction of Hierarchical Hollow $Co_9S_8/ZnIn_2S_4$ Tubular Heterostructures for Highly Efficient Solar Energy Conversion and Environmental Remediation. *Angew. Chem. Int. Ed.* **2020**, *59*, 8255–8261. [CrossRef] [PubMed]
43. Lakhera, S.K.; Vijayarajan, V.S.; Rishi Krishna, B.S.; Veluswamy, P.; Neppolian, B. Cobalt phosphate hydroxide loaded $g-C_3N_4$ photocatalysts and its hydrogen production activity. *Int. J. Hydrogen Energy* **2020**, *45*, 7562–7573. [CrossRef]
44. Liu, Z.-G.; Wei, Y.; Xie, L.; Chen, H.-Q.; Wang, J.; Yang, K.; Zou, L.-X.; Deng, T.; Lu, K.-Q. Decorating CdS with cobaltous hydroxide and graphene dual cocatalyst for photocatalytic hydrogen production coupled selective benzyl alcohol oxidation. *Mol. Catal.* **2024**, *553*, 113738. [CrossRef]
45. Wei, Y.; Hao, J.-G.; Zhang, J.-L.; Huang, W.-Y.; Ouyang, S.-B.; Yang, K.; Lu, K.-Q. Integrating $Co(OH)_2$ nanosheet arrays on graphene for efficient noble-metal-free EY-sensitized photocatalytic H_2 evolution. *Dalton Trans.* **2023**, *52*, 13923–13929. [CrossRef]
46. Ai, G.; Mo, R.; Li, H.; Zhong, J. Cobalt phosphate modified TiO_2 nanowire arrays as co-catalysts for solar water splitting. *Nanoscale* **2015**, *7*, 6722–6728. [CrossRef]
47. Jiang, Q.; Sun, L.; Bi, J.; Liang, S.; Li, L.; Yu, Y.; Wu, L. MoS_2 Quantum Dots-Modified Covalent Triazine-Based Frameworks for Enhanced Photocatalytic Hydrogen Evolution. *ChemSusChem* **2018**, *11*, 1108–1113. [CrossRef]
48. Li, X.-X.; Liu, X.-C.; Liu, C.; Zeng, J.-M.; Qi, X.-P. Co_3O_4/stainless steel catalyst with synergistic effect of oxygen vacancies and phosphorus doping for overall water splitting. *Tungsten* **2022**, *5*, 100–108. [CrossRef]
49. Mu, P.; Zhou, M.; Yang, K.; Chen, X.; Yu, Z.; Lu, K.; Huang, W.; Yu, C.; Dai, W. $Cd_{0.5}Zn_{0.5}S/CoWO_4$ Nanohybrids with a Twinning Homojunction and an Interfacial S-Scheme Heterojunction for Efficient Visible-Light-Induced Photocatalytic CO_2 Reduction. *Inorg. Chem.* **2021**, *60*, 14854–14865. [CrossRef]
50. Jiang, X.; Gong, H.; Liu, Q.; Song, M.; Huang, C. In situ construction of $NiSe/Mn_{0.5}Cd_{0.5}S$ composites for enhanced photocatalytic hydrogen production under visible light. *Appl. Catal. B* **2020**, *268*, 118439. [CrossRef]
51. Li, M.; Zhang, D.; Zhou, h.; Sun, K.; Ma, X.; Dong, M. Construction of hollow tubular $Co_9S_8/ZnSe$ S-scheme heterojunctions for enhanced photocatalytic H_2 evolution. *Int. J. Hydrogen Energy* **2023**, *48*, 5126–5137. [CrossRef]
52. Li, J.-Y.; Qi, M.-Y.; Xu, Y.-J. Efficient splitting of alcohols into hydrogen and C–C coupled products over ultrathin Ni-doped $ZnIn_2S_4$ nanosheet photocatalyst. *Chin. J. Catal.* **2022**, *43*, 1084–1091. [CrossRef]
53. Chong, W.-K.; Ng, B.-J.; Lee, Y.J.; Tan, L.-L.; Putri, L.K.; Low, J.; Mohamed, A.R.; Chai, S.-P. Self-activated superhydrophilic green $ZnIn_2S_4$ realizing solar-driven overall water splitting: Close-to-unity stability for a full daytime. *Nat. Commun.* **2023**, *14*, 7676. [CrossRef]
54. Jiang, J.; Xiong, Z.; Wang, H.; Liao, G.; Bai, S.; Zou, J.; Wu, P.; Zhang, P.; Li, X. Sulfur-doped $g-C_3N_4/g-C_3N_4$ isotype step-scheme heterojunction for photocatalytic H_2 evolution. *J. Mater. Sci. Technol.* **2022**, *118*, 15–24. [CrossRef]
55. Yan, W.; Zhang, Y.; Bi, Y. Subnanometric Bismuth Clusters Confined in Pyrochlore-$Bi_2Sn_2O_7$ Enable Remarkable CO_2 Photoreduction. *Angew. Chem. Int. Ed.* **2023**, *63*, e202316459. [CrossRef] [PubMed]
56. Wang, X.-K.; Liu, J.; Zhang, L.; Dong, L.-Z.; Li, S.-L.; Kan, Y.-H.; Li, D.-S.; Lan, Y.-Q. Monometallic Catalytic Models Hosted in Stable Metal–Organic Frameworks for Tunable CO_2 Photoreduction. *ACS Catal.* **2019**, *9*, 1726–1732. [CrossRef]
57. Lu, K.-Q.; Li, Y.-H.; Zhang, F.; Qi, M.-Y.; Chen, X.; Tang, Z.-R.; Yamada, Y.M.A.; Anpo, M.; Conte, M.; Xu, Y.-J. Rationally designed transition metal hydroxide nanosheet arrays on graphene for artificial CO_2 reduction. *Nat. Commun.* **2020**, *11*, 5181. [CrossRef]

58. Guan, X.; Qian, Y.; Zhang, X.; Jiang, H.L. Enaminone-Linked Covalent Organic Frameworks for Boosting Photocatalytic Hydrogen Production. *Angew. Chem. Int. Ed.* **2023**, *62*, e202306135. [CrossRef]
59. Gao, J.-X.; Tian, W.-J.; Zhang, H.-Y. Progress of Nb-containing catalysts for carbon dioxide reduction: A minireview. *Tungsten* **2022**, *4*, 284–295. [CrossRef]
60. Zou, J.; Wu, S.; Liu, Y.; Sun, Y.; Cao, Y.; Hsu, J.-P.; Shen Wee, A.T.; Jiang, J. An ultra-sensitive electrochemical sensor based on 2D g-C_3N_4/CuO nanocomposites for dopamine detection. *Carbon* **2018**, *130*, 652–663. [CrossRef]
61. Hu, M.; Wu, C.; Feng, S.; Hua, J. A High Crystalline Perylene-Based Hydrogen-Bonded Organic Framework for Enhanced Photocatalytic H_2O_2 Evolution. *Molecules* **2023**, *28*, 6850. [CrossRef] [PubMed]
62. Lu, K.-Q.; Chen, Y.; Xin, X.; Xu, Y.-J. Rational utilization of highly conductive, commercial Elicarb graphene to advance the graphene-semiconductor composite photocatalysis. *Appl. Catal. B* **2018**, *224*, 424–432. [CrossRef]
63. Su, B.; Kong, Y.; Wang, S.; Zuo, S.; Lin, W.; Fang, Y.; Hou, Y.; Zhang, G.; Zhang, H.; Wang, X. Hydroxyl-Bonded Ru on Metallic TiN Surface Catalyzing CO_2 Reduction with H_2O by Infrared Light. *J. Am. Chem. Soc.* **2023**, *145*, 27415–27423. [CrossRef]
64. Luo, D.; Peng, L.; Wang, Y.; Lu, X.; Yang, C.; Xu, X.; Huang, Y.; Ni, Y. Highly efficient photocatalytic water splitting utilizing a WO_{3-x}/$ZnIn_2S_4$ ultrathin nanosheet Z-scheme catalyst. *J. Mater. Chem. A* **2021**, *9*, 908–914. [CrossRef]
65. Tang, C.; Bao, T.; Li, S.; Wang, X.; Rao, H.; She, P.; Qin, J.-S. Bioinspired 3D penetrating structured micro-mesoporous NiCoFe-LDH@$ZnIn_2S_4$ Z-scheme heterojunction for simultaneously photocatalytic H_2 evolution coupled with benzylamine oxidation. *Appl. Catal. B* **2024**, *342*, 123384. [CrossRef]
66. Li, J.; Li, M.; Jin, Z. Rational design of a cobalt sulfide/bismuth sulfide S-scheme heterojunction for efficient photocatalytic hydrogen evolution. *J. Colloid Interface Sci.* **2021**, *592*, 237–248. [CrossRef]
67. Li, M.; Li, J.; Jin, Z. Synergistic effect of MoS_2 over WP photocatalyst for promoting hydrogen production. *J. Solid State Chem.* **2020**, *288*, 121419. [CrossRef]
68. Wu, Z.; Yuan, X.; Zeng, G.; Jiang, L.; Zhong, H.; Xie, Y.; Wang, H.; Chen, X.; Wang, H. Highly efficient photocatalytic activity and mechanism of Yb^{3+}/Tm^{3+} codoped In_2S_3 from ultraviolet to near infrared light towards chromium (VI) reduction and rhodamine B oxidative degradation. *Appl. Catal. B* **2018**, *225*, 8–21. [CrossRef]

Disclaimer/Publisher's Note: The statements, opinions and data contained in all publications are solely those of the individual author(s) and contributor(s) and not of MDPI and/or the editor(s). MDPI and/or the editor(s) disclaim responsibility for any injury to people or property resulting from any ideas, methods, instructions or products referred to in the content.

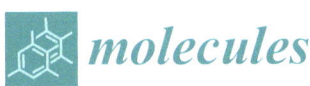

Article

Pd:In-Doped TiO$_2$ as a Bifunctional Catalyst for the Photoelectrochemical Oxidation of Paracetamol and Simultaneous Green Hydrogen Production

Nicolás Sacco [1], Alexander Iguini [2], Ilaria Gamba [2], Fernanda Albana Marchesini [1] and Gonzalo García [2,*]

1. Instituto de Investigaciones en Catálisis y Petroquímica, INCAPE (UNL-CONICET), Facultad de Ingeniería Química, Santiago del Estero 2829, Santa Fe 3000, Argentina; nsacco@fiq.unl.edu.ar (N.S.); albana.marchesini@gmail.com (F.A.M.)
2. Departamento de Química, Instituto Universitario de Materiales y Nanotecnología, Universidad de La Laguna (ULL), P.O. Box 456, 38200 La Laguna, Spain; alu0101100890@ull.edu.es (A.I.); ilgamba@ull.edu.es (I.G.)
* Correspondence: ggarcia@ull.edu.es

Citation: Sacco, N.; Iguini, A.; Gamba, I.; Marchesini, F.A.; García, G. Pd:In-Doped TiO$_2$ as a Bifunctional Catalyst for the Photoelectrochemical Oxidation of Paracetamol and Simultaneous Green Hydrogen Production. *Molecules* **2024**, *29*, 1073. https://doi.org/10.3390/molecules29051073

Academic Editors: Stefano Falcinelli and Sugang Meng

Received: 22 January 2024
Revised: 24 February 2024
Accepted: 27 February 2024
Published: 29 February 2024

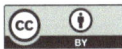

Copyright: © 2024 by the authors. Licensee MDPI, Basel, Switzerland. This article is an open access article distributed under the terms and conditions of the Creative Commons Attribution (CC BY) license (https://creativecommons.org/licenses/by/4.0/).

Abstract: The integration of clean energy generation with wastewater treatment holds promise for addressing both environmental and energy concerns. Focusing on photocatalytic hydrogen production and wastewater treatment, this study introduces PdIn/TiO$_2$ catalysts for the simultaneous removal of the pharmaceutical contaminant paracetamol (PTM) and hydrogen production. Physicochemical characterization showed a high distribution of Pd and In on the support as well as a high interaction with it. The Pd and In deposition enhance the light absorption capability and significantly improve the hydrogen evolution reaction (HER) in the absence and presence of paracetamol compared to TiO$_2$. On the other hand, the photoelectroxidation of PTM at TiO$_2$ and PdIn/TiO$_2$ follows the full mineralization path and, accordingly, is limited by the adsorption of intermediate species on the electrode surface. Thus, PdIn-doped TiO$_2$ stands out as a promising photoelectrocatalyst, showcasing enhanced physicochemical properties and superior photoelectrocatalytic performance. This underscores its potential for both environmental remediation and sustainable hydrogen production.

Keywords: PdIn-doped TiO$_2$ catalyst; green H$_2$ production; photoelectrochemical oxidation; paracetamol; pharmaceutical removal from water

1. Introduction

Energy production and water availability pose significant challenges for future generations. The global consumption of both resources is experiencing substantial growth, driven by population increases and improved living standards. The combustion of fossil fuels releases greenhouse gases and other pollutants into the atmosphere, resulting in critical consequences for the environment. On the other hand, water availability is threatened by the presence of contaminants in wastewater and the lack of water sanitation solutions.

The Sustainable Development Goals (SDGs) set forth by the United Nations for 2030 include specific objectives related to energy consumption (SDG 7: Affordable and Clean Energy) and water pollution (SDG 6: Clean Water Sanitation). Renewable energies could be a key part of the solution for sustainable energy production if electricity storage is ensured. Hydrogen has emerged as a highly promising renewable fuel due to its high energy content, lack of environmental hazards, and, most importantly, its ability to be produced from water [1,2]. The production of green hydrogen is a promising way to supply and distribute intermittently generated energy through fuel cells. However, its production through water splitting is not cost-effective due to the large amounts of energy required for the oxygen evolution reaction (OER) at the anode. It is important to consider that in the case of water splitting, the thermodynamic potential needed to break down water into oxygen and hydrogen is 1.23 V. However, high overpotentials are usually employed to overcome the slow kinetics of the OER [3]. Photoelectrocatalytic production of hydrogen by oxidizing organic or inorganic compounds at the anode can be achieved without the need for electrical input, but current catalysts do not meet the requirements to approach viability goals. On the other hand, the potential required for the degradation of contaminants depends on the nature and concentration of the contaminants, the nature of the photoelectrocatalyst, and the efficiency of the process used [4].

Electrocatalytic hydrogen production has emerged as a popular method for hydrogen generation [5]. However, there are several issues, including cost-effectiveness, associated with these techniques. To address the dual challenges of the energy crisis and environmental pollution, sustainable photocatalytic hydrogen production has shown promise [6,7]. However, efficient photocatalytic hydrogen generation typically requires the use of external sacrificial agents or donors, such as alcohols or organic acids, to scavenge holes and reduce recombination [8]. The addition of these sacrificial agents increases the cost of hydrogen evolution, making it economically viable but less practical in the long run [9]. Thus, for sustainable and efficient hydrogen production, there are two main requirements to achieve. Firstly, the photocatalyst must possess efficient electron–hole separation, numerous active reaction sites, and high visible light activity [10,11], which is crucial for effective hydrogen generation. The second challenge involves the recovery or generation of hydrogen energy from wastewater, enabling environmentally friendly and sustainable energy production combined with water treatment on a larger scale. This integrated approach holds promise for addressing both energy and environmental concerns.

Various catalysts for efficient photocatalytic H_2 generation have been synthesized by different authors. Meng et al. [12] developed $Ni_{12}P_5/ZnIn_2S_4$ (NP/ZIS) heterostructures using a hydrothermal method, demonstrating visible-light-driven photocatalytic splitting of benzyl alcohol into H_2 and benzaldehyde. The use of 7% NP/ZIS significantly improved the thermodynamics and kinetics of H_2 production compared to pure water splitting and individual ZIS, attributed to increased surface area, porous structure, creation of defect states (zinc vacancies), and the enhancement of the NP co-catalyst. Amorphous TiO_2 and $Co-ZnIn_2S_4$ were combined to form a heterojunction, improving photocarrier separation efficiency and catalyst stability. The introduction of amorphous TiO_2 induced oxygen vacancies, enhancing carrier density. Additionally, MoP nanoparticles were introduced as co-catalysts, serving as hydrogen production sites and achieving efficient hydrogen production [13].

Long et al. [14] investigated nanostructured polymeric carbon nitride (PCN) for visible-light-driven photocatalytic hydrogen evolution, attributing improved activity to increased BET specific surface area, higher active site quantity, and accelerated transfer and separation of photo-excited charge carriers. Additionally, Zheng et al. [15] demonstrated the excellent photocatalytic activity of Au/ZnO nanomaterial in bisphenol A degradation and photoelectrochemical water splitting. The enhanced activities were linked to heightened light absorption and unique charge transfer of photogenerated electrons, effectively reducing the recombination rate and prolonging the lifetime of photo-excited carriers.

Contaminants of emerging concern (CECs) are increasingly being detected in water sources worldwide, posing significant challenges to water quality and human health. These CECs include a wide range of pollutants, such as pharmaceuticals, personal care products, pesticides, industrial chemicals, and microplastics, which can enter water bodies through various pathways [16,17]. The presence of CECs in water raises concerns for both ecological and human health. These contaminants can have adverse effects on aquatic ecosystems, including the disruption of endocrine systems, alteration of reproductive behaviors, and changes in the composition of microbial communities. In terms of human health, exposure to CECs through drinking water consumption or recreational activities in contaminated water bodies can pose risks, particularly for vulnerable populations such as children and pregnant women [18].

Paracetamol, also known as acetaminophen, is a widely used over-the-counter medication for pain relief and fever reduction. Like many pharmaceuticals, it can enter the environment through various pathways, including improper disposal, excretion, and wastewater treatment plant effluents. While it is generally considered safe for human use when taken at recommended doses, the presence of PTM in water bodies as a CEC is a topic of growing interest and research. The presence of acetaminophen in aquatic environments can have adverse effects on aquatic organisms. Even at low concentrations, it can disrupt the endocrine systems of fish and other aquatic organisms, affecting their reproductive capabilities [19].

Thus, utilizing PTM as a sacrificial agent in photocatalytic hydrogen evolution serves the purposes of both clean energy generation and wastewater treatment.

Photoelectrochemical oxidation (PECO) is indeed a promising technique for the removal of PTM from water. PECO involves the use of a photoactive electrode, typically a semiconductor material, which generates reactive oxygen species (ROS) upon exposure to light. These ROS, such as hydroxyl radicals, play a crucial role in the degradation of organic contaminants like PTM [20].

Since the discovery of TiO_2's ability for water-splitting and photocatalytic degradation of organic compounds, numerous semiconductors have been studied for environmental and energy applications. TiO_2 is the most extensively investigated due to its chemical stability, low cost, and good photocatalytic efficiency [21]. However, TiO_2 does have a limitation in its optical response. With a large band gap (E.g., ~3.2 eV), TiO_2 primarily responds to UV light, which accounts for only 5% of solar energy [22]. To address this issue, various modifications of TiO_2 have been extensively studied to enhance its wavelength range response, promote charge generation, and facilitate efficient charge separation to minimize recombination [23]. Techniques for TiO_2 modifications include metal loading, ion doping, semiconductor coupling, and dye sensitization. Depositing precious metals or rare-earth metals onto semiconductors is a widely investigated approach to enhance the photocatalytic properties of TiO_2 [24]. This method offers two main advantages: the formation of a Schottky junction for efficient charge separation and the localized surface plasmon resonance (LSPR) effect, which promotes enhanced charge generation through the absorption of visible light.

Pd and Pd-In catalysts have been widely reported in the catalytic reduction and electrochemical reduction of inorganic ions present in water [25]. It has been demonstrated that the Pd-In combination can hydrogenate nitrate ions into nitrites in water [26]. On the other hand, Pd has attracted significant attention as it is one of the platinum-group metals with high catalytic activity for the HER [27]. It is important to note that most of the catalysts, either mono- or bimetallic, based on Pd for the electrocatalytic production of H_2 imply the use of high metal loadings, which considerably increases the cost of these technologies. This work evaluates the catalytic performance of PdIn-doped TiO_2 catalysts (Pd, 1 wt.%, In 0.25 wt.%) in the photoelectrochemical oxidation of PTM and the simultaneous HER. The reaction mechanism, both for PTM oxidation and HER, and the stability of the catalyst are discussed.

2. Results and Discussion

2.1. Characterization

2.1.1. UV-DRS Analysis

To evaluate the absorbance properties of TiO_2 and $PdIn/TiO_2$ synthesized in this study, UV–Vis diffuse reflectance spectra (DRS) were measured (Figure 1). The absorption band edge of TiO_2 occurs at approximately 400 nm. The addition of PdIn leads to an increase in absorption at longer wavelengths within the visible range. The band gap values of TiO_2 and $PdIn/TiO_2$ were 3.67 and 3.47 eV, respectively. The lowest band gap value obtained after the impregnation of PdIn onto TiO_2 would indicate that the Pd and In deposition enhances the light absorption capability, resulting in a possible higher catalytic activity when compared to TiO_2 alone. This behavior could be related to the Fermi levels of Pd, which are lower than those of TiO$_2$, facilitating the efficient transfer of photogenerated electrons from the conduction band of TiO$_2$ to the metal particles. This process of electron trapping greatly diminishes the rate of electron–hole recombination, leading to enhanced photocatalytic reactions.

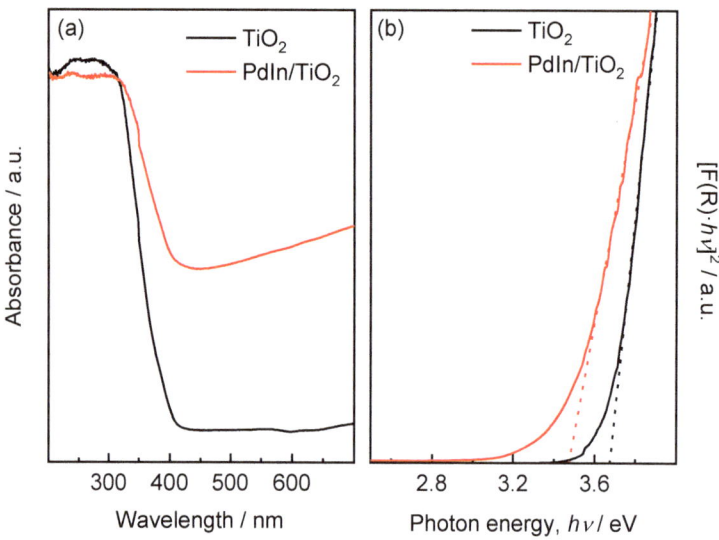

Figure 1. (**a**) UV–vis absorption spectra and (**b**) bandgap energy plot (Kubelka–Munk function) of TiO$_2$ (black line) and PdIn/TiO$_2$ (red line) materials.

2.1.2. Physicochemical Properties

Morphology and elemental analysis of PdIn/TiO$_2$ were studied through SEM–EDS and HRTEM techniques, respectively. Figure 2a shows an SEM–EDS micrograph of the PdIn/TiO$_2$ catalyst and the corresponding mappings. A homogeneous distribution of the materials was obtained. Indeed, a high distribution of Pd and In on the TiO$_2$ particles is perceived, with an average wt.% composition of 0.85 ± 0.07 and 0.22 ± 0.04, respectively, and a Pd:In atomic ratio close to the nominal value was detected. Figure 2b shows the HRTEM micrograph of the PdIn/TiO$_2$ catalyst. Particles with an average size of 18 nm are observed and depicted in the particle size distribution graph (Figure S1). Furthermore, particles with smaller sizes (~5 nm) are discerned and may be ascribed to Pd and/or In-based species.

The surface area and pore volume of PdIn/TiO$_2$, obtained from BET analysis, were 48.84 m^2/g and 0.0015 cm^3/g, respectively. For commercial TiO$_2$, a surface area of 48.47 m^2/g was reported, a similar value [28]. Therefore, no diminution of the surface area is perceived after metal deposition onto TiO$_2$ material. Figure S2 shows nitrogen adsorption isotherms of TiO$_2$ and PdIn/TiO$_2$ materials. N$_2$ adsorption isotherms align with type II, as per the IUPAC classification. These isotherms are indicative of non-porous or macroporous solids, exhibiting low or negligible microporosity and unrestricted multilayer adsorption.

XRD patterns of PdIn/TiO$_2$ and the bare support were assayed to elucidate the crystalline phases present. Figure 3 shows the corresponding diffractograms, respectively. Anatase (JCPDS 00-021-1272) and rutile (JCPDS 00-021-1276) phases were detected in both TiO$_2$ and PdIn/TiO$_2$ catalysts. No crystalline phases corresponding to Pd or In were detected, which could be due to the low metal loading, the high dispersion of the material on the support, and/or the amorphous nature of the dispersed species. The crystallite size of both phases, anatase (plane 1 0 1, 2θ = 25.281°) and rutile (plane 1 1 0, 2θ = 27.477°), for PdIn/TiO$_2$ and TiO$_2$ were calculated using the Scherrer equation. Crystallite sizes of 20.93 nm were obtained for the anatase phase of both catalysts. For the rutile phase of

TiO$_2$ and PdIn/TiO$_2$, crystallite sizes of 25.6 and 31.4 nm, respectively, were obtained. This change of crystallite size in the rutile phase could be due to a strong interaction with Pd and In species or to their introduction into its crystalline network since the doping of the material could affect its electronic and structural properties and consequently the crystallite size [29–31].

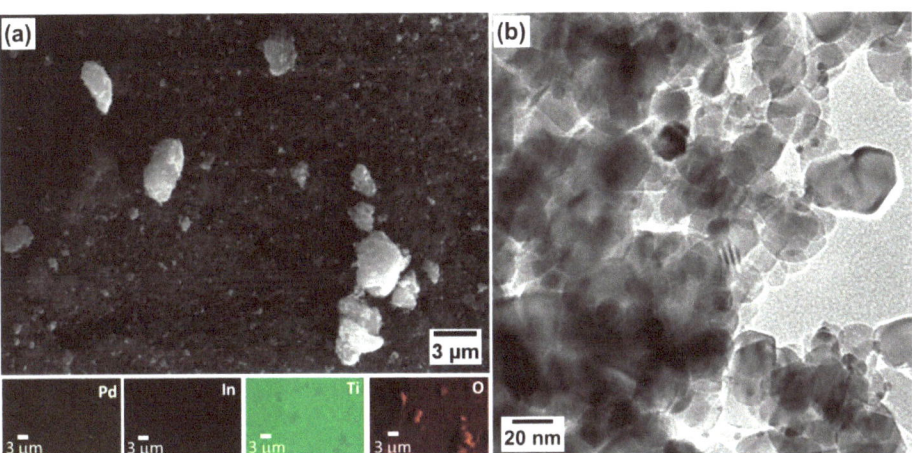

Figure 2. (**a**) SEM micrograph of PdIn/TiO$_2$ catalyst and corresponding mappings of Pd, In, O, and Ti species. (**b**) HRTEM micrograph of PdIn/TiO$_2$ catalyst.

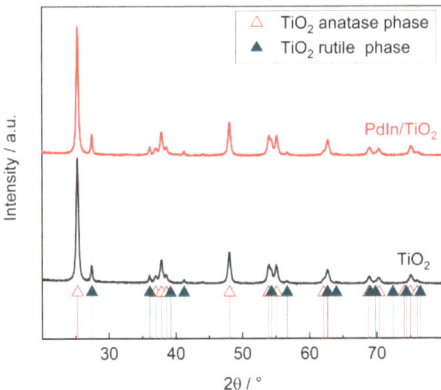

Figure 3. XRD patterns of PdIn/TiO$_2$ (red line) and TiO$_2$ (black line) samples.

The electroactive surface area was calculated by performing CVs at different scan rates in a potential range where no faradaic reaction occurs (i.e., capacitive currents are employed) by plotting the anodic and cathodic current densities at a fixed potential versus the scanning rate (see Figure S3 as an example for GC in the Supplementary Material). The same procedure was performed for TiO$_2$ and PdIn/TiO$_2$. The corresponding values of anodic and cathodic electrochemical double-layer capacitances (EDLC$_A$ and EDLC$_V$, respectively) and electroactive surface areas for different electrodes, calculated using Equations (14) and (15) (see Experimental section), are summarized in Table 1. Considering the slopes obtained for each material, it can be observed that the PdIn/TiO$_2$ catalyst reveals a higher ECSA than GC and TiO$_2$.

Table 1. Double-layer capacitance and electroactive surface area for the photoelectrocatalysts prepared.

Photocatalyst	EDLC$_A$ (mF/cm^2)	EDLC$_C$ (mF/cm^2)	Electroactive Surface Area (cm^2)
GC	0.00003	−0.00003	0.6
TiO$_2$	0.00011	−0.0001	2.5
PdIn/TiO$_2$	0.0004	−0.0004	8.24

2.2. Hydrogen Evolution Reaction

Figure 4 shows cyclic voltammograms performed at GC (black line), TiO$_2$ (red line), and PdIn/TiO$_2$ (blue line) between −0.3 V and 1.5 V in the electrolyte solution. As expected, the GC electrode reveals only capacitive currents in the potential range under study. On the other hand, TiO$_2$ and PdIn/TiO$_2$ catalysts show an increment of the cathodic current at potentials more negative than 0.0 V, which is associated with the HER. Interestingly, the presence of PdIn significantly improves the HER in the electrolyte solution. Indeed, PdIn/TiO$_2$ develops double the current at −0.25 V compared with TiO$_2$.

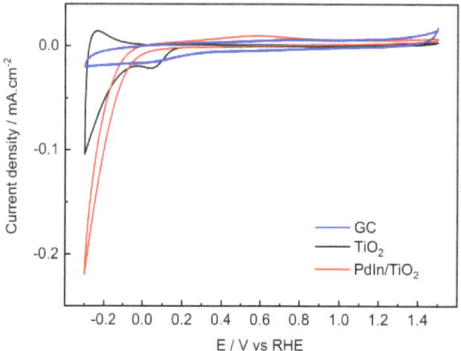

Figure 4. Cyclic voltammograms of GC (blue line), TiO$_2$ (black line), and PdIn/TiO$_2$ (red line). Sweep rate = 20 mV·s^{-1}, in 0.1 M phosphate buffer solution, pH = 7.

The photoelectrocatalytic performance of TiO$_2$ (black lines) and PdIn/TiO$_2$ (red lines) catalysts toward the HER was evaluated through chronoamperometry technique in the presence (light on) and absence (light of) of radiation at 0 and −0.1 V with an irradiation intermittence of 30 s (Figure 5).

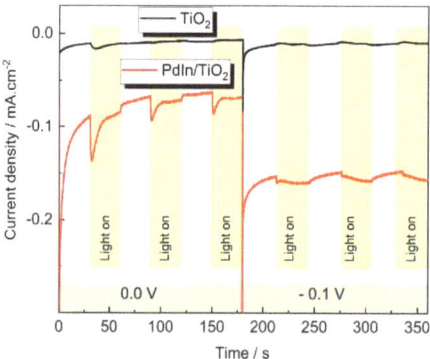

Figure 5. Current transients of TiO$_2$ (black line) and PdIn/TiO$_2$ (red line) recorded at 0.0 and −0.1 V in 0.1 M phosphate buffer solution, pH = 7, under the absence and presence of light.

TiO$_2$ material develops low cathodic current and photocurrents at both studied potentials. Oppositely, the PdIn/TiO$_2$ catalyst reveals high cathodic current values at both applied potentials and suitable photoactivity at 0.0 V. The decrease of the photoactivity of PdIn/TiO$_2$ at -0.1 V suggests that the flat band potential is close. In addition, the PdIn/TiO$_2$ catalyst develops similar cathodic current values over time, which indicates an appropriate photoelectrochemical stability and, thus, a suitable photoelectrocatalytic performance toward the HER.

A Tafel plot was employed to better understand the reaction kinetics and mechanism of the HER at the best catalyst developed in the current work. For this purpose, linear sweep voltammetry (LSV) was performed between 0.2 and -0.2 V at a sweep speed of 5 mV·s^{-1}. Two reaction mechanisms are commonly discussed in the literature [32,33], denoted as Volmer–Heyrovsky and Volmer–Tafel. Both mechanisms have in common that hydrogen is adsorbed (H$_{ad}$) on the electrode through the electrochemical Volmer step but differ in the second stage. For the Volmer–Heyrovsky mechanism (Equation (1)), the Heyrovsky step (Equation (2)) involves the adsorbed hydrogen recombining with another proton from the solution to release an H$_2$ molecule. On the other hand, the Volmer–Tafel mechanism consists of two consecutive Volmer steps and the Tafel step (Equation (3)) in a recombination step of two adjacent hydrogen adsorbates to form H$_2$.

$$\text{Volmer} : H_2O + e^- \rightleftharpoons H_{ad} + OH^-, \tag{1}$$

$$\text{Heyrovsky} : H_{ad} + H_2O + e^- \rightleftharpoons H_2 + OH^-, \tag{2}$$

and

$$\text{Tafel} : H_{ad} + H_{ad} \rightleftharpoons H_2 \tag{3}$$

Tafel slope (TS) values were employed to discern which reaction mechanism follows the HER at the PdIn/TiO$_2$ catalyst. TS values of 120, 30, and 40 mV·dec^{-1} are associated with Volmer, Tafel, and Heyrovsky as the rate-determining step (RDS), respectively. Figure 6a shows the LSV recorded for PdIn/TiO$_2$ performed at 5 mv·s^{-1} from 0.2 V to -0.2 V in the electrolyte solution. Figure 6b shows a TS close to 120 mV·dec^{-1}, which is attributed to the Volmer step as the RDS during the HER at the PdIn/TiO$_2$ catalyst. In this sense, the high TS may be attributed to the high amount of surface oxygenated species of TiO$_2$, which may inhibit the first electron transfer step.

2.3. Paracetamol Oxidation Reaction

The photoelectrocatalytic activity of GCE, PdIn/TiO$_2$, and TiO$_2$ support towards the oxidation of PTM (100 ppm) was evaluated using cyclic voltammetry under irradiation and in the absence of irradiation. Figure 7 shows CV profiles of PTM electro-oxidation in the dark at GCE, TiO$_2$, and PdIn/TiO$_2$. As discussed above (see Figure 4), the presence of PTM does not change the catalytic performance toward the HER at PdIn/TiO$_2$, and consequently, the catalytic active sites for the HER are not compromised.

PTM oxidation on GCE (blue line) exhibits an anodic current generation with an anodic peak at 1.1V, and an onset potential of 1.0 V. A quasi-reversible process with a peak-to-peak separation of $\Delta V = 250$ mV was determined, as reported by Nematollahi et al. [34] for the same material and similar pH conditions. At more positive potentials than the anodic current peak, a large drop in current density is observed, showing a Cottrell behavior, indicating that the process is limited by diffusion of the species towards the electrode surface.

On the other hand, TiO$_2$ (black line) and PdIn/TiO$_2$ (red line) show an irreversible behavior toward the PTM oxidation with onset potentials of 1.0 V and $\Delta V = 750$ and 420 mV, respectively. Evidently, at higher potentials than the anodic peak current, the oxidation behavior is different for GCE compared with TiO$_2$-based materials. This suggests that the reaction mechanism at TiO$_2$-based materials is limited by adsorbed species.

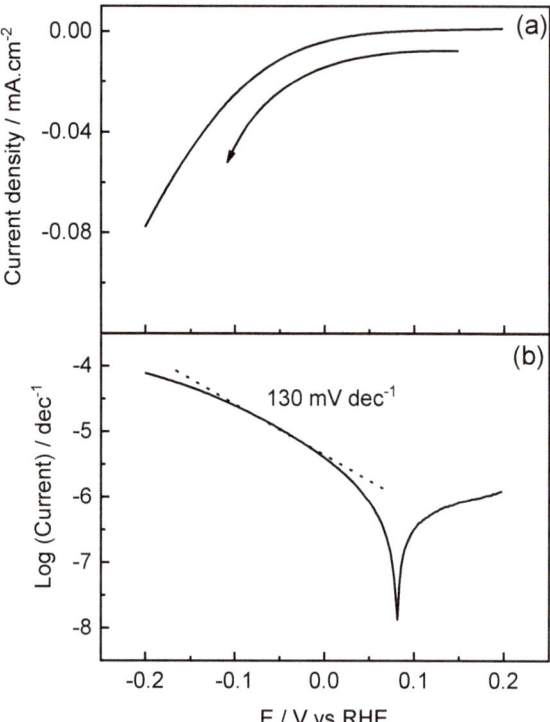

Figure 6. Linear sweep voltammogram recorded at 5 mV·s^{-1} (**a**) and Tafel plot (**b**) for PdIn/TiO$_2$ in 0.1 M phosphate buffer solution, pH = 7.

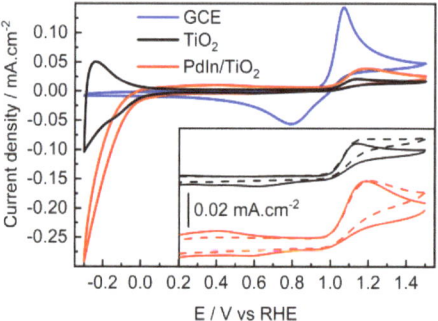

Figure 7. Cyclic voltammograms of GC (blue line), TiO$_2$ (black line), and PdIn/TiO$_2$ (red line) in a 100 ppm PTM solution in 0.1 M phosphate buffer solution. Sweep rate = 20 mV·s^{-1}, pH = 7. Inset (For the sake of clarity, the CVs were vertically translated): TiO$_2$ and PdIn/TiO$_2$ in the absence (solid lines) and the presence of light (dashed lines) in a 100 ppm PTM solution in 0.1 M phosphate buffer solution. Sweep rate = 20 mV·s^{-1}, pH = 7.

The same CV experiments were performed on TiO$_2$ and PdIn/TiO$_2$ but in the presence of light. The inset plot in Figure 7 compares voltammograms corresponding to the PTM oxidation at TiO$_2$ and PdIn/TiO$_2$ catalysts under the absence (solid lines) and the presence (dashed lines) of light. During the oxidation of PTM in the absence of light, at more positive potentials than the anodic peak, the current density slightly decreases (i.e., non-Cottrell behavior) with the rise of the applied potential, suggesting that the current is limited by kinetic. Conversely, in the presence of light, the current density remained almost constant at more positive potentials than the anodic peak, which implies that the current is limited by kinetics and suggests that adsorbed species are responsible. On the other hand, during the reverse scan, the presence of light made the system completely irreversible, i.e., no cathodic currents were discerned.

To better understand the kinetics and reaction mechanism of the PTM oxidation at all materials studied in the current work, rotating disk experiments at different rotational speeds were performed.

Figure 8a,b compares CV profiles of PTM oxidation at GCE performed at different sweep rates and rotational rates, respectively. These experiments demonstrate that the PTM oxidation process is diffusion-limited on the GCE since, as shown in Figure 8, the anodic current density reaches a constant diffusion value (I_{DIF}), which increases with the growth of the rotational speed.

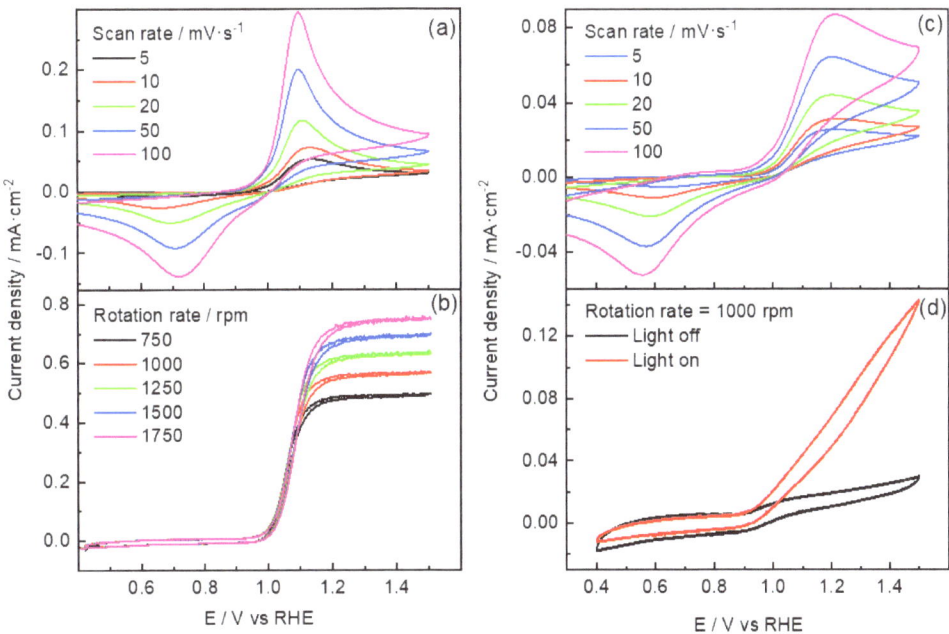

Figure 8. Cyclic voltammograms at diverse sweep rates at (**a**) GCE and (**c**) PdIn/TiO$_2$. Steady-state polarization curves recorded at 10 mV·s^{-1} at several rotation rates at (**b**) GCE and (**d**) at the PdIn/TiO$_2$ electrode in the presence (red line) and the absence (black line) of radiation. All assays were performed in a 100 ppm PTM solution in 0.1 M phosphate buffer, pH = 7.

For GCE, Randles–Sevsick and Koutecky–Levich plots with the corresponding slope value are shown in Figure S4, respectively. Koutecky–Levich equation is shown in Equation (4), where I_{DIF} is the limit current (A), I_k the kinetic current, and I_{lev} is expressed using Equation (5):

$$\frac{1}{I_{DIF}} = \frac{1}{I_{lev}} + \frac{1}{I_k} \quad (4)$$

and

$$I_{lev} = 0.62nFAD^{2/3}\omega^{1/2}\nu^{-1/6}C, \quad (5)$$

where v is the kinematic viscosity, w is the angular frequency of rotation (rad·s^{-1}), A is the disk electrode area (cm^2), and other symbols have their conventional meanings. By plotting $\frac{1}{I_{DIF}}$ vs $\omega^{-1/2}$ and obtaining from the literature for the kinematic viscosity of the electrolyte (0.012 cm^2·s^{-1}) [35] and the diffusion coefficient D (6.1 × 10^{-6} cm^2·s^{-1}) [36], the number of electrons transferred involved in the reaction yielded a value of 2, as reported by Nematollahi et al. [34]. Thus, this process could be associated with the reversible transformation of PTM into N-acetyl-p-benzoquinone amine (NAPQI) [34]:

$$C_8H_9NO_2 \rightleftharpoons C_8H_7NO_2 + 2H^+ + 2e^-. \quad (6)$$

Figure 8c,d compares CV profiles of PTM oxidation at PdIn/TiO$_2$ performed at different sweep rates and rotational rates, respectively. On the other hand, the anodic peak potential for TiO$_2$ and PdIn/TiO$_2$ was plotted as a function of the scan rate, and a linear trend was discerned, which suggests that the process is limited by the adsorption of species on the electrode surface. The number of electrons (n) transferred to the surface of the electrode was calculated through the Laviron equation for an irreversible process, where α is the electron-transfer coefficient (0.5), and n is the number of electrons involved in the redox process [37]:

$$E_{pA} = \frac{RT}{(1-\alpha)nF} log(v). \quad (7)$$

For both TiO$_2$-based electrodes, the number of transferred electrons was 1, and the subsequent reaction is the most plausible to occur:

$$C_8H_9NO_2 \rightleftharpoons (C_8H_8NO_2)_{ad} + H^+ + 1e^-. \quad (8)$$

Then, the adsorbed species may follow subsequent reactions at more positive potentials:

$$(C_8H_8NO_2)_{ad} \rightleftharpoons (C_8H_7NO_2)_{ad} + H^+ + 1e^-, \quad (9)$$

$$(C_8H_7NO_2)_{ad} \rightleftharpoons C_8H_7NO_2, \quad (10)$$

and

$$(C_8H_7NO_2)_{ad} + 14H_2O \rightarrow 8CO_2 + \frac{1}{2}N_2 + 35H^+ + 35e^-. \quad (11)$$

Equation (10) seems to be facile at GCE, while the opposite happens at TiO$_2$-based electrodes, and accordingly, the adsorbate path is favored. In this sense, Equation (11) indicates the global reaction toward the total mineralization of paracetamol, which is expected to follow the adsorbate route via deprotonation processes. In this context, it is important to note that the presence of radiation at TiO$_2$-based electrodes completely inhibits the pathway toward soluble species (i.e., Equation (10)), and consequently, no cathodic peaks are detected during the reverse sweep.

In this regard, Figure 8d suggests the aforementioned phenomenon, as a subsequent increment in the anodic current is perceived with the rise of applied potential in the presence of light. Remarkably, the same current values were obtained at rotation rates higher than 750 rpm, and no inhibition was discerned in the subsequent cycles. Therefore, the adsorbate route seems to predominate in TiO$_2$-based catalysts. Furthermore, the addition of a small amount of PdIn into TiO$_2$ not only increases the catalytic efficiency toward PTM oxidation but also intensely raises the HER, which is not inhibited in the presence of the organic molecule.

Finally, to test the catalytic stability of PdIn/TiO$_2$ toward the degradation of PTM in the absence and presence of light, a current transient was recorded at 1.2 V and depicted in Figure 9. An initial decrease in the anodic current density in the absence of light is observed, which rises and remains almost constant when the system is exposed to light. This indicates an improved catalyst performance toward PTM photoelectroxidation.

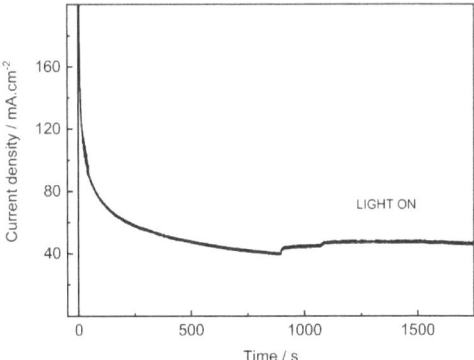

Figure 9. Photo/current transients of PdIn/TiO$_2$ recorded at 1.2 V and 1000 rpm, under the absence and the presence of light in a 100 ppm PTM solution in 0.1 M phosphate buffer solution, pH = 7.

3. Experimental

3.1. Catalyst Synthesis

The bimetallic catalyst supported on titania was prepared using the conventional wet impregnation method by co-impregnating Pd:In in a 1:0.25 wt.% ratio relative to the support (TiO$_2$), followed by calcination and reduction.

A solution of PdCl$_2$ (Sigma Aldrich, St. Louis, MO, USA, p.a.) and InCl$_3$ (Sigma Aldrich, 99.9%) was utilized to achieve the desired bimetallic catalyst. The process involved the addition of a specific mass of TiO$_2$ support (Degussa, Zürich, Germany, P25, 48 m^2/g) to a container containing water, along with a volume of concentrated Pd and In solutions, to attain the desired weight percentages of the metals, namely 1.00% Pd and 0.25% In.

Once the mixture was homogeneous and the solvent was evaporated, the material was dried overnight at 80 °C, and then calcined at 500 °C for 4 h. Finally, it was reduced using a 0.2 M solution of hydrazine hydrate and washed several times with deionized water. The material was left to dry overnight at 80 °C and named PdIn/TiO$_2$.

3.2. Physicochemical Characterization

X-ray diffraction (XRD), energy-dispersive X-ray spectroscopy (EDX), N$_2$ adsorption–desorption isotherms, scanning electron microscopy (SEM), and transmission electron microscopy (TEM) were employed for the physicochemical characterization of catalysts.

XRD powder spectra were generated utilizing the X'Pert PRO X-ray diffractometer (PANalytical, Tokyo, Japan) to ascertain the crystal structure. The measurements were conducted using CuKα radiation (λ = 1.5405 Å) and the X'pert high score plus diffraction software, version 1.0f. The 2θ data were collected in the range of 20° to 100° with a scanning rate of 0.04° s^{-1}. The identification of crystalline phases was achieved by comparing the experimental diffraction patterns with those in the Joint Committee on Powder Diffraction Standards (JCPDS).

Morphological characterization of the synthesized catalysts was performed using SEM images recorded with a ZEISS EVO 15 SEM with a 2 nm resolution and Oxford X-MAX 50 mm^2 EDX.

TEM studies were conducted using a JEOL JEM 2100 electron microscope operating at 100 kV. The samples were diluted in ethanol and placed in a conventional TEM copper grid with a thin holey carbon film.

N$_2$ adsorption–desorption isotherms of the carbon supports were measured at −196 °C using Micromeritics ASAP 2020 equipment. The total surface area was calculated from the BET (Brunauer, Emmett, and Teller) equation, and the total pore volume was determined using the single-point method at P/P$_0$ = 0.99. Pore size distribution (PSD) curves were obtained from the analysis of the desorption branch of the N$_2$ isotherm using the BJH (Barrett, Joyner, and Halenda) method.

3.3. Photochemical Properties

The materials were initially characterized using diffuse reflectance to obtain the band-gap values of the catalysts and narrow down the spectrum of catalysts to be studied. The band-gap values of each material were obtained using the Kubelka–Munk method (K–M or $F(R)$), as shown in Equation (12):

$$F(R) = \frac{(1-R)^2}{2R}, \tag{12}$$

where R is the reflectance, and $F(R)$ is proportional to the extinction coefficient (α). A modified K–M function can be obtained by multiplying the $F(R)$ function by hν, using the corresponding coefficient (n) associated with an electronic transition (Equation (13)):

$$(F(R) \times h\nu)^n. \tag{13}$$

Graphing Equation (12) as a function of energy in eV yields the value of the material's band gap. The band gap refers to the energy difference between the valence band (the highest energy level filled with electrons) and the conduction band (the lowest empty energy level) in a material. The size of the band gap determines a material's ability to absorb light and participate in photochemical reactions. Therefore, materials with smaller band gaps are usually more efficient at utilizing a wider range of light energy, requiring less energy to promote electrons to the conduction band.

3.4. Electrochemical Characterization

A temperature of 20 °C was chosen to assess the electrochemical performance of the catalysts in a three-electrode cell controlled via a GAMRY Reference 620–45080 Potentiostat/Galvanostat. The reference electrode used was a reversible hydrogen electrode (RHE), and all potentials mentioned below are presented relative to this electrode. The counter electrode (CE) consisted of a glassy carbon (GC) rod, while the working electrode (WE) was applied as ink onto a GC disk. Assays in a rotating disk electrode (RDE) AUTOLAB RDE-2 were carried out under the same conditions. Current density values were obtained from the geometrical area of the WE.

For the preparation of the inks to be deposited on the GC disk, 2 mg of the catalyst was placed in an Eppendorf tube. Subsequently, 15 µL of NAFION and 500 µL of isopropyl alcohol were introduced into the tube, and the blend was subjected to 30 min of sonication for homogenization. After achieving homogeneity, the dispersed ink (40 µL) was applied onto a polished GC disk (10 mm diameter). The ink was then dried under an inert atmosphere before being utilized in the electrochemical cell. For assays in the RDE, 12 µL of the dispersed ink was applied onto the polished GC disk (3 mm diameter).

The electrochemical behavior of the catalyst powders in a phosphate buffer solution with and without PTM (100 mg·L^{-1}), purged with pure N$_2$ before each measurement, was examined using cyclic voltammetry (CV) and chronoamperometry techniques.

Electrolytic solutions were prepared using potassium phosphates salts (H$_2$KPO$_4$ and HK$_2$PO$_4$) and milli-Q water to form a solution of 0.1 mol·L^{-1} with pH = 7.

Electroactive surface area was estimated from the CV curves of the catalyst at different scan rates in the electrolyte support. CVs were performed for each material, including the bare electrode (i.e., glassy carbon), at different scan rates (5, 10, 20, 50, and 100 mV·s^{-1}) in the double-layer region to obtain the electroactive surface area (ECSA). The calculation of ECSA (Equation (14)) from the CV data involves the use of the electrochemical double-layer capacitance (EDLC), which can be obtained from the slope of the current density versus scan rate:

$$ECSA = R_f \times S \tag{14}$$

Assuming that S is the geometric area of 0.785 cm^2, and R_f is the roughness factor obtained through Equation (15):

$$R_f = {C_{dl}} \Big/ {40 \ \mu\text{F}\cdot\text{cm}^{-2}} \qquad (15)$$

Hydrodynamic voltammetry employing Rotating Disk Electrode (RDE) techniques was conducted. The rotation rate of the disk ranged from 750 rpm to 1750 rpm.

3.5. Photoelectrochemical Characterization

A Light source, Xe lamp XSS-5XD (Power 150 to 320 W, Radiant Output: 50 W), was used to assess the photoelectrochemical characterization of the materials. A light intensity of 57,500 lux (lumen/m^2) was used for the experiments.

Photoelectrochemical properties were evaluated using chronoamperometry and CV techniques, both in the presence and absence of irradiation. The tests were carried out in a system as shown in the design shown in Figure S5. The temperature of the working solution was monitored throughout the experiments, and no variations were discerned.

4. Conclusions

A small amount of Pd (1.00 wt.%) and In (0.25 wt.%) deposition into TiO$_2$ enhanced the light absorption capacity and led to a notable improvement of the hydrogen evolution reaction (HER). This improvement is observed not only in the electrolyte but also in the presence of paracetamol (PTM). In the context of PTM oxidation, both TiO$_2$ and PdIn/TiO$_2$ exhibit irreversible behavior, primarily hindered by the adsorption of species on the electrode surface. The presence of radiation at TiO$_2$-based electrodes completely inhibits the pathway toward soluble species, resulting in a fully irreversible process and improving the catalyst performance toward PTM photoelectroxidation.

Thus, a small amount of Pd and In into TiO$_2$ not only increases the (photo)electrocatalytic efficiency toward the PTM oxidation but also intensely raises the HER, which is not inhibited in the presence of the organic molecule, highlighting its capability for both environmental remediation and sustainable hydrogen production.

Consequently, PdIn-doped TiO$_2$ emerges as a promising catalyst, showcasing heightened physicochemical properties and superior catalytic performance. This highlights its potential for applications in both environmental remediation and sustainable hydrogen production.

Supplementary Materials: The following supporting information can be downloaded at https://www.mdpi.com/article/10.3390/molecules29051073/s1, Figure S1. Particle size distribution of TiO$_2$ and Pd obtained from counts of different regions and TEM micrographs. Figure S2. (a) Nitrogen adsorption/desorption isotherms of TiO$_2$ and PdIn/TiO$_2$. (b) BET surface area plot of TiO$_2$ and PdIn/TiO$_2$. Figure S3. (a) Cyclic voltammograms recorded at different sweep rates 5 (black line), 10 (red line), 20 (green line), 50 (blue line) and 100 (pink line) mV·s^{-1} at GC electrode in 0.1 M phosphate buffer solution. (b) Current density (mA·cm^{-2}) as a function of scan rate (V·s^{-1}). Data acquired from Figure S3a at 0.3 V. Figure S4. Linear fit of current peak vs square root of scan rate (a) and diffusion current vs the inverse of square root rotation rate (b). Data acquired from Figure 8a,b, respectively. Figure S5. Illustration of the system (not to scale) used for photoelectrochemical assays. (A) Photoelectrochemical cell with four holes for RE, WE, AE, and recirculation of inert gas. (B) Arrangement of cell and lamp spaced 2 cm apart. (C) Arrangement for the RDE system.

Author Contributions: Conceptualization, G.G., N.S., F.A.M. and I.G.; Methodology, N.S., A.I. and I.G.; Formal analysis, G.G., N.S. and F.A.M.; data curation, N.S. and A.I.; writing-review and editing, G.G. and N.S., funding acquisition, G.G. and F.A.M. All authors have read and agreed to the published version of the manuscript.

Funding: Ministry of Science, Technology, and Innovation (MinCyT). In addition, this work has been supported by the Ministerio de Ciencia e Innovación (MCIN) under projects PCI2020-112249 and PID2020-117586RB-I00 funded by MCIN/AEI/10.13039/501100011033 and by the Agencia Canaria de Investigación, Innovación y Sociedad de la Información (ACIISI, ProID2021010098).

Institutional Review Board Statement: Not applicable.

Informed Consent Statement: Not applicable.

Data Availability Statement: The data presented in this study are available in article and Supplementary Materials.

Acknowledgments: G.G. acknowledges NANOtec, INTech, Cabildo de Tenerife, and ULL for laboratory facilities.

Conflicts of Interest: The authors declare no conflicts of interest.

References

1. Feng, C.; Chen, Z.; Jing, J.; Sun, M.; Tian, J.; Lu, G.; Ma, L.; Li, X.; Hou, J. Significantly Enhanced Photocatalytic Hydrogen Production Performance of G-C_3N_4/CNTs/CdZnS with Carbon Nanotubes as the Electron Mediators. *J. Mater. Sci. Technol.* **2021**, *80*, 75–83. [CrossRef]
2. Kim, D.; Yong, K. Boron Doping Induced Charge Transfer Switching of a C_3N_4/ZnO Photocatalyst from Z-Scheme to Type II to Enhance Photocatalytic Hydrogen Production. *Appl. Catal. B* **2021**, *282*, 119538. [CrossRef]
3. Fernandez-Ibanez, P.; McMichael, S.; Rioja Cabanillas, A.; Alkharabsheh, S.; Tolosana Moranchel, A.; Byrne, J.A. New Trends on Photoelectrocatalysis (PEC): Nanomaterials, Wastewater Treatment and Hydrogen Generation. *Curr. Opin. Chem. Eng.* **2021**, *34*, 100725. [CrossRef]
4. Truong, H.B.; Bae, S.; Cho, J.; Hur, J. Advances in Application of g-C_3N_4-Based Materials for Treatment of Polluted Water and Wastewater via Activation of Oxidants and Photoelectrocatalysis: A Comprehensive Review. *Chemosphere* **2022**, *286*, 131737. [CrossRef]
5. Xie, L.; Wang, L.; Zhao, W.; Liu, S.; Huang, W.; Zhao, Q. WS2 Moiré Superlattices Derived from Mechanical Flexibility for Hydrogen Evolution Reaction. *Nat. Commun.* **2021**, *12*, 5070. [CrossRef]
6. Yang, Z.Z.; Zhang, C.; Zeng, G.M.; Tan, X.F.; Huang, D.L.; Zhou, J.W.; Fang, Q.Z.; Yang, K.H.; Wang, H.; Wei, J.; et al. State-of-the-Art Progress in the Rational Design of Layered Double Hydroxide Based Photocatalysts for Photocatalytic and Photoelectrochemical H_2/O_2 Production. *Coord. Chem. Rev.* **2021**, *446*, 214103. [CrossRef]
7. Wang, L.; Xie, L.; Zhao, W.; Liu, S.; Zhao, Q. Oxygen-Facilitated Dynamic Active-Site Generation on Strained MoS_2 during Photo-Catalytic Hydrogen Evolution. *Chem. Eng. J.* **2021**, *405*, 127028. [CrossRef]
8. Chen, Z.; Li, S.; Peng, Y.; Hu, C. Tailoring Aromatic Ring-Terminated Edges of g-C_3N_4 nanosheets for Efficient Photocatalytic Hydrogen Evolution with Simultaneous Antibiotic Removal. *Catal. Sci. Technol.* **2020**, *10*, 5470–5479. [CrossRef]
9. Kumar, A.; Sharma, G.; Kumari, A.; Guo, C.; Naushad, M.; Vo, D.V.N.; Iqbal, J.; Stadler, F.J. Construction of Dual Z-Scheme g-C_3N_4/$Bi_4Ti_3O_{12}$/$Bi_4O_5I_2$ Heterojunction for Visible and Solar Powered Coupled Photocatalytic Antibiotic Degradation and Hydrogen Production: Boosting via I^-/I^{3-} and Bi^{3+}/Bi^{5+} Redox Mediators. *Appl. Catal. B* **2021**, *284*, 119808. [CrossRef]
10. Sharma, G.; Dionysiou, D.D.; Sharma, S.; Kumar, A.; Al-Muhtaseb, A.H.; Naushad, M.; Stadler, F.J. Highly Efficient Sr/Ce/Activated Carbon Bimetallic Nanocomposite for Photoinduced Degradation of Rhodamine B. *Catal. Today* **2019**, *335*, 437–451. [CrossRef]
11. Zhang, S.; Wang, L.; Liu, C.; Luo, J.; Crittenden, J.; Liu, X.; Cai, T.; Yuan, J.; Pei, Y.; Liu, Y. Photocatalytic Wastewater Purification with Simultaneous Hydrogen Production Using MoS_2 QD-Decorated Hierarchical Assembly of $ZnIn_2S_4$ on Reduced Graphene Oxide Photocatalyst. *Water Res.* **2017**, *121*, 11–19. [CrossRef]
12. Meng, S.; Chen, C.; Gu, X.; Wu, H.; Meng, Q.; Zhang, J.; Chen, S.; Fu, X.; Liu, D.; Lei, W. Efficient Photocatalytic H_2 Evolution, CO_2 Reduction and N_2 Fixation Coupled with Organic Synthesis by Cocatalyst and Vacancies Engineering. *Appl. Catal. B* **2021**, *285*, 119789. [CrossRef]
13. Wu, K.; Shang, Y.; Li, H.; Wu, P.; Li, S.; Ye, H.; Jian, F.; Zhu, J.; Yang, D.; Li, B.; et al. Synthesis and Hydrogen Production Performance of MoP/a-TiO_2/Co-$ZnIn_2S_4$ Flower-like Composite Photocatalysts. *Molecules* **2023**, *28*, 4350. [CrossRef]
14. Long, B.; He, H.; Yu, Y.; Cai, W.; Gu, Q.; Yang, J.; Meng, S. Bifunctional Hot Water Vapor Template-Mediated Synthesis of Nanostructured Polymeric Carbon Nitride for Efficient Hydrogen Evolution. *Molecules* **2023**, *28*, 4862. [CrossRef]
15. Zheng, X.; Zhang, Z.; Meng, S.; Wang, Y.; Li, D. Regulating Charge Transfer over 3D Au/ZnO Hybrid Inverse Opal toward Efficiently Photocatalytic Degradation of Bisphenol A and Photoelectrochemical Water Splitting. *Chem. Eng. J.* **2020**, *393*, 124676. [CrossRef]
16. Priyadarshini, M.; Sathe, S.M.; Ghangrekar, M.M. Hybrid Treatment Solutions for Removal of Micropollutant from Wastewaters. In *Microconstituents in the Environment*; Wiley: Hoboken, NJ, USA, 2023; pp. 491–512.
17. Babuji, P.; Thirumalaisamy, S.; Duraisamy, K.; Periyasamy, G. Human Health Risks Due to Exposure to Water Pollution: A Review. *Water* **2023**, *15*, 2532. [CrossRef]

18. Inostroza, P.A.; Carmona, E.; Arrhenius, Å.; Krauss, M.; Brack, W.; Backhaus, T. Target Screening of Chemicals of Emerging Concern (CECs) in Surface Waters of the Swedish West Coast. *Data* **2023**, *8*, 93. [CrossRef]
19. Talaat, A.; Elgendy, Y.A.; Mohamed, H.F.; Saed, N.M.; Abd Elrouf, N.A.; Elgendy, H.A.; Elbalakousy, H.H.; Elmezaien, M.S.; Sayed, Y.M.; Hekal, Y.E.; et al. Ameliorative Effects of Frankincense Oil on Rats Treated with a Minimum Toxic Dose of Paracetamol. *J. Med. Life Sci.* **2023**, *5*, 155–175. [CrossRef]
20. Zhang, C.; Li, T.; Zhang, J.; Yan, S.; Qin, C. Degradation of P-Nitrophenol Using a Ferrous-Tripolyphosphate Complex in the Presence of Oxygen: The Key Role of Superoxide Radicals. *Appl. Catal. B* **2019**, *259*, 118030. [CrossRef]
21. Hashimoto, K.; Irie, H.; Fujishima, A. TiO_2 Photocatalysis: A Historical Overview and Future Prospects. *Jpn. J. Appl. Phys.* **2005**, *44*, 8269–8285. [CrossRef]
22. Daghrir, R.; Drogui, P.; Robert, D. Modified TiO_2 for Environmental Photocatalytic Applications: A Review. *Ind. Eng. Chem. Res.* **2013**, *52*, 3581–3599. [CrossRef]
23. Ni, M.; Leung, M.K.H.; Leung, D.Y.C.; Sumathy, K. A Review and Recent Developments in Photocatalytic Water-Splitting Using TiO_2 for Hydrogen Production. *Renew. Sustain. Energy Rev.* **2007**, *11*, 401–425. [CrossRef]
24. Yilmaz, P.; Lacerda, A.M.; Larrosa, I.; Dunn, S. Photoelectrocatalysis of Rhodamine B and Solar Hydrogen Production by TiO_2 and Pd/TiO_2 Catalyst Systems. *Electrochim. Acta* **2017**, *231*, 641–649. [CrossRef]
25. Marchesini, F.A.; Mendow, G.; Picard, N.P.; Zoppas, F.M.; Aghemo, V.S.; Gutierrez, L.B.; Querini, C.A.; Miró, E.E. PdIn Catalysts in a Continuous Fixed Bed Reactor for the Nitrate Removal from Groundwater. *Int. J. Chem. React. Eng.* **2019**, *17*, 1–17. [CrossRef]
26. Marchesini, F.A.; Gutierrez, L.B.; Querini, C.A.; Miró, E.E. Pt,In and Pd,In Catalysts for the Hydrogenation of Nitrates and Nitrites in Water. FTIR Characterization and Reaction Studies. *Chem. Eng. J.* **2010**, *159*, 203–211. [CrossRef]
27. Sarkar, S.; Peter, S.C. An Overview on Pd-Based Electrocatalysts for the Hydrogen Evolution Reaction. *Inorg. Chem. Front.* **2018**, *5*, 2060–2080. [CrossRef]
28. Merino-Garcia, I.; García, G.; Hernández, I.; Albo, J. An Optofluidic Planar Microreactor with Photoactive $Cu_2O/Mo_2C/TiO_2$ heterostructures for Enhanced Visible Light-Driven CO_2 conversion to Methanol. *J. CO2 Util.* **2023**, *67*, 102340. [CrossRef]
29. Yang, Y.-K.; Jiao, C.-Q.; Meng, Y.-S.; Yao, N.-T.; Jiang, W.-J.; Liu, T. Substituent Effect on Metal-to-Metal Charge Transfer Behavior of Cyanide-Bridged {Fe_2Co_2} Square. *Inorg. Chem. Commun.* **2021**, *130*, 108712. [CrossRef]
30. Chavez Zavaleta, R.; Fomichev, S.; Khaliullin, G.; Berciu, M. Effects of Reduced Dimensionality, Crystal Field, Electron-Lattice Coupling, and Strain on the Ground State of a Rare-Earth Nickelate Monolayer. *Phys. Rev. B* **2021**, *104*, 205111. [CrossRef]
31. Dehury, T.; Kumar, S.; Rath, C. Structural Transformation and Bandgap Engineering by Doping Pr in HfO_2 Nanoparticles. *Mater. Lett.* **2021**, *302*, 130413. [CrossRef]
32. Bazan-Aguilar, A.; García, G.; Pastor, E.; Rodríguez, J.L.; Baena-Moncada, A.M. In-Situ Spectroelectrochemical Study of Highly Active Ni-Based Foam Electrocatalysts for Hydrogen Evolution Reaction. *Appl. Catal. B* **2023**, *336*, 122930. [CrossRef]
33. López, M.; Exner, K.S.; Viñes, F.; Illas, F. Theoretical Study of the Mechanism of the Hydrogen Evolution Reaction on the V2C MXene: Thermodynamic and Kinetic Aspects. *J. Catal.* **2023**, *421*, 252–263. [CrossRef]
34. Nematollahi, D.; Shayani-Jam, H.; Alimoradi, M.; Niroomand, S. Electrochemical Oxidation of Acetaminophen in Aqueous Solutions: Kinetic Evaluation of Hydrolysis, Hydroxylation and Dimerization Processes. *Electrochim. Acta* **2009**, *54*, 7407–7415. [CrossRef]
35. Chenlo, F.; Moreira, R.; Pereira, G.; Vázquez, M.J. Viscosity of Binary and Ternary Aqueous Systems of NaH_2PO_4, Na_2HPO_4, Na_3PO_4, KH_2PO_4, K_2HPO_4, and K_3PO_4. *J. Chem. Eng. Data* **1996**, *41*, 906–909. [CrossRef]
36. Pournaghi-Azar, M.H.; Kheradmandi, S.; Saadatirad, A. Simultaneous Voltammetry of Paracetamol, Ascorbic Acid, and Codeine on a Palladium-Plated Aluminum Electrode: Oxidation Pathway and Kinetics. *J. Solid State Electrochem.* **2010**, *14*, 1689–1695. [CrossRef]
37. Zoubir, J.; Bakas, I.; Assabbane, A. A Simple Platform for the Electro-Catalytic Detection of the Dimetridazole Using an Electrochemical Sensor Fabricated by Electro-Deposition of Ag on Carbon Graphite: Application: Orange Juice, Tomato Juice and Tap Water. *Heliyon* **2021**, *7*, e07542. [CrossRef]

Disclaimer/Publisher's Note: The statements, opinions and data contained in all publications are solely those of the individual author(s) and contributor(s) and not of MDPI and/or the editor(s). MDPI and/or the editor(s) disclaim responsibility for any injury to people or property resulting from any ideas, methods, instructions or products referred to in the content.

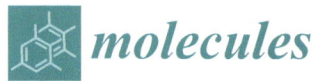

Article

Unveiling the Low-Lying Spin States of [Fe₃S₄] Clusters via the Extended Broken-Symmetry Method

Shibing Chu * and Qiuyu Gao

School of Physics and Electronic Engineering, Jiangsu University, Zhenjiang 212013, China; gaoqiuyuuu@gmail.com
* Correspondence: c@ujs.edu.cn

Abstract: Photosynthetic water splitting, when synergized with hydrogen production catalyzed by hydrogenases, emerges as a promising avenue for clean and renewable energy. However, theoretical calculations have faced challenges in elucidating the low-lying spin states of iron–sulfur clusters, which are integral components of hydrogenases. To address this challenge, we employ the Extended Broken-Symmetry method for the computation of the cubane–[Fe₃S₄] cluster within the [FeNi] hydrogenase enzyme. This approach rectifies the error caused by spin contamination, allowing us to obtain the magnetic exchange coupling constant and the energy level of the low-lying state. We find that the Extended Broken-Symmetry method provides more accurate results for differences in bond length and the magnetic coupling constant. This accuracy assists in reconstructing the low-spin ground state force and determining the geometric structure of the ground state. By utilizing the Extended Broken-Symmetry method, we further highlight the significance of the geometric arrangement of metal centers in the cluster's properties and gain deeper insights into the magnetic properties of transition metal iron–sulfur clusters at the reaction centers of hydrogenases. This research illuminates the untapped potential of hydrogenases and their promising role in the future of photosynthesis and sustainable energy production.

Keywords: iron–sulfur clusters; density functional theory; Extended Broken-Symmetry method; magnetic coupling constant; low-lying spin state

---

Citation: Chu, S.; Gao, Q. Unveiling the Low-Lying Spin States of [Fe₃S₄] Clusters via the Extended Broken-Symmetry Method. *Molecules* **2024**, *29*, 2152. https://doi.org/10.3390/molecules29092152

Academic Editor: Franck Rabilloud

Received: 7 April 2024
Revised: 29 April 2024
Accepted: 2 May 2024
Published: 6 May 2024

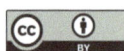

Copyright: © 2024 by the authors. Licensee MDPI, Basel, Switzerland. This article is an open access article distributed under the terms and conditions of the Creative Commons Attribution (CC BY) license (https://creativecommons.org/licenses/by/4.0/).

1. Introduction

In the face of the energy crisis and the imperative of climate change mitigation, societal growth and development have increasingly depended on fossil energy. However, as we continue to exploit these resources, their depletion is becoming inevitable. Moreover, the use of fossil fuels results in substantial greenhouse gas emissions, which contribute to the greenhouse effect and global warming [1,2]. Consequently, in order to align with the principles of green chemistry and clean technology, it is essential to intensify research and development in renewable energy, like hydrogen. Today, more than 95% of hydrogen is produced from hydrocarbons through steam reforming or partial oxidation. These methods are energy-consuming, and they are still dependent on fossil fuels, generating CO_2, black carbon particles, and climate-relevant reactive gases as by-products. The establishment of a hydrogen-based economy remains a challenging task, and there is much one can learn from nature. Nowadays, there are several pathways to solve this problem by using different ways to produce and apply hydrogen, like making electrolytic devices [3], chemical fuel cells [4], artificial hydrogenases [5], and nanomaterials made of transition metal oxides [6]. The application of solar energy and hydrogenases is also a possible way, which is called photosynthesis. At present, photosynthesis is the only process that can gently split water into electrons and hydrogen [7,8]. However, the conversion efficiency of natural photosynthetic systems remains low [9–11]. Therefore, enhancing this conversion efficiency through artificial means is of significant importance.

In the photosynthetic system, the catalytic conversion reaction is primarily facilitated by hydrogenase [12]. Hydrogenase is the enzyme catalyzing the interconversion of hydrogen into protons and electrons (hydrogen ↔2H$^+$+2e$^-$) in bacteria, archaea, and eukaryotes [13]. Even though several microorganisms using hydrogen as an energy source attracted the attention of scientists in the 1800s, Stephenson and Stickland [14] were the first to propose the existence of hydrogenases and report the kinetic properties, as well as the oxygen sensitivity, of these enzymes. More recently, several crystal structures of hydrogenase have helped to unveil the geometry and mode of action of their active site [15], and extensive phylogenetic analyses have revealed that microorganisms harboring genes encoding hydrogenases encompass the three domains of the tree of life and are ubiquitous in the environment [16]. These enzymes are utilized to generate energy, disperse reducing equivalents produced during fermentation, or generate reduced cofactors involved in several reactions of cellular metabolism. In general, microorganisms utilize hydrogen under a mixotrophic lifestyle, which confers the ability to proliferate and survive in environments lacking readily available organic substrates. From an ecological perspective, hydrogen is viewed as a universal energy source, supporting a seed bank of hydrogen-oxidizing microorganisms that provide a broad range of ecosystem services [17]. Advances in our understanding of the biochemistry, diversity, and functions of hydrogenases contribute to the development of new biotechnologies and a better understanding of the hydrogen cycle and the ecological role of hydrogen-oxidizing microorganisms.

The catalytic conversion carried out by hydrogenase predominantly occurs in transition metal clusters at its core. These clusters can serve as catalysts, continually providing protons or hydrogen [18]. A comprehensive understanding of these transition metal clusters within hydrogenases will aid in elucidating their catalytic processes, and this is crucial for the design of transition metal complexes that serve as potentially sustainable proton reduction or H$_2$ oxidation catalysts. Hydrogenases can be classified into several types based on the differences in the central transition metal cluster, including [NiFe] hydrogenases, [FeFe] hydrogenases, and [Fe] hydrogenases [19]. Among these, [NiFe] hydrogenases represent a crucial category and can be further divided into two types: oxygen-tolerant [NiFe] hydrogenases and oxygen-sensitive [NiFe] hydrogenases [20]. However, oxygen-sensitive [NiFe] hydrogenases become inactive when exposed to oxygen, thus limiting their practical applications [21]. Consequently, the development of oxygen-tolerant [NiFe] hydrogenases presents a significant area of research.

Within the protein fragment of oxygen-tolerant [NiFe] hydrogenases, there exists a catalytic conversion pathway in which the [NiFe] cluster serves as the central active site. The active site of the [NiFe] hydrogenases features a nickel tetrathiolate (four cysteines) with two S bridges to an Fe(CN)$_2$(CO) center [22]. Four key states in the catalytic cycle are Ni-SI$_a$ (Ni^{II}Fe^{II}), Ni–L (Ni^{I}Fe^{II}), Ni–C (Ni^{III}μ(H)Fe^{II}), and Ni–R (Ni^{II}μ(H)Fe^{II}) [23]. During the catalytic process, in the process of valence changes of iron and nickel, three electrons are required, which are supplied by [Fe$_4$S$_3$], [Fe$_3$S$_4$], and [Fe$_4$S$_4$] [24]. The relative positions and distances between these clusters are depicted in Figure 1. Existing studies indicate that the [Fe$_3$S$_4$] cluster plays a pivotal role in oxygen-tolerant [NiFe] hydrogenases [25,26]. Therefore, research focusing on [Fe$_3$S$_4$] clusters could represent a significant breakthrough in the development of oxygen-tolerant hydrogenases.

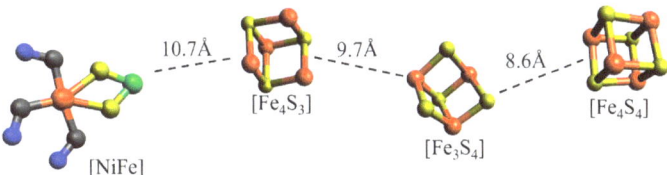

Figure 1. The diagram illustrates the [NiFe], [Fe$_4$S$_3$], [Fe$_3$S$_4$], and [Fe$_4$S$_4$] clusters involved in the catalytic pathway, as well as the distances between each cluster.

Currently, calculations of transition metal clusters, such as [Fe$_3$S$_4$] clusters, primarily rely on density functional theory (DFT) [27,28]. The Broken-Symmetry (BS) method is a common approach within DFT. This method calculates the energy difference between the high-spin state and the BS state, allowing for an estimation of the magnetic coupling constant, J, between spin centers [29]. However, because the BS state is not an eigenstate of the total spin operator $\hat{S}^2$ [30], some errors may occur when using the BS method to calculate the magnetic coupling constant J. Additionally, due to the strong magnetism of transition metal clusters and the high degree of dynamic and static correlation among the 3d orbital electrons of the central atom [31], clusters exhibit multiple degenerate states, with the ground state (GS) typically being a low-spin state. Concerning the static correlation, we may distinguish two different effects: the local static correlation necessary to correctly describe the nature of the bonds between each metal atom and its ligands and the global static correlation among the spin centers due to the interactions between localized unpaired electrons. This latter contribution is crucial to guaranteeing the correct overall spin symmetry of the wave function [32]. In the DFT method, the open-shell single-determinant wavefunction utilized in the Kohn–Sham equation fails to deliver the correct spin symmetry [33]; therefore, the DFT method cannot correctly describe the low-spin GS of the cluster, nor can it correctly calculate the cluster's magnetic properties.

Previous studies have conducted a series of computational analyses on transition metal clusters, specifically those involving iron (Fe), manganese (Mn), and cobalt (Co) complexes within photosynthetic systems [34–37]. However, due to the limitations of the DFT method previously discussed, the calculated values of system energy and magnetic coupling constants J for multicenter transition metal clusters significantly deviate from experimental data. This discrepancy underscores the need to refine our computational methods to more accurately characterize the properties of transition metal clusters.

To rectify the errors resulting from the issues mentioned above, in this study, we will apply the Extended Broken-Symmetry (EBS) method [38] to perform calculations on the cubane–[Fe$_3$S$_4$] cluster. Through the Heisenberg–Dirac–van Vleck (HDvV) Hamiltonian, we aim to derive a low-spin ground state (GS) with correct symmetry for a cluster with an arbitrary number of spin centers. Based on preliminary calculations [39], for the low-spin GS, we will carry out multiple iterative optimizations on the geometric structure until the program converges. We will then obtain the magnetic exchange coupling constant J, energy levels, and energy spectral distribution of the final cluster structure. By comparing the EBS method with the BS method and the high-spin (HS) method, we find that the EBS method yields a bond length and magnetic coupling constant data that are closer to the experimental data, indicating a better description of the system. We anticipate that the EBS method will yield more accurate properties and structures of the low-lying state, which is closest to the eigenstate of transition metal clusters. As these clusters are the core catalytic oxidation reaction centers of hydrogenases, and the function of hydrogenase is carried out by the redox process of these clusters, obtaining more precise information on their magnetic properties and structure can lead to a deeper understanding of the nature of the hydrogenases in which they are incorporated.

2. Results and Discussion

2.1. Structure and Spin State

The object of our calculation is the [[Fe$_3$S$_4$](CH$_3$CH$_2$S)$_3$(CH$_3$CH$_2$SH)]$^{3-}$ cluster, with its central cluster being [Fe$_3$S$_4$]$^{1+}$. In this cluster, all three Fe centers are Fe(III), and the 3d orbital contains five electrons.

Initially, we characterized the clusters using the BS method. The central [Fe$_3$S$_4$]$^{1+}$ cluster contains three Fe spin centers and four different BS states. We assume that the outermost electrons of each Fe atom have spins in the same direction at each spin center, implying that the spin at each spin center is $s = 5/2$; Therefore, the spins of the four different BS states are presented in Table 1. The clusters we selected were from existing research [40], and the cluster model is illustrated in Figure 2.

Table 1. Different spin states of the $[Fe_3S_4]^{1+}$ cluster.

BS_k	Spin State	$|s_1, s_2, s_3\rangle$	S_{tot}
BS_1	↑↑↑	$\left|\frac{5}{2}, \frac{5}{2}, \frac{5}{2}\right\rangle$	$\frac{15}{2}$
BS_2	↓↑↑	$\left|-\frac{5}{2}, \frac{5}{2}, \frac{5}{2}\right\rangle$	$\frac{5}{2}$
BS_3	↑↓↑	$\left|\frac{5}{2}, -\frac{5}{2}, \frac{5}{2}\right\rangle$	$\frac{5}{2}$
BS_4	↑↑↓	$\left|\frac{5}{2}, \frac{5}{2}, -\frac{5}{2}\right\rangle$	$\frac{5}{2}$

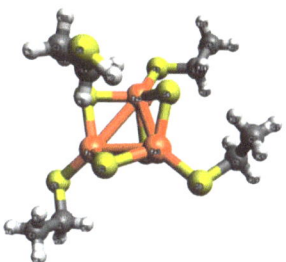

Figure 2. The structure of the $[Fe_3S_4(CH_3CH_2SH)_3]^{2-}$ complex. Iron is represented in orange, sulfur in yellow, carbon in black, and hydrogen in gray.

2.2. Bond Lengths between Spin Centers

We employed three methods—the HS method, the BS method, and the EBS method—to calculate the structure of the cluster and compared the results. The HS method calculates the geometry of the high-spin state of the cluster. The BS method calculates the four different BS states of the cluster. The details of EBS method can be found in Section 3.

The bond lengths of the cluster's Fe–Fe bonds obtained from these calculations are presented in Table 2, where the unit of the bond length is Å.

Table 2. Bond length of the $[[Fe_3S_4](CH_3CH_2S)_3(CH_3CH_2SH)]^{2-}$ cluster. The experimental data are from the X-ray structure analysis [41]. Errors are calculated according to the differences between the experimental value and the calculated value.

Hybrid Function	Method	Fe_1-Fe_2/Å	Fe_2-Fe_3/Å	Fe_1-Fe_3/Å	Error/%
	Exp [41]	2.71	2.67	2.73	
B3LYP	HS	3.05	3.07	3.06	12%~15%
	BS	2.88	3.03	2.90	6%~13%
	EBS	2.85	2.79	2.87	4%~5%
TPSSh	HS	2.99	3.02	2.99	10%~13%
	BS	2.76	2.95	2.79	2%~8%
	EBS	2.73	2.78	2.78	0.7%~4%

From the table, it is evident that the B3LYP functional calculations using the HS method generally have a large deviation from the experimental data of approximately 0.3~0.4 Å, with an error of around 15%. The bond length error is about 0.2~0.3 Å, and the error percentage is roughly 10%. The discrepancy between the bond length data calculated using the EBS method and the experimental structure is approximately 0.1 Å, and the deviation percentages from the experimental data are 5% and 4%, respectively.

Similar conclusions were reached in the calculations using the TPSSh functional on clusters. We observed that the bond lengths calculated using the HS method have large discrepancies from the experimental values, resulting in a loose cluster structure. The cluster structure has been optimized to some extent using the BS method, but there is still a significant error in some bond lengths. However, the EBS structure optimization yielded a structure closest to the experimental data. Therefore, we believe that the results obtained using the EBS method are more accurate than those obtained using the HS and BS methods. Based on the above results, the HS, BS, and EBS methods, which give the smallest deviation, underestimate the bond length between spin centers. Bond lengths from the X-ray diffraction method were obtained for the solid phase, where the structure is distorted by intermolecular interactions. Meanwhile, the bond lengths from the HS, BS, and EBS methods were obtained for free molecular systems. Therefore, these methods fail to consider that the field generated by the external ligands and external molecules could be the reason for this underestimation.

Figure 3a,b illustrate the comparison of the bond length difference, Δr, which represents the differences between the experimental value and calculated value using the HS, BS, and EBS methods with the B3LYP and TPSSh functionals, respectively.

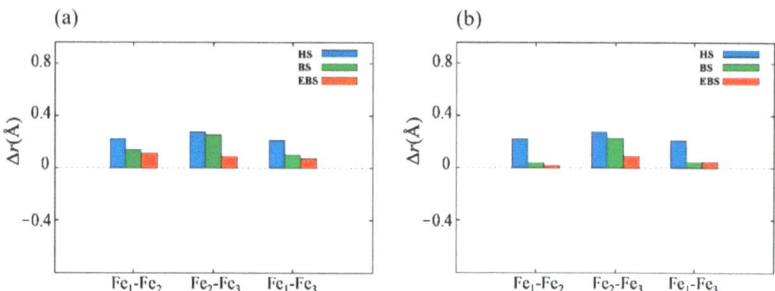

Figure 3. (**a**) Shows the comparison of Δr using HS, BS, and EBS methods with the B3LYP hybrid functional. (**b**) Shows the same comparison using the TPSSh hybrid functional.

2.3. Exchange Coupling Constants

The magnetic coupling constants J calculated using the BS method and the EBS method are shown in Table 3, where J_1 represents the magnetic coupling between Fe_1 and Fe_2, J_2 represents the magnetic coupling between Fe_2 and Fe_3, and J_3 represents the magnetic coupling between Fe_1 and Fe_3. In the EBS method, each structure optimization provides a new optimized structure and outputs its corresponding magnetic coupling constant J. For the optimized geometry obtained using the B3LYP functional, the corresponding J values are -109.5 cm^{-1}, -119.8 cm^{-1}, and -100.9 cm^{-1}; For the converged geometry obtained using the TPSSh functional, the J values were -155.7 cm^{-1}, -149.6 cm^{-1}, and -124.3 cm^{-1}, respectively.

Table 3. Magnetic spin coupling J/cm^{-1} between spin centers calculated using the BS and EBS methods with B3LYP and TPSSh hybrid functionals. The experimental data are from the X-ray structure analysis [42].

Hybrid Function	Method	J_1/cm^{-1}	J_2/cm^{-1}	J_3/cm^{-1}
B3LYP	BS	-65.4	-67.5	-62.1
	EBS	-109.5	-119.8	-100.9
TPSSh	BS	-94.0	-89.0	-88.5
	EBS	-155.7	-149.6	-124.3
Exp [42]		$-(200\sim300)$, $J_1 \approx J_2 \approx J_3$		

In contrast with the range provided by experimental values, we observe that the magnetic coupling constants (J values) obtained using both the B3LYP and TPSSh functionals are smaller. From the Fe–Fe bond lengths in Table 2, it is suggested that as the Fe–Fe distance increases, the antiferromagnetic coupling becomes weaker. Therefore, we believe that the obtained J coupling constant aligns with the bond length data.

The J values calculated using the BS and EBS methods revealed that the J coupling constants given by the BS method generally deviate significantly from the experimental values. After optimization using the EBS method, the J value is noticeably closer to the range provided by experimental values, reducing the error by approximately 15% compared to the BS method with the same functional. Furthermore, a comparison of the J coupling constants and bond lengths indicates that the EBS-optimized structure is denser and has shorter bond lengths than the one optimized using the BS method, leading to stronger magnetic coupling. In summary, we believe that the EBS method reduces the calculation error to a certain extent, and the structure obtained using the BS method, once optimized through the EBS method, yields a compact cluster structure closer to the experimental data. Based on the calculations we have performed, we believe that the best results can be obtained by using the EBS method and the TPSSh hybrid function.

Compared to the linear–[Fe$_3$S$_4$] [38] cluster, which has two similar exchange coupling constants, the cubane–[Fe$_3$S$_4$] cluster in this study provides three similar exchange coupling constants, as shown in Table 3. This could generate more nearly degenerate states and enrich the properties of the cluster as a catalyst. The spatial configuration of the transition metal atoms in a cluster plays an important role in determining its electron conductivity and magnetic properties.

2.4. Energy Spectrum

The energy spectral distributions of the HS state and the GS state after EBS optimization using the B3LYP functional are depicted in Figure 4. The energy spectral distribution reveals multiple degeneracies in the low-spin GS of the [[Fe$_3$S$_4$](CH$_3$CH$_2$S)$_3$(CH$_3$CH$_2$SH)]$^{2-}$ cluster. The small gap between energy levels suggests that the cluster is susceptible to redox reactions when perturbed. Additionally, upon comparing the cluster energies calculated using the two methods, the cluster energy calculated using the HS method is -7294.034 Eh, while the cluster energy calculated using the EBS method is -7294.056 Eh. We found that structure optimization through EBS can achieve a lower energy, with an energy difference of 0.022 Eh (4828.44 cm^{-1}).

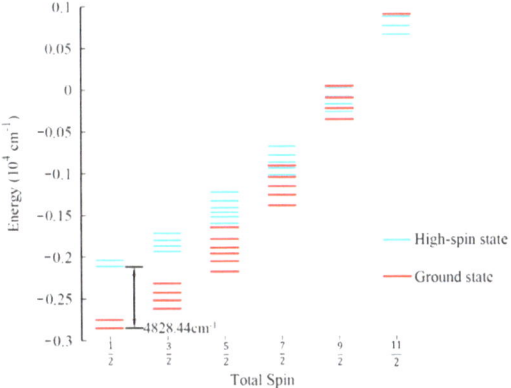

Figure 4. Comparison of the spin ladder of the GS and high−spin state calculated using the B3LYP functional. The blue lines represent the spin ladder of the high−spin state, and the red lines represent the spin ladder of the GS. After the optimization of the structure using the EBS method, the calculated energy difference between GS and HS states is 4828.44 cm^{-1}.

The energy spectral distributions of the HS state and the GS state after EBS optimization using the TPSSh functional are depicted in Figure 5. The cluster energy calculated using the HS method is -7295.034 Eh, and the cluster energy calculated using the EBS method is -7295.144 Eh. We find that the structure optimization of the cluster using the

EBS method can achieve a lower energy. The energy difference between them is 0.034 Eh (7498.35 cm^{-1}).

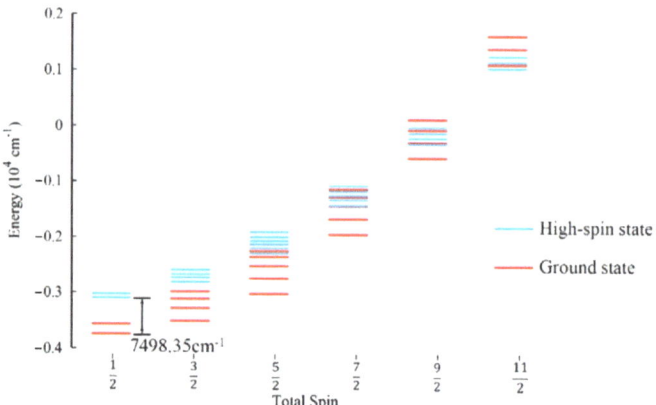

Figure 5. Comparison of the spin ladder of the GS and high–spin state calculated using the TPSSh functional. The blue lines represent the spin ladder of the high–spin state, and the red lines represent the spin ladder of the GS. After the optimization of the structure with the EBS method, the calculated energy difference between GS and HS states is 7498.35 cm^{-1}.

3. Computational Method

In this calculation, ORCA [43] software was used. The all-electronic Ahlrichs TZVP [44] and Def2-TZVP [45] basis sets were chosen. The self-consistent field (SCF) convergence criterion was set to TightSCF and Grid4. The B3LYP and TPSSh hybrid functionals were chosen for this study. In addition to the B3LYP hybrid function, which is most commonly used in the calculation of transition metal clusters, we also selected the TPSSh hybrid function benchmarked on transition metal diatomics. This choice was motivated by findings that the TPSSh functional produces structures of comparable quality to those obtained using other commonly used hybrid and non-hybrid functionals, such as B3LYP and BP86. Moreover, the inclusion of 10% exact exchange in TPSSh can eliminate the large systematic component of the error, providing an advantage over other functionals [46].

In this study, we used the Extended Broken-Symmetry (EBS) calculation method to compute the properties of clusters. The detailed derivation has been described in a previous study [38]. Our primary results include the magnetic coupling constant J and the optimized energy spectral distribution of the cluster structure. The calculation process consists of several main steps.

In the first step, we calculate the energy ε^{BS} of each BS state using the BS method. Furthermore, we apply the EBS method using the results we obtained from the BS method, as follows. We construct the matrix $A_{kp} = \langle s_i \cdot s_j \rangle$, and a linear equations system is defined in Equation (1):

$$\begin{pmatrix} \varepsilon_1^{BS} \\ \varepsilon_2^{BS} \\ \varepsilon_3^{BS} \\ \vdots \\ \varepsilon_{N_k}^{BS} \end{pmatrix} = -2 \begin{pmatrix} A_{11} & A_{12} & \cdots & A_{1N_p} \\ A_{21} & A_{21} & \cdots & A_{2N_p} \\ A_{31} & A_{31} & \cdots & A_{3N_p} \\ \vdots & \vdots & \ddots & \vdots \\ A_{N_k1} & A_{N_k2} & \cdots & A_{N_kN_p} \end{pmatrix} \begin{pmatrix} J_1 \\ J_2 \\ J_3 \\ \vdots \\ J_{N_p} \end{pmatrix} \quad (1)$$

After rewriting the above equations as matrix A, we obtain the inverse matrix A^{-1} of the matrix A_{kp} via singular value decomposition (SVD) [39]. The magnetic coupling constant J is then obtained from Equation (2).

$$J = -\frac{1}{2} A^{-1} \cdot \varepsilon^{BS} \qquad (2)$$

Secondly, the Hamiltonian matrices $\langle b_l |$ and $| b_r \rangle$ are constructed, where $\langle b_l |$ represents the left basis vector of each eigenstate and $| b_r \rangle$ represents the right basis vector of each eigenstate. Using the J coupling constant obtained from Equation (2) and the Clebsch–Gordan (CG) coefficient [47], we can diagonalize the Hamiltonian, as indicated in Equation (3). The CG coefficient essentially functions as a transformation matrix for representations grounded in group theory, and it is capable of converting an uncoupled representation into a coupled one [48]. In the case of the cubane–[Fe$_3$S$_4$] cluster, we can describe the low-spin GS through the combination of the CG coefficients and each BS state.

$$\begin{aligned}
\langle b_l | \hat{H} | b_r \rangle &= -2 \sum_{i<j} \langle b_l | J_{ij} \hat{s}_i \cdot \hat{s}_j | b_r \rangle \\
&= -\sum_{i<j} J_{ij} \langle b_l | \hat{S}_{ij}^2 | b_r \rangle + \sum_{i<j} J_{ij} \langle b_l | \hat{s}_i^2 \cdot \hat{s}_j^2 | b_r \rangle \\
&= -\sum_{i<j} J_{ij} \times CG_{ij}^l \times CG_{ij}^r \times S_{ij}(S_{ij}+1) \\
&\quad + \sum_{i<j} J_{ij} \times (s_i(s_i+1) + s_j(s_j+1))
\end{aligned} \qquad (3)$$

Through the above two steps, we can obtain the GS structure and its corresponding energy spectral distribution of the cluster, as shown in Figure 6.

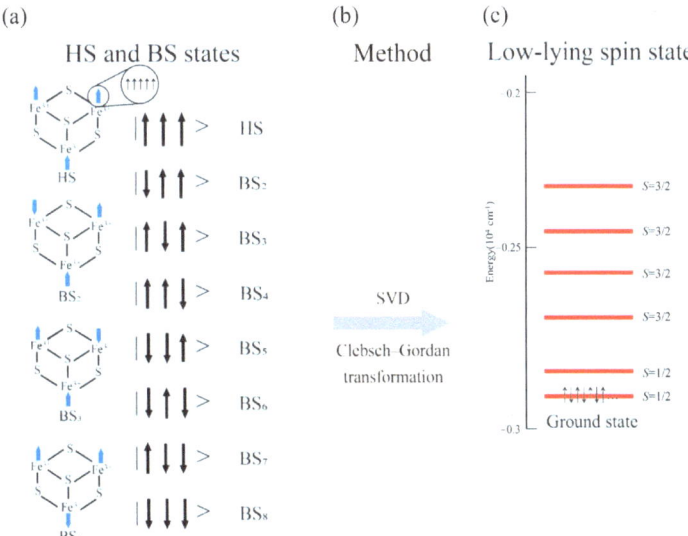

Figure 6. (**a**) Depicts the 8 broken symmetry states of the cubane–[Fe$_3$S$_4$] cluster, complete with spin details. The energy level of the low-lying state (LS state) is illustrated in (**c**), where the total spins S_{tot} of 1/2 and 3/2 are shown. This implies that there are 7 pairs of electrons and 1 single electron in the state with $S = 1/2$ and 6 pairs of electrons and 3 spin-up electrons in the state with $S = 3/2$. The energy in (**c**) is derived from calculations of cubane–[Fe$_3$S$_4$] clusters using the B3LYP functional. The magnetic coupling constant J can be extracted from the SVD matrix. The Clebsch–Gordan transformation, represented in (**b**), enables the description of the cluster's GS.

Having completed all of the calculations above, we have obtained the energy of all BS states, the magnetic coupling constant J, and the optimized structure, along with its GS. Once we have these preliminary results, we can perform geometry optimization using the EBS method, a FORTRAN code generated by interfacing the external optimizer features available in ORCA. Figure 7 provides a schematic diagram of the entire calculation process.

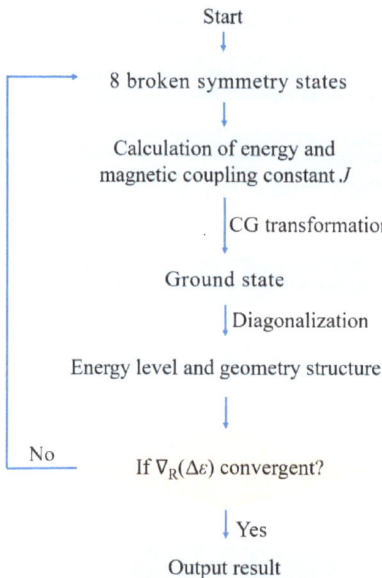

Figure 7. Flow chart of the geometric optimization of clusters using the EBS method.

We investigated the energy gradient, denoted as $\nabla_R(\Delta\varepsilon)$, with further details provided in the previous study [38].

When $\nabla_R(\Delta\varepsilon)$ becomes less than the convergence value, it indicates that the optimized GS geometry has achieved our required accuracy. At this point, the program terminates, and the final GS geometry, magnetic coupling constant J, and energy spectral distribution are output.

4. Conclusions

We calculated the energies of all BS states of the cubane–[Fe$_3$S$_4$] cluster via the DFT method and obtained the GS energy spectrum structure via the SVD method and CG transformation. Based on this ground-state energy surface, we further optimized the geometry and energy spectral distribution of the low-spin GS. We find that compared to those obtained through the BS method, the geometric parameters calculated using the EBS method can match better with the experimental data. Therefore, we believe that the EBS method compensates for the shortcomings of the BS method used in the DFT method and that it reduces the errors caused by the static correlation and spin contamination. From the energy spectrum, it is evident that the [Fe$_3$S$_4$] cluster possesses rich magnetic properties, suggesting that [Fe$_3$S$_4$] clusters could serve as exceptional mediators of electron conductivity. Furthermore, the nearly equal J values of the three magnetic coupling constants in [Fe$_3$S$_4$] clusters could be a crucial factor contributing to the robust oxygen tolerance of [NiFe] hydrogenase. These J values are determined according to the spatial configuration of the transition metal atoms within the cluster, further highlighting the significance of the metal center's geometric arrangement in the cluster's properties. The EBS method represents an important step toward the precise study of transition metal clusters. We believe that for multiple magnetic clusters, it is necessary to consider the static correlation effect and perform quantitative comparisons with the experimental data to deepen the understanding of the clusters. We hope that the study of magnetic properties and energy spectral distributions can help us better understand transition metal clusters and their functions and properties in hydrogenases.

Author Contributions: Conceptualization, S.C.; methodology, S.C. and Q.G.; software, S.C. and Q.G.; validation, S.C. and Q.G.; formal analysis, S.C. and Q.G.; investigation, S.C. and Q.G.; resources, S.C.; data curation, S.C. and Q.G.; writing—original draft preparation, Q.G.; writing—review and editing, S.C. and Q.G.; visualization, Q.G.; supervision, S.C.; project administration, S.C.; funding acquisition, S.C. All authors have read and agreed to the published version of the manuscript.

Funding: This work was supported by the National Natural Science Foundation of China (funding Nos. 11904137 and 11747081) and funding No. 4111190003 from Jiangsu University (JSU).

Institutional Review Board Statement: Not applicable.

Informed Consent Statement: Not applicable.

Data Availability Statement: Data are contained within the article.

Conflicts of Interest: The authors declare no conflicts of interest.

References

1. Manahan, S.E. *Environmental Chemistry*; CRC Press: Boca Raton, FL, USA, 2022.
2. Montzka, S.A.; Dlugokencky, E.J.; Butler, J.H. Non-CO_2 greenhouse gases and climate change. *Nature* **2011**, *476*, 43–50. [CrossRef] [PubMed]
3. Sharmila, V.G.; Banu, J.R.; Kim, S.H.; Kumar, G. A review on evaluation of applied pretreatment methods of wastewater towards sustainable H2 generation: Energy efficiency analysis. *Int. J. Hydrogen Energy* **2020**, *45*, 8329–8345. [CrossRef]
4. Ogo, S.; Ando, T.; Mori, Y.; Matsumoto, T.; Yatabe, T.; Yoon, K.S.; Sato, Y.; Hibino, T.; Kaneko, K. A NiRhS fuel cell catalyst–lessons from hydrogenase. *Chem. Commun.* **2020**, *56*, 11787–11790. [CrossRef] [PubMed]
5. Esmieu, C.; Raleiras, P.; Berggren, G. From Protein Engineering to Artificial Enzymes-Biological and Biomimetic Approaches towards Sustainable Hydrogen Production. *Sustain. Energy Fuels* **2018**, *2*, 724–750. [CrossRef] [PubMed]
6. Sun, Y.; Ma, Y.; Zhang, B.; Sun, H.; Wang, N.; Wang, L.; Zhang, J.; Xue, R. Comparison of magnetite/reduced graphene oxide nanocomposites and magnetite nanoparticles on enhancing hydrogen production in dark fermentation. *Int. J. Hydrogen Energy* **2022**, *47*, 22359–22370. [CrossRef]
7. Bockris, J.O.M. The Hydrogen Economy: Its History. *Int. J. Hydrogen Energy*, 2013; 38, 2579–2588.
8. Tachibana, Y.; Vayssieres, L.; Durrant, J.R. Artificial photosynthesis for solar water-splitting. *Nat. Photonics* **2012**, *6*, 511–518. [CrossRef]
9. Zhang, J.Z.; Reisner, E. Advancing photosystem II photoelectrochemistry for semi-artificial photosynthesis. *Nat. Rev. Chem.* **2020**, *4*, 6–21. [CrossRef]
10. Lv, J.; Xie, J.; Mohamed, A.G.A.; Zhang, X.; Feng, Y.; Jiao, L.; Zhou, F.; Yuan, D.; Wang, Y. Solar utilization beyond photosynthesis. *Nat. Rev. Chem.* **2023**, *7*, 91–105. [CrossRef] [PubMed]
11. Zhang, L.; Morello, G.; Carr, S.B.; Armstrong, F.A. Aerobic photocatalytic H2 production by a [NiFe] hydrogenase engineered to place a silver nanocluster in the electron relay. *J. Am. Chem. Soc.* **2020**, *142*, 12699–12707. [CrossRef]
12. Land, H.; Senger, M.; Berggren, G.; Stripp, S.T. Current state of [FeFe]-hydrogenase research: Biodiversity and spectroscopic investigations. *ACS Catal.* **2020**, *10*, 7069–7086. [CrossRef]
13. Grinter, R.; Kropp, A.; Venugopal, H.; Senger, M.; Badley, J.; Cabotaje, P.R.; Jia, R.; Duan, Z.; Huang, P.; Stripp, T.P. Structural basis for bacterial energy extraction from atmospheric hydrogen. *Nature* **2023**, *615*, 541–547. [CrossRef] [PubMed]
14. Stephenson, M.; Stickland, L.H. Hydrogenase: A bacterial enzyme activating molecular hydrogen. *J. Biochem.* **1931**, *25*, 205–214. [CrossRef] [PubMed]
15. Fontecilla-Camps, J.C.; Volbeda, A.; Cavazza, C.; Nicolet, Y. Structure/function relationships of [NiFe]- and [FeFe]-hydrogenases. *Chem. Rev.* **2007**, *107*, 4273–4303.
16. Greening, C.; Biswas, A.; Carere, C.R.; Jackson, C.J.; Taylor, M.C.; Stott, M.B.; Cook, G.M.; Morales, S.E. Genomic and meta-genomic surveys of hydrogenase distribution indicate hydrogen is a widely utilised energy source for microbial growth and survival. *ISME J.* **2016**, *10*, 761–777. [CrossRef] [PubMed]
17. Morita, R.Y. Is hydrogen the universal energy source for long-term survival? *Microb. Ecol.* **1999**, *38*, 307–320. [CrossRef] [PubMed]
18. Ji, W.Q.; Zhang, K.; Zhan, K.; Wang, P. Advances in research on antiviral activities of sulfated polysaccharides from seaweeds. *Chin. J. Struct. Chem.* **2022**, *5*, 15–29.
19. Lacasse, M.J.; Zamble, D.B. [NiFe]-hydrogenase maturation. *Biochemistry* **2016**, *55*, 1689–1701. [CrossRef] [PubMed]
20. Schilter, D.; Camara, J.M.; Huynh, M.T.; Hammes-Schiffer, S.; Rauchfuss, T.B. Hydrogenase enzymes and their synthetic models: The role of metal hydrides. *Chem. Rev.* **2016**, *116*, 8693–8749. [CrossRef] [PubMed]

21. Kim, D.H.; Kim, M.S. Hydrogenases for biological hydrogen production. *Bioresour. Technol.* **2011**, *8423*, 8431. [CrossRef] [PubMed]
22. Barber, J. A Mechanism for Water Splitting and Oxygen Production in Photosynthesis. *Nat. Plants* **2017**, *3*, 17041. [CrossRef] [PubMed]
23. Tai, H.; Hirota, S. Mechanism and application of the catalytic reaction of [NiFe] hydrogenase: Recent developments. *ChemBioChem* **2020**, *21*, 1573–1581. [CrossRef]
24. Bachmeier, A.S.J.L. *Metalloenzymes as Inspirational Electrocatalysts for Artificial Photosynthesis: From Mechanism to Model Devices*; Springer: Cham, Switzerland, 2017; pp. 193–206.
25. Shafaat, H.S.; Rüdiger, O.; Ogata, H.; Lubitz, W. [NiFe] hydrogenases: A common active site for hydrogen metabolism un-der diverse conditions. *Biochim. Biophys. Acta Bioenerg.* **2013**, *1827*, 986–1002. [CrossRef] [PubMed]
26. Fritsch, J.; Lenz, O.; Friedrich, B. Structure, function and biosynthesis of O_2-tolerant hydrogenases. *Nat. Rev. Microbiol.* **2013**, *11*, 106–114. [CrossRef] [PubMed]
27. Sholl, D.S.; Steckel, J.A. *Density Functional Theory: A Practical Introduction*; John Wiley & Sons: Hoboken, NJ, USA, 2022.
28. Cramer, C.J.; Truhlar, D.G. Density functional theory for transition metals and transition metal chemistry. *Phys. Chem. Chem. Phys.* **2009**, *11*, 10757–10816. [PubMed]
29. Ramos, P.; Pavanello, M. Static correlation density functional theory. *arXiv* **2019**, arXiv:1906.06661.
30. Qu, Z.; Ma, Y. Variational multistate density functional theory for a balanced treatment of static and dynamic correlations. *J. Chem. Theory Comput.* **2020**, *16*, 4912–4922. [CrossRef] [PubMed]
31. Schlimgen, A.W.; Mazziotti, D.A. Static and dynamic electron correlation in the ligand noninnocent oxidation of nickel dithiolates. *J. Phys. Chem. A* **2017**, *121*, 9377–9384. [CrossRef] [PubMed]
32. Martin, J.M.L.; Santra, G.; Semidalas, E. An exchange-based diagnostic for static correlation. *AIP Conf. Proc.* **2022**, *2611*, 020014.
33. Sandala, G.M.; Hopmann, K.H.; Ghosh, A.; Noodleman, L. Calibration of DFT Functionals for the Prediction of [57]Fe Mössbauer Spectral Parameters in Iron–Nitrosyl and Iron–Sulfur Complexes: Accurate Geometries Prove Essential. *J. Chem. Theory Comput.* **2011**, *7*, 3232–3247. [CrossRef] [PubMed]
34. David, G.; Ferré, N.; Le Guennic, B. Consistent Evaluation of Magnetic Exchange Couplings in Multicenter Compounds in KS-DFT: The Recomposition Method. *J. Chem. Theory Comput.* **2022**, *19*, 157–173. [CrossRef] [PubMed]
35. Pantazis, D.A. Meeting the challenge of magnetic coupling in a triply-bridged chromium dimer: Complementary broken-symmetry density functional theory and multireference density matrix renormalization group perspectives. *J. Chem. Theory Comput.* **2019**, *15*, 938–948. [CrossRef] [PubMed]
36. Sharma, S.; Sivalingam, K.; Neese, F.; Chan, G.K.L. Low-energy spectrum of iron–sulfur clusters directly from many-particle quantum mechanics. *Nat. Chem.* **2014**, *6*, 927–933. [CrossRef] [PubMed]
37. Ames, W.; Pantazis, D.A.; Krewald, V.; Cox, N.; Messinger, J.; Lubitz, W.; Neese, F. Theoretical evaluation of structural models of the S2 state in the oxygen evolving complex of photosystem II: Protonation states and magnetic interactions. *J. Am. Chem. Soc.* **2011**, *133*, 19743–19757. [CrossRef] [PubMed]
38. Chu, S.; Bovi, D.; Cappelluti, F.; Orellana, A.G.; Martin, H.; Guidoni, L. Effects of static correlation between spin centers in multicenter transition metal complexes. *J. Chem. Theory Comput.* **2017**, *13*, 4675–4683. [CrossRef] [PubMed]
39. Bisgard, J. *Analysis and Linear Algebra: The Singular Value Decomposition and Applications*; American Mathematical Society: Providence, RI, USA, 2020.
40. Lauterbach, L.; Gee, L.B.; Pelmenschikov, V.; Jenney, F.E.; Kamali, S.; Yoda, Y.; Adams, M.W.W.; Cramer, S.P. Characterization of the [3Fe–4S]$^{0/1+}$ cluster from the D14C variant of *Pyrococcus furiosus* ferredoxin via combined NRVS and DFT analyses. *Dalton Trans.* **2016**, *45*, 7215–7219. [CrossRef] [PubMed]
41. Zhou, J.; Hu, Z.; Münck, E.; Holm, R.H. The cuboidal Fe_3S_4 cluster: Synthesis, stability, and geometric and electronic structures in a non-protein environment. *J. Am. Chem. Soc.* **1996**, *118*, 1966–1980. [CrossRef]
42. Yoo, S.J.; Hu, Z.; Goh, C.; Bominaar, E.L.; Holm, R.H.; Münck, E. Determination of the Exchange-Coupling Constant of an Fe^{3+}–Fe^{3+} Pair in a Cubane-Type Iron$^-$ Sulfur Cluster. *J. Am. Chem. Soc.* **1997**, *119*, 8732–8733. [CrossRef]
43. Neese, F. The ORCA program system. *WIREs Comput. Mol. Sci.* **2012**, *2*, 73–78. [CrossRef]
44. Schäfer, A.; Horn, H.; Ahlrichs, R. Fully optimized contracted Gaussian basis sets for atoms Li to Kr. *J. Chem. Phys.* **1992**, *97*, 2571–2577. [CrossRef]
45. Weigend, F.; Ahlrichs, R. Balanced basis sets of split valence, triple zeta valence and quadruple zeta valence quality for H to Rn: Design and assessment of accuracy. *Phys. Chem. Chem. Phys.* **2005**, *7*, 3297–3305. [CrossRef] [PubMed]
46. Jensen, K.P. Bioinorganic Chemistry Modeled with the TPSSh Density Functional. *Inorg. Chem.* **2008**, *47*, 10357–10365. [CrossRef] [PubMed]
47. Pain, J.C. Group theory and the link between expectation values of powers of r and Clebsch-Gordan coefficients. *arXiv* **2021**, arXiv:2101.07872.
48. Simon, A. *Numerical Table of the Clebsch-Gordan Coefficiencts*; Oak Ridge National Laboratory: Oak Ridge, TN, USA, 1954.

Disclaimer/Publisher's Note: The statements, opinions and data contained in all publications are solely those of the individual author(s) and contributor(s) and not of MDPI and/or the editor(s). MDPI and/or the editor(s) disclaim responsibility for any injury to people or property resulting from any ideas, methods, instructions or products referred to in the content.

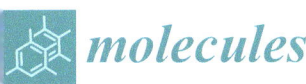

Article

One-Step Synthesis of Ag$_2$O/Fe$_3$O$_4$ Magnetic Photocatalyst for Efficient Organic Pollutant Removal via Wide-Spectral-Response Photocatalysis–Fenton Coupling

Chuanfu Shan [1], Ziqian Su [1], Ziyi Liu [1], Ruizheng Xu [1], Jianfeng Wen [1], Guanghui Hu [1], Tao Tang [1], Zhijie Fang [2], Li Jiang [1,*] and Ming Li [1,*]

[1] College of Science & Key Laboratory of Low-Dimensional Structural Physics and Application, Education Department of Guangxi Zhuang Autonomous Region, Guilin University of Technology, Guilin 541004, China
[2] School of Electronics Engineering, Guangxi University of Science and Technology, Liuzhou 545006, China
* Correspondence: jiangli1515@glut.edu.cn (L.J.); 2006017@glut.edu.cn (M.L.)

Abstract: Photocatalysis holds great promise for addressing water pollution caused by organic dyes, and the development of Ag$_2$O/Fe$_3$O$_4$ aims to overcome the challenges of slow degradation efficiency and difficult recovery of photocatalysts. In this study, we present a novel, environmentally friendly Ag$_2$O/Fe$_3$O$_4$ magnetic nanocomposite synthesized via a simple coprecipitation method, which not only constructs a type II heterojunction but also successfully couples photocatalysis and Fenton reaction, enhancing the broad-spectrum response and efficiency. The Ag$_2$O/Fe$_3$O$_4$ (10%) nanocomposite demonstrates exceptional degradation performance toward organic dyes, achieving 99.5% degradation of 10 mg/L methyl orange (MO) within 15 min under visible light irradiation and proving its wide applicability by efficiently degrading various dyes while maintaining high stability over multiple testing cycles. Magnetic testing further highlighted the ease of Ag$_2$O/Fe$_3$O$_4$ (10%) recovery using magnetic force. This innovative approach offers a promising strategy for constructing high-performance photocatalytic systems for addressing water pollution caused by organic dyes.

Keywords: photocatalysis; Ag$_2$O/Fe$_3$O$_4$; heterosuperstructure; Fenton reaction; magnetic separation

1. Introduction

With the acceleration of global industrialization, water pollution caused by organic dyes has become an increasingly urgent issue of public concern. Photocatalytic technology has been widely researched owing to its advantages, such as high efficiency and the absence of secondary pollution [1–8] Among them, silver oxide (Ag$_2$O) nanoparticles are extensively employed to degrade water pollutants due to their simple preparation, stable properties, and environmental friendliness [9–12]. However, the narrow bandgap and low photogenerated carrier-separation efficiency of Ag$_2$O limit its application in water treatment [13–16]. Furthermore, using Ag$_2$O as a powder photocatalyst makes it challenging to recycle. Therefore, it is practically significant to develop a magnetic material to couple with Ag$_2$O through heterojunctions to enhance the photogenerated carrier separation efficiency and fabricate an efficient and magnetically recoverable Ag$_2$O-based photocatalyst.

Fe$_3$O$_4$ nanoparticles possess unique magnetic properties and nanoscale characteristics, which make them highly versatile for various potential applications, including drug delivery, MRI contrast agents, biomolecule separation, biosensing, and catalysis, due to their magnetism and biocompatibility [17–22]. Additionally, Fe$_3$O$_4$ nanoparticles demonstrate strong light-absorption ability, absorbing most of the light in the UV–visible range [23]. Furthermore, the Fe^{2+} ions in Fe$_3$O$_4$ can react with hydrogen peroxide (H$_2$O$_2$) through the Fenton reaction to generate a large number of free radical groups, which can oxidize many known organic compounds, such as carboxylic acids, alcohols, and esters, into

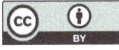

inorganic forms, exhibiting a significant oxidation ability to remove refractory organic pollutants [24–27]. It is known that the Fenton reaction can produce a large number of oxygen-related species through the following reactions:

$$2Fe^{2+} + H_2O_2 + O_2 \rightarrow 2Fe^{3+} + \cdot O_2^- + (OH)^- + \cdot OH \quad (1)$$

$$H_2O_2 + 2Fe^{3+} \rightarrow 2Fe^{2+} + O_2 + 2H^+ \quad (2)$$

Additionally, Fe_3O_4 is a magnetic material that can be recycled and reused by an external magnetic field, thereby reducing the cost of recovery treatment [28–30]. In contrast, the use of Fe_3O_4 in the Fenton reaction to oxidize organic pollutants in water has significant limitations, including the need to consume externally provided H_2O_2 in the reaction and the requirement of an acidic environment to generate free radicals through the Fenton reaction. However, when Fe_3O_4 is coupled with a photocatalyst, the H_2O_2 generated at the interface of the photocatalyst can be used for the Fenton reaction with Fe_3O_4. Another advantage of selecting Fe_3O_4 is that it contains both Fe^{2+} and Fe^{3+} ions, facilitating the continuous progress of the Fenton reaction. Consequently, numerous researchers have employed Fe_3O_4 as a cocatalyst in the photocatalyst system [31–34].

In this article, the Ag_2O/Fe_3O_4 binary magnetic nanoparticles were synthesized using a simple chemical coprecipitation method with $FeCl_2 \cdot 4H_2O$, $FeCl_3 \cdot 6H_2O$, and $AgNO_3$ as raw materials, and they were applied to degrade the organic dyes in water. The results showed that the introduction of Fe_3O_4 to load Ag_2O could generate a type II heterojunction at the contact interface, facilitating the fast transfer of photogenerated carriers. At the same time, the photocatalysis–Fenton combined reaction was also constructed to improve the utilization efficiency of photogenerated carriers, further enhancing the degradation efficiency of the photocatalyst. The Ag_2O/Fe_3O_4 nanoparticles exhibited very high efficiency in degrading dyes, such as methyl orange (MO), under visible light irradiation.

2. Results and Discussion

2.1. TEM Analysis

Transmission electron microscopy (TEM) was used to characterize the microstructure of the samples. Figure 1 shows the results. Firstly, TEM analysis was performed on Fe_3O_4 nanoparticles, and the average particle size was found to be 15 ± 5 nm with a typical spherical morphology, as shown in Figure 1a. Due to the large surface area, the Fe_3O_4 nanoparticles exhibited obvious aggregation in the image. Figure 1b shows the TEM image of the Ag_2O nanoparticles, which had a particle size distribution ranging from 30 to 80 nm and a polyhedral morphology that differed greatly from Fe_3O_4. The nanoparticles of the two materials could be easily distinguished. Figure 1c shows the TEM image of binary Ag_2O/Fe_3O_4 (10%) nanoparticles, which demonstrates that Fe_3O_4 nanoparticles with smaller size and spherical morphology could encapsulate Ag_2O nanoparticles with larger size and polyhedral morphology, indicating good compatibility between Fe_3O_4 and Ag_2O. A high-resolution TEM (HRTEM) analysis was performed on a circular region indicated in Figure 1c to confirm the successful formation of Ag_2O/Fe_3O_4 (10%). Figure 1d shows the results. The clear interface between Fe_3O_4 nanoparticles and Ag_2O nanoparticles was observed with lattice spacing of 0.25 nm (corresponding to the (311) plane of/Fe_3O_4) and 0.29 nm (corresponding to the (220) plane of Ag_2O), respectively, further demonstrating the successful formation of Ag_2O/Fe_3O_4 (10%).

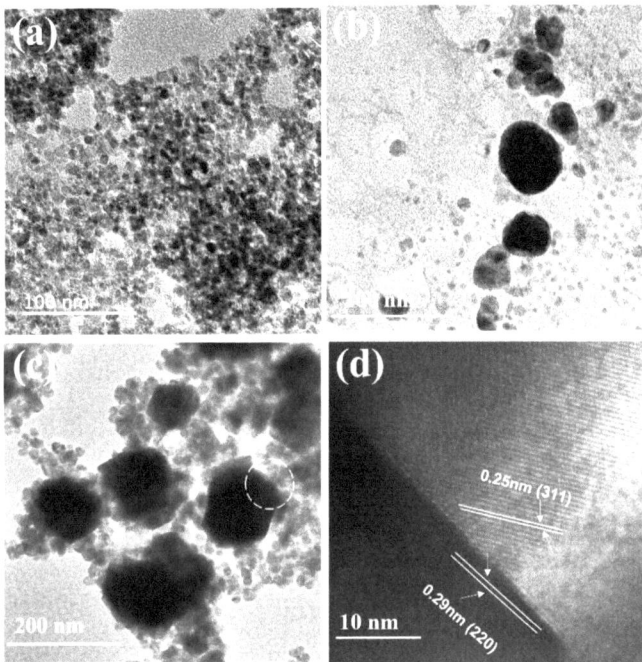

Figure 1. (**a**) TEM image of Fe$_3$O$_4$ nanoparticles; (**b**) TEM image of Ag$_2$O nanoparticles; (**c**) TEM image of Ag$_2$O/Fe$_3$O$_4$ (10%); (**d**) HRTEM image of Ag$_2$O/Fe$_3$O$_4$ (10%).

2.2. SEM and EDS Analysis

Ag$_2$O/Fe$_3$O$_4$ (10%) was analyzed through scanning electron microscopy to better verify the successful coupling of Ag$_2$O and Fe$_3$O$_4$ to form Ag$_2$O/Fe$_3$O$_4$ binary nanoparticles, as shown in Figure 2. A relatively large size was selected for characterization to better analyze the overall morphology and surface element distribution of the binary nanoparticles. As shown in Figure 2a, it can be observed that the smaller Fe$_3$O$_4$ nanoparticles with approximately spherical shape were well loaded onto the surface of larger-sized Ag$_2$O nanoparticles with polyhedral shape, forming a compact structure of binary nanoparticles with good structural stability, which is consistent with the conclusion obtained from the TEM image analysis. Additionally, the loading of Fe$_3$O$_4$ increased the number of reaction sites. Note that almost no Fe$_3$O$_4$ spherical nanoparticles were present in unoccupied areas on the surface of Ag$_2$O, indicating that Ag$_2$O has a good ability to capture Fe$_3$O$_4$. EDS analysis was performed in this area to analyze the surface element distribution of Ag$_2$O/Fe$_3$O$_4$ (10%) binary nanoparticles. Figure 2b–e shows the results, where all Fe elements of Fe$_3$O$_4$ are uniformly distributed on the surface of Ag$_2$O, indicating that Fe$_3$O$_4$ was successfully loaded onto the surface of Ag$_2$O to form Ag$_2$O/Fe$_3$O$_4$ binary nanoparticles. EDS data statistics were conducted to further demonstrate the contents of Fe$_3$O$_4$ and Ag$_2$O. Table 1 presents the results. It can be seen that ratio of the number of Ag atoms and Fe atoms is approximately 6:1, indicating that the mass ratio of Ag$_2$O to Fe$_3$O$_4$ is approximately 9:1, and Fe$_3$O$_4$ accounts for 10% of the total mass.

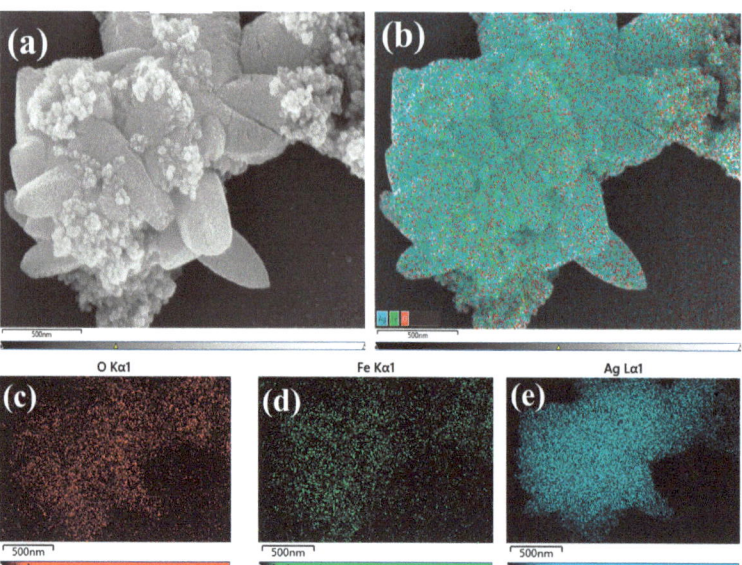

Figure 2. SEM images and element distributions of Ag$_2$O/Fe$_3$O$_4$ (10%) nanoparticles, including (**a**) SEM image, (**b**) element distribution, and (**c–e**) O, Fe, and Ag element distributions.

Table 1. EDS data statistics of Ag$_2$O/Fe$_3$O$_4$ (10%) nanoparticles.

Element	Line Type	wt%	wt% Sigma	at%
O	K series	21.33	0.46	63.01
Fe	K series	6.17	0.23	5.22
Ag	L series	72.49	0.47	31.76
Total		100.00		100.00

2.3. XRD Analysis

X-ray diffraction (XRD) was used to characterize the pure Ag$_2$O and Fe$_3$O$_4$ nanoparticles as well as Ag$_2$O/Fe$_3$O$_4$ (10%) nanocomposites to investigate their crystal structure. Figure 3 shows the results. The diffraction peaks of Ag$_2$O nanoparticles at X-ray diffraction angles (2θ) of 26.9°, 33.0°, 38.3°, 55.1°, 65.7°, and 68.7° were indexed to the (110), (111), (200), (220), (311), and (222) crystal planes of Ag$_2$O, respectively, which were consistent with the JCPDS card (PDF#75 1532) for Ag$_2$O. The diffraction peaks of Fe$_3$O$_4$ nanoparticles at X-ray diffraction angle (2θ) of 28.26°, 34.53°, 44.01° and 61.88° were indexed to the (220), (311), (400), and (440) crystal planes of Fe$_3$O$_4$, respectively, which were consistent with the JCPDS card (PDF#19-0629) for Fe$_3$O$_4$. The XRD pattern of Ag$_2$O/Fe$_3$O$_4$ (10%) nanocomposites showed the same diffraction peaks at 26.9°, 33.0°, 38.3°, 55.1°, 65.7°, and 68.7° for Ag$_2$O and at 28.26°, 34.53°, 44.01°, and 61.88° for Fe$_3$O$_4$, indicating a good coupling of Ag$_2$O and Fe$_3$O$_4$ and showing no change in their crystal structure. Additionally, no other impurity phases were observed, indicating that Ag$_2$O/Fe$_3$O$_4$ (10%) is a two-phase composite.

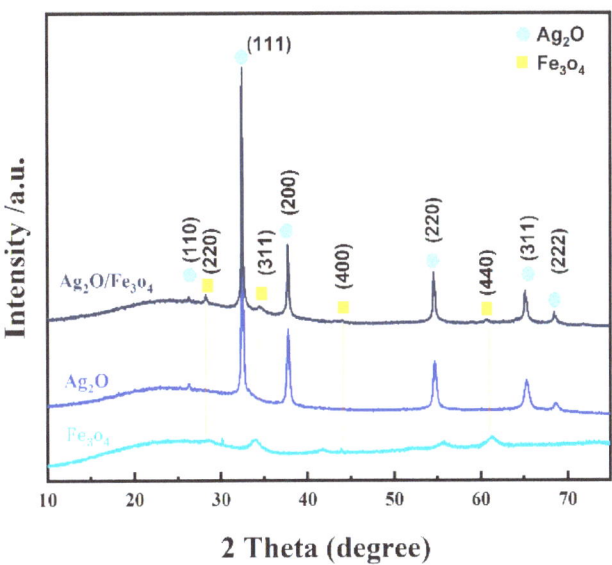

Figure 3. XRD characterization patterns of Ag_2O/Fe_3O_4 (10%) nanoparticles, Ag_2O nanoparticles, and Fe_3O_4 nanoparticles.

2.4. XPS Elemental Analysis

X-ray photoelectron spectroscopy (XPS) was used to investigate the chemical composition of the Ag_2O/Fe_3O_4 (10%) sample. Figure 4a shows the XPS spectrum of the sample, exhibiting distinct peaks at around 285.2 eV (C 1s), 368.8 eV (Ag 3d), 530.08 eV (O 1s), and 711.08 eV (Fe 2p), which indicate the presence of four elements, namely C, Ag, O, and Fe. The presence of C is attributed to the fixation of CO_2 from air during the preparation of the binary composite material. XPS fine-spectrum measurement was performed to investigate the elemental state in detail. Figure 4b shows the Ag 3d fine spectrum, exhibiting binding energies of 368.2 eV and 374.0 eV for Ag 3d5/2 and Ag 3d3/2, respectively. These binding energies correspond to the orbit peaks of Ag^+ in Ag_2O, confirming the existence of Ag_2O in the compound. As depicted in Figure 4c, the Fe 2p XPS spectrum reveals two spin–orbit doublets. The first doublet, attributed to Fe^{2+}, is observed at 710.58 eV (Fe 2p3/2) and 723.78 eV (Fe 2p1/2), while the second doublet, assigned to Fe^{3+}, is observed at 712.18 eV (Fe 2p3/2) and 726.12 eV (Fe 2p1/2). This mixed phase confirms the formation of Fe_3O_4. Figure 4d shows the O 1s fine spectrum, in which the peak at 532.11 eV is attributed to external −OH groups or adsorbed water molecules on the surface, the peak at 531.11 eV corresponds to the lattice oxygen atoms in Ag_2O, and the peak at 529.39 eV is attributed to the Fe-O bond [35,36]. Therefore, XPS analysis confirms the presence of Ag_2O and Fe_3O_4 in the Ag_2O/Fe_3O_4 (10%) binary nanocomposite material and their successful composition.

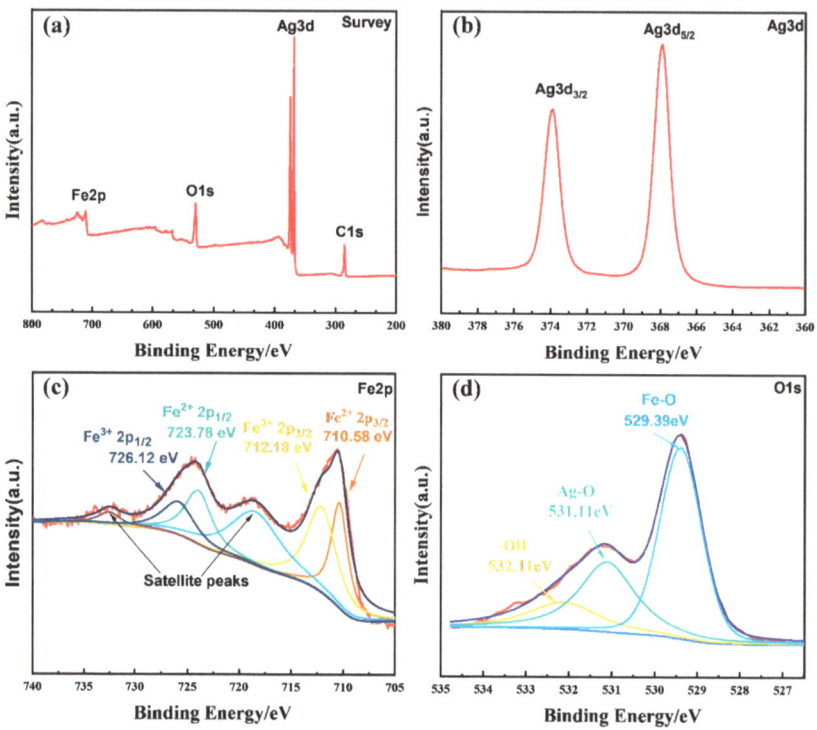

Figure 4. XPS spectra of Ag$_2$O/Fe$_3$O$_4$ (10%), including (**a**) full-spectrum, (**b**) Ag3d high-resolution spectrum, (**c**) Fe2p high-resolution spectrum, and (**d**) O1s high-resolution spectrum.

2.5. UV–Vis and PL Analysis

UV–vis and PL tests were conducted to determine the optical properties of the synthesized nanomaterials. UV–vis testing was used to measure the absorbance of the synthesized nanomaterials. Figure 5a shows the results. Ag$_2$O exhibits strong absorption in the ultraviolet and near-ultraviolet regions, with a peak at a wavelength of 500 nm [13–15]. Fe$_3$O$_4$ exhibits a strong optical response across the whole examined spectral range, indicating that the strong visible light-absorption capability of Ag$_2$O/Fe$_3$O$_4$ binary composite catalysts is undoubtedly due to the optical properties of Fe$_3$O$_4$ [23,31–33]. Furthermore, compared with Ag$_2$O, a gradual redshift was observed at the absorption edge of Ag$_2$O/Fe$_3$O$_4$ binary composite catalysts, and a significant increase in absorption was observed in the near-infrared region of 600–800 nm, indicating a strong interaction between Ag$_2$O and Fe$_3$O$_4$ in the binary composite catalyst. It is worth noting that as the loading amount of Fe$_3$O$_4$ increases, the light absorption ability of Ag$_2$O/Fe$_3$O$_4$ binary photocatalysts in the UV–visible spectral range also increases. Ag$_2$O/Fe$_3$O$_4$ (15%) exhibits the best light-absorption ability, followed by Ag$_2$O/Fe$_3$O$_4$ (10%) and Ag$_2$O/Fe$_3$O$_4$ (5%). The Kubelka–Munk equation was used to calculate the bandgap energy of the semiconductor:

$$(ahv)^{\frac{2}{n}} = A(hv - E_g) \qquad (3)$$

where α represents the absorption coefficient of the semiconductor, h is a constant and stands for the Planck constant, v represents the frequency of light, A is a constant and represents a constant term, and n is closely related to the semiconductor transition process. The indirect semiconductors Ag$_2$O and Fe$_3$O$_4$ both have n values of 4. The Kubelka-Munk function was used to derive the absorption spectra of all the synthesized catalysts, which were then used to generate Tauc plots. As shown in Figure 5b, the results of Tauc plots show that the optical bandgaps of Ag_2O and Fe_3O_4 are 2.0 eV and 1.2 eV, respectively, while the bandgaps of Ag_2O/Fe_3O_4 (5%), Ag_2O/Fe_3O_4 (10%), and Ag_2O/Fe_3O_4 (15%) are 1.6 eV, 1.5 eV, and 1.4 eV, respectively. These results are in good agreement with the increasing trend in the redshift observed at the absorption edge with the increase in the Fe_3O_4 loading amount shown in Figure 5a.

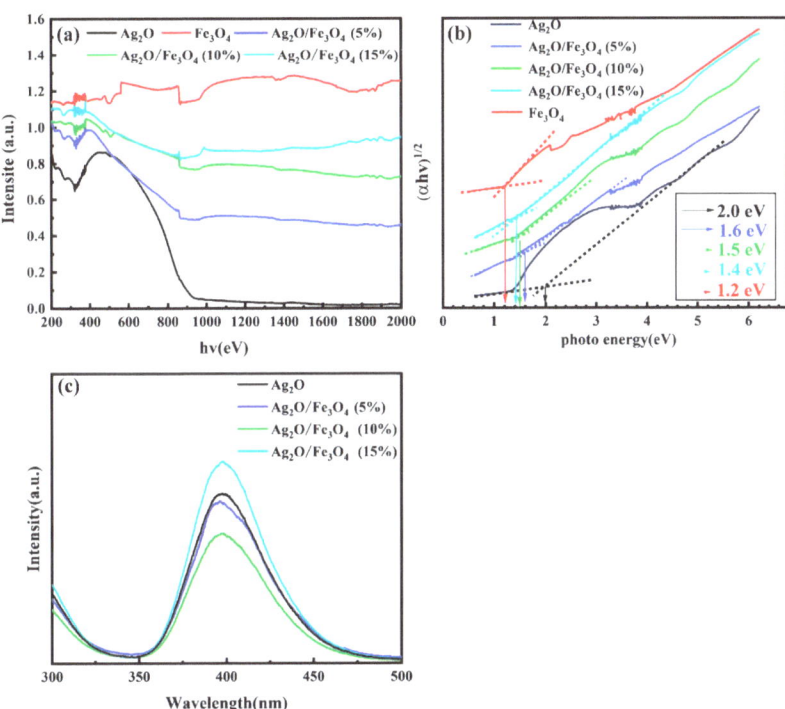

Figure 5. Ag_2O, Fe_3O_4, Ag_2O/Fe_3O_4 (5%), Ag_2O/Fe_3O_4 (10%), and Ag_2O/Fe_3O_4 (15%) of (**a**) UV–vis spectra and (**b**) Tauc plots. (**c**) PL spectra of Ag_2O, Ag_2O/Fe_3O_4 (5%), Ag_2O/Fe_3O_4 (10%), and Ag_2O/Fe_3O_4 (15%).

When Ag_2O and Fe_3O_4 are exposed to light, valence band electrons absorb photon energy and transition to the conduction band, forming photogenerated electron–hole pairs. PL emission occurs when conduction band electrons recombine with valence band holes. Therefore, PL intensity is proportional to the separation of photogenerated charge carriers; lower PL intensity reflects a reduction in recombination probability. As shown in Figure 5c, when the samples of Ag_2O, Ag_2O/Fe_3O_4 (5%), Ag_2O/Fe_3O_4 (10%), and Ag_2O/Fe_3O_4 (15%) were subjected to PL testing under 260nm excitation light, their emission peak positions were all at 400 nm. Although the emission peak intensity of Ag_2O was higher, it decreased with the loading of Fe_3O_4. Compared with Ag_2O, the emission peak intensity of Ag_2O/Fe_3O_4 (5%) decreased to 90%, while that of Ag_2O/Fe_3O_4 (10%) decreased significantly to 60%. However, as the loading of Fe_3O_4 continued to increase, the emission peak intensity of Ag_2O/Fe_3O_4 (15%) was higher than that of the original Ag_2O. Therefore, it can be concluded that photogenerated electron–hole pairs are generated when light is irradiated onto the surface of Ag_2O. When Fe_3O_4 with a low loading is coupled to the surface of Ag_2O, they enhance the separation efficiency of photogenerated electron–hole pairs generated by Ag_2O. However, when the loading of Fe_3O_4 exceeds 15% of the total mass, an excess Fe_3O_4 forms a thick covering layer on the surface of Ag_2O. Under light irradiation, Fe_3O_4 absorbs photons, causing the electrons on the valence band to be excited to the conduction band, generating photogenerated electron–hole pairs. Due to the low optical bandgap of Fe_3O_4, which is only 1.6 eV, photogenerated electrons and holes are prone to recombine, producing strong light emission.

2.6. Electrochemical Characterization Analysis

Mott–Schottky analysis, photocurrent response analysis, and EIS were performed to determine the electrochemical properties of the prepared samples. The Mott–Schottky plot is the most commonly used method to distinguish between n-type and p-type semiconductors [37]. A positive slope and a negative slope indicate an n-type and a p-type semiconductor, respectively. Additionally, the Mott–Schottky plot can be extrapolated to estimate the flat-band potential (Efb) of the semiconductor, which can be used to estimate the position of the Fermi level [38]. Assuming that the Fermi level is very close to the band edge, the extrapolated flat-band potential (Efb) can be utilized as the position of the edge of either the n-type semiconductor (E_{CB}) or the p-type semiconductor (E_{VB}). Figure 6a,b shows the Mott–Schottky plots of Ag_2O and Fe_3O_4 with Ag/AgCl as the reference electrode. It can be seen that both Ag_2O and Fe_3O_4 have positive slopes, indicating that they are p-type semiconductors. By extrapolation, the Mott–Schottky plots of Ag_2O and Fe_3O_4 intersect the x-axis at 1.84 eV and 1.95 eV, respectively. Considering the difference between the reference electrode (Ag/AgCl) and the standard value of 0.19 eV (relative to the normal hydrogen electrode), the Evb values of Ag_2O and Fe_3O_4 are estimated to be 2.03 eV and 2.14 eV, respectively. Furthermore, based on the previously obtained data, the optical bandgaps of Ag_2O and Fe_3O_4 are 2.0 eV and 1.2 eV, respectively. Therefore, the E_{VB} of Ag_2O and Fe_3O_4 can be calculated using the following equation:

$$E_{VB} = E_g + E_{CB} \qquad (4)$$

where E_g represents the optical bandgap energy. By substituting the values of E_g as 2.0 eV and E_{VB} as 2.03 eV for Ag_2O in the formula, the value of E_{CB} is calculated as -0.03 eV. Similarly, by substituting the values of E_g as 1.2 eV and E_{VB} as 2.14 eV for Fe_3O_4 in the formula, the value of E_{CB} is calculated as 0.94 eV. The photogenerated current response analysis can be used to verify the efficiency of the photogenerated carriers in the samples. The research results show that when a small amount of Fe_3O_4 is loaded on the surface of Ag_2O, the photocurrent intensity of the sample is significantly improved, and the photocurrent intensity of Ag_2O/Fe_3O_4 (10%) is the highest, as shown in Figure 6c. However, when the loading amount of Fe_3O_4 reaches 15%, the photocurrent intensity of the formed Ag_2O/Fe_3O_4 (15%) is lower than that of Ag_2O. This indicates that too much Fe_3O_4 loading will reduce the utilization efficiency of photogenerated carriers. In addition, EIS measurements were also conducted to study the charge-transfer resistance and transfer efficiency of photogenerated carriers. As shown in Figure 6d, it can be observed that the Nyquist semicircle diameters of the Ag_2O/Fe_3O_4 (5%) and Ag_2O/Fe_3O_4 (10%) nanocomposites are smaller than those of Ag_2O and Ag_2O/Fe_3O_4 (15%). The Nyquist semicircle diameter of Ag_2O/Fe_3O_4 (10%) is the lowest, indicating that its resistance is lower than that of Ag_2O and the other samples. Therefore, loading a small amount of Fe_3O_4 can improve the transfer efficiency of photogenerated carriers in Ag_2O, which is a favorable condition for enhancing the photocatalytic activity. However, when the loading amount of Fe_3O_4 reaches 15%, the Nyquist semicircle diameter of Ag_2O/Fe_3O_4 (15%) is larger than that of Ag_2O, indicating that too much Fe_3O_4 loading will reduce the available surface area of oxidized silver, leading to an increase in the resistance encountered by electrons and holes during transmission and a decrease in the transfer efficiency of photogenerated carriers.

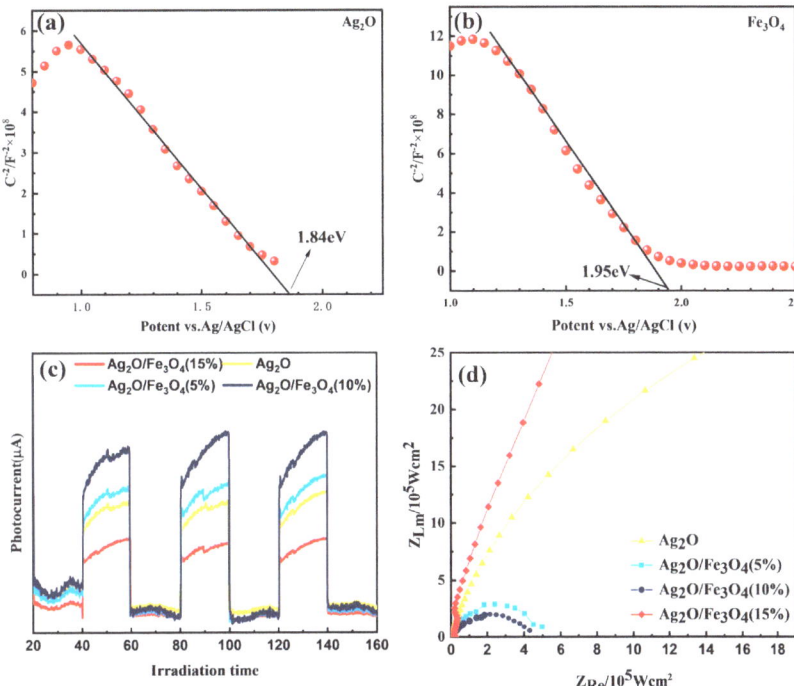

Figure 6. Mott–Schottky curves of (**a**) Ag$_2$O and (**b**) Fe$_3$O$_4$; (**c**) sample photocurrent response profiles; (**d**) sample EIS test graph.

2.7. Photocatalytic Performance Analysis

Fe$_3$O$_4$, Ag$_2$O, Ag$_2$O/Fe$_3$O$_4$ (5%), Ag$_2$O/Fe$_3$O$_4$ (10%), and Ag$_2$O/Fe$_3$O$_4$ (15%) were placed under a xenon lamp light source (λ > 420nm) to simulate visible light in sunlight and to photocatalyze a 10 mol/L MO solution to better demonstrate the visible light photocatalytic performance of different samples. Figure 7a shows the results. When pure Fe$_3$O$_4$ was placed in the MO solution and irradiated with visible light, no MO degradation was observed, indicating that Fe$_3$O$_4$ alone does not have the ability to degrade the MO solution under visible light. When pure Ag$_2$O was placed in the MO solution and irradiated with visible light, MO was significantly degraded. Approximately 80% of the MO solution was degraded in 15 min of light irradiation, and 99.1% of the MO solution was degraded in 30 min of light irradiation, indicating that Ag$_2$O can absorb photon energy and produce photocatalytic reactions under visible light, which is a considerable catalytic rate for the MO solution.

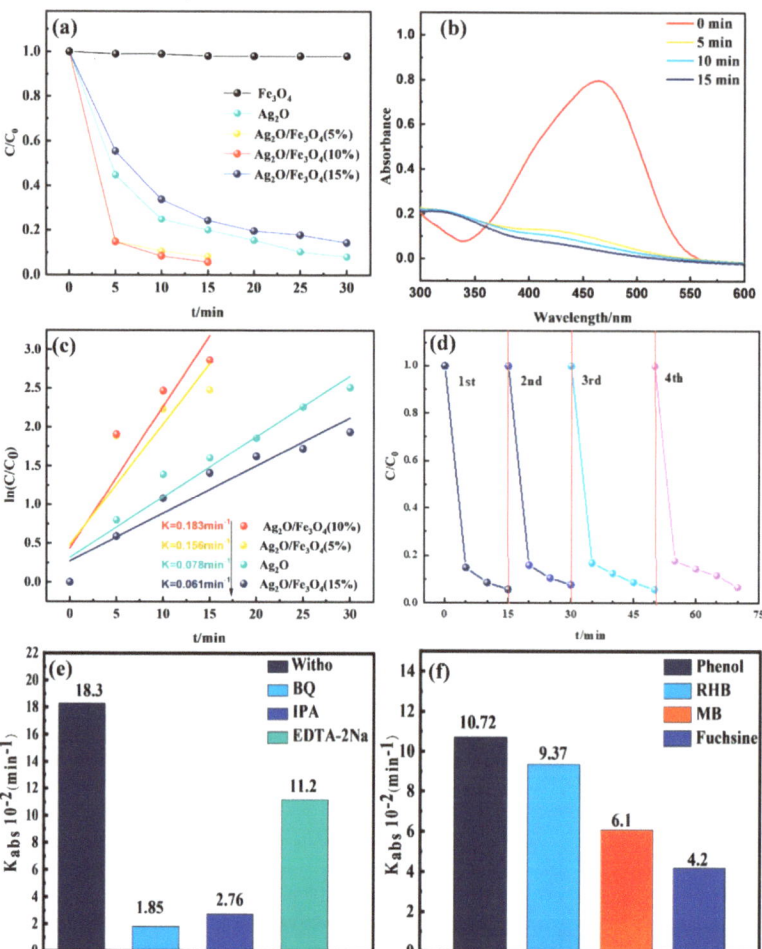

Figure 7. (**a**) Degradation rate of the MO solution by different photocatalyst samples; (**b**) UV–vis absorption spectra of the MO solution degraded by Ag_2O/Fe_3O_4 (10%); (**c**) pseudo-first-order kinetic model diagram of the MO solution degradation; (**d**) cycle test of the Ag_2O/Fe_3O_4 (10%) sample degradation; (**e**) kinetics rate of the MO solution degradation using Ag_2O/Fe_3O_4 (10%) with different scavengers; (**f**) kinetics of different water pollutants degradation using Ag_2O/Fe_3O_4 (10%).

The photocatalytic rate of Ag_2O changed significantly after Fe_3O_4 was loaded onto its surface. When the Fe_3O_4 loading amount was 5wt% of the overall weight, the Ag_2O/Fe_3O_4 (5%) binary catalyst was formed, degrading 99.1% of the MO solution after 15 min of visible light irradiation. When the Fe_3O_4 loading amount was 10wt% of the overall weight, the Ag_2O/Fe_3O_4 (10%) binary catalyst was formed, degrading 99.5% of the MO solution after 15 min of visible light irradiation. It is worth noting that when the Fe_3O_4 loading amount continued to increase to 15wt% of the overall weight, the Ag_2O/Fe_3O_4 (15%) binary catalyst did not increase but decreases the degradation rate of the MO solution. Moreover, it only degraded 75.1% and 85.2% of the MO solution after 15 min and 30 min of visible light irradiation, respectively. This indicates that during the Fe_3O_4 loading, a coverage layer forms on the surface of Ag_2O, and Fe_3O_4 absorb photons and produce electron–hole pairs under light irradiation, which are then be transferred from type-II heterojunction to the electrode of Ag_2O to participate in the reaction. However, when there is too much Fe_3O_4 loading, the thicker coverage layer it forms reduces the available surface area of

Ag$_2$O, blocks the entry of photons, and shields the surface of Ag$_2$O from light, thereby reducing the generation of photoinduced carriers. In addition, in photocatalytic reactions, electrons and holes are transmitted through the surface conductor, thereby participating in redox reactions. The reduction in the available surface area of oxidized silver increases the resistance encountered by electrons and holes during transmission, resulting in a slower charge transfer rate and reduced reaction efficiency under visible light irradiation. Figure 7b shows the UV–vis absorption spectra during the photocatalytic degradation of the MO solution using Ag$_2$O/Fe$_3$O$_4$ (10%). It can be observed that the absorption peak at 464 nm of MO decreases significantly with the irradiation time, and the peak intensity almost reaches zero after 15 min of irradiation. No new absorption peaks were generated, indicating that MO was completely degraded into inorganic substances without the formation of other organic compounds. Figure 7c shows the degradation of MO by different photocatalysts using a pseudo-first-order kinetics model. It can be seen that the degradation rate of Ag$_2$O/Fe$_3$O$_4$ (10%) is the fastest, reaching 0.183 min^{-1}, which is 2.3 times higher than that of pure Ag$_2$O (0.078 min^{-1}), 3 times higher than that of Ag$_2$O/Fe$_3$O$_4$ (15%) (0.061 min^{-1}), and 1.17 times higher than that of Ag$_2$O/Fe$_3$O$_4$ (5%) (0.156 min^{-1}). Four photocatalytic cycling tests were conducted to verify the structural stability of the Ag$_2$O/Fe$_3$O$_4$ (10%) sample. Figure 7d shows the results. After four cycles, the catalytic rate of Ag$_2$O/Fe$_3$O$_4$ (10%) slightly decreased but still exhibited a fast catalytic rate, indicating good structural stability.

In general, the reactive species in photocatalytic processes are often considered to be holes (h$^+$), hydroxyl radicals (·OH), and superoxide ion radicals (·O$_2^-$). Therefore, EDTA-2Na, isopropyl alcohol (IPA), and benzene quinone (BQ) were selected as the capture agents to study the capture of these reactive species, as shown in Figure 7e. Through the photodegradation experiment of MO using the Ag$_2$O/Fe$_3$O$_4$ (10%) photocatalyst under visible light, in which the original photocatalytic degradation was 18.3×10^{-2} min^{-1}, it was observed that the degree of inhibition of the photocatalytic degradation rate decreased in the following order: BQ (1.85×10^{-2} min^{-1}), IPA (2.76×10^{-2} min^{-1}), and EDTA-2Na (11.2×10^{-2} min^{-1}). This reveals that ·O$_2^-$ and ·OH have a significant impact on the degradation of MO in the Ag$_2$O/Fe$_3$O$_4$ photocatalytic reaction, while h$^+$ has a relatively small degree of participation.

The catalytic rates of phenol, rhodamine B, methyl blue, and basic fuchsin were tested under visible light irradiation to verify the applicability of the Ag$_2$O/Fe$_3$O$_4$ (10%) photocatalyst for the degradation of organic pollutants in water. As shown in Figure 7f, the degradation rates of basic fuchsin, rhodamine B, and methyl blue were 10.72×10^{-2} min^{-1}, 9.37×10^{-2} min^{-1}, and 6.1×10^{-2} min^{-1}, respectively. This demonstrates that the Ag$_2$O/Fe$_3$O$_4$ (10%) photocatalyst has a good applicability and a good catalytic effect on various types of organic pollutants in water.

2.8. Magnetic Properties Analysis

Vibrating sample magnetometer (VSM) measurements were performed on Ag$_2$O/Fe$_3$O$_4$ (5%), Ag$_2$O/Fe$_3$O$_4$ (10%), and Ag$_2$O/Fe$_3$O$_4$ (15%) to determine the magnetic properties of the samples. Figure 8a–c show the results. As shown in Figure 8a, the magnetic properties of the Ag$_2$O/Fe$_3$O$_4$ binary nanocomposites gradually increase with the increase in Fe$_3$O$_4$ surface loading content. Ag$_2$O/Fe$_3$O$_4$ (15%) exhibited the strongest magnetism, with a maximum saturation magnetization of 1.01 emu/g and a hysteresis loop showing a clear bent shape without a saturation region. In contrast, Ag$_2$O/Fe$_3$O$_4$ (10%) and Ag$_2$O/Fe$_3$O$_4$ (5%) exhibited the maximum saturation magnetization of 0.31 emu/g and 0.15 emu/g, respectively. Figure 8b,c show the hysteresis loop characteristics of Ag$_2$O/Fe$_3$O$_4$ (5%) and Ag$_2$O/Fe$_3$O$_4$ (10%), respectively. It can be observed that although the size of the magnetic moment increases with the external magnetic field, its maximum value is much smaller than the saturation magnetization of ferromagnetic materials. Therefore, the hysteresis loop shows a curve similar to paramagnetism. Since the magnetic moment is very small, the hysteresis loop of Ag$_2$O/Fe$_3$O$_4$ nanocomposites is smoother and more symmetrical than that of paramagnetic materials. Therefore, due to the introduction of Fe$_3$O$_4$, it was confirmed that Ag$_2$O/Fe$_3$O$_4$ (5%), Ag$_2$O/Fe$_3$O$_4$ (10%), and Ag$_2$O/Fe$_3$O$_4$ (15%) all have superparamagnetic properties [39].

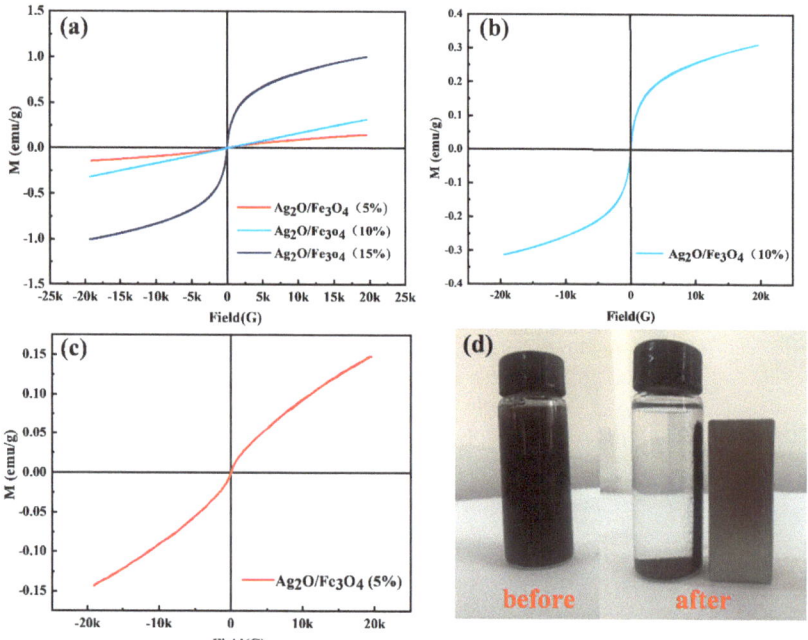

Figure 8. VSM curves of the (**a**) overall magnetic samples, (**b**) Ag$_2$O/Fe$_3$O$_4$ (5%) composite, (**c**) Ag$_2$O/Fe$_3$O$_4$ (10%) composite, and (**d**) test of Ag$_2$O/Fe$_3$O$_4$ (10%) composite under Nd magnet adsorption.

A neodymium magnet adsorption experiment was performed to verify whether Ag$_2$O/Fe$_3$O$_4$ (10%) can be magnetically recovered. Figure 8d shows the results. Specifically, a neodymium magnet was placed next to the Ag$_2$O/Fe$_3$O$_4$ (10%) suspension and was allowed to stand still for 20 min. It was observed that the neodymium magnet clearly adsorbed the gray-brown catalyst powder. Therefore, it was confirmed that magnetic adsorption can recover Ag$_2$O/Fe$_3$O$_4$ (10%).

2.9. Photocatalytic Reaction Mechanism Analysis

First, under visible light irradiation, Ag$_2$O and Fe$_3$O$_4$ on the surface of Ag$_2$O/Fe$_3$O$_4$ are excited from the valence band to the conduction band, generating photogenerated electrons (e$^-$) and leaving behind holes (h$^+$). As the E_{CB} of Ag$_2$O is -0.67 eV, which is more negative than that of Fe$_3$O$_4$, i.e., 0.54 eV, and the E_{VB} of Ag$_2$O is 2.03 eV, which is more negative than that of Fe$_3$O$_4$, i.e., 2.14 eV, a type-II heterojunction is formed due to the band offset when the two are coupled. The h$^+$ on the Fe$_3$O$_4$ valence band transfers to the Ag$_2$O valence band, and the e$^-$ on the Ag$_2$O conduction band transfers to the Fe$_3$O$_4$ conduction band, thus improving the separation efficiency of the photogenerated electrons and holes. These electrons and holes then participate in other reactions. The e$^-$ on the Fe$_3$O$_4$ conduction band reacts with the dissolved oxygen and water in the liquid to form H$_2$O$_2$ and OH$^-$. H$_2$O$_2$ can then further participate in the Fenton reaction, while the h$^+$ on the Ag$_2$O valence band reacts with H$_2$O to generate ·OH free radicals and H$^+$.

Second, the Fenton reaction occurs on Fe$_3$O$_4$. Fe^{2+} in Fe$_3$O$_4$, H$_2$O$_2$ generated in the photocatalytic reaction, and dissolved O$_2$ in water react to generate Fe^{3+}, ·O$_2^-$, and ·OH, respectively. Next, H$_2$O$_2$ can reduce Fe^{3+} to replenish the consumed Fe^{2+} and O$_2$ and generate H$^+$, so the reaction can be cycled. The large amounts of ·OH, and ·O$_2^-$

generated by the combined photocatalytic and Fenton reactions can further participate in the oxidation and degradation of organic compounds, decomposing them into smaller harmless compounds, as shown in Figure 9. The specific reaction process is as follows:

$$Ag_2O/Fe_3O_4 + h\nu \rightarrow e^- + h^+ \quad (5)$$

$$h^+ + H_2O \rightarrow \cdot OH + H^+ \quad (6)$$

$$2e^- + O_2 + 2H_2O \rightarrow H_2O_2 + 2OH^- \quad (7)$$

$$\cdot O_2 + MO \rightarrow \text{Degraded products} \quad (8)$$

$$H_2O_2 + 2Fe^{3+} \rightarrow 2Fe^{2+} + O_2 + 2H^+ \quad (9)$$

$$\cdot O_2 + MO \rightarrow \text{Degraded products} \quad (10)$$

$$\cdot OH + MO \rightarrow \text{Degraded products} \quad (11)$$

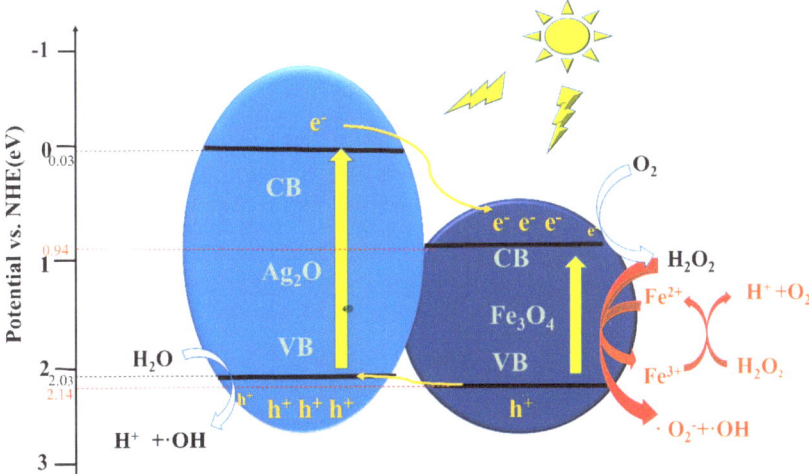

Figure 9. Schematic of the possible photocatalytic reaction mechanism of Ag_2O/Fe_3O_4 under visible light irradiation.

3. Materials and Methods

3.1. Material

Silver nitrate ($AgNO_3$, 99%) was purchased from National Pharmaceutical Group Co., Ltd. (Shanghai, China). Iron(II) chloride tetrahydrate ($FeCl_2 \cdot 4H_2O$, ≥92.0%), Iron(III) chloride hexahydrate ($FeCl_3 \cdot 6H_2O$, ≥98.1%), sodium hydroxide (NaOH, ≥96.0%), and methyl orange (MO) were purchased from Xilong Science Co., Ltd. (Guangdong, China). All the raw materials were of analytical grade and used without any additional purification. Deionized water was used for all the experiments.

3.2. Preparation of Fe_3O_4

Approximately 0.198 g of $FeCl_3 \cdot 6H_2O$ and 0.072 g of $FeCl_2 \cdot 4H_2O$ were dissolved in 200 mL of deionized water by ultrasonication for 30 min. Approximately 20 mL of NaOH solution (1 M) was then added. The mixture was sonicated for 1 h, centrifuged, washed three times with deionized water, and then freeze-dried to obtain Fe_3O_4.

3.3. Preparation of Ag_2O

Approximately 0.5 g of $AgNO_3$ was dissolved in 200 mL of deionized water, and 20 mL of NaOH solution (1 M) was then added. The mixture was sonicated for 1 h, centrifuged, washed three times with deionized water, and then freeze-dried to obtain Ag_2O.

3.4. Preparation of Ag_2O/Fe_3O_4

The Ag_2O/Fe_3O_4 catalyst was prepared using a one-step coprecipitation method. First, 0.5 g of $AgNO_3$ was dissolved ultrasonically in 200 mL of deionized water, and 0.041, 0.088, and 0.119 g of $FeCl_3 \cdot 6H_2O$ were dissolved with 0.015, 0.032, and 0.044 g of $FeCl_2 \cdot 4H_2O$, respectively, in 200 mL of deionized water as different precursors of Fe_3O_4. The precursor of the Ag_2O solution was then added into the Fe_3O_4 precursor solutions and treated ultrasonically for 1 h. Next, a 1 M NaOH solution was continuously dripped into the quickly stirred precursor solution until no further color change was observed. Finally, the product was washed three times by centrifugation, freeze-dried, and obtained as Ag_2O/Fe_3O_4 (5%, 10%, 15%) binary photocatalysts.

3.5. Characterization

The samples were subjected to various analytical techniques to investigate their morphologies, chemical environments, structures, microstructures, surface composition, optical features, bandgap, and magnetic performance. Specifically, scanning electron microscopy (SEM, TESCAN, MIRA) equipped with an electron-dispersive spectroscopy (EDS) detector was used to observe the morphologies and chemical environments, while X-ray diffraction (XRD, MiniFlex-600, Rigaku, Tokyo, Japan) and high-resolution transmission electron microscopy (HRTEM, JEM-2100F, JEOL) were used to analyze the structures and microstructures, respectively. X-ray photoelectronic spectroscopy (XPS, ESCALAB-250XI, Thermo Fisher, Waltham, MA, USA) was used to study the surface composition. A photoluminescence spectroscopy (PL, Cary Eclipse, Varian, Cheadle, UK) and UV–vis spectrometer (UV, PerkinElmer (Houston, TX, USA), Lambda 950) were used to analyze the optical features and bandgap, respectively. A vibrating sample magnetometer (VSM, Lake Shore (Westerville, OH, USA), 7404) was used to evaluate the magnetic performance.

3.6. Photocatalytic Measurement

The photocatalytic performance test was conducted under a xenon lamp source (PLS-SXE300) with a power of 300 W for the degradation of MO (10 mg/L) by Ag_2O/Fe_3O_4. In the experiment, 100 mg of Ag_2O/Fe_3O_4 was dispersed in 100 mL MO solution. After mixing, the mixture was stirred in the dark for 30 min to allow the catalyst to reach adsorption–desorption equilibrium with MO. The mixture containing the photocatalyst was then placed 10 cm away from the xenon lamp source and stirred at a speed of 200 r/min. During the light irradiation, 3 mL of the solution was taken out every 5 min and transferred to a centrifuge tube, and the catalyst powder was removed using a needle filter with a 0.22 µm pore size. A UV–visible spectrophotometer was used to measure the filtered MO concentration. The degradation rate of MO can be expressed as (C0-C)/C0, where C represents the MO concentration after xenon lamp irradiation, C0 represents the original concentration before irradiation, and the concentration of undegraded MO can be expressed as C/C0.

3.7. Photoelectrochemical Measurement

The experiment was conducted using an electrochemical analyzer (CHI660E, Shanghai) equipped with a standard three-electrode system. A 100 mL Na_2SO_4 solution (0.1 M) was used as the electrolyte, with a platinum (Pt) foil as the counter electrode, Ag/AgCl as the reference electrode, and the loading samples on FTO glass as working electrodes.

Electrochemical impedance spectroscopy (EIS), a Mott–Schottky curve, and photocurrent response tests were performed.

4. Conclusions

In summary, a novel type of environmentally friendly magnetic nanocomposite, i.e., Ag_2O/Fe_3O_4, has been synthesized and characterized as a high-performance visible-light-responsive photocatalyst. According to the XRD, SEM, TEM, XPS, UV–vis, PL, and electrochemical characterization, it has been confirmed that Ag_2O and Fe_3O_4 are well compounded and exhibit a good synergistic effect. Loading Fe_3O_4 onto the surface of Ag_2O not only constructs the type II heterojunction but also successfully couples the photocatalysis and Fenton reaction, enhancing its broad-spectrum response and efficiency. Under simulated sunlight irradiation, the Ag_2O/Fe_3O_4 (10%) exhibited the fastest MO degradation rate, rapidly degrading 99.5% of 10 mg/L MO within 15 min, which was 2.4 times higher than that of pure Ag_2O. Furthermore, after four cycles of testing, the sample still exhibited a fast degradation rate, indicating high stability. Magnetic testing emphasized the ease of material recovery using magnetic force, making the nanocomposite suitable for practical applications in water treatment and environmental remediation. Therefore, Ag_2O/Fe_3O_4 exhibits magnetic properties, wide spectral response, and high oxidative degradation performance, and its preparation method provides a new approach for the development of future photocatalysts.

Author Contributions: Conceptualization, J.W., G.H. and T.T.; Methodology, Z.S. and Z.L.; Software, R.X.; Formal analysis, Z.F.; Investigation, L.J.; Writing—original draft, C.S.; Supervision, M.L. All authors have read and agreed to the published version of the manuscript.

Funding: This work was financially supported by the National Natural Science Foundation of China (12164013), the Natural Science Foundation of Guangxi Province (2020GXNSFBA297125), the Science and Technology Base and Talent Special Project of Guangxi Province (AD21220029), Research Foundation of Guilin University of Technology (GUTQDJJ2019011), and innovation Project of Guangxi Graduate Education (YCSW2022331).

Institutional Review Board Statement: Not applicable.

Informed Consent Statement: Not applicable.

Data Availability Statement: The data can be made available upon reasonable request.

Conflicts of Interest: The authors declare no conflict of interest.

Sample Availability: Not applicable.

References

1. Nuengmatcha, P.; Chanthai, S.; Mahachai, R.; Oh, W.-C. Sonocatalytic performance of ZnO/graphene/TiO$_2$ nanocomposite for degradation of dye pollutants (methylene blue, texbrite BAC-L, texbrite BBU-L and texbrite NFW-L) under ultrasonic irradiation. *Dye. Pigment.* **2016**, *134*, 487–497. [CrossRef]
2. Portillo-Vélez, N.S.; Hernández-Gordillo, A.; Bizarro, M. Morphological effect of ZnO nanoflakes and nanobars on the photocatalytic dye degradation. *Catal. Today* **2017**, *287*, 106–112. [CrossRef]
3. Vijayan, P.; Mahendiran, C.; Suresh, C.; Shanthi, K. Photocatalytic activity of iron doped nanocrystalline titania for the oxidative degradation of 2, 4, 6-trichlorophenol. *Catal. Today* **2009**, *141*, 220–224. [CrossRef]
4. Wen, X.-J.; Shen, C.-H.; Fei, Z.-H.; Fang, D.; Liu, Z.-T.; Dai, J.-T.; Niu, C.-G. Recent developments on AgI based heterojunction photocatalytic systems in photocatalytic application. *Chem. Eng. J.* **2020**, *383*, 123083. [CrossRef]
5. Liu, B.; Zhao, X.; Terashima, C.; Fujishima, A.; Nakata, K. Thermodynamic and kinetic analysis of heterogeneous photocatalysis for semiconductor systems. *Phys. Chem. Chem. Phys.* **2014**, *16*, 8751–8760. [CrossRef]
6. Zhang, Y.; Zhang, W. Research progress on the photocatalysis of TiO$_2$ under visible light. *Rare Met. Mater. Eng.* **2007**, *36*, 1299–1303.
7. Liu, L.; Zhang, X.; Yang, L.; Ren, L.; Wang, D.; Ye, J. Metal nanoparticles induced photocatalysis. *Nat. Sci. Rev.* **2017**, *4*, 761–780. [CrossRef]
8. Long, Z.; Li, Q.; Wei, T.; Zhang, G.; Ren, Z. Historical development and prospects of photocatalysts for pollutant removal in water. *J. Hazard. Mater.* **2020**, *395*, 122599. [CrossRef]

9. Chen, F.; Ren, Z.; Gong, S.; Li, X.; Shen, G.; Han, G. Selective Deposition of Silver Oxide on Single-Domain Ferroelectric Nanoplates and Their Efficient Visible-Light Photoactivity. *Chem. Eur. J.* **2016**, *22*, 12160–12165. [CrossRef]
10. Torabi, S.; Mansoorkhani, M.J.K.; Majedi, A.; Motevalli, S. Synthesis, medical and photocatalyst applications of nano-Ag$_2$O. *J. Coord. Chem.* **2020**, *73*, 1861–1880. [CrossRef]
11. Khattak, R.; Begum, B.; Qazi, R.A.; Gul, H.; Khan, M.S.; Khan, S.; Bibi, N.; Han, C.; Rahman, N.U. Green Synthesis of Silver Oxide Microparticles Using Green Tea Leaves Extract for an Efficient Removal of Malachite Green from Water: Synergistic Effect of Persulfate. *Catalysts* **2023**, *13*, 227.
12. Yu, K.; Yang, S.; Liu, C.; Chen, H.; Li, H.; Sun, C.; Boyd, S.A. Degradation of organic dyes via bismuth silver oxide initiated direct oxidation coupled with sodium bismuthate based visible light photocatalysis. *Environ. Sci. Technol.* **2012**, *46*, 7318–7326. [CrossRef]
13. Liu, G.; Wang, G.; Hu, Z.; Su, Y.; Zhao, L. Ag$_2$O nanoparticles decorated TiO$_2$ nanofibers as a pn heterojunction for enhanced photocatalytic decomposition of RhB under visible light irradiation. *Appl. Surf. Sci.* **2019**, *465*, 902–910. [CrossRef]
14. Wang, X.; Li, S.; Yu, H.; Yu, J.; Liu, S. Ag$_2$O as a new visible-light photocatalyst: Self-stability and high photocatalytic activity. *Chem. Eur. J.* **2011**, *17*, 7777–7780. [CrossRef] [PubMed]
15. Yang, H.; Tian, J.; Li, T.; Cui, H. Synthesis of novel Ag/Ag$_2$O heterostructures with solar full spectrum (UV, visible and near-infrared) light-driven photocatalytic activity and enhanced photoelectrochemical performance. *Catal. Commun.* **2016**, *87*, 82–85. [CrossRef]
16. Suo, J.; Jiao, K.; Fang, D.; Bu, H.; Liu, Y.; Li, F.; Ruzimuradov, O. Visible photocatalytic properties of Ag–Ag$_2$O/ITO NWs fabricated by mechanical injection-discharge-oxidation method. *Vacuum* **2022**, *204*, 111338. [CrossRef]
17. Nordin, A.H.; Ahmad, Z.; Husna, S.M.N.; Ilyas, R.A.; Azemi, A.K.; Ismail, N.; Nordin, M.L.; Ngadi, N.; Siti, N.H.; Nabgan, W. The State of the Art of Natural Polymer Functionalized Fe$_3$O$_4$ Magnetic Nanoparticle Composites for Drug Delivery Applications: A Review. *Gels* **2023**, *9*, 121. [CrossRef]
18. Zhao, S.; Yu, X.; Qian, Y.; Chen, W.; Shen, J. Multifunctional magnetic iron oxide nanoparticles: An advanced platform for cancer theranostics. *Theranostics* **2020**, *10*, 6278. [CrossRef]
19. Wu, W.; Jiang, C.Z.; Roy, V.A. Designed synthesis and surface engineering strategies of magnetic iron oxide nanoparticles for biomedical applications. *Nanoscale* **2016**, *8*, 19421–19474. [CrossRef]
20. Yu, S.; Tang, Y.; Yan, M.; Aguilar, Z.P.; Lai, W.; Xu, H. A fluorescent cascade amplification method for sensitive detection of Salmonella based on magnetic Fe$_3$O$_4$ nanoparticles and hybridization chain reaction. *Sens. Actuators B Chem.* **2019**, *279*, 31–37. [CrossRef]
21. Hudson, R.; Feng, Y.; Varma, R.S.; Moores, A. Bare magnetic nanoparticles: Sustainable synthesis and applications in catalytic organic transformations. *Green Chem.* **2014**, *16*, 4493–4505. [CrossRef]
22. Serga, V.; Burve, R.; Maiorov, M.; Krumina, A.; Skaudžius, R.; Zarkov, A.; Kareiva, A.; Popov, A.I. Impact of gadolinium on the structure and magnetic properties of nanocrystalline powders of iron oxides produced by the extraction-pyrolytic method. *Materials* **2020**, *13*, 4147. [CrossRef] [PubMed]
23. Lee, D.-E.; Devthade, V.; Moru, S.; Jo, W.-K.; Tonda, S. Magnetically sensitive TiO$_2$ hollow sphere/Fe$_3$O$_4$ core-shell hybrid catalyst for high-performance sunlight-assisted photocatalytic degradation of aqueous antibiotic pollutants. *J. Alloys Compd.* **2022**, *902*, 163612. [CrossRef]
24. Wang, C.; Jiang, R.; Yang, J.; Wang, P. Corrigendum: Enhanced Heterogeneous Fenton Degradation of Organic Pollutants by CRC/Fe3O4 Catalyst at Neutral pH. *Front. Chem.* **2022**, *10*, 892424. [CrossRef]
25. Liu, Y.; Sun, C.; Chen, L.; Yang, H.; Ming, Z.; Bai, Y.; Feng, S.; Yang, S.-T. Decoloration of methylene blue by heterogeneous Fenton-like oxidation on Fe$_3$O$_4$/SiO$_2$/C nanospheres in neutral environment. *Mat. Chem. Phys.* **2018**, *213*, 231–238. [CrossRef]
26. Cleveland, V.; Bingham, J.-P.; Kan, E. Heterogeneous Fenton degradation of bisphenol A by carbon nanotube-supported Fe$_3$O$_4$. *Sep. Purif. Technol.* **2014**, *133*, 388–395. [CrossRef]
27. Jiao, Y.; Wan, C.; Bao, W.; Gao, H.; Liang, D.; Li, J. Facile hydrothermal synthesis of Fe$_3$O$_4$@ cellulose aerogel nanocomposite and its application in Fenton-like degradation of Rhodamine B. *Carbohydr. Polym.* **2018**, *189*, 371–378. [CrossRef]
28. Zhang, L.; Li, P.; Mi, W.; Jiang, E.; Bai, H. Positive and negative magnetoresistance in Fe$_3$O$_4$-based heterostructures. *J. Magn. Magn. Mater.* **2012**, *324*, 3731–3736. [CrossRef]
29. Takahashi, H.; Soeya, S.; Hayakawa, J.; Ito, K.; Kida, A.; Asano, H.; Matsui, M. Half-metallic Fe$_3$O$_4$ films for high-sensitivity magnetoresistive devices. *IEEE Trans. Magn.* **2004**, *40*, 313–318. [CrossRef]
30. Choi, J.; Han, S.; Kim, H.; Sohn, E.-H.; Choi, H.J.; Seo, Y. Suspensions of hollow polydivinylbenzene nanoparticles decorated with Fe$_3$O$_4$ nanoparticles as magnetorheological fluids for microfluidics applications. *ACS Appl. Nano Mater.* **2019**, *2*, 6939–6947. [CrossRef]
31. Liu, J.; Liu, G.; Yuan, C.; Chen, L.; Tian, X.; Fang, M. Fe$_3$O$_4$/ZnFe$_2$O$_4$ micro/nanostructures and their heterogeneous efficient Fenton-like visible-light photocatalysis process. *N. J. Chem.* **2018**, *42*, 3736–3747. [CrossRef]
32. Kucukcongar, S.; Alwindawi, A.G.J.; Turkyilmaz, M.; Ozaytekin, I. Reactive Dye Removal by Photocatalysis and Sonophotocatalysis Processes Using Ag/TiO$_2$/Fe$_3$O$_4$ Nanocomposite. *Water Air Soil Pollut.* **2023**, *234*, 103. [CrossRef]
33. Banić, N.; Šojić Merkulov, D.; Despotović, V.; Finčur, N.; Ivetić, T.; Bognár, S.; Jovanović, D.; Abramović, B. Rapid Removal of Organic Pollutants from Aqueous Systems under Solar Irradiation Using ZrO$_2$/Fe$_3$O$_4$ Nanoparticles. *Molecules* **2022**, *27*, 8060. [CrossRef]

34. Tseng, W.J.; Chuang, Y.-C.; Chen, Y.-A. Mesoporous Fe_3O_4@Ag@TiO_2 nanocomposite particles for magnetically recyclable photocatalysis and bactericide. *Adv. Powder Technol.* **2018**, *29*, 664–671. [CrossRef]
35. Cai, A.; Sun, Y.; Du, L.; Wang, X. Hierarchical Ag_2O–ZnO–Fe_3O_4 composites with enhanced visible-light photocatalytic activity. *J. Alloys Compd.* **2015**, *644*, 334–340. [CrossRef]
36. Atta, A.M.; El-Faham, A.; Al-Lohedan, H.A.; Othman, Z.A.A.; Abdullah, M.M.; Ezzat, A.O. Modified triazine decorated with Fe_3O_4 and Ag/Ag_2O nanoparticles for self-healing of steel epoxy coatings in seawater. *Prog. Org. Coat.* **2018**, *121*, 247–262. [CrossRef]
37. Tong, Y.; Liu, W.; Li, C.; Liu, X.; Liu, J.; Zhang, X. A metal/semiconductor contact induced Mott–Schottky junction for enhancing the electrocatalytic activity of water-splitting catalysts. *Sustain. Energy Fuels* **2023**, *7*, 12–30. [CrossRef]
38. Guo, Z.; Wu, H.; Li, M.; Tang, T.; Wen, J.; Li, X. Phosphorus-doped graphene quantum dots loaded on TiO_2 for enhanced photodegradation. *Appl. Surf. Sci.* **2020**, *526*, 146724. [CrossRef]
39. Kumar, A.P.; Bilehal, D.; Desalegn, T.; Kumar, S.; Ahmed, F.; Murthy, H.A.; Kumar, D.; Gupta, G.; Chellappan, D.K.; Singh, S.K. Studies on synthesis and characterization of Fe_3O_4@SiO_2@Ru hybrid magnetic composites for reusable photocatalytic application. *Adsorpt. Sci. Technol.* **2022**, *2022*, 1–18. [CrossRef]

Disclaimer/Publisher's Note: The statements, opinions and data contained in all publications are solely those of the individual author(s) and contributor(s) and not of MDPI and/or the editor(s). MDPI and/or the editor(s) disclaim responsibility for any injury to people or property resulting from any ideas, methods, instructions or products referred to in the content.

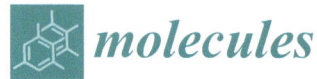

Article

Boosted Photocatalytic Performance for Antibiotics Removal with Ag/PW$_{12}$/TiO$_2$ Composite: Degradation Pathways and Toxicity Assessment

Hongfei Shi [1,*], Haoshen Wang [1], Enji Zhang [1], Xiaoshu Qu [1], Jianping Li [1,*], Sisi Zhao [2], Huajing Gao [1] and Zhe Chen [1]

[1] Institute of Petrochemical Technology, Jilin Institute of Chemical Technology, Jilin City 132022, China; 18638813901@163.com (H.W.); 13664448948@163.com (E.Z.); xiaoshuqu@jlict.edu.cn (X.Q.); huajing_gao@163.com (H.G.); chenzhecz999@163.com (Z.C.)
[2] Institute of Catalysis for Energy and Environment, College of Chemistry & Chemical Engineering, Shenyang Normal University, Shenyang 110034, China; zhaoss0905@163.com
* Correspondence: shihf813@nenu.edu.cn (H.S.); lijp156@nenu.edu.cn (J.L.)

Citation: Shi, H.; Wang, H.; Zhang, E.; Qu, X.; Li, J.; Zhao, S.; Gao, H.; Chen, Z. Boosted Photocatalytic Performance for Antibiotics Removal with Ag/PW$_{12}$/TiO$_2$ Composite: Degradation Pathways and Toxicity Assessment. *Molecules* 2023, 28, 6831. https://doi.org/10.3390/molecules28196831

Academic Editor: Sugang Meng

Received: 7 September 2023
Revised: 22 September 2023
Accepted: 25 September 2023
Published: 27 September 2023

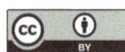

Copyright: © 2023 by the authors. Licensee MDPI, Basel, Switzerland. This article is an open access article distributed under the terms and conditions of the Creative Commons Attribution (CC BY) license (https://creativecommons.org/licenses/by/4.0/).

Abstract: Photocatalyst is the core of photocatalysis and directly determines photocatalytic performance. However, low quantum efficiency and low utilization of solar energy are important technical problems in the application of photocatalysis. In this work, a series of polyoxometalates (POMs) [H$_3$PW$_{12}$O$_{40}$] (PW$_{12}$)-doped titanium dioxide (TiO$_2$) nanofibers modified with various amount of silver (Ag) nanoparticles (NPs) were prepared by utilizing electrospinning/photoreduction strategy, and were labelled as x wt% Ag/PW$_{12}$/TiO$_2$ (abbr. x% Ag/PT, x = 5, 10, and 15, respectively). The as-prepared materials were characterized with a series of techniques and exhibited remarkable catalytic activities for visible-light degradation tetracycline (TC), enrofloxacin (ENR), and methyl orange (MO). Particularly, the 10% Ag/PT catalyst with a specific surface area of 155.09 m^2/g and an average aperture of 4.61 nm possessed the optimal photodegradation performance, with efficiencies reaching 78.19% for TC, 93.65% for ENR, and 99.29% for MO, which were significantly higher than those of PW$_{12}$-free Ag/TiO$_2$ and PT nanofibers. Additionally, various parameters (the pH of the solution, catalyst usage, and TC concentration) influencing the degradation process were investigated in detail. The optimal conditions are as follows: catalyst usage: 20 mg; TC: 20 mL of 20 ppm; pH = 7. Furthermore, the photodegradation intermediates and pathways were demonstrated by HPLC-MS measurement. We also investigated the toxicity of products generated during TC removal by employing quantitative structure-activity relationship (QSAR) prediction through a toxicity estimation software tool (T.E.S.T. Version 5.1.2.). The mechanism study showed that the doping of PW$_{12}$ and the modification of Ag NPs on TiO$_2$ broadened the visible-light absorption, accelerating the effective separation of photogenerated carriers, therefore resulting in an enhanced photocatalytic performance. The research provided some new thoughts for exploiting efficient and durable photocatalysts for environmental remediation.

Keywords: Ag nanoparticles; PW$_{12}$/TiO$_2$ nanofibers; degradation of antibiotics; degradation pathways; toxicity assessment

1. Introduction

In recent years, photocatalysis technology, which can use solar energy for environmental purification and energy conversion, has received worldwide attention [1,2]. Photocatalytic technology has a wide range of applications in pollutants degradation, CO$_2$ reduction, water splitting to produce hydrogen and nitrogen fixation, etc. [3]. The core of photocatalysis is designing and developing the photocatalysts with visible-light response, prominent catalytic activity, and recyclability. Among the various photocatalysts, TiO$_2$ has received a lot of attention due to its low synthesis cost, lack of toxicity, and high catalytic activity [4]. However, the wide band gap and low utilization efficiency of carriers limit its practical applications [5]. Therefore, it is urgent to enhance the visible-light absorption and the driving force for the separation of photoinduced carriers. Many strategies have been made to improve its catalytic activity, including dye sensitization [6], construction of heterojunction [7], morphology engineering [8], and metal/non-metal element doping, etc. [9].

POMs are identified as a promising candidate to embellish TiO_2 for addressing this challenge. POMs demonstrate semiconductor-like characteristics with their tunable electronic structures and energy levels. They also possess high negative charge and excellent solubility and are endowed with favorable processing properties [10,11]. Therefore, POMs are easily encapsulated or dispersed within various semiconductors, which can constantly enhance the redox property, modulate the band gap structure, and facilitate the separation efficiency of photoproduced carriers [12–14]. Among various POMs, $H_3PW_{12}O_{40}$ (abbr. PW_{12}), as a Keggin-type POM, has demonstrated important applications in photocatalysis fields such as water splitting and contaminants removal [15,16].

Besides, the strategy of noble metals (such as Ag, Pd, Pt, and Au) modifying semiconductors has been extensively investigated to expand spectral absorption and accelerate the separation of photon-generated carriers [17–19]. Typically, a Schottky junction is formed at the interface between a metal and a semiconductor to create a built-in electric region that enhances the surface plasmon resonance (SPR) effect. Among these noble metals, Ag has been extensively applied in SPR photocatalysis due to the excellent electrical conductivity, relatively cheap price, wide SPR absorption, and intense local electromagnetic fields caused by SPR [20,21]. For instance, Ag@TiO_2 composites with core-shell nanostructures were prepared, applying the one-step solvothermal method by Zeng et al., which displayed enhanced light absorption range and enabled the effective separation of e^--h^+ pairs, resulting in an improved photocatalytic performance [22]. Moreover, the electrostatic spinning technology has been considered as a versatile technology capable of adjusting the composition, diameter, and orientation of materials according to the intended function and application [23], which is employed extensively in the fabrication of metal oxides (TiO_2, ZnO, Fe_2O_3, WO_3, etc.) nanofibers for photocatalytic degradation of pollutants [24], hydrogen production [25], and CO_2 reduction [26], etc.

Based on the above considerations, we prepared a novel Ag/PW_{12}/TiO_2 (abbr. Ag/PT) composite by electrospinning/photoreduction methods, according to the literature [11,19]. Firstly, the electrospinning/calcination method was used to obtain PW_{12}/TiO_2 material; then, the Ag NPs were loaded on PW_{12}/TiO_2 using the photoreduction method, obtaining the Ag/PT composite. Moreover, these as-prepared Ag/PT nanofibers exhibited remarkable photocatalytic activities for the degradation of multiple pollutants. The 10% Ag/PT catalyst possessed the optimal photodegradation performance, whose efficiency reached 78.19% for TC, 93.65% for ENR, and 99.29% for MO, which was significantly higher than those of PW_{12}-free Ag/TiO_2 and PT. Furthermore, the influence parameters, including the pH of the solution, catalyst usage, and the concentration of TC, were studied in detail. The degradation intermediates and pathways were revealed by LC-MS data. QSAR prediction was employed to investigate the toxicity of products in TC photodegradation. Ultimately, the photocatalytic mechanism was investigated with radical capture analysis and band gap structures.

2. Results and Discussion

2.1. Characterization of Ag/PT Composites

The microstructure and morphology of PT nanofibers are presented in Figure 1a. The surface of the nanofibers after calcination at 550 °C is relatively rough and porous, and the fiber diameter is about 80 ± 20 nm. Figure 1b,c show the SEM and TEM images for 10% Ag/PT, respectively. Distinctly, these Ag NPs are equally deposited on the surface of PT with an average diameter of 10 ± 5 nm. The HRTEM images of 10% Ag/PT verify the latticed coexistence of TiO_2 and Ag in these samples (Figure 1d). The observed lattice spacing of 0.233 nm corresponds to the (112) crystal plane of the anatase phase TiO_2 (JCPDS no. 21-1272), and the lattice spacing of 0.145 nm corresponds to the Ag (220) plane (JCPDS no. 04-0783). As shown in Figure 1e–j, the elemental mapping images of 10% Ag/PT and the EDS data (Figure S1) further indicated the uniform distribution of Ag, P, W, Ti, and O elements in the sample.

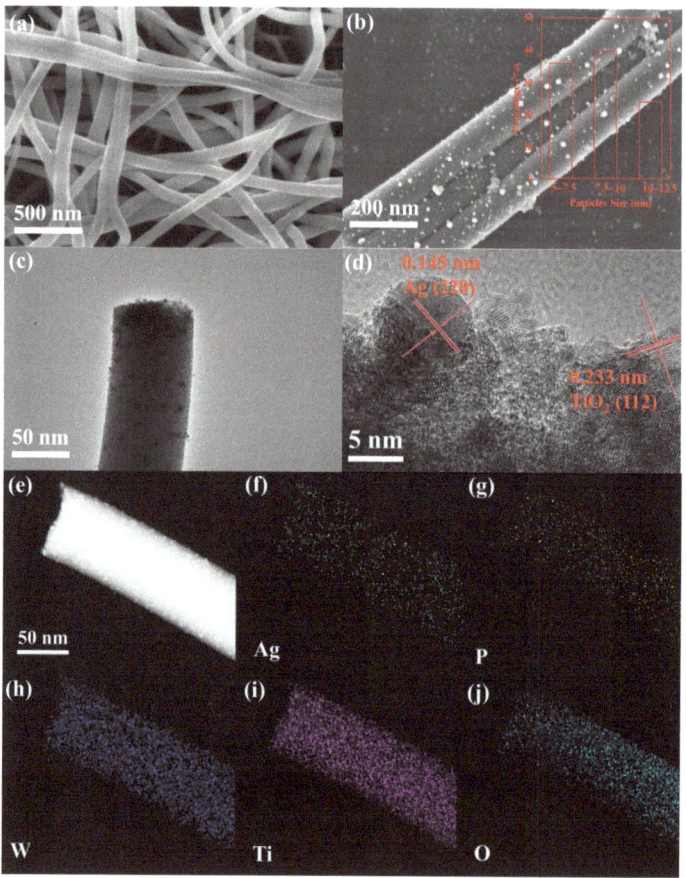

Figure 1. SEM images of PT (**a**) and 10% Ag/PT (**b**); TEM (**c**) and HRTEM (**d**) images of 10% Ag/PT; (**e–j**) Elemental mapping images of 10% Ag/PT sample: (**f**) Ag; (**g**) P; (**h**) W; (**i**) Ti; (**j**) O.

The phase composition and purity of the prepared catalysts were investigated with XRD (Figure 2a). For TiO_2, these characteristic diffraction peaks at 25.3°, 36.9°, 37.8°, 38.5°, 48.0°, 53.9°, 55.0°, and 62.7° are attributed to the (101), (103), (004), (112), (200), (105), (211), and (204) crystal plane of anatase phase TiO_2 (JCPDS no. 21-1272), respectively [27,28]. With the introduction of PW_{12} into TiO_2, no peaks of PW_{12} are found in the diffraction peaks of PT, demonstrating the doping of PW_{12} in TiO_2. When Ag NPs are deposited on PT, the main diffraction peaks of Ag/PT composite are similar to those of PT. Additionally, the main diffraction peak at 38.1°, belonging to Ag (111) phase (JCPDS no. 04-0783), is not obviously found, which might be attributed to the cover effect with diffraction peak of PT [29]. The obtained results certify the presence of PT and Ag NPs in these Ag/PT composites.

Figure 2b displays the FT-IR spectra of various samples. TiO_2 has no obvious characteristic vibration peak, and the PW_{12} exhibits four characteristic infrared absorption peaks in 700~1100 cm^{-1}, including the peaks at 1075, 975, 882, and 830 cm^{-1}, respectively. Concretely, the peak at 1075 cm^{-1} is caused by the vibration of the P-O bond, the peak at 975 cm^{-1} is assigned to the vibration of the W=O bond, and the two peaks at

882 and 830 cm^{-1} are attributable to the vibration of the two kinds of W-O$_{c/e}$-W bridge bonds [30,31]. Besides, the peak of PW$_{12}$ near 1600 cm^{-1} may belong to the adsorbed H$_2$O molecules [32]. These peaks can be also observed in the PT and Ag/PT materials, indicating the integrity of the PW$_{12}$ Keggin unit in these composites. However, a shift in the vibrational frequencies (1060, 961, 868, and 815 cm^{-1}) is detected for Ag/PT, manifesting the presence of interaction between PT and Ag [19]. The aforementioned results certify that the Ag/PT materials have been fabricated successfully.

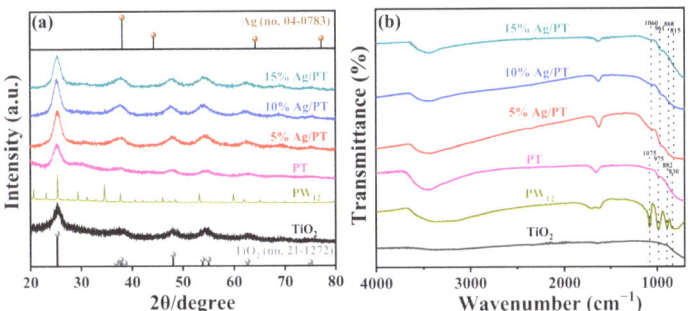

Figure 2. (**a**) XRD and (**b**) FT-IR of the constructed specimens.

A UV-Vis diffuse reflectance spectra (DRS) measurement was performed to evaluate the light absorption properties of the obtained specimens. According to Figure 3a, the light absorption edge of TiO$_2$, PW$_{12}$ catalysts appeared around 400 and 380 nm. For PT photocatalysts, the light absorption intensity was increased due to the adulteration of PW$_{12}$. In particular, the strongest optical absorption ability in the Ag/PT composites can be attributed to the introduction of Ag NPs [33], which would be beneficial to produce more photogenerated charge carriers to participate in the reaction [34]. We found that the SPR absorption band of Ag NPs ranges from 480 nm to 550 nm (Figure S2) [35]. Furthermore, as shown in Figure 3b, the band gaps of various catalysts were calculated by the following equation: $\alpha h\nu = A(h\nu - E_g)^{1/2}$, in which A, $h\nu$, and α represent the constant, photon energy, and absorption coefficient, respectively [36].

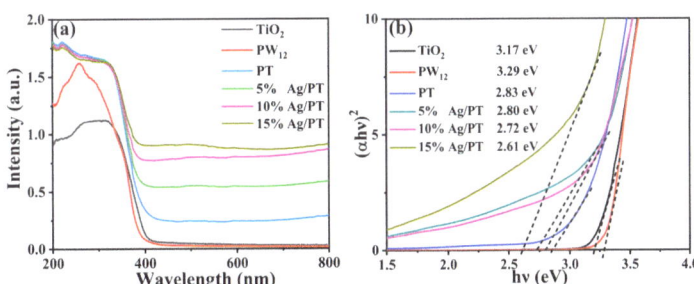

Figure 3. (**a**) UV-Vis absorption spectra and (**b**) the corresponding Tauc plots of obtained specimens.

The band gap values were 3.17, 3.29, 2.83, 2.80, 2.72, and 2.61 eV for TiO$_2$, PW$_{12}$, PT, and x% Ag/PT (x = 5, 10 and 15), respectively. The doping of H$_3$PW$_{12}$O$_{40}$ introduces additional electronic states and energy levels into the band structure of TiO$_2$. These additional electronic states can interact with the electron energy levels of TiO$_2$, leading to adjustments in the band structure, thereby reducing the band gap [11,27]. Obviously, in comparison with PT, the band gap of Ag/PT was reduced, which suggests that Ag might introduce a local energy level to the band gap of PT, resulting in a reduced energy gap [37].

The composition and chemical state information of as-prepared specimens were probed with X-ray photoelectron spectroscopy (XPS). The elemental composition of

10% Ag/PT was demonstrated by the signal detection of P, W, O, Ti, and Ag elements in the full XPS spectra (Figure 4a). Figure 4b–f shows the high resolution XPS profiles for Ag 3d, P 2p, W 4f, Ti 2p, and O 1s of PT and 10% Ag/PT, confirming the successful preparation of the composites. As presented in Figure 4b, the 10% Ag/PT composite showed two peaks at Ag 3d, located at 367.61 eV and 373.59 eV, belonging to Ag^0 $3d_{5/2}$ and Ag^0 $3d_{3/2}$ metallic silver monomers, respectively [38,39]. The P 2p XPS profile for PT (Figure 4c) has a peak at 133.70 eV, and this binding energy was considered to be the presence of P^{5+} [40]. The P 2p peak of 10% Ag/PT was shifted towards the lower binding energy region in comparison with PT. In the PT material, the high-resolution XPS spectrum of the W 4f region (Figure 4d) showed two peaks at 35.58 eV and 37.63 eV for the W $4f_{7/2}$ and W $4f_{5/2}$ binding energies, respectively, and, in 10% Ag/PT, W 4f was shifted toward the lower binding energy with binding energies of 35.28 eV and 37.32 eV [41,42]. Figure 4e shows the presence of Ti $2p_{3/2}$ and Ti $2p_{1/2}$ characteristic peaks observed at 458.49 eV and 464.16 eV in PT, which are features of Ti^{4+} in TiO_2 [43]. Notably, the binding energies of Ti 2p XPS for 10% Ag/PT were shifted to 458.45 eV and 464.13 eV, providing evidence of the interaction between PT and Ag [44]. Figure 4f shows the XPS spectra of O 1s. Two peaks, at 529.57 eV (PT) and 529.48 eV (10% Ag/PT), were found, which were considered as Ti-O [45]; meanwhile, two peaks are found at 531.21 eV and 532.12 eV (PT) and 531.11 eV and 532.01 eV (10% Ag/PT), corresponding to W-O and P-O, respectively [46]. Notably, these peaks in 10% Ag/PT composites shifted to lower binding energies compared to PT, which indicated the presence of interfacial interaction between Ag and PT [47].

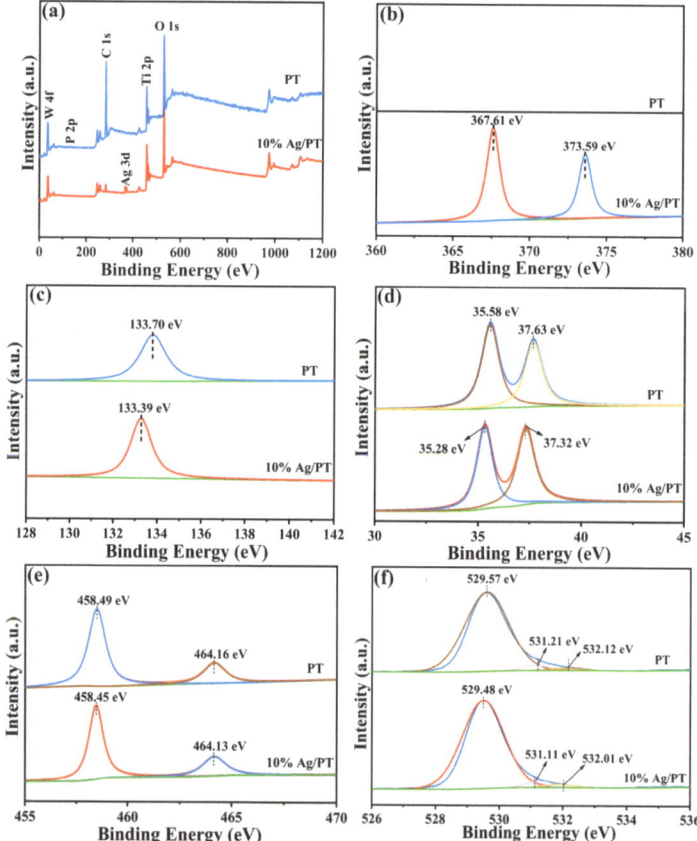

Figure 4. The XPS profiles: (**a**) full spectra; (**b**) Ag 3d; (**c**) P 2p; (**d**) W 4f; (**e**) Ti 2p; (**f**) O 1s.

Figure 5a demonstrates that the N_2 adsorption and desorption isotherms of different specimens conform to type IV, while the hysteresis line follows type H1, indicating the presence of a mesoporous structure [48,49]. The specific surface areas (SSA) were 30.39, 146.85, 156.42, 155.09, and 166.91 m^2/g for TiO_2, PT and x% Ag/PT (x = 5, 10 and 15), respectively. The result suggested that the introduce of PW_{12} is beneficial to enhance the SSA of TiO_2, which would demonstrate an improved catalytic performance. Figure 5b presents the pore size distributions of as-obtained samples. The average pore volumes were 11.57, 5.32, 4.25, 4.61, and 4.40 nm for TiO_2, PT, and x% Ag/PT (x = 5, 10 and 15), respectively. It is clear that the average pore volume of Ag/PT composites decreased, which might be due to the accumulation of Ag NPs on the PT surface.

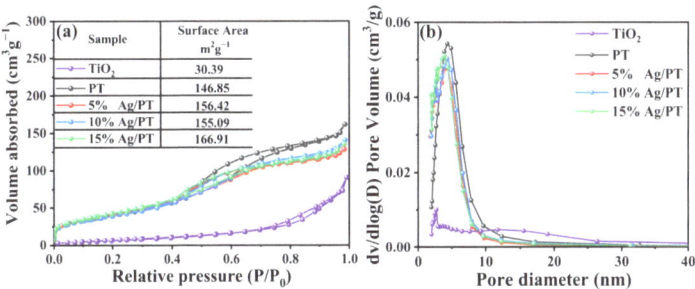

Figure 5. (a) N_2 adsorption-desorption isotherms and (b) pore size distributions of as-synthesized samples.

2.2. Catalytic Activity Assessment of Ag/PT Composites

2.2.1. Photocatalytic Removal of TC

TC was chosen as an organic pollutant to explore the photocatalytic capacity of obtained samples [50,51]. As presented in Figure 6a, the adsorption-desorption equilibrium was reached between the catalyst and TC under dark conditions within 20 min. The control experiment was designed and demonstrated that the self-photolysis process of TC can be excluded. TiO_2 exhibits a negative effect on the TC degradation. The degradation efficiencies of TC on PT and 10% Ag/TiO_2 were significantly higher compared to pure TiO_2, which reached 26.53% and 43.52% within 60 min, respectively. This indicates that the photocatalytic activity of TiO_2 can be improved with the proper introduction of $H_3PW_{12}O_{40}$ or Ag NPs. Moreover, the photocatalytic property of Ag/PT was further boosted, benefiting from the remarkable contribution of the SPR effect originating from the Ag NPs. The 10% Ag/PT composite shows the optimal degradation efficiency of 78.19% (Figure S3a), which exhibits better performance compared to numerous other catalysts, in terms of TC removal (Table S1). Besides, the removal of total organic carbon (TOC) for TC degradation reached 60.08% within 1 h using 10% Ag/PT material (Figure S4), which implies that the TC degradation was incomplete. Nevertheless, when more Ag was deposited on the PT, the TC removal rate of the synthesized 15% Ag/PT composite reduced to 71.12%. Because excessive Ag occupies a part of the active sites of PT, the adsorption capacity and degradation rate of Ag/PT composite towards TC molecules is reduced.

As presented in Figure 6b, the fitting results of the TC degradation rate indicate that it was in accordance with the first-order kinetic model. Distinguishingly, the reaction rate constant k for TC degradation with 10% Ag/PT was 0.0227 min^{-1}, which was about 29- and 8-times higher than those of TiO_2 and PT, respectively. Therefore, the doping of PW_{12} and the modification of Ag NPs are effective methods to boost the photocatalytic performance of TiO_2.

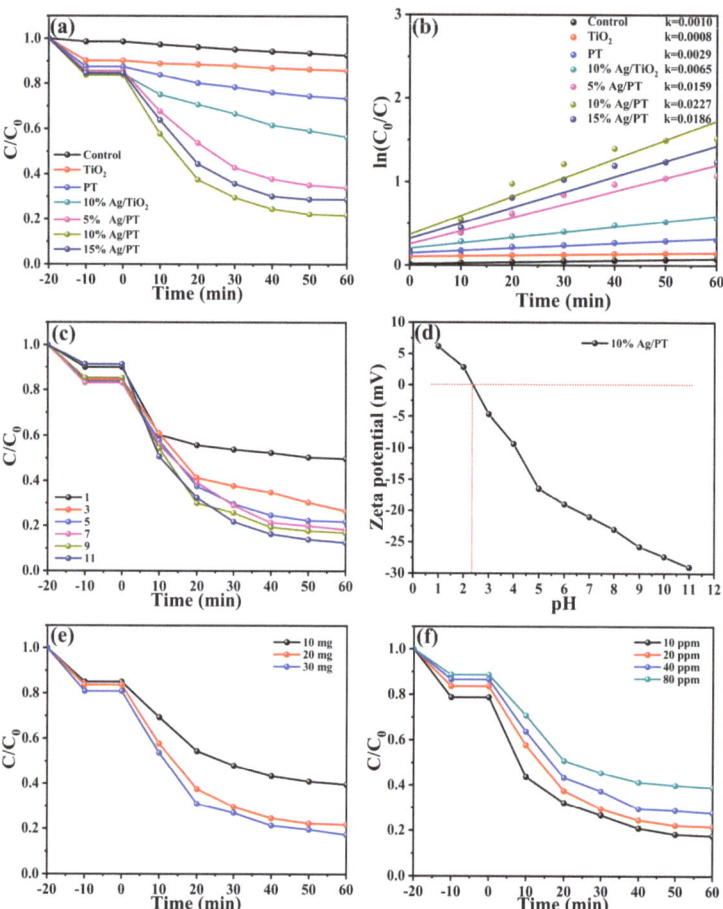

Figure 6. (**a**) The visible-light (λ > 420 nm) degradation of TC utilizing various specimens (catalyst usage: 20 mg; TC: 20 mL of 20 ppm; pH = 7); (**b**) The pseudo-first-order kinetic study for TC degradation; Degradation of TC with 10% Ag/PT with various conditions: (**c**) Different pH values (TC: 20 mL of 20 ppm; catalyst usage: 20 mg); (**d**) Zeta potential of 10% Ag/PT at different pH values; (**e**) Diverse catalyst amount (TC: 20 mL of 20 ppm; pH = 7); (**f**) Different concentration of TC (TC: 20 mL; pH = 7; catalyst amount: 20 mg). Light source: 300 W Xe light (CEL-HXF300, AULIGI IT).

Effect of different pH values: The degradation of TC in aqueous solution undergoes protonation and deprotonation reactions, and the pH of the solution will lead to different charge states, which affects the decomposition of TC. As shown in Figure 6c, the TC degradation efficiency gradually increased with the increase of pH, which achieved the optimal value of 87.42% at pH 11. The alkaline environment favors the generation of $\bullet O_2^-$, which is one kind of active species during the pollutant degradation process [52]. Besides, TC molecules exhibit a high susceptibility to photolysis in alkaline conditions, benefiting from the transition from the π to π* states of the (HOMO-1 to LUMO) chromophore [53]. At neutral pH, the TC removal rate was 78.19% after 60 min of light exposure. However, under acidic conditions, the degradation efficiency of TC further decreased. In Figure 6c, the adsorption removal efficiency of TC by 10% Ag/PT at different pH conditions were 10.04% (pH 1.0), 15.41% (pH 3.0), 16.28% (pH 5.0), 16.78% (pH 7.0), 14.61% (pH 9.0), and 8.67% (pH 11.0). This may be related to the zeta potential of the catalyst, which was examined for 10% Ag/PT at different pH conditions (Figure 6d). Obviously, the zeta potential of 10% Ag/PT was positive at pH < 2.4 and negative at pH > 2.4. Moreover, when pH < 3.3, TC appeared as a cation (TCH_3^+); when pH = 3.3~7.7, TC existed as an ampholyte (TCH_2^0); when pH was greater than 7.7, TC appeared as an anion (TCH_3^-) [54]. Therefore, when pH = 1.0, the surface of 10% Ag/PT was positively charged and the TC molecules were present in the protonated (TCH_3^+, pH < 3.3), which generated an intense electrostatic repulsion and weak adsorption ability. With the increase of pH from 3 to 7, the positive surface charge of 10% Ag/PT decreased from −4.64 mV to −21.07 mV, and the TC molecules were in neutral (TCH_2^0, pH 3.3–7.7), indicating that the electrostatic repulsion was suppressed, thus promoting the adsorption capacity. When the pH was 9.0 and 11.0, the electrostatic repulsion existed between the catalyst with a negative charge and TC (TCH_3^-, pH > 7.7). Furthermore, the excess OH^- could occupy the adsorption sites of the catalyst, generating a slight reduction of adsorption ability [55].

Influence of catalyst dosage: As shown in Figure 6e, the degradation efficiency was significantly enhanced from 60.35% to 78.19%, with the catalyst quantity from 10 to 20 mg, which could be assigned to the increase of active sites [56]. However, the TC degradation rate increased indistinctively (78.19% to 82.64%) upon further increasing the catalyst usage from 20 to 30 mg, which may be due to the poor light transmission of the solution applying too much catalyst [57].

Effects of initial TC concentration: Figure 6f provides the effect of TC concentration on the photodegradation performance. The TC degradation rate decreased continuously, with the TC concentration ranging from 10 to 80 ppm. The explanation may be that the limited number of photogenerated carriers lead to restrict TC degradation when the initial TC concentration was too high. In addition, the higher TC concentration affected the penetration ability of photons and, thus, negatively affects the photocatalytic activity [58].

2.2.2. Photocatalytic Degradation of ENR and MO

The catalytic performance for Ag/PT composites were further evaluated by degrading ENR and MO in visible-light. During the dark reaction, the pollutants molecules were adsorbed on the photocatalyst surface for 20 min to obtain the adsorption-desorption equilibrium. As presented in Figure 7a, the photocatalytic degradation efficiencies of ENR with control, TiO_2, 10% Ag/TiO_2, PT, 5% Ag/PT, 10% Ag/PT, and 15% Ag/PT were 1.99%, 20.17%, 58.84%, 63.09%, 87.93%, 93.65%, and 89.98%. Specially, 10% Ag/PT had the best photocatalytic activity of 93.65% (k = 0.0194) (Figures 7b and S3b), which was 4.64-, 1.48-, and 1.59-times higher than that of TiO_2, 10% Ag/TiO_2, and PT, respectively. Similarly, the degradation profiles in Figure 7c manifesting 10% Ag/PT also displayed an excellent MO degradation rate of 99.29% (k = 0.1549) (Figures 7d and S3c). The influencing parameters of catalyst dosage and MO concentration were also studied in Figure S6. Moreover, the degradation efficiencies of Ag/PT composites are superior to other catalysts for ENR and MO removal (Tables S2 and S3). These data verify that as-prepared Ag/PT is one kind of multi-functional material in the field of environmental remediation.

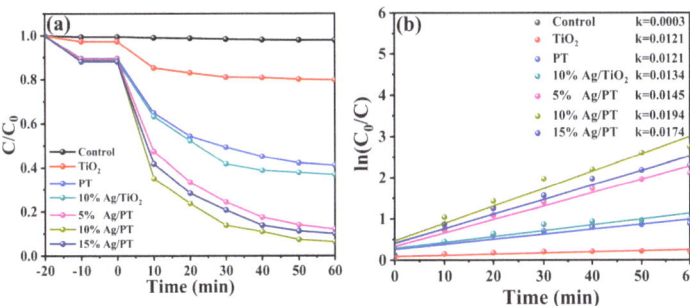

Figure 7. Cont.

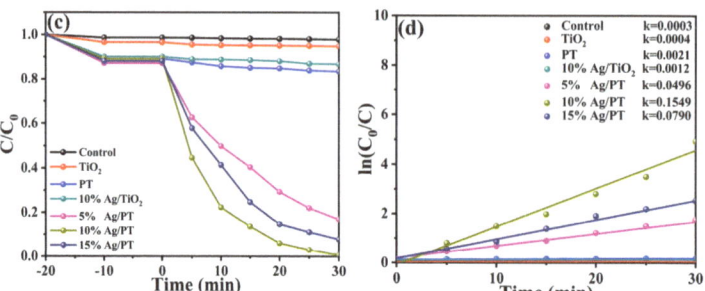

Figure 7. (**a**) Visible-light removal curses of ENR by different specimens; (**b**) Reaction rate constant k; The degradation profiles (**c**) and reaction rate constant k (**d**) of MO degradation.

2.3. Stability Test of Photocatalyst

Figure 8a shows the cycling experiments of 10% Ag/PT as a visible-light catalyst for the degradation of various contaminants. After 20 cycles of reuse, the degradation efficiency of MO, ENR, and TC exhibited a slight decrease, and by using ICP-6000 test, the leaching amount of Ag after degradation was 2.1 ppm, indicating that the as-obtained Ag/PT composites had good reuse performance. Moreover, the photocatalytic stability of Ag/PT materials was confirmed with XRD and FT-IR. As shown in Figure 8b,c, the XRD diffraction peaks and FT-IR spectra of the used 10% Ag/PT remained unchanged in comparison with the fresh sample, verifying the good structural stability of these materials. Furthermore, the TEM image after TC removal (Figure 8d) also demonstrated the good cycling stability of the catalyst.

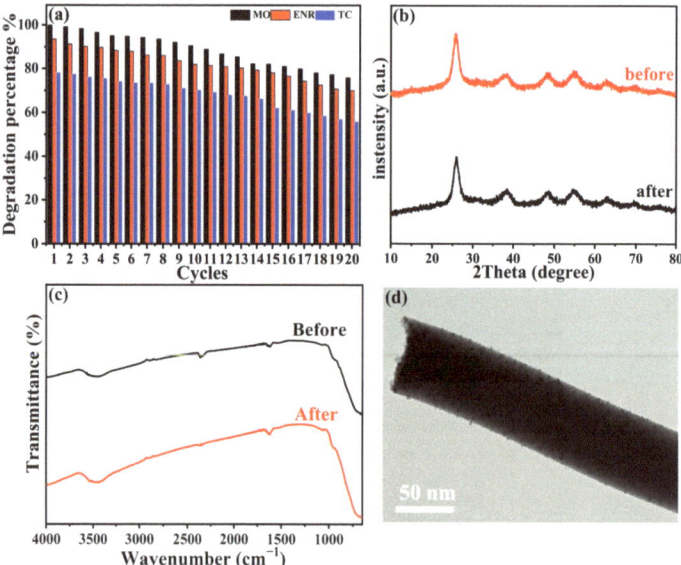

Figure 8. (**a**) The cyclic experiments for removing TC, ENR, and MO by 10% Ag/PT; XRD (**b**), FT-IR (**c**) TEM image (**d**) for 10% Ag/PT before and after use in TC degradation.

2.4. Photocatalytic Mechanism Investigation

2.4.1. Photogenerated Carriers Behavior Analysis

The photoluminescence (PL) spectra were measured to reflect the separation efficiency of photoinduced carriers from the synthesized catalysts. As demonstrated in Figure 9a, these materials exhibited similar peaks at 425 nm. The fluorescence intensity for

Ag/PT composite exhibited a significant decrease compared to TiO_2, PT, and 10% Ag/TiO_2, implying that the recombination of photogenerated charge carriers was effectively suppressed [59,60]. In addition, the 10% Ag/PT catalyst had the lowest peak intensity, implying a higher separation rate of electron-hole pairs and better catalytic capacity compared to the remaining specimens. The fluorescence lifetimes of PT and 10% Ag/PT were determined by time-resolved fluorescence attenuation spectrometry (TRPL). As revealed in Figure 9b, the fluorescence intensity of PT and 10% Ag/PT both decreased exponentially. The average fluorescence lifetime τ_{ave} of PT and 10% Ag/PT were calculated to be 0.18 ns and 0.06 ns, respectively (Table S4). The result shows that 10% Ag/PT has a shorter average decay time than PT, which indicates that the deposition of Ag nanoparticles is beneficial to delay the recombination of photoinduced carriers [61]. The corresponding quenching and lifetime reduction of TRPL implies a high non-radiative decay rate at 10% Ag/PT, and the establishment of a fast electron transfer pathway for accumulated photoproduced electrons is conducive to the enhancement of catalytic capacity [62].

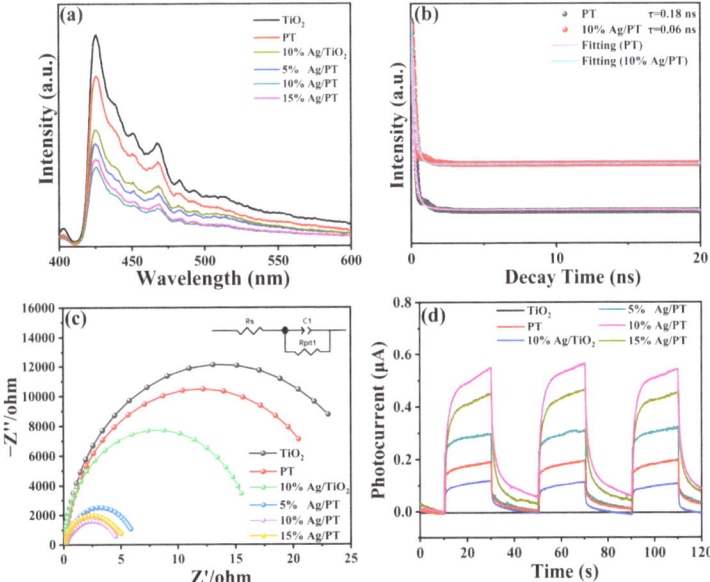

Figure 9. The steady PL (**a**), transient PL (**b**), EIS (Insert: impedance equivalent circuit diagram) (**c**) and photocurrent (**d**) of various samples.

The electrochemical impedance spectroscopy (EIS) and instantaneous photocurrent have been employed for examining the separation and migration ability of photogenerated electron-hole pairs. Figure 9c illustrates the EIS Nyquist plots form distinct electrodes, and the equivalent circuit are provided as an insert. Generally, the small EIS radian of the electrochemical impedance corresponds to the low charge transfer resist [63]. It is clear that the radius of these Ag/PT materials were much smaller than those of TiO_2, PT, and 10% Ag/TiO_2. Specially, 10% Ag/PT has the smallest radius, which strongly manifested that the composite possessed fastest transfer and migration ability of carriers [64]. Additionally, Figure S7 presents the Bode plots of PT and 10% Ag/PT, which confirmed a prolonged lifetime of photoinduced electrons for 10% Ag/PT in comparison to PT. The photocurrents of obtained specimens were measured in Figure 9d. The photocurrent was found to be stable and reproducible in three cycles. The photocurrent density obeyed the following order: 10% Ag/PT > 15% Ag/PT > 5% Ag/PT > 10% Ag/TiO_2 > PT > TiO_2. Specifically, the photocurrent density of 10% Ag/PT (0.23 $\mu A/cm^2$) was much larger than that of PT (0.09 $\mu A/cm^2$) and 10% Ag/TiO_2 (0.05 $\mu A/cm^2$), which would lead to a remarkable enhancement in photocatalytic capability [65]. The results of various measurements collectively demonstrated that the Ag/PT composites have low charge transfer resistance and high separation efficiency of photogenerated carriers, which would reveal an outstanding catalytic performance.

2.4.2. Active Species in Photocatalytic Reactions

To elucidate the degradation mechanism of TC, the radical capture experiments were performed, and the results were presented in Figure 10a. Herein, 4-hydroxymethylpropane (TEMPO, $\cdot O_2^-$ quencher), triethanolamine (TEOA, h^+ quencher), and isopropyl alcohol (IPA, $\cdot OH$ quencher) were employed as free radical trapping agents [66,67]. Distinctly, the addition of TEOA to the reaction system significantly inhibited the degradation efficiency, and the addition of TEMPO also reduced the degradation activity to some extent, verifying the important function of h^+ and $\cdot O_2^-$ in TC degradation. Meanwhile, the degradation rate was almost unchanged with the addition of IPA, implying that $\cdot OH$ was not the dominating active substance.

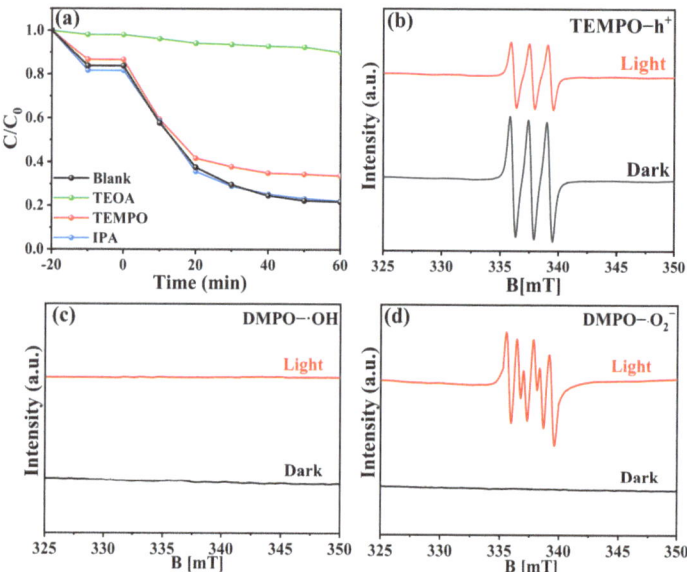

Figure 10. (a) The degradation of TC with diverse scavenges by 10% Ag/PT sample; (b) ESR spectra of TEMPO-h^+; ESR signals of (c) DMPO-$\cdot OH$ and (d) DMPO-$\cdot O_2^-$.

To directly verify the reactive species involved in the reaction process, electron spin resonance (ESR) measurement was conducted, applying 5,5-dimethyl-1-pyrroline N-oxide (DMPO) and 2,2,6,6-Tetramethyl-1-piperidinyloxy (TEMPO) as spin-trapping agents [68]. TEMPO can trap the photogenerated holes and form⁺ TEMPO-h^+ spin-products, which exhibit silent ESR signals. As displayed in Figure 10b, under dark conditions, three distinctive peaks corresponding to the TEMPO were identified, which were obviously declined under visible-light, demonstrating the production of TEMPO-h^+ spin-products [69]. Meanwhile, $\cdot OH$ and $\cdot O_2^-$ can be captured with DMPO, generating evident ESR signals. In Figure 10c, no characteristic peaks were found under both dark and light conditions in the $\cdot OH$ test, indicating that $\cdot OH$ did not play a role in the catalytic reaction. In Figure 10d, in the $\cdot O_2^-$ test, no characteristic peaks were detected under dark conditions; nevertheless, the characteristic peaks corresponding to DMPO-$\cdot O_2^-$ were clearly observed upon visible-light irradiation, authenticating successful generation of $\cdot O_2^-$ radicals. These results indicated that the photodegradation of TC was primarily driven with the involvement of $\cdot O_2^-$ radicals and h^+.

2.4.3. Degradation Pathways of TC and Toxicity Assessment

As revealed in Figures 11 and S5, the pathways of TC photodegradation were explored by HPLC-MS. The molecular weight of TC is expressed as the product $m/z = 444$. Figure 11 summarizes and illustrates two possible degradation pathways. In pathway 1, the intermediate of T1 ($m/z = 463$) may be derived from the dehydroxylation of TC, after which T1 forms T2 ($m/z = 403$) through the deamidation process. Intermediate with T3 ($m/z = 357$) is resulted from loss of one N-2 methyl group. The product T4 ($m/z = 259$) is obtained by the ring-opening reaction of T3. Pathway 2 is the transition from TC to T5 ($m/z = 427$) after deamination. Then, T5 is dehydroxylated and dedimethylated to T6 ($m/z = 398$), which is deaminated and demethylated to T7 ($m/z = 318$). After T4, T8 is formed by the break of double-bond oxygen, and T7 is formed by ring-opening and dehydroxylation. After continuous ring-opening reactions, T8 forms T9 ($m/z = 228$), T10 ($m/z = 182$), T11 ($m/z = 100$), and T12 ($m/z = 74$). Further degradation of intermediates can produce small molecules such as CO_2, H_2O, and inorganic ions. According to the above analysis, it can be inferred that photocatalytic degradation of tetracycline involves deamidation, dehydroxylation, and ring-opening reactions [3,70].

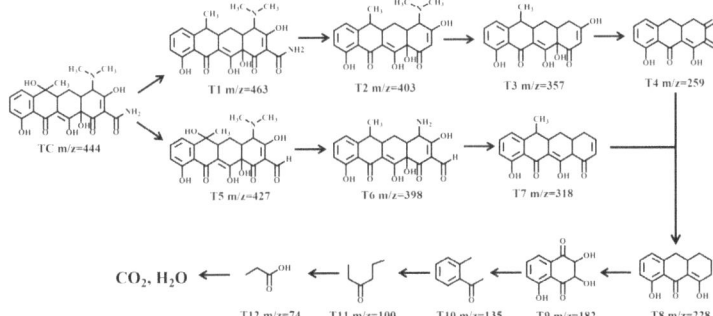

Figure 11. The probable catalytic degradation pathways for TC.

Furthermore, we investigated the toxicity of TC and its 12 intermediates using QSAR prediction with a toxicity estimation software tool (T.E.S.T. Version 5.1.2) [71]. Figure 12a,b show that TC was "developmentally toxic" and "mutagenic positive" [72]. One developmentally non-toxic TC intermediate (T10) and four mutagenic-negative TC intermediates (T7, T10, T11, T12) were produced after light treatment. Furthermore, most intermediates were less toxic than TC. As illustrated in Figure 12c, the bioaccumulation factors of intermediates T9 and T6 were lower than those of TC, and the photodegradation process could reduce the bioaccumulation factor for TC, which was primarily attributed to the hydroxylation reaction [73].

In Figure 12d–f, three evaluation indicators were used to evaluate the acute toxicity of TC and its intermediates: (i) Fathead minnow LC50 (96 h) represents the concentration at which 50% of fathead minnows are killed after 96 h; (ii) Daphnia magna LC50 (48 h) represents the concentration at which 50% of Daphnia magna are killed after 48 h; and (iii) Oral rats LD50 represents the concentration at which 50% of rats are killed after 48 h of oral ingestion. The LC50 values of 0.90 mg/L for blackhead minnow, 12.70 mg/L for Daphnia magna, and 1105.75 mg/kg for TC in rats were defined as "highly toxic", "harmful", and "toxic" compounds, respectively [74]. Obviously, T1, T6, T7, and T8 intermediates all showed low LD50 values (Figure 12d). Daphnia magna showed lower LC50 values than TC intermediates, except for T6, T7, T1, T2, T3, and T8 (Figure 12e). With the exception of intermediates T5 and T11, rats exhibited lower toxicity to TC intermediates (Figure 12f). According to the aforementioned toxicity prediction results, the toxicity of several intermediates still exists, which could be reduced by extending the reaction time.

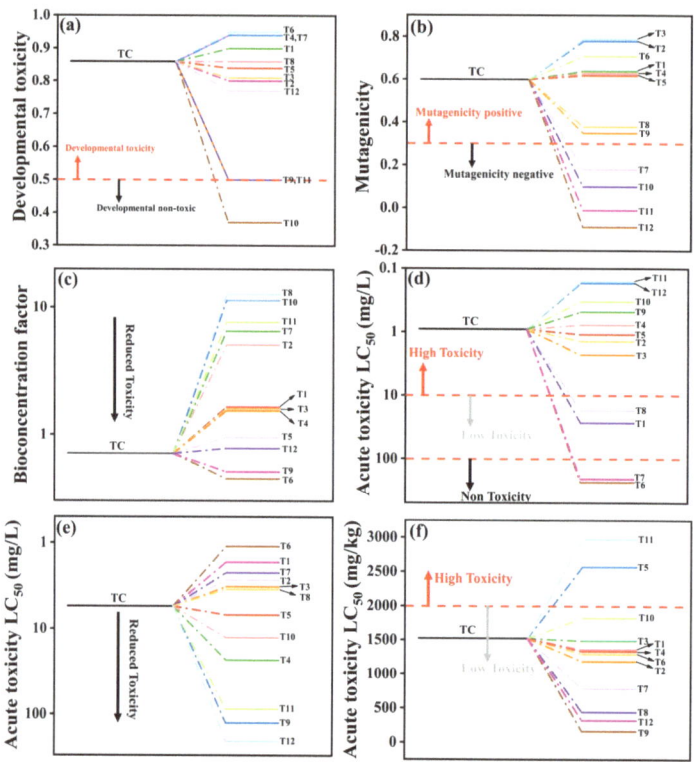

Figure 12. (**a**) Developmental toxicity; (**b**) mutagenicity; (**c**) bioconcentration factor; (**d**) fathead minnow, (**e**) Daphnia magna (**f**), and oral rat for these products in TC degradation.

2.4.4. Possible Photocatalytic Mechanism

In Figure S9, the tangent slope of the Mott-Schottky profile reflects that PT belongs to n-type semiconductor. The E_{fb} of PT relative to Hg/Hg_2Cl_2 was found to be −0.17 eV. Given that the conduction band energy (E_{CB}) of n-type semiconductor is approximately 0.2 eV higher than the flat band potential (E_{fb}) [75], the E_{CB} for PT could be determined as −0.13 eV (vs. NHE), according to $E_{NHE} = E_{Hg/Hg_2Cl_2} + 0.242$ eV. From the $(\alpha h\nu)^2$ vs. $h\nu$ plot (Figure 3b), the band gap energy (E_g) of PT is calculated to be 2.83 eV. Therefore, the VB (valence band) edge position of PT ($E_{VB} = E_{CB} + E_g$) is determined to be 2.70 eV [76]. Based on the aforementioned results, the catalytic mechanism for TC degradation by Ag/PT system with visible-light was proposed (Figure 13). The PT was photoexcited to generate electrons and holes under visible-light irradiation (Equation (1)). Meanwhile, a large number of hot electrons are produced, due to the surface plasmon resonance (SPR) effect of Ag NPs [77,78]. The Ag NPs serving as electron traps could effectively capture photoinduced electrons on the CB of PT, while the Schottky barrier established by Ag^0 could promote the transfer of SPR-excited electrons, further accelerating the charge separation (Equation (2)). These electrons on Ag NPs react with O_2 to form $\cdot O_2^-$ participating in oxidation reaction (Equations (3) and (4)). Moreover, the photoinduced holes in PT directly oxidize TC according to the result of ESR measurements and capturing tests (Equation (5)). Ultimately, TC was efficiently removed with the help of h^+ and $\cdot O_2^-$ active species (Equation (6)).

$$Ag/PT + h\nu \rightarrow Ag/PT\ (h^+ + e^-) \quad (1)$$

$$Ag/PT\ (h^+ + e^-) \rightarrow PT\ (h^+) + Ag\ (e^-) \quad (2)$$

$$O_2 + Ag\ (e^-) \rightarrow \bullet O_2^- + Ag \tag{3}$$

$$\bullet O_2^- + TC \rightarrow CO_2 + H_2O \tag{4}$$

$$PT\ (h^+) + TC \rightarrow PT + H_2O + CO_2 \tag{5}$$

$$h^+/\bullet O_2^- + TC \rightarrow intermediate\ products \rightarrow CO_2 + H_2O \tag{6}$$

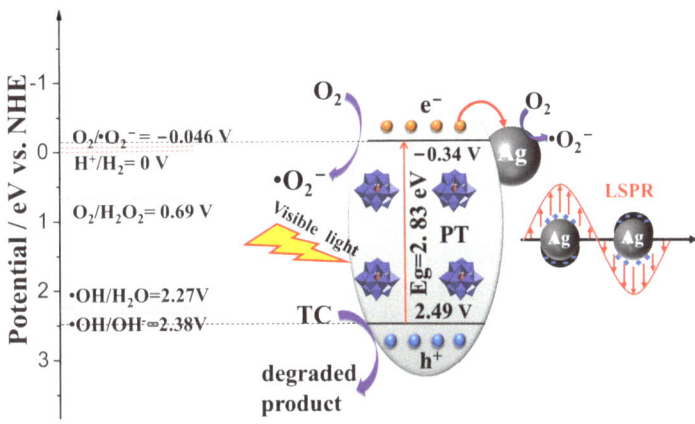

Figure 13. The photocatalytic mechanism of TC degradation using Ag/PT system.

3. Experiments and Characterizations

Construction of Ag/PT Photocatalysts

As shown in Scheme 1, Ag/PT composite nanofibers were prepared employing electrospinning/photoreduction methods. First of all, PT nanofibers were synthesized by the electrospinning/calcination method. Briefly, PVP was dissolved in a mixture of anhydrous ethanol, acetic acid, and tetrabutyl titanate, and stirred for 1 h. PW_{12} was then added and stirred until complete dissolution. The homogeneous precursor solution was subjected to electrostatic spinning operation, followed by calcination, to prepare PT nanofibers. Secondly, Ag NPs were modified on the PT nanofibers by photoreduction. PT nanofibers powder was added to the solution of $V_{water}:V_{isoprobanol} = 1:1$, which was then sonicated for 30 min. Then, the solution was evacuated, and the suspension was illuminated for 1 h using a 300 W xenon lamp with full spectrum light. Then, $AgNO_3$ solution was added and stirred for 60 min. The Ag/PT composite was prepared.

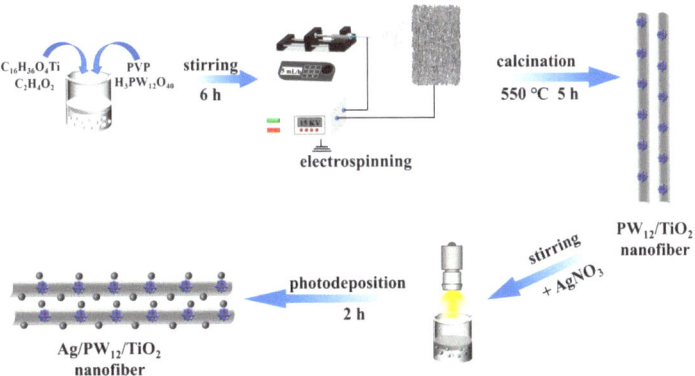

Scheme 1. Schematic diagram for the fabrication process of Ag/PT composite.

The fabrication and characterization methods of Ag/PT composites are displayed in the Supplementary Material.

4. Conclusions

Herein, a novel Ag/PT composite material has been constructed utilizing electrospinning/photoreduction methods, which exhibited remarkable photocatalytic activities for degradation TC, ENR, and MO. The results of mechanism investigation showed that the excellent catalytic property could be due to the following two reasons: (1) the doping of PW_{12} to TiO_2 can enhance the utilization of visible spectrum and redox reaction activity of titanium dioxide; (2) the precious metal Ag possesses the LSPR effect, which can improve the utilization of sunlight and generate more charge carriers. Besides, the LSPR effect will have a high-intensity small range electromagnetic field, which will greatly improve the separation rate of photogenerated electron-hole pairs. Moreover, the degradation intermediates and pathways were revealed through HPLC-MS. The toxicity of TC degradation products was also investigated using QSAR prediction. This current work offers novel thoughts for developing efficient and stable catalysts for environmental remediation.

Supplementary Materials: The following supporting information can be downloaded at: https://www.mdpi.com/article/10.3390/molecules28196831/s1, Figure S1: EDX data of 10% Ag/PT sample; Figure S2: UV-Vis absorption spectra of 5%, 10% and 15% Ag/PT sample; Figure S3: The profiles of photocatalytic degradation of TC (a), ENR (b) and MO (c) by 10% Ag/PT under visible-light irradiation ($\lambda > 420$ nm); Figure S4: The TOC removal (%) for TC degradation by 10% Ag/PT sample; Figure S5: Photodegradation of TC with 10% Ag/PT under Diverse water quality (catalyst amount: 20 mg; TC: 20 mL of 20 ppm; pH = 7). Figure S6: Degradation of MO with 10% Ag/PT with various conditions: (a) Diverse catalyst amount (MO: 20 mL of 20 ppm; pH = 1) and (b) Different concentration of MO (MO: 20 mL; pH = 1; catalyst amount: 20 mg). Figure S7: The Bode plots of PT and 10% Ag/PT composite; Figure S8: The main intermediate products generated during the photocatalytic TC degradation process: (a) 0 min; (b) 30 min; (c) 60 min with 10% Ag/PT as catalyst; Figure S9: The E_{fb} of PT (V vs. Hg/Hg_2Cl_2). Table S1: The comparison of TC degradation activity of 10% Ag/PT with previous literatures; Table S2: The comparison of ENR degradation activity of 10% Ag/PT with previous literatures; Table S3: The comparison of MO degradation activity of 10% Ag/PT with previous literatures; Table S4: Fitted parameters of the TRPL decay profiles. References [79–122] are cited in the Supplementary Materials.

Author Contributions: Conceptualization, H.S.; methodology, H.W.; validation, H.W., E.Z., S.Z. and H.G.; investigation, E.Z. and H.G.; resources, H.S. and J.L.; writing—original draft preparation, H.W. and E.Z.; writing—review and editing, H.S.; funding acquisition, H.S., X.Q., J.L., S.Z. and Z.C.; supervision, Z.C.; Software, H.W. All authors have read and agreed to the published version of the manuscript.

Funding: The work was financially supported with the Natural Science Foundation of Jilin Province (YDZJ202201ZYTS360, YDZJ202201ZYTS358, YDZJ202201ZYTS591), the Project of Jilin Provincial Department of Education (JJKH20210233KJ) and the National Natural Science Foundation of China (22309061, 22278172, 22071080, 22109105).

Institutional Review Board Statement: Not applicable.

Informed Consent Statement: Not applicable.

Data Availability Statement: Data are contained within the article and Supplementary Materials.

Acknowledgments: The authors would like to acknowledge the technical support from JLICT CCA.

Conflicts of Interest: The authors declare no conflict of interest.

Sample Availability: Samples of the compounds are available from the authors.

References

1. Wu, Z.; Wang, M.Y.; Bai, Y.; Song, H.; Lv, J.X.; Mo, X.F.; Li, X.Q.; Lin, Z. Upcycling of nickel iron slags to hierarchical self-assembled flower-like photocatalysts for highly efficient degradation of high-concentration tetracycline. *Chem. Eng. J.* **2023**, *464*, 142532. [CrossRef]
2. Miao, Y.X.; Zhao, Y.X.; Zhang, S.; Shi, R.; Zhang, T.R. Strain engineering: A boosting strategy for photocatalysis. *Adv. Mater.* **2022**, *34*, 2200868. [CrossRef] [PubMed]
3. Li, B.; Tong, F.X.; Lv, M.; Wang, Z.Y.; Liu, Y.Y.; Wang, P.; Cheng, H.F.; Dai, Y.; Zheng, Z.K.; Huang, B.B. In situ monitoring charge transfer on topotactic epitaxial heterointerface for tetracycline degradation at the single-particle level. *ACS Catal.* **2022**, *12*, 9114–9124. [CrossRef]
4. Liccardo, L.; Bordin, M.; Sheverdyaeva, P.M.; Belli, M.; Moras, P.; Vomiero, A.; Moretti, E. Surface defect engineering in colored TiO_2 hollow spheres toward efficient photocatalysis. *Adv. Funct. Mater.* **2023**, *33*, 2212486. [CrossRef]
5. Cao, H.; Liu, F.Y.; Tai, Y.T.; Wang, W.; Li, X.Y.; Li, P.Y.; Zhao, H.Z.; Xia, Y.Q.; Wang, S.J. Promoting photocatalytic performance of TiO_2 nanomaterials by structural and electronic modulation. *Chem. Eng. J.* **2023**, *466*, 143219. [CrossRef]
6. Zhu, Y.; Wang, D.; Huang, Q.; Du, J.; Sun, L.; Li, F.; Meyer, T.J. Stabilization of a molecular water oxidation catalyst on a dye-sensitized photoanode by apyridyl anchor. *Nat. Commun.* **2020**, *11*, 4610. [CrossRef]
7. Xing, F.Y.; Wang, C.Z.; Liu, S.Q.; Jin, S.H.; Jin, H.B.; Li, J.B. Interfacial chemical bond engineering in a direct Z-Scheme g-C_3N_4/MoS_2 heterojunction. *ACS Appl. Mater. Interface* **2023**, *15*, 11731–11740. [CrossRef]
8. Sun, G.T.; Tai, Z.G.; Li, F.; Ye, Q.; Wang, T.; Fang, Z.Y.; Jia, L.C.; Liu, W.; Wang, H.Q. Construction of $ZnIn_2S_4$/CdS/PdS S-Scheme heterostructure for efficient photocatalytic H_2 production. *Small* **2023**, *19*, 2207758. [CrossRef]
9. Zhao, X.Y.; Zhang, Y.; Zhao, Y.N.; Tan, H.Q.; Zhao, Z.; Shi, H.F.; Wang, E.B.; Li, Y.G. $Ag_xH_{3-x}PMo_{12}O_{40}$/Ag nanorods/g-$C_3N_4$ 1D/2D Z-scheme heterojunction for highly efficient visible-light photocatalysis. *Dalton Trans.* **2019**, *48*, 6484–6491. [CrossRef]
10. Horn, M.R.; Singh, A.; Alomari, S.; Goberna-Ferrón, S.; Benages-Vilau, R.; Chodankar, N.; Motta, N.; Ostrikov, K.; MacLeod, J.; Sonar, P.; et al. Polyoxometalates (POMs): From electroactive clusters to energy materials. *Energy Environ. Sci.* **2021**, *14*, 1652–1700. [CrossRef]
11. Shi, H.F.; Yu, Y.C.; Zhang, Y.; Feng, X.J.; Zhao, X.Y.; Tan, H.Q.; Khan, S.U.; Li, Y.G.; Wang, E.B. Polyoxometalate/TiO_2/Ag composite nanofibers with enhanced photocatalytic performance under visible light. *Appl. Catal. B-Environ.* **2018**, *221*, 280–289. [CrossRef]
12. Chen, L.; Chen, W.L.; Wang, X.L.; Li, Y.G.; Su, Z.M.; Wang, E.B. Polyoxometalates in dye-sensitized solar cells. *Chem. Soc. Rev.* **2019**, *48*, 260–284. [CrossRef] [PubMed]
13. Mirzaei, M.; Eshtiagh-Hosseini, H.; Alipour, M.; Frontera, A. Recent developments in the crystal engineering of diverse coordination modes (0–12) for Keggin-type polyoxometalates in hybrid inorganic-organic architectures. *Coord. Chem. Rev.* **2014**, *275*, 1–18. [CrossRef]
14. Xing, F.S.; Zeng, R.Y.; Cheng, C.C.; Liu, Q.W.; Huang, C.J. POM-incorporated $ZnIn_2S_4$ Z-scheme dual-functional photocatalysts for cooperative benzyl alcohol oxidation and H_2 evolution in aqueous solution. *Appl. Catal. B Environ.* **2022**, *306*, 121087. [CrossRef]
15. Yu, B.; Zhang, S.M.; Wang, X. Helical microporous nanorods assembled by polyoxometalate clusters for the photocatalytic oxidation of toluene. *Angew. Chem. Int. Ed.* **2021**, *60*, 17404–17409. [CrossRef] [PubMed]
16. Li, Y.S.; Liu, M.X.; Chen, L. Polyoxometalate built-in conjugated microporous polymers for visible-light heterogeneous photocatalysis. *J. Mater. Chem. A* **2017**, *5*, 13757–13762. [CrossRef]
17. He, B.W.; Luo, C.; Wang, Z.L.; Zhang, L.Y.; Yu, J.G. Synergistic enhancement of solar H_2O_2 and HCOOH production over TiO_2 by dual co-catalyst loading in a tri-phase system. *Appl. Catal. B-Environ.* **2023**, *323*, 122200. [CrossRef]
18. Pellejero, I.; Clemente, A.; Reinoso, S.; Cornejo, A.; Navajas, A.; Vesperinas, J.J.; Urbiztondo, M.A.; Gandía, L.M. Innovative catalyst integration on transparent silicone microreactors for photocatalytic applications. *Catal. Today* **2022**, *383*, 164–172. [CrossRef]
19. Shi, H.F.; Zhao, T.T.; Zhang, Y.; Tan, H.Q.; Shen, W.H.; Wang, W.D.; Li, Y.G.; Wang, E.B. Pt/POMs/TiO_2 composite nanofibers with enhanced visible-light photocatalytic performance for environmental remediation. *Dalton Trans.* **2019**, *48*, 13353–13359. [CrossRef]
20. Chen, X.; Wang, Z.P.; Shen, X.C.; Zhang, Y.; Lou, Y.; Pan, C.S.; Zhu, Y.F.; Xu, J. A plasmonic Z-scheme Ag@AgCl/PDI photocatalyst for the efficient elimination of organic pollutants, antibiotic resistant bacteria and antibiotic resistance genes. *Appl. Catal. B-Environ.* **2023**, *324*, 122220. [CrossRef]
21. Xu, Z.Y.; Guo, C.Y.; Liu, X.; Li, L.; Wang, L.; Xu, H.L.; Zhang, D.K.; Li, C.H.; Li, Q.; Wang, W.T. Ag nanoparticles anchored organic/inorganic Z-scheme 3DOMM-TiO_{2-x}-based heterojunction for efficient photocatalytic and photoelectrochemical water splitting. *Chin. J. Catal.* **2022**, *43*, 1360–1370. [CrossRef]
22. Zeng, Q.L.; Xie, X.F.; Wang, X.; Wang, Y.; Lu, G.H.; Pui, D.Y.H.; Sun, J. Enhanced photocatalytic performance of Ag@TiO_2 for the gaseous acetaldehyde photodegradation under fluorescent lamp. *Chem. Eng. J.* **2018**, *341*, 83–92. [CrossRef]
23. Kumar, P.S.; Sundaramurthy, J.; Sundarrajan, S.; Babu, V.J.; Singh, G.; Allakhverdiev, S.I.; Ramakrishna, S. Hierarchical electrospun nanofibers for energy harvesting, production and environmental remediation. *Energy Environ. Sci.* **2014**, *7*, 3192–3222. [CrossRef]
24. Li, C.X.; Zhao, Y.X.; Song, Y.X.; Qiu, X.J.; Wang, S.Z.; Sun, P.Z. Optimization of electron transport pathway: A novel strategy to solve the photocorrosion of Ag-based photocatalysts. *Environ. Sci. Technol.* **2023**. [CrossRef] [PubMed]

25. Zhang, J.M.; Jiang, X.Y.; Huang, J.D.; Lu, W.; Zhang, Z.Y. Plasmon-enhanced photocatalytic overall water-splitting over Au nanoparticle-decorated $CaNb_2O_6$ electrospun nanofibers. *J. Mater. Chem. A* **2022**, *10*, 20048–20058. [CrossRef]
26. Le, T.T.; Lee, M.; Chae, K.H.; Moon, G.H.; Kim, S.H. Control of copper element in mesoporous iron oxide photocatalysts towards UV light-assisted superfast mineralization of isopropyl alcohol with peroxydisulfate. *Chem. Eng. J.* **2023**, *451*, 139048. [CrossRef]
27. Shi, H.F.; Zhao, T.T.; Wang, J.B.; Wang, Y.T.; Chen, Z.; Liu, B.L.; Ji, H.F.; Wang, W.D.; Zhang, G.L.; Li, Y.G. Fabrication of g-C_3N_4/PW_{12}/TiO_2 composite with significantly enhanced photocatalytic performance under visible light. *J. Alloys Compd.* **2021**, *860*, 157924. [CrossRef]
28. Mahadadalkar, M.A.; Park, N.; Yusuf, M.; Nagappan, S.; Nallal, M.; Park, K.H. Electrospun Fe doped TiO_2 fiber photocatalyst for efficient wastewater treatment. *Chemosphere* **2023**, *330*, 138599. [CrossRef]
29. Ni, J.X.; Liu, D.M.; Wang, W.; Wang, A.W.; Jia, J.L.; Tian, J.Y.; Xing, Z.P. Hierarchical defect-rich flower-like BiOBr/Ag nanoparticles/ultrathin g-C_3N_4 with transfer channels plasmonic Z-scheme heterojunction photocatalyst for accelerated visible-light-driven photothermal-photocatalytic oxytetracycline degradation. *Chem. Eng. J.* **2021**, *419*, 129969. [CrossRef]
30. Huang, X.Y.; Liu, X. Highly polymerized linear polyimide/$H_3PW_{12}O_{40}$ photocatalyst with full visible light region absorption. *Chemosphere* **2021**, *283*, 131230. [CrossRef]
31. You, Y.L.J.; Gao, S.Y.; Yang, Z.; Cao, M.N.; Cao, R. Facile synthesis of polyoxometalate-thionine composite via direct precipitation method and its photocatalytic activity for degradation of rhodamine B under visible light. *J. Colloid Interface Sci.* **2012**, *365*, 198–203. [CrossRef] [PubMed]
32. Song, Y.B.; Guo, Y.M.; Qi, S.P.; Zhang, K.; Yang, J.F.; Li, B.N.; Chen, J.X.; Zhao, Y.X.; Lou, Y.B. Cu_7S_4/$MnIn_2S_4$ heterojunction for efficient photocatalytic hydrogen generation. *J. Alloys Compd.* **2021**, *884*, 161035. [CrossRef]
33. Gao, B.Q.; Tao, K.K.; Xi, Z.H.; El-Sayed, M.M.H.; Shoeib, T.; Yang, H. Fabrication of 3D lignosulfonate composited sponges impregnated by $BiVO_4$/polyaniline/Ag ternary photocatalyst for synergistic adsorption-photodegradation of fluoroquinolones in water. *Chem. Eng. J.* **2022**, *446*, 137282. [CrossRef]
34. Kong, W.H.; Wang, S.L.; Wu, D.; Chen, C.R.; Luo, Y.S.; Pei, Y.T.; Tian, B.Z.; Zhang, J.L. Fabrication of 3D sponge@AgBr-AgCl/Ag and tubular photoreactor for continuous wastewater purification under sunlight irradiation. *ACS Sustain. Chem. Eng.* **2019**, *7*, 14051–14063. [CrossRef]
35. Tamilselvan, S.; Soniya, R.M.; Vasantharaja, R.; Kannan, M.; Supriya, S. Silver nanoparticles based spectroscopic sensing of eight metal ions in aqueous solutions. *Environ. Res.* **2022**, *212*, 113585. [CrossRef]
36. Shi, H.F.; Jin, T.; Li, J.P.; Li, Y.L.; Chang, Y.Q.; Jin, Z.H.; Jiang, W.; Qu, X.S.; Chen, Z. Construction of Z-scheme $Cs_3PMo_{12}O_{40}$/g-C_3N_4 composite photocatalyst with highly efficient photocatalytic performance under visible light irradiation. *J. Solid State Chem.* **2022**, *311*, 123069. [CrossRef]
37. Devi, L.G.; Kavitha, R. A review on plasmonic metal–TiO_2 composite for generation, trapping, storing and dynamic vectorial transfer of photogenerated electrons across the Schottky junction in a photocatalytic system. *Appl. Surf. Sci.* **2016**, *360*, 601–622. [CrossRef]
38. Mu, F.H.; Liu, C.X.; Xie, Y.; Zhou, S.J.; Dai, B.L.; Xia, D.H.; Huang, H.B.; Zhao, W.; Sun, C.; Kong, Y.; et al. Metal-organic framework-derived rodlike AgCl/Ag/In_2O_3: A plasmonic Z-scheme visible light photocatalyst. *Chem. Eng. J.* **2021**, *415*, 129010. [CrossRef]
39. Basumatary, B.; Basumatary, R.; Ramchiary, A.; Konwar, D. Evaluation of Ag@TiO_2/WO_3 heterojunction photocatalyst for enhanced photocatalytic activity towards methylene blue degradation. *Chemosphere* **2022**, *286*, 131848. [CrossRef]
40. Yang, R.X.; Zhong, S.; Zhang, L.S.; Liu, B.J. PW_{12}/CN@Bi_2WO_6 composite photocatalyst prepared based on organic-inorganic hybrid system for removing pollutants in water. *Sep. Purif. Technol.* **2020**, *235*, 116270. [CrossRef]
41. Lu, N.; Wang, Y.Q.; Ning, S.Q.; Zhao, W.J.; Qian, M.; Ma, Y.; Wang, J.; Fan, L.Y.; Guan, J.N.; Yuan, X. Design of plasmonic Ag-TiO_2/$H_3PW_{12}O_{40}$ composite film with enhanced sunlight photocatalytic activity towards o-chlorophenol degradation. *Sci. Rep.* **2017**, *7*, 17298. [CrossRef] [PubMed]
42. Yang, X.; Li, M.H.; Xu, L.; Li, F.Y. Limitation of WO_3 in Zn-Co_3O_4 nanopolyhedra by the pyrolysis of $H_3PW_{12}O_{40}$@BMZIF: Synergistic effect of heterostructure and oxygen vacancies for enhanced nitrogen fixation. *Inorg. Chem.* **2023**, *62*, 8710–8718. [CrossRef] [PubMed]
43. Chen, Z.; Chen, H.X.; Wang, K.; Chen, J.; Li, M.; Wang, Y.; Tsiakaras, P.; Song, S.Q. Enhanced TiO_2 photocatalytic 2 e$^-$ oxygen reduction reaction via interfacial microenvironment regulation and mechanism analysis. *ACS Catal.* **2023**, *13*, 6497–6508. [CrossRef]
44. Gao, Y.T.; Chen, F.; Chen, Z.; Shi, H.F. $Ni_xCo_{1-x}S$ as an effective noble metal-free cocatalyst for enhanced photocatalytic activity of g-C_3N_4. *J. Mater. Sci. Technol.* **2020**, *56*, 227–235. [CrossRef]
45. Guo, J.; Gan, W.; Ding, C.S.; Lu, Y.Q.; Li, J.R.; Qi, S.H.; Zhang, M.; Sun, Z.Q. Black phosphorus quantum dots and Ag nanoparticles co-modified TiO_2 nanorod arrays as powerful photocatalyst for tetracycline hydrochloride degradation: Pathways, toxicity assessment, and mechanism insight. *Sep. Purif. Technol.* **2022**, *297*, 121454. [CrossRef]
46. Li, J.H.; Kang, W.L.; Yang, X.; Yu, X.D.; Xu, L.L.; Guo, Y.H.; Fang, H.B.; Zhang, S.D. Mesoporous titania-based $H_3PW_{12}O_{40}$ composite by a block copolymer surfactant-assisted templating route: Preparation, characterization, and heterogeneous photocatalytic properties. *Desalination* **2010**, *255*, 107–116. [CrossRef]
47. Yang, C.D.; Feng, S.; Ma, C.C.; Zhou, Y.; Dai, X.J.; Ye, Z.W.; Wang, Y. $Bi_2Sn_2O_7$/UiO-66-NH_2 heterojunction photocatalyst simultaneously adsorbed and photodegraded tetracycline. *J. Environ. Chem. Eng.* **2023**, *11*, 109664. [CrossRef]

48. Wang, S.J.; Chen, L.; Zhao, X.L.; Zhang, J.Q.; Ao, Z.M.; Liu, W.R.; Wu, H.; Shi, L.; Yin, Y.; Xu, X.Y.; et al. Efficient photocatalytic overall water splitting on metal-free 1D SWCNT/2D ultrathin C_3N_4 heterojunctions via novel non-resonant plasmonic effect. *Appl. Catal. B-Environ.* **2020**, *278*, 119312. [CrossRef]
49. Li, S.Y.; Niu, Z.W.; Pan, D.Q.; Cui, Z.P.; Shang, H.W.; Lian, J.; Wu, W.S. Efficient photoreduction strategy for uranium immobilization based on graphite carbon nitride/activated carbon nanocomposites. *Chin. Chem. Lett.* **2022**, *33*, 3581–3584. [CrossRef]
50. Wu, C.; Dai, J.N.; Ma, J.; Zhang, T.Y.; Qiang, L.S.; Xue, J.Q. Mechanistic study of B-TiO_2/$BiVO_4$ S-scheme heterojunction photocatalyst for tetracycline hydrochloride removal and H_2 production. *Sep. Purif. Technol.* **2023**, *312*, 123398. [CrossRef]
51. Zhu, L.D.; Zhou, Y.X.; Fei, L.Y.; Cheng, X.L.; Zhu, X.X.; Deng, L.Q.; Ma, X. Z-scheme CuO/Fe_3O_4/GO heterojunction photocatalyst: Enhanced photocatalytic performance for elimination of tetracycline. *Chemosphere* **2022**, *309*, 136721. [CrossRef] [PubMed]
52. Wan, Y.; Wang, H.J.; Liu, J.J.; Liu, X.; Song, X.H.; Zhou, W.Q.; Zhang, J.S.; Huo, P.W. Enhanced degradation of polyethylene terephthalate plastics by CdS/CeO_2 heterojunction photocatalyst activated peroxymonosulfate. *J. Hazard. Mater.* **2023**, *452*, 131375. [CrossRef] [PubMed]
53. Santos, H.F.D.; Xavier, É.S.; Zerner, M.C.; Almeida, W.B.D. Spectroscopic investigation of the Al(III)-anhydrotetracycline complexation process. *J. Mol. Struct.* **2000**, *527*, 193–202. [CrossRef]
54. Yang, J.H.; Sun, J.L.; Chen, S.; Lan, D.Q.; Li, Z.H.; Li, Z.J.; Wei, J.W.; Yu, Z.B.; Zhu, H.X.; Wang, S.F.; et al. S-scheme 1 T phase $MoSe_2$/AgBr heterojunction toward antibiotic degradation: Photocatalytic mechanism, degradation pathways, and intermediates toxicity evaluation. *Sep. Purif. Technol.* **2022**, *290*, 120881. [CrossRef]
55. Gao, P.; Li, Z.X.; Feng, L.; Liu, Y.Z.; Du, Z.W.; Zhang, L.Q. Construction of novel MWCNTs/$Bi_4O_5I_2$ nanosheets with enhanced adsorption and photocatalytic performance for the degradation of tetracycline: Efficiency, mechanism and regeneration. *Chem. Eng. J.* **2022**, *429*, 132398. [CrossRef]
56. Abilarasu, A.; Kumar, P.S.; Vo, D.V.N.; Krithika, D.; Ngueagni, P.T.; Joshiba, G.J.; Carolin, C.F.; Prasannamedha, G. Enhanced photocatalytic degradation of diclofenac by $Sn_{0.15}Mn_{0.85}Fe_2O_4$ catalyst under solar light. *J. Environ. Chem. Eng.* **2021**, *9*, 104875. [CrossRef]
57. Shi, H.F.; Zhu, H.W.; Jin, T.; Chen, L.; Zhang, J.Y.; Qiao, K.Y.; Chen, Z. Construction of Bi/Polyoxometalate doped TiO_2 composite with efficient visible-light photocatalytic performance: Mechanism insight, degradation pathway and toxicity evaluation. *Appl. Surf. Sci.* **2023**, *615*, 156310. [CrossRef]
58. Chen, D.D.; Yi, X.H.; Zhao, C.; Fu, H.F.; Wang, P.; Wang, C.C. Polyaniline modified MIL-100(Fe) for enhanced photocatalytic Cr(VI) reduction and tetracycline degradation under white light. *Chemosphere* **2020**, *245*, 125659. [CrossRef]
59. Wang, H.X.; Liao, B.; Lu, T.; Ai, Y.L.; Liu, G. Enhanced visible-light photocatalytic degradation of tetracycline by a novel hollow BiOCl@CeO_2 heterostructured microspheres: Structural characterization and reaction mechanism. *J. Hazard. Mater.* **2020**, *385*, 12155. [CrossRef]
60. Chen, Z.; Gao, Y.T.; Chen, F.; Shi, H.F. Metallic NiSe cocatalyst decorated g-C_3N_4 with enhanced photocatalytic activity. *Chem. Eng. J.* **2023**, *413*, 127474. [CrossRef]
61. Liu, C.; He, X.X.; Xu, Q.X.; Chen, M. A general way to realize the bi-directional promotion effects on the photocatalytic removal of heavy metals and organic pollutants in real water by a novel S-scheme heterojunction: Experimental investigations, QSAR and DFT calculations. *J. Hazard. Mater.* **2023**, *445*, 130551. [CrossRef] [PubMed]
62. Liu, C.; Han, Z.T.; Feng, Y.; Dai, H.L.; Zhao, Y.F.; Han, N.; Zhang, Q.F.; Zou, Z.G. Ultrathin Z-scheme 2D/2D N-doped $HTiNbO_5$ nanosheets/g-C_3N_4 porous composites for efficient photocatalytic degradation and H_2 generation under visible light. *J. Colloid Interface Sci.* **2021**, *583*, 58–70. [CrossRef] [PubMed]
63. Shi, H.F.; Yan, G.; Zhang, Y.; Tan, H.Q.; Zhou, W.Z.; Ma, Y.Y.; Li, Y.G.; Chen, W.L.; Wang, E.B. Ag/$Ag_xH_{3-x}PMo_{12}O_{40}$ nanowires with enhanced visible light-driven photocatalytic performance. *ACS Appl. Mater. Interface* **2017**, *9*, 422–430. [CrossRef] [PubMed]
64. Chen, Z.; Gao, Y.T.; Mu, D.Z.; Shi, H.F.; Lou, D.W.; Liu, S.Y. Recyclable magnetic $NiFe_2O_4$/C yolk-shell nanospheres with excellent visible-light-Fenton degradation performance of tetracycline hydrochloride. *Dalton Trans.* **2019**, *48*, 3038–3044. [CrossRef] [PubMed]
65. Shi, H.F.; Tan, H.Q.; Zhu, W.B.; Sun, Z.C.; Ma, Y.J.; Wang, E.B. Electrospun Cr-doped $Bi_4Ti_3O_{12}$/$Bi_2Ti_2O_7$ heterostructure fibers with enhanced visible-light photocatalytic properties. *J. Mater. Chem. A* **2015**, *3*, 6586–6591. [CrossRef]
66. Wang, Y.H.; Han, D.M.; Wang, Z.H.; Gu, F.B. Efficient photocatalytic degradation of tetracycline under visible light by an all-solid-state Z-Scheme Ag_3PO_4/MIL-101(Cr) heterostructure with metallic Ag as a charge transmission bridge. *ACS Appl. Mater. Interface* **2023**, *15*, 22085–22100. [CrossRef] [PubMed]
67. Feng, S.; Xie, T.P.; Wang, J.K.; Yang, J.W.; Kong, D.S.; Liu, C.W.; Chen, S.L.; Yang, F.L.; Pan, M.J.; Yang, J.; et al. Photocatalytic activation of PMS over magnetic heterojunction photocatalyst $SrTiO_3$/$BaFe_{12}O_{19}$ for tetracycline ultrafast degradation. *Chem. Eng. J.* **2023**, *470*, 143900. [CrossRef]
68. Li, S.J.; Yan, R.Y.; Cai, M.J.; Jiang, W.; Zhang, M.Y.; Li, X. Enhanced antibiotic degradation performance of $Cd_{0.5}Zn_{0.5}S$/Bi_2MoO_6 S-scheme photocatalyst by carbon dot modification. *J. Mater. Sci. Technol.* **2023**, *164*, 59–67. [CrossRef]
69. Li, X.L.; Yang, G.Q.; Li, S.S.; Xiao, N.; Li, N.; Gao, Y.Q.; Lv, D.; Ge, L. Novel dual co-catalysts decorated Au@HCS@PdS hybrids with spatially separated charge carriers and enhanced photocatalytic hydrogen evolution activity. *Chem. Eng. J.* **2020**, *379*, 122350. [CrossRef]
70. Li, S.J.; Cai, M.J.; Wang, C.C.; Liu, Y.P. Ta_3N_5/CdS core–shell S-scheme heterojunction nanofibers for efficient photocatalytic removal of antibiotic tetracycline and Cr(VI): Performance and mechanism insights. *Adv. Fiber Mater.* **2023**, *5*, 994–1007. [CrossRef]

71. Li, S.J.; Wang, C.C.; Dong, K.X.; Zhang, P.; Chen, X.B.; Li, X. MIL-101(Fe)/BiOBr S-scheme photocatalyst for promoting photocatalytic abatement of Cr(VI) and enrofloxacin antibiotic: Performance and mechanism. *Chin. J. Catal.* **2023**, *51*, 101–112. [CrossRef]
72. Cai, Z.Q.; Song, Y.G.; Jin, X.B.; Wang, C.C.; Ji, H.D.; Liu, W.; Sun, X.B. Highly efficient AgBr/h-MoO$_3$ with charge separation tuning for photocatalytic degradation of trimethoprim: Mechanism insight and toxicity assessment. *Sci. Total. Environ.* **2021**, *781*, 146754. [CrossRef] [PubMed]
73. Fan, S.L.; Chen, J.; Tian, L.; Fan, C.; Xu, W.T.; Zhang, Y.J.; Gan, T.; Hu, H.Y.; Huang, Z.Q.; Qin, Y.B. Construction of a recyclable chitosan-based aerogel-supported TiO$_2$ catalyst for treating high-concentration surfactants. *Compos. Part. B-Eng.* **2023**, *251*, 110475. [CrossRef]
74. Zhou, Q.; Zhang, L.H.; Zhang, L.F.; Jiang, B.; Sun, Y.L. In-situ constructed 2D/2D ZnIn$_2$S$_4$/Bi$_4$Ti$_3$O$_{12}$ S-scheme heterojunction for degradation of tetracycline: Performance and mechanism insights. *J. Hazard. Mater.* **2022**, *438*, 129438. [CrossRef] [PubMed]
75. Liu, J.; Wang, H.; Li, W.J.; Xie, H.X.; Li, X.; Ge, B.; Yang, L.Q.; Chang, M.J.; Du, H.L.; Song, S.J. Controllable fabrication of Bi$_4$Ti$_3$O$_{12}$/C/Bi$_2$S$_3$/MoS$_2$ heterojunction with effective suppression of Bi$_2$S$_3$ assisted by amorphous carbon interlayer for significantly enhanced photocatalysis. *J. Taiwan Inst. Chem. E* **2023**, *146*, 104882. [CrossRef]
76. Shi, H.F.; Fu, J.C.; Jiang, W.; Wang, Y.T.; Liu, B.L.; Liu, J.X.; Ji, H.F.; Wang, W.D.; Chen, Z. Construction of g-C$_3$N$_4$/Bi$_4$Ti$_3$O$_{12}$ hollow nanofibers with highly efficient visible-light-driven photocatalytic performance. *Colloid Surf. A* **2021**, *615*, 126063. [CrossRef]
77. Sayed, M.; Yu, J.G.; Liu, G.; Jaroniec, M. Non-noble plasmonic metal-based photocatalysts. *Chem. Rev.* **2022**, *122*, 10484–10537. [CrossRef]
78. Jin, Z.Z.; Li, J.R.; Zhang, Y.M.; Liu, D.; Ding, M.; Mamba, B.B.; Kuvarega, A.T.; Gui, J.Z. Rational design of efficient visible-light photocatalysts (1D@2D/0D) ZnO@Ni-doped BiOBr/Bi heterojunction: Considerations on hierarchical structures, doping and SPR effect. *J. Mater. Sci. Technol.* **2022**, *125*, 38–50. [CrossRef]
79. He, D.; Chen, Y.; Situ, Y.; Zhong, L.; Huang, H. Synthesis of ternary g-C$_3$N$_4$/Ag/-FeOOH photocatalyst: An integrated heterogeneous fenton-like system for effectively degradation of azo dye methyl orange under visible light. *Appl. Surf. Sci.* **2017**, *425*, 862–872. [CrossRef]
80. Liang, J.X.; Hou, Y.P.; Zhu, H.X.; Xiong, J.H.; Huang, W.Y.; Yu, Z.B.; Wang, S.F. Levofloxacin degradation performance and mechanism in the novel electro-Fenton system constructed with vanadium oxide electrodes under neutral pH. *Chem. Eng. J.* **2021**, *433*, 133574. [CrossRef]
81. Gong, Y.N.; Wang, Y.; Tang, M.M.; Zhang, H.; Wu, P.; Liu, C.J.; He, J.; Jiang, W. A two-step process coupling photocatalysis with adsorption to treat tetracycline-Copper(II) hybrid wastewaters, degradation mechanism, pathways and biotoxicity evaluation. *J. Water. Process. Eng.* **2022**, *47*, 102710. [CrossRef]
82. Chen, L.J.; Li, Y.H.; Zhang, J.W.; Li, M.X.; Yin, W.Y.; Chen, X. Oxidative degradation of tetracycline hydrochloride by Mn$_2$O$_3$/Bi$_2$O$_3$ photocatalysis activated peroxymonosulfate. *Inorg. Chem. Commun.* **2022**, *140*, 109414. [CrossRef]
83. Zhang, X.M.; Wang, H.; Gao, M.M.; Zhao, P.F.; Xia, W.L.; Yang, R.L.; Huang, Y.C.; Wang, L.; Liu, M.X.; Wei, T.; et al. Template-directed synthesis of pomegranate-shaped zinc oxide/zeolitic imidazolate framework for visible light photocatalytic degradation of tetracycline. *Chemosphere* **2022**, *294*, 133782. [CrossRef] [PubMed]
84. Yin, W.Q.; Cao, X.J.; Wang, B.; Jiang, Q.; Chen, Z.G.; Xia, J.X. In-situ synthesis of MoS$_2$/BiOBr material via mechanical ball milling for boosted photocatalytic degradation pollutants performance. *ChemistrySelect* **2021**, *6*, 928–936. [CrossRef]
85. Wu, S.Q.; Li, X.Y.; Tian, Y.Q.; Lin, Y.; Hu, Y.H. Excellent photocatalytic degradation of tetracycline over black anatase-TiO$_2$ under visible light. *Chem. Eng. J.* **2021**, *406*, 126747. [CrossRef]
86. Li, S.Y.; Tang, Y.W.; Wang, M.; Kang, J.; Jin, C.Y.; Liu, J.Y.; Li, Z.L.; Zhu, J.W. NiO/g-C$_3$N$_4$ 2D/2D heterojunction catalyst as efficient peroxymonosulfate activators toward tetracycline degradation: Characterization, performance and mechanism. *J. Alloys Compd.* **2021**, *880*, 160547. [CrossRef]
87. Shen, X.F.; Zhang, Y.; Shi, Z.; Shan, S.D.; Liu, J.S.; Zhang, L.S. Construction of C$_3$N$_4$/CdS nanojunctions on carbon fiber cloth as a filter-membrane-shaped photocatalyst for degrading flowing wastewater. *J. Alloys Compd.* **2021**, *851*, 156743. [CrossRef]
88. Ghoreishian, S.M.; Ranjith, K.S.; Lee, H.; Park, B.; Norouzi, M.; Nikoo, S.Z.; Kim, W.S.; Han, Y.K.; Huh, Y.S. Tuning the phase composition of 1D TiO$_2$ by Fe/Sn co-doping strategy for enhanced visible-light-driven photocatalytic and photoelectrochemical performances. *J. Alloys Compd.* **2021**, *851*, 156826. [CrossRef]
89. Jiang, H.; Wang, Q.; Chen, P.; Zheng, H.; Shi, J.; Shu, H.; Liu, Y. Photocatalytic degradation of tetracycline by using a regenerable (Bi)BiOBr/rGO composite. *J. Clean. Prod.* **2022**, *339*, 130771. [CrossRef]
90. Chen, Z.J.; Guo, H.; Liu, H.Y.; Niu, C.G.; Huang, D.W.; Yang, Y.Y.; Liang, C.; Li, L.; Li, J.C. Construction of dual S-scheme Ag$_2$CO$_3$/Bi$_4$O$_5$I$_2$/g-C$_3$N$_4$ heterostructure photocatalyst with enhanced visible-light photocatalytic degradation for tetracycline. *Chem. Eng. J.* **2022**, *438*, 135471. [CrossRef]
91. Cestaro, R.; Philippe, L.; Serrà, A.; Gómez, E.; Schmutz, P. Electrodeposited manganese oxides as efficient photocatalyst for the degradation of tetracycline antibiotics pollutant. *Chem. Eng. J.* **2023**, *462*, 142202. [CrossRef]
92. Mahmoodi, M.; Rafiee, E.; Eavani, S. Photocatalytic removal of toxic dyes, liquorice and tetracycline wastewaters by a mesoporous photocatalyst under irradiation of different lamps and sunlight. *J. Environ. Manag.* **2022**, *313*, 115023. [CrossRef] [PubMed]
93. Chen, Z.G.; Chen, X.L.; Di, J.; Liu, Y.L.; Yin, S.; Xia, J.X.; Li, H.M. Graphene-like boron nitride modified bismuth phosphate materials for boosting photocatalytic degradation of enrofloxacin. *J. Colloid Interface Sci.* **2017**, *492*, 51–60. [CrossRef] [PubMed]

94. Liu, Y.C.; Li, G.B.; Wang, D.; Zhong, Z.C.; Hu, K.B.; Zhang, C.Q.; Hu, G.P.; Li, X.W.; Wan, Y.H. Lanthanide-doped upconversion glass-ceramic photocatalyst fabricated from fluorine-containing waste for the degradation of organic pollutants. *J. Colloid Interface Sci.* **2023**, *638*, 461–473. [CrossRef]
95. Huang, J.X.; Li, D.G.; Li, R.B.; Chen, P.; Zhang, Q.X.; Liu, H.J.; Lv, W.Y.; Liu, G.G.; Feng, Y.P. One-step synthesis of phosphorus/oxygen co-doped g-C_3N_4/anatase TiO_2 Z-scheme photocatalyst for significantly enhanced visible-light photocatalysis degradation of enrofloxacin. *J. Hazard. Mater.* **2020**, *386*, 12. [CrossRef]
96. Wen, X.J.; Niu, C.G.; Zhang, L.; Liang, C.; Zeng, G.M. A novel Ag_2O/CeO_2 heterojunction photocatalysts for photocatalytic degradation of enrofloxacin: Possible degradation pathways; mineralization activity and an in depth mechanism insight. *Appl. Catal. B-Environ.* **2018**, *221*, 701–714. [CrossRef]
97. Cai, M.J.; Liu, Y.P.; Wang, C.C.; Lin, W.; Li, S.J. Novel $Cd_{0.5}Zn_{0.5}S/Bi_2MoO_6$ S-scheme heterojunction for boosting the photodegradation of antibiotic enrofloxacin: Degradation pathway; mechanism and toxicity assessment. *Sep. Purif. Technol.* **2023**, *304*, 11. [CrossRef]
98. Li, T.C.; Liu, J.X.; Shi, F.; Zhang, H.Y.; Zhang, H.J.; Ma, C.C.; Wasim, M. A novel S-type $Cs_xWO_3/BiOI$ heterojunction photocatalyst constructed in graphene aerogel with high degradation efficiency for enrofloxacin: Degradation mechanism and DFT calculation. *J. Environ. Chem. Eng.* **2023**, *11*, 109301. [CrossRef]
99. Xiao, L.Q.; Zhang, S.Y.; Chen, B.Q.; Wu, P.P.; Feng, N.D.; Deng, F.; Wang, Z. Visible-light photocatalysis degradation of enrofloxacin by crawfish shell biochar combined with g-C_3N_4: Effects and mechanisms. *J. Environ. Chem. Eng.* **2023**, *11*, 109693. [CrossRef]
100. Huang, P.Q.; Luan, J.F. Synthesis of a GaOOH/$ZnBiTaO_5$ heterojunction photocatalyst with enhanced photocatalytic performance toward enrofloxacin. *RSC Adv.* **2020**, *10*, 4286–4292. [CrossRef]
101. Sciscenko, I.; Mestre, S.; Climent, J.; Valero, F.; Escudero-Onate, C.; Oller, I.; Arques, A. Magnetic Photocatalyst for Wastewater Tertiary Treatment at Pilot Plant Scale: Disinfection and Enrofloxacin Abatement. *Water* **2021**, *13*, 12. [CrossRef]
102. Su, Y.H.; Chen, P.; Wang, F.L.; Zhang, Q.X.; Chen, T.S.; Wang, Y.F.; Yao, K.; Lv, W.Y.; Liu, G.G. Decoration of TiO_2/g-C_3N_4 Z-scheme by carbon dots as a novel photocatalyst with improved visible-light photocatalytic performance for the degradation of enrofloxacin. *RSC Adv.* **2017**, *7*, 34096–34103. [CrossRef]
103. Huang, P.Q.; Luan, J.F. Dispersed GaOOH rods loaded on the surface of $ZnBiNbO_5$ particles with enhanced photocatalytic activity toward enrofloxacin. *RSC Adv.* **2019**, *9*, 32027–32033. [CrossRef]
104. Yu, Y.Q.; Yan, L.; Cheng, J.M.; Jing, C.Y. Mechanistic insights into TiO_2 thickness in $Fe_3O_4@TiO_2$-GO composites for enrofloxacin photodegradation. *Chem. Eng. J.* **2017**, *325*, 647–654. [CrossRef]
105. Mahjoub, A.R.; Rahmani, H.; Khazaee, Z. Bimetallic CuAg alloyed nanoparticles anchored on CdS nanorods for the photocatalytic degradation of enrofloxacin. *ACS Appl. Nano. Mater.* **2023**, *6*, 4554–4566. [CrossRef]
106. Luan, J.F.; Liu, W.L.; Yao, Y.; Ma, B.B.; Niu, B.W.; Yang, G.M.; Wei, Z.J. Synthesis and Property Examination of $Er_2FeSbO_7/BiTiSbO_6$ Heterojunction Composite Catalyst and Light-Catalyzed Retrogradation of Enrofloxacin in Pharmaceutical Waste Water under Visible Light Irradiation. *Materials* **2022**, *15*, 26. [CrossRef] [PubMed]
107. Zhao, Y.J.; Liu, X.T.; Gu, S.N.; Liu, J.M. Enhanced photocatalytic performance of rhodamine B and enrofloxacin by Pt loaded $Bi_4V_2O_{11}$: Boosted separation of charge carriers; additional superoxide radical production; and the photocatalytic mechanism. *RSC Adv.* **2021**, *11*, 9746–9755. [CrossRef] [PubMed]
108. Tian, J.L.; Wu, S.; Liu, S.X.; Zhang, W. Photothermal enhancement of highly efficient photocatalysis with bioinspired thermal radiation balance characteristics. *Appl. Surf. Sci.* **2022**, *592*, 153304. [CrossRef]
109. Sane, P.K.; Rakte, D.; Tambat, S.; Bhalinge, R.; Sontakke, S.M.; Nemade, P. Enhancing solar photocatalytic activity of Bi_5O_7I photocatalyst with activated carbon heterojunction. *Adv. Powder. Technol.* **2022**, *33*, 103357. [CrossRef]
110. Harikumar, B.; Okla, M.K.; Alaraidh, I.A.; Mohebaldi, A.; Soufa, W.; Abdel-Maksoud, M.A.; Aufy, M.; Thomas, A.M.; Raju, L.L.; Khan, S. Robust visible light active $CoNiO_2$–$BiFeO_3$–NiS ternary nanocomposite for photo-fenton degradation of rhodamine B and methyl orange: Kinetics; degradation pathway and toxicity assessment. *J. Environ. Manag.* **2022**, *317*, 115321. [CrossRef] [PubMed]
111. Bi, H.F.; Liu, J.S.; Wu, Z.Y.; Zhu, K.J.; Suo, H.; Lv, X.L.; Fu, Y.L.; Jian, R.; Sun, Z.B. Construction of $Bi_2WO_6/ZnIn_2S_4$ with Z-scheme structure for efficient photocatalytic performance. *Chem. Phys. Lett.* **2021**, *769*, 138449. [CrossRef]
112. Van, N.U.; Thuy, N.P.; Hanh, V.N.; Loan, D.T.; Vuong, D.B.; Thao, T.T. Low-temperature designing of $BiVO_4$ nanocubes with coexposed {010}/{110} facets for solar light photocatalytic degradation of methyl orange and diazinon. *Inorg. Chem. Commun.* **2022**, *136*, 109136. [CrossRef]
113. Hieu, V.Q.; Phung, T.K.; Nguyen, T.; Khan, A.; Doan, V.D.; Tran, V.A.; Le, V.T. Photocatalytic degradation of methyl orange dye by Ti_3C_2-eTiO_2 heterojunction under solar light. *Chemosphere* **2021**, *276*, 130154. [CrossRef] [PubMed]
114. Wang, L.; Li, T.; Tao, L.L.; Lei, H.W.; Ma, P.Y.; Liu, J. A novel copper-doped porous carbon nanospheres film prepared by onestep ultrasonic spray pyrolytic of sugar for photocatalytic degradation of methyl orange. *Process. Saf. Environ.* **2022**, *158*, 79–86. [CrossRef]
115. Menon, S.G.; Bedyala, A.K.; Pathakc, T.; Kumara, V.; Swart, H.C. $Sr_4Al_{14}O_{25}$: Eu^{2+}, Dy^{3+}@ZnO nanocomposites as highly efficient visible light photocatalysts for the degradation of aqueous methyl orange. *J. Alloys Compd.* **2021**, *860*, 158370. [CrossRef]
116. Li, J.W.; He, M.Z.; Yan, J.K.; Liu, J.H.; Zhang, J.X.; Ma, J.J. Room temperature engineering crystal facet of Cu_2O for photocatalytic degradation of methyl orange. *Nanomaterials* **2022**, *10*, 1697. [CrossRef]

117. Kanakaraju, D.; Jasni, M.A.A.; Lim, Y.C. A highly photoresponsive and efficient molybdenum modifiedtitanium dioxide photocatalyst for the degradation of methyl orange. *Int. J. Environ. Sci. Technol.* **2022**, *19*, 5579–5594. [CrossRef]
118. Lu, G.F.; Liu, X.D.; Zhang, P.; Xu, S.T.; Gao, Y.J.; Yu, S.Y. Preparation and Photocatalytic Studies on Nanocomposites of 4-Hydroxylphenyl-Substituted Corrole/TiO$_2$ towards Methyl Orange Photodegradation. *ChemistrySelect* **2021**, *6*, 6841–6846. [CrossRef]
119. Kourab, P.; Mukherjee, S.P. CsPbBr$_3$/Cs$_4$PbBr$_6$ perovskite@COF nanocomposites for visible-light-driven photocatalytic applications in water. *J. Mater. Chem. A.* **2021**, *9*, 6819–6826.
120. Arumugam, M.; Seralathan, K.; Praserthdam, S.; Tahir, M.P. Synthesis of novel graphene aerogel encapsulated bismuth oxyiodide composite towards effective removal of methyl orange azo-dye under visible light. *Chemosphere* **2022**, *303*, 135121. [CrossRef]
121. Tang, H.D.; Zhang, W.J.; Meng, Y.; Xie, B.; Ni, Z.M.; Xia, S.J. Investigation onto the performance and mechanism of visible light photodegradation of methyl orange catalyzed by M/CeO$_2$ (M = Pt; Ag; Au). *Mater. Res. Bull.* **2021**, *144*, 111497. [CrossRef]
122. Aadnan, I.; Zegaoui, O.; Mragui, A.E.; Silva, J.C.G.E. Physicochemical and photocatalytic properties under visible light of ZnO-Bentonite/Chitosan hybrid-biocompositefor water remediation. *Nanomaterials* **2022**, *12*, 102. [CrossRef] [PubMed]

Disclaimer/Publisher's Note: The statements, opinions and data contained in all publications are solely those of the individual author(s) and contributor(s) and not of MDPI and/or the editor(s). MDPI and/or the editor(s) disclaim responsibility for any injury to people or property resulting from any ideas, methods, instructions or products referred to in the content.

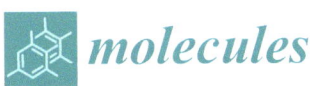

Article

In Situ Decoration of Bi$_2$S$_3$ Nanosheets on Zinc Oxide/Cellulose Acetate Composite Films for Photodegradation of Dyes under Visible Light Irradiation

Yixiao Dan [1,†], Jialiang Xu [1,†], Jian Jian [1,*], Lingxi Meng [1], Pei Deng [1], Jiaqi Yan [2,*], Zhengqiu Yuan [1], Yusheng Zhang [1] and Hu Zhou [1]

[1] Hunan Engineering Research Center for Functional Film Materials, School of Chemistry and Chemical Engineering, Hunan University of Science and Technology, Xiangtan 411201, China; dyx13536505551@gmail.com (Y.D.); isxujialiang@163.com (J.X.); lingximengqr@163.com (L.M.); dengpei0901@163.com (P.D.); yuanzhengqiu@126.com (Z.Y.); zys_2002@hotmail.com (Y.Z.); hnustchemzhou@163.com (H.Z.)

[2] Furong College, Hunan University of Arts and Science, Changde 415000, China

* Correspondence: jianjianjqr@126.com (J.J.); theyjq@outlook.com (J.Y.)

† These authors contributed equally to this work.

Abstract: A novel Bi$_2$S$_3$-zinc oxide/cellulose acetate composite film was prepared through a blending-wet phase conversion and in situ precipitate method. The results revealed that the incorporation of Bi$_2$S$_3$ in the film increased the cavity density and uniformity, which provided additional space for the growth of active species and improved the interaction between dye pollutants and active sites. Zinc oxide acted as a mediator to facilitate the separation of electron–hole pairs effectively preventing their recombination, thus reducing the photo-corrosion of Bi$_2$S$_3$. As a result, the Bi$_2$S$_3$-ZnO/CA composite film exhibited favorable photocatalytic activity in the degradation of various dyes. Additionally, the composite film displayed effortless separation and recovery without the need for centrifugation or filtration, while maintaining its exceptional catalytic performance even after undergoing various processes.

Keywords: cellulose acetate; ZnO; Bi$_2$S$_3$; photocatalytic; dye degradation

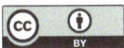

1. Introduction

The advancement of the textile industry has yielded economic affluence and societal equilibrium for humanity. Nevertheless, due to its highly polluting nature, the textile industry generates approximately 1.6 million liters of dyes per day [1–3]. This substantial dye consumption has resulted in a significant volume of dye wastewater, posing severe threats to both the ecological environment and human well-being [4,5]. Consequently, individuals have implemented diverse approaches, including biological, physical, and chemical methods, to effectively and safely treat dye wastewater [6]. The efficacy of conventional treatment methods is frequently constrained by the considerable persistence and solubility of synthetic dyes in water. There is a pressing need to establish economically viable and ecologically sound treatment approaches that can effectively address dye wastewater prior to its ultimate release into the environment. Photocatalytic technology, characterized by its straightforward procedural nature, gentle operating conditions, and environmentally friendly attributes, offers a viable solution by facilitating the degradation of organic pollutants in aqueous solutions into H$_2$O, CO$_2$, or other diminutive molecules [7–9]. However, the powdered photocatalyst tends to agglomerate during the process of photocatalysis, resulting in a challenge to separating and recycling. Additionally, this agglomeration can lead to secondary pollution in the water system, thereby limiting its effectiveness in degrading organic pollutants [10–12]. Therefore, it becomes imperative to develop an appropriate support substrate that can address these issues by facilitating the deposition of the catalyst [13].

Cellulose acetate (CA) is classified as a biopolymer, possessing notable attributes such as exceptional biocompatibility, biodegradability, robust mechanical strength, hydrophilicity, and film-forming capabilities. Consequently, it has found extensive applications in diverse sectors including medical care, packaging, textile, filtration, and various other domains [14–16]. However, the practical application of CA is impeded by its susceptibility to microbial attack, which poses a significant challenge. Despite the potential limitation of biofouling on CA films in water purification, the integration of nanotechnology and membrane loading technology presents a promising solution to overcome the drawbacks associated with cellulose acetate. Fu et al. [17] conducted a one-step coagulation process in Na_2SO_4 aqueous solutions to produce cellulose-based ZnO nanocomposite films. These films demonstrated remarkable UV-blocking properties and antibacterial activities. Similarly, Abad et al. [18] employed a phase inversion and co-precipitation method to create a CA/Au/ZnO film, which exhibited high photocatalytic activity and achieved a 95.28% degradation rate of Eosin Y pollutant. The incorporation of nanocomposite technology into fiber films can enhance their characteristics, thereby addressing their limitations and enabling their use as catalyst support substrates.

Bismuth sulfide (Bi_2S_3) is a promising candidate for contaminant removal, electrochemical energy conversion, and storage due to its electrical and optical properties [19–21]. Additionally, Bi_2S_3 possesses advantageous characteristics including an appropriate band gap (1.33 eV), strong visible light absorption capability, high carrier mobility, and non-toxicity [22]. Furthermore, Bi_2S_3 can be easily synthesized through a straightforward solution method at room temperature. However, the utilization of Bi_2S_3 as a sole photocatalyst encounters challenges due to its rapid recombination as a photogenerated electron–hole pair and photoinduced corrosion [23]. One approach to enhance the photocatalytic efficiency of Bi_2S_3 involves combining it with another photocatalytic semiconductor possessing suitable band positioning to mitigate the recombination efficiency of its photogenerated carriers. Sang et al. [24] constructed nanoflower-like Bi_2O_3/Bi_2S_3 heterojunctions that were fabricated through a one-step hydrothermal method, and obtained a removal rate of 99.72% for rhodamine B (RhB) and 91.80% for Cr(VI), respectively. Similarly, Lu et al. [25] synthesized nuclear-shell structure TiO_2/Bi_2S_3 heterojunctions using the coprecipitation method, and the results indicated that an optimal quantity of Bi_2S_3 could enhance the photocatalytic activity of TiO_2. The removal rate of methyl orange (MO) for TiO_2/Bi_2S_3 can reach 99% within 10 min under UV irradiation. Zinc oxide (ZnO) is a typical n-type semiconductor due to its wide band gap (3.37 eV) and the low cost of raw materials that have attracted people's attention in the field of ultraviolet detection [26,27]. The effective detection of UV light by a single ZnO is limited due to the rapid recombination of electron–hole pairs under illumination, which hinders its practical application [28,29]. It is possible to form a type-II band structure by matching the band positions between Bi_2S_3 and ZnO. Yuan et al. [30] successfully prepared a ZnO/Bi_2S_3 photocatalyst with a heterojunction structure using a solvothermal method for Cr(VI) removal and obtained a removal rate of 96% within 120 min under visible-light irradiation. It can be seen that the coupling of Bi_2S_3 with ZnO to form a heterostructure and stably loading it on the CA composite film present a novel and significant research idea for supported photocatalysts.

In this study, a novel stable Bi_2S_3-ZnO/CA composite film was successfully prepared by the blending-wet phase conversion and in situ synthesis method. SEM, XRD, XPS, and PL were used to characterize the morphology, phase structure, element valence, and electron–hole pair recombination ability of the prepared composite materials. The photocatalytic performance and stability of RhB as a model pollutant were evaluated in the presence of visible light. In addition, different dyes were tested under different conditions to determine the photocatalytic activity of the composite film, and the photocatalytic mechanism was speculated through the active species capture experiment.

2. Results and Discussion
2.1. Structural Characterization

The surface and internal structures of pure CA, ZnO/CA, Bi_2S_3/CA, and Bi_2S_3-ZnO/CA composite films were observed by FE-SEM characterization, and the results are shown in Figure 1. The surface images reveal a thickness of approximately 200 μm for the composite films. Figure 1(a_1–a_3) illustrate that the pure CA composite film exhibits a characteristic asymmetric structure comprising of sponge-like hollow fiber skin and irregular cavities [31,32]. Upon loading ZnO onto the CA film, as depicted in Figure 1(b_1–b_3), the surface of the composite film becomes smoother and the number of pores decreases significantly. Additionally, the rod-shaped ZnO is observed to extend from the interior to the exterior of the thin film, indicating a favorable integration between ZnO and CA [33]. As demonstrated in Figure 1(c_1–c_3), the Bi_2S_3 within the Bi_2S_3/CA composite film is observed to form a granular cluster on the film's surface. Furthermore, the incorporation of Bi_2S_3 enhances the density and uniformity of the cavities within the composite film. These cavities provide additional space for the growth of active species and enhance the contact efficiency between water pollutants and photocatalysts [34]. Figure 1(d_1–d_3) depict the notable alterations in the morphology and distribution of Bi_2S_3 within the Bi_2S_3-ZnO/CA composite film in the presence of ZnO. The incorporation of ZnO into the composite film leads to a notable improvement in surface smoothness and a significant reduction in pore density. Consequently, the ingress of S^{2-} ions generated by thioacetamide into the pores is impeded, resulting in a lower concentration of S^{2-} ions within the ZnO/CA composite compared to the pure CA film. The elevated concentration of S^{2-} ions would promote the formation of numerous crystal nuclei and facilitate rapid crystal growth, thereby favoring the aggregation of Bi_2S_3 into granular clusters under high S^{2-} ion concentrations. Conversely, Bi_2S_3 would gradually grow at low S^{2-} ion concentrations, giving rise to the formation of flaky Bi_2S_3 nanosheets. Similar results have been verified in the relevant literature [35,36]. Therefore, the Bi_2S_3-ZnO/CA composite film displays uniform Bi_2S_3 micro-nano flakes (thickness of 10 nm and width of approximately 70 nm) and is evenly distributed within the fibers of the composite film. The EDS map of the Bi_2S_3/ZnO-CA composite film, depicted in Figure 1(e_1–e_6), illustrates a homogeneous distribution of Zn, O, Bi, and S elements throughout the composite film. This finding further confirms the attachment of nanostructured Bi_2S_3 and ZnO to the internal surface of the composite film.

The composition and crystal structure of ZnO/CA and Bi_2S_3-ZnO/CA composite films were determined by XRD characterization. As shown in Figure 2, the strong diffraction peaks appearing at 31.77°, 34.42°, 36.25°, 47.54°, 56.60°, 62.86°, 67.96°, and 69.01° in the ZnO/CA composite film corresponded to the (100), (002), (101), (102), (110), (103), (112), and (201) crystal planes, respectively. These characteristic peaks corresponded to the body-centered cubic structure of ZnO (JCPDS No. 36-1451) [37]. The addition of Bi_2S_3 resulted in a weakening of the intensity of the ZnO diffraction peaks, particularly as the Bi_2S_3 load increased. The Bi_2S_3-containing composites have quite broad diffraction peaks; this may be due to the incorporation of Bi_2S_3 in the film which increased the cavity density and uniformity, resulting in the ZnO and Bi_2S_3 being evenly distributed inside the film. Especially Bi_2S_3 coated the surface of ZnO, leading to a reduction in the diffraction peak intensity of ZnO. Furthermore, extremely weak diffraction peaks at 24.93° were observed, which corresponded to the (130) crystal planes of Bi_2S_3 [38]. The fact that the diffraction peak of Bi_2S_3 was very weak might be due to the high distribution and small size of Bi_2S_3 particles, which was consistent with findings reported in the literature [39]. These results confirmed the successful synthesis of ZnO and Bi_2S_3 in CA composite film using the in situ precipitate method.

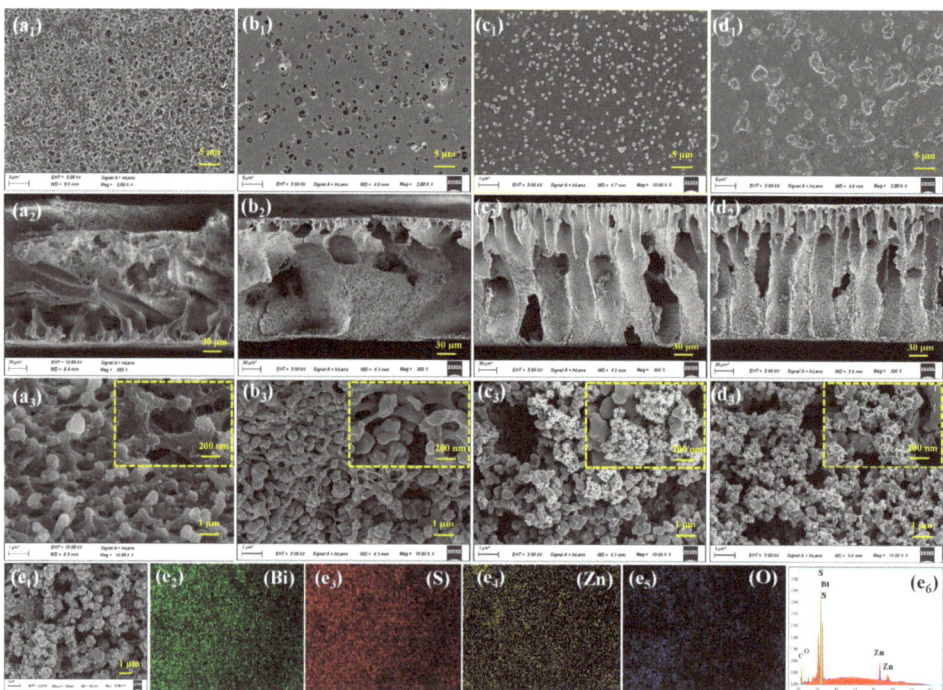

Figure 1. Surface and cross-sectional SEM images of CA (a_1–a_3), ZnO/CA (b_1–b_3), Bi_2S_3/CA (c_1–c_3), and Bi_2S_3-ZnO/CA (d_1–d_3) composite films, and EDS images of Bi_2S_3-ZnO/CA (e_1–e_6).

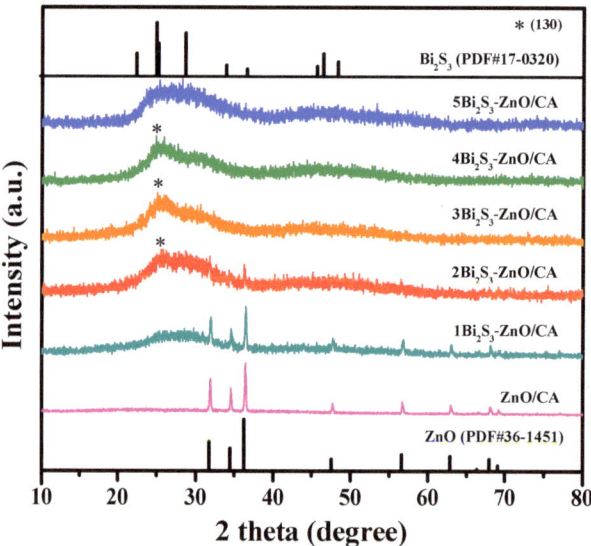

Figure 2. Typical XRD patterns of ZnO/CA and Bi_2S_3-ZnO/CA films.

Figure 3 displays the spectra of the pure CA, ZnO/CA, and Bi_2S_3-ZnO/CA composite films. The ZnO/CA spectrum exhibits characteristic peaks at 1747 cm^{-1}, 1237 cm^{-1}, 1371 cm^{-1}, and 1044 cm^{-1}, which correspond to N-H stretching vibration, C-H stretching vibration, -CH$_2$ symmetric stretching vibration, and free C=O stretching vibration and partial H-bonded carbonyl stretching vibration, respectively [40,41]. The absorption peak at 482 cm^{-1} is attributed to ZnO, while the peak at 3442 cm^{-1} is associated with the O-H stretching mode [42,43]. The FTIR spectra of the pure CA film exhibit a marked resemblance to those of the Bi$_2$S$_3$-ZnO/CA and the ZnO/CA composite film, suggesting that the incorporation of bismuth sulfide and zinc oxide does not result in the formation of novel bonds with the CA film, nor does it compromise the integrity of the film's structure.

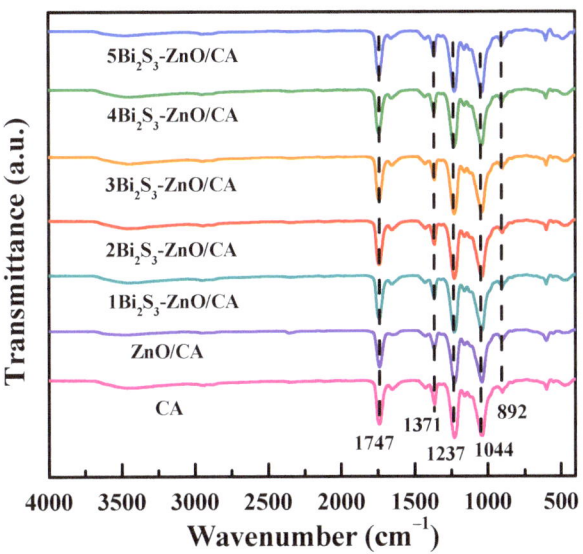

Figure 3. FTIR spectra of ZnO/CA and Bi$_2$S$_3$-ZnO/CA composite films.

The utilization of XPS spectroscopy facilitated the examination of the surface composition and chemical state of the Bi$_2$S$_3$-ZnO/CA sample, as depicted in Figure 4. The composite material is shown to contain Zn, Bi, S, O, and C elements, as demonstrated by the comprehensive spectrum presented in Figure 4a. Figure 4b displays two prominent peaks that are concentrated at 1043.65 and 1020.28 eV, with a binding energy difference of 23.37 eV, which corresponds to Zn 2p$_{1/2}$ and Zn 2p$_{3/2}$, respectively. These values align with the established reference values for ZnO [44]. In Figure 4c, the high-resolution X-ray photoelectron spectroscopy spectrum of oxygen is analyzed and fitted with two distinct peaks. The weaker peak observed at 530.98 eV is attributed to the solid-state lattice oxygen present in ZnO, while the stronger peak at 531.58 eV is assigned to the interaction between carbonyl oxygen atoms in CA [37]. The Bi 4f$_{7/2}$ and Bi 4f$_{5/2}$ orbitals corresponding to Bi^{3+} are also observed at 156.78 eV and 162.17 eV, respectively [29]. The XPS peak of sulfur observed in Figure 4e at 162.47 eV is consistent with the standard S 2p peak, providing evidence for the formation of Bi$_2$S$_3$. In Figure 4f, the spectra associated with C can be effectively modeled with four distinct peaks at 283.58 eV, 285.07 eV, 286.12 eV, and 287.59 eV, respectively, which correspond to H$_3$C(C=O), C-H, C-OH, and C-C-O in the CA structure [45,46]. These results not only confirm the successful synthesis of Bi2S3 but also suggest no alterations have occurred in ZnO. Additionally, the absence of any other impurities on the surface of the composite film indicates the relatively high purity of the synthesized Bi$_2$S$_3$ nanosheets.

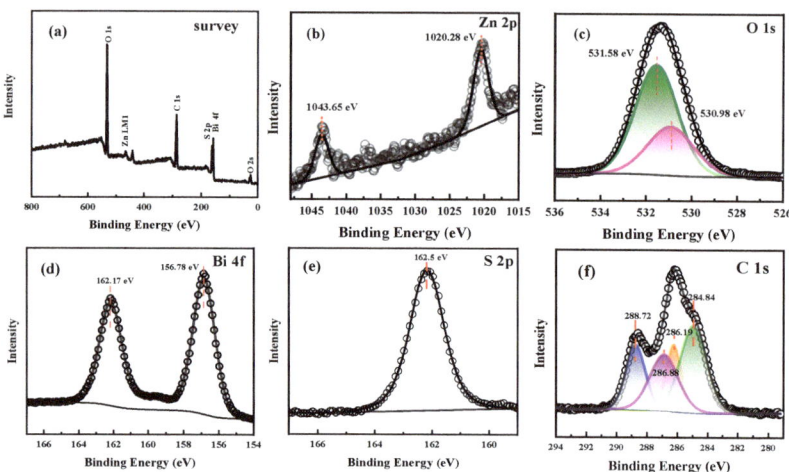

Figure 4. XPS spectra of 4Bi$_2$S$_3$-ZnO/CA composite: (**a**) survey, (**b**) Zn 2p, (**c**) O 1s, (**d**) Bi 4f, (**e**) S 2p, and (**f**) C 1s.

The optical properties of these composite films were investigated by UV-vis DRS. As illustrated in Figure 5a, both ZnO and Bi$_2$S$_3$ sensitization considerably broadened the spectrum of light absorption [47]. Notably, the Bi$_2$S$_3$ film with co-modification of ZnO and Bi$_2$S$_3$ exhibited superior visible light harvesting capabilities compared to the single Bi$_2$S$_3$ deposition, potentially due to the modulation of the bandgap by the sensitizer. The band gap width of Bi$_2$S$_3$-ZnO/CA composite film was calculated by the Tauc formula ($ahv = A(hv - E_g)^n$, where α, hv, A, and E_g were defined as the absorption coefficient, photonic energy, constant, and band gap, respectively. The n value was 1 because ZnO and Bi$_2$S$_3$ belong to direct bandgap semiconductors [48]. In Figure 5b, the calculated bandgap widths for ZnO/CA and Bi$_2$S$_3$/CA were 3.17 eV and 1.78 eV, respectively [49,50]. Additionally, the valence band (VB) and conduction band (CB) edge potentials of the ZnO/CA and Bi$_2$S$_3$/CA composite films were calculated using the empirical equations $E_{VB} = X - E_e + 0.5E_g$ and $E_{CB} = E_{VB} - E_g$. Here, E_{VB} and E_{CB} are the VB and CB edge potentials, respectively. E_e is the energy of the free electron versus hydrogen (4.5 eV), and E_g is the bandgap width. The X was the Mulliken electronegativity of the ZnO and Bi$_2$S$_3$ semiconductors, and was selected as 5.75 eV and 5.27 eV, respectively, according to the literature [49,50]. Therefore, the E_{VB} and E_{CB} values were approximately 2.84 eV and −0.34 eV (vs. NHE) for the ZnO/CA film, and 1.66 eV and −0.12 eV (vs. NHE) for the Bi$_2$S$_3$/CA film.

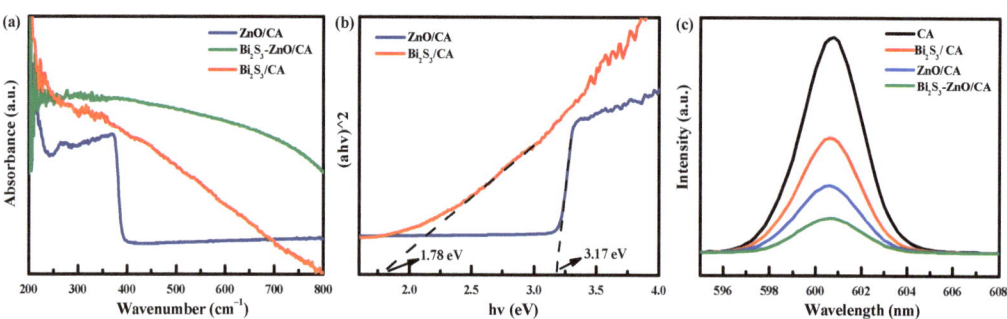

Figure 5. UV-vis DRS spectra (**a**,**b**) and PL spectra (**c**) of CA, CA/Bi$_2$S$_3$, ZnO/CA, and Bi$_2$S$_3$-ZnO/CA composite films.

Photoluminescence spectroscopy (PL) was also utilized to examine the efficacy of electron–hole pair recombination and separation in composite films. Generally, greater fluorescence intensity denotes accelerated electron–hole pair recombination rates, whereas lower fluorescence intensity signifies heightened separation efficiency [51]. Elevated electron recombination rates are disadvantageous for photocatalytic reactions. The photoluminescence spectra of pure CA, ZnO/CA, Bi_2S_3/CA, and Bi_2S_3-ZnO/CA composite films are presented in Figure 5c. ZnO/CA and Bi_2S_3/CA films exhibit an absorption peak at approximately 601 nm, while Bi_2S_3-ZnO/CA displays a lower resolution exciton absorption peak. The results suggest that the combination of ZnO and Bi_2S_3 mitigates the recombination of photo-induced electron–hole pairs and enhances the efficiency of charge separation, thereby augmenting the photocatalytic activity of the catalyst.

2.2. Photocatalytic Efficiency

The photocatalytic performance of Bi_2S_3-ZnO/CA composite films was evaluated through the degradation of RhB as a model pollutant, as depicted in Figure 6a. The absence of a photocatalyst and the sole use of a pure CA film resulted in a negligible degradation of RhB, indicating that the self-degradation effect of RhB and the adsorption effect of the CA film can be disregarded. The degradation rate of single-component ZnO/CA composite film was 26.51%, which might be attributed to the good hydrophilicity of ZnO improving the adsorption capacity of RhB. The single-component $4Bi_2S_3$/CA composite film exhibited a higher degradation rate of 50.26%, indicating that Bi_2S_3 has a favorable photocatalytic activity for RhB. The addition of ZnO and Bi_2S_3 to the CA composite film can significantly improve the photocatalytic performance, and the catalytic performance is gradually increased with the increase in the Bi_2S_3 loading. The highest degradation rate of 90.2% was achieved with the $4Bi_2S_3$-ZnO/CA film as the catalyst. Notably, a further increase in Bi_2S_3 loading led to a decline in photocatalytic efficiency. The possible reason might be that the particle aggregation at high loading resulted in a reduction in the effective active species on the composite film and a subsequent decrease in photocatalytic performance. In the Bi_2S_3-ZnO/CA catalyst, Bi_2S_3 is deemed as the primary active constituent due to its superior photocatalytic activity compared to ZnO/CA. However, ZnO acts as a mediator to facilitate the separation of electron–hole pairs, effectively preventing their recombination, thus reducing the photo-corrosion of Bi_2S_3. Consequently, this mechanism significantly enhances the overall photocatalytic efficiency.

To further investigate the degradation kinetics of RhB, a pseudo-first-order kinetic model has been employed for exploration, as illustrated in Equation (3.2): $\ln(C_0/C) = kt$ (3.2). In this equation, C_0 and C denote the initial concentration and real-time concentration of RhB, respectively, while k represents the apparent reaction rate constant under irradiation. The results of the fitting indicated that it conformed to a quasi-first-order kinetic equation. The kinetic curves of ZnO/CA, $4Bi_2S_3$/CA, and Bi_2S_3-ZnO/CA composite films are presented in Figure 6b. The apparent reaction rate constant of the $4Bi_2S_3$-ZnO/CA composite film was determined to be 0.0175 min^{-1}, which exhibited 8.8 and 4.7 times higher values compared to the single-phase ZnO/CA (0.00198 min^{-1}) and $4Bi_2S_3$/CA (0.00372 min^{-1}) films, respectively. These results suggested that the synergistic effect of ZnO and Bi_2S_3 could significantly augment the photocatalytic efficiency of the composite film. Figure 6c depicts the dynamic absorbance spectra of the RhB solution on the $4Bi_2S_3$-ZnO/CA composite film under visible light irradiation. The absorbance at the maximum absorption wavelength (553 nm) of the RhB solution was gradually diminished over time and reached a negligible level after 120 min, indicating the degradation of RhB in the solution without any production of other derivatives during the photocatalysis process. Figure 6d displays the durability of the Bi_2S_3-ZnO/CA composite film in the photodegradation of RhB. The results indicated that the Bi_2S_3-ZnO/CA composite film exhibited excellent performance stability, as evidenced by the sustained degradation rate of RhB at 88% over five cycles. Additionally, the composite film can be retrieved from the aqueous phase without the requirement of centrifugal filtration, thereby preventing the loss of nanoparticles and minimizing the risk of secondary pollution, which is advantageous for the practical implementation of photocatalysis technology.

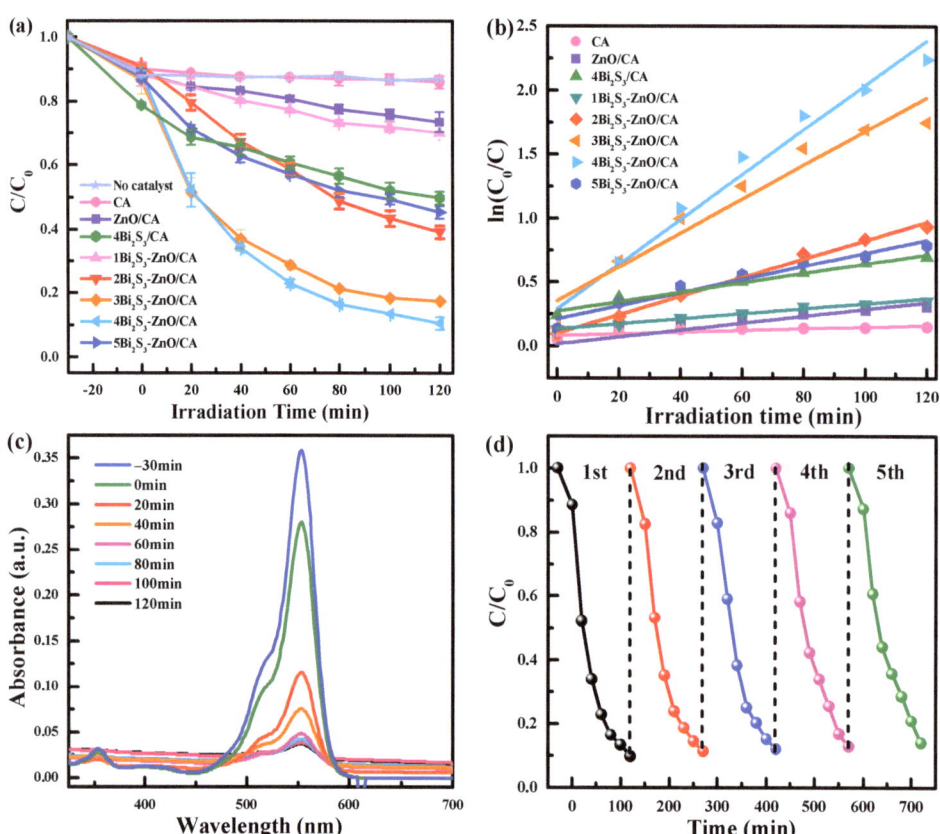

Figure 6. Photocatalytic performance of CA, ZnO/CA, Bi$_2$S$_3$/CA, and Bi$_2$S$_3$-ZnO/CA composite films with different Bi$_2$S$_3$ loading for the degradation of RhB under visible light irradiation (**a**); related degradation rate (ln(C$_0$/C) = kt) plots (**b**); absorption spectrum of RhB solution in the presence of 4Bi$_2$S$_3$-ZnO/CA composite film (**c**); and cycle runs over 4Bi$_2$S$_3$-ZnO/CA degradation of RhB under visible light irradiation (**d**).

Figure 7a illustrates the degradation rate of RhB by a Bi$_2$S$_3$-ZnO/CA composite film under visible light conditions and varying pH levels. The photocatalytic removal rates for RhB were determined to be 91.98%, 90.16%, and 90.35% in acidic, neutral, and alkaline solutions, respectively, which suggested that the Bi$_2$S$_3$-ZnO/CA composite film exhibited commendable photocatalytic performance for RhB degradation across a broad pH range. The photodegradation of various dyes in the Bi$_2$S$_3$-ZnO/CA composite film was also investigated and the results are presented in Figure 7b. The removal rates of RhB, malachite green (MG), methylene blue (MB), and crystal violet (CV) were 90.16%, 88.85%, 86.88%, and 87.20%, respectively. These results suggested that the Bi$_2$S$_3$-ZnO/CA composite film exhibited a universal capacity for dye pollutant treatment. Furthermore, the aforementioned dyes demonstrated commendable photocatalytic efficacy in the presence of natural light (the sunlight between 2:00 p.m. and 4:00 p.m. on a sunny day with a PM 2.5 of 26 micrograms per cubic meter in Xiangtan, Hunan, China). The solar insolation was measured and recorded by an optical power meter. Notably, RhB and CV exhibited a degradation efficiency reduction of merely 2% and 4% in comparison to simulating visible light. In addition, the photocatalytic activity of the Bi_2S_3-ZnO/CA composite film is slightly lower than that reported in other related studies (Table 1). This may be due to the better mass transfer effect of the powder compared to the film. However, composite film materials have better practical application prospects because of their easy separation and recovery in dye wastewater treatment.

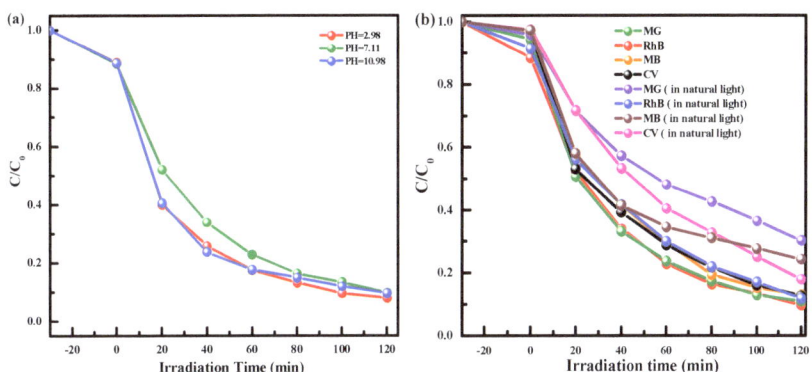

Figure 7. Effect of pH for the photodegradation of RhB on the 4Bi_2S_3-ZnO/CA composite film (**a**); degradation of different dyes by the 4Bi_2S_3-ZnO/CA composite film under a xenon lamp and natural light conditions (**b**).

Table 1. Performance of different Bi_2S_3-based composites for the photodegradation of dyes under visible light.

Photocatalyst	Photocatalyst Form	Catalyst Dosage /(g/L)	Dye Concentration /(mg/L)	Time /min	pH Levels	Degradation Rate/min	Ref.
Bi_2S_3-BiOI	powder	1.0	10.0-RhB	60	8–9	>99.0	[21]
SnO_2/Bi_2S_3-Bi25	powder	0.33	10.0-RhB	180	8–9	>80.0	[23]
Bi_2O_3-Bi_2S_3	powder	0.5	20.0-RhB	90	8–9	>99.0	[24]
TiO_2-Bi_2S_3	powder	5.0	20.0-MO	10	3–4	>99.0	[25]
Bi_2S_3-BiOBr/TiO_2 NTA	powder	0.05	20.0-RhB	180	8–9	>98.0	[35]
Bi_2S_3-ZnO/CA	film	1.0	10.0-RhB	120	3–11	>90.0	This work

To ascertain the photocatalytic degradation mechanism, radical-trapping experiments were conducted utilizing isopropanol (IPA), triethanolamine (TEOA), and 4-hydroxy-TEMPO (TEMPO) as scavengers for hydroxyl groups (•OH), holes (h^+), and superoxide radicals (•O_2^-), respectively [52,53]. Figure 8 demonstrates that the inclusion of IPA had negligible impact on the degradation of RhB, thereby suggesting that •OH played a minor role in the photodegradation of RhB by the Bi_2S_3-ZnO/CA composite film. Conversely, the presence of TEOA and TEMPO resulted in a substantial inhibition of the RhB degradation, indicating that h^+ and •O_2^- were the primary active components responsible for the photocatalytic degradation of RhB by the Bi_2S_3-ZnO/CA composite film.

Based on the aforementioned results, the potential mechanism for the photodegradation of RhB by the Bi_2S_3/ZnO-CA composite film was hypothesized, as illustrated in Scheme 1. When exposed to visible light, both the ZnO and Bi_2S_3 particles present in the film were stimulated to generate electrons and holes in their respective conduction and valence bands. Due to the more negative conduction band (CB) energy of ZnO (−0.34 eV/NHE) compared to that of Bi_2S_3 (−0.12 eV/NHE), the photogenerated electrons in ZnO readily migrated to the CB of Bi_2S_3, where they were scavenged by the available surface O_2 to produce $\bullet O_2^-$ radicals [54]. Simultaneously, the photogenerated holes in ZnO migrated to the valence band (VB) of Bi_2S_3 due to the higher VB energy of ZnO (+2.84 eV/NHE) compared to Bi_2S_3 (+1.66 eV/NHE). The abundant concentration of reactive holes in the Bi_2S_3 VB effectively oxidizes the dye [55]. The strong oxidation ability of these holes and $\bullet O_2^-$ radicals can over-decompose RhB into harmless molecules such as CO_2 and H_2O. As a result, the separation of electron–hole pairs is efficiently achieved, leading to a significant reduction in charge recombination and an enhancement in the photocatalytic activity of the composite film.

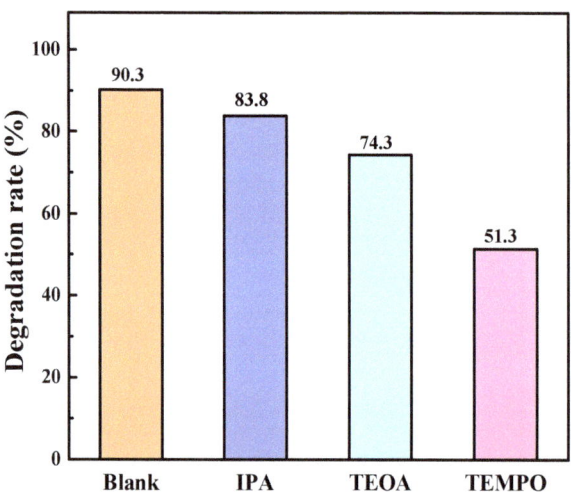

Figure 8. Trapping experiment of the active species over the Bi_2S_3-ZnO/CA composite film for RhB degradation.

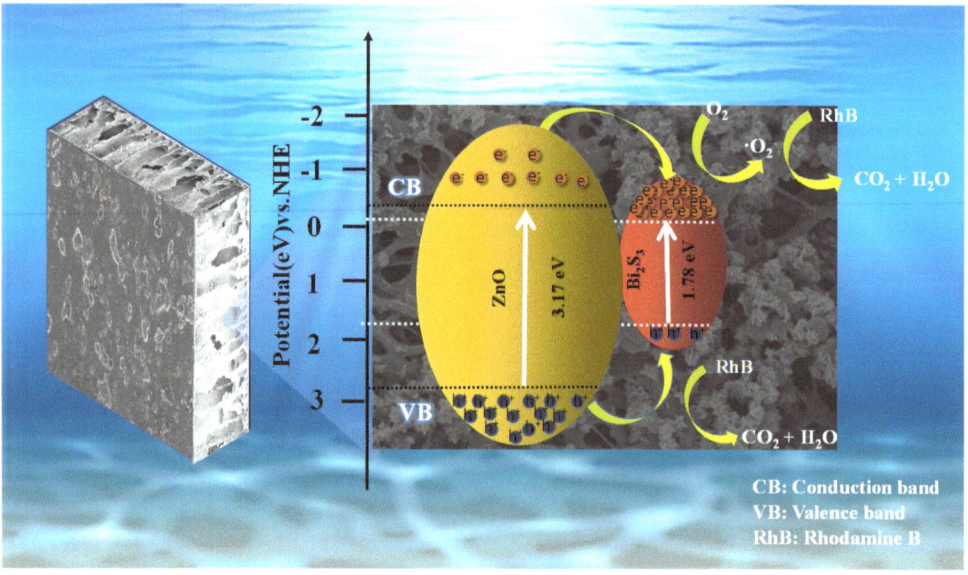

Scheme 1. Catalytic mechanism of RhB degradation by Bi_2S_3-ZnO/CA composite film.

3. Experimental Section

3.1. Synthesis of Bi_2S_3-ZnO/CA Composite Films

The Bi_2S_3-ZnO/CA composite films were prepared by blending-wet phase conversion and in situ precipitate method [53,56]; the detailed steps are presented in Scheme 2. Typically, 2 g CA, 1 g ZnO, and $Bi(NO_3)_3 \cdot 5H_2O$ at different quantities (1, 2, 3, 4, and 5 g) were successively added to the 20 g DMF solvent with vigorous stirring at room temperature for 2 h. The obtained uniformly mixed solution was held in the air for 30 min to eliminate bubbles. Subsequently, the mixture was cast evenly on the glass mold, and quickly immersed in thioacetamide solutions (equimolar with $Bi(NO_3)_3 \cdot 5H_2O$) for 8 h to the in situ synthesis of Bi_2S_3-ZnO/CA composite films [35]. Afterward, the resultant composite films were rinsed with ethanol and deionized water several times, and subsequently dried overnight at −40 °C in a freeze-drying oven. Based on the content of $Bi(NO_3)_3 \cdot 5H_2O$, the acquired films were labeled as $1Bi_2S_3$-ZnO/CA, $2Bi_2S_3$-ZnO/CA, $3Bi_2S_3$-ZnO/CA, $4Bi_2S_3$-ZnO/CA, and $5Bi_2S_3$-ZnO/CA, respectively. By comparison, the pure CA, ZnO/CA, and Bi_2S_3/CA films were also prepared using the same methods.

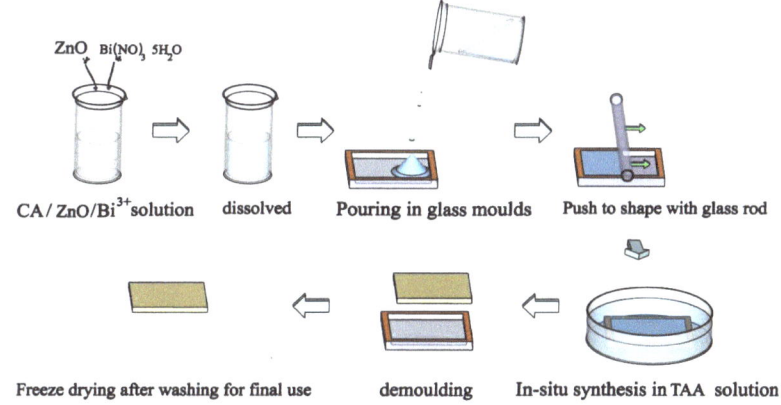

Scheme 2. The preparation process for the synthesis of Bi_2S_3-ZnO/CA composite films.

3.2. Characterization

The crystal structures of the composite films were analyzed using the X-ray diffraction (XRD) measurement on a Brucker AXS D8-Advance with Cu-Kα irradiation. The morphology of the samples was observed by Field Emission Scanning Electron Microscopy (FE-SEM, Zeiss Sigma 300). FT-IR spectra were recorded using a Brucker TENSORII FT-IR spectrometer from 4000 to 400 cm^{-1}. Surface electronic states were detected using X-ray photoelectron spectroscopy (XPS) using a K-Alpha 1063, and all binding energies were corrected by a C1s peak at 284.8 eV. The composite films' UV-vis diffuse reflectance spectra (DRS) were obtained using a Shimadzu UV-2550 spectrophotometer. The recombination of electron–hole pairs was explored using photoluminescence spectroscopy (PL) on HitachiF-2700.

3.3. Evaluation of Photocatalytic Activity

The photocatalytic activities of composite films were evaluated by the degradation of dyes under visible light illumination using a 300W Xe lamp equipped with a UV cutoff filter (λ between 420 and 800 nm). Generally, 0.2 g of catalyst was added to a condensation reactor containing 200 mL of RhB (10 mg/L). The suspension was continuously stirred for 30 min in the dark to achieve an adsorption–desorption equilibrium between the composite film and RhB-simulated liquid. Then, the mixture was subjected to photocatalysis using a xenon-mercury parallel light source. During the photocatalytic reaction, 10 mL of the reaction solution was sampled every 20 min. The residual concentration of RhB was measured using a UV-visible spectrophotometer at the maximum absorption wavelength. In addition, hydroxyl (•OH), holes (h^+), and superoxide radicals (•O_2^-) were detected with IPA, TEOA, and TEMPO in this photocatalytic reaction, respectively.

4. Conclusions

In summary, a novel Bi_2S_3/ZnO-CA composite film was successfully prepared through the blending-wet phase conversion and in situ precipitate techniques. The results indicated that the incorporation of ZnO induced a notable modification in the configuration and dispersion of Bi_2S_3 particles, transitioning from clustered nanospheres to evenly distributed nanosheets. Furthermore, ZnO acted as a mediator for the separation of electron–hole pairs, effectively impeding the recombination of photo-generated electron–hole pairs and mitigating the photo-corrosion of sulfides. Among the catalysts, the 4Bi_2S_3/ZnO-CA composite film showed the best photocatalytic activity with a 90.16% RhB degradation rate. More importantly, the composite film presented advantages in terms of operational simplicity, facile recovery, and the elimination of secondary pollution compared to powder-type photocatalysts, rendering it an efficient and versatile material for wastewater treatment.

Author Contributions: Y.D.: writing—original draft preparation and software. J.X.: investigation and formal analysis. J.J.: writing—review and editing, funding acquisition, and resources. L.M.: data curation. P.D.: methodology. J.Y.: conceptualization and supervision. Z.Y.: visualization. Y.Z.: validation. H.Z.: project administration. All authors have read and agreed to the published version of the manuscript.

Funding: This work was funded by the National Natural Science Foundation of China (22202068), the Natural Science Foundation in Hunan Province (2021JJ30239), and the Natural Science Foundation for Distinguished Young Scholars in Hunan Province (2020JJ2014).

Institutional Review Board Statement: Not applicable.

Informed Consent Statement: Not applicable.

Data Availability Statement: The data in this study are available from the corresponding author upon reasonable request.

Conflicts of Interest: The authors declare that they have no known competing financial interests or personal relationships that could have appeared to influence the work reported in this paper.

Sample Availability: Samples of some compounds may be available from the authors.

References

1. Uddin, F. Environmental hazard in textile dyeing wastewater from local textile industry. *Cellulose* **2021**, *28*, 10715–10739. [CrossRef]
2. Zhang, L.; Meng, Y.; Xie, B.; Ni, Z.; Xia, S. Br doping promotes the transform of Cu_2O (100) to Cu_2O (111) and facilitates efficient photocatalytic degradation of tetracycline. *Mol. Catal.* **2023**, *548*, 113431. [CrossRef]
3. Zhang, L.; Chen, L.; Xia, Y.; Liang, Z.; Huang, R.; Liang, R.; Yan, G. Modification of polymeric carbon nitride with Au–CeO_2 hybrids to improve photocatalytic activity for hydrogen evolution. *Molecules* **2022**, *27*, 7489. [CrossRef] [PubMed]
4. Kesraoui, A.; Selmi, T.; Seffen, M.; Brouers, F. Influence of alternating current on the adsorption of indigo carmine. *Environ. Sci. Pollut. Res.* **2017**, *24*, 9940–9950. [CrossRef]
5. Sarma, G.K.; Gupta, S.S.; Bhattacharyya, K.G. RETRACTED: Adsorption of Crystal violet on raw and acid-treated montmorillonite, K10, in aqueous suspension. *J. Environ. Manag.* **2016**, *171*, 1–10. [CrossRef]
6. Barisci, S.; Inan, H.; Turkay, O.; Dimoglo, A.; Erol, D. Degradation of toxic indigo carmine dye by electrosynthesized ferrate (VI). *J. Appl. Solut. Chem. Model.* **2017**, *6*, 75–83. [CrossRef]
7. Ibrahim, Y.O.; Gondal, M. Visible-light-driven photocatalytic performance of a Z-scheme based TiO_2/WO_3/g-C_3N_4 ternary heterojunctions. *Mol. Catal.* **2021**, *505*, 111494. [CrossRef]
8. Gupta, V.K.; Jain, R.; Mittal, A.; Saleh, T.A.; Nayak, A.; Agarwal, S.; Sikarwar, S. Photo-catalytic degradation of toxic dye amaranth on TiO_2/UV in aqueous suspensions. *Mater. Sci. Eng. C* **2012**, *32*, 12–17. [CrossRef]
9. Yu, Z.; Qian, L.; Zhong, T.; Ran, Q.; Huang, J.; Hou, Y.; Li, F.; Li, M.; Sun, Q.; Zhang, H. Enhanced visible light photocatalytic activity of CdS through controllable self-assembly compositing with ZIF-67. *Mol. Catal.* **2020**, *485*, 110797. [CrossRef]
10. Wu, G.; Liang, R.; Ge, M.; Sun, G.; Zhang, Y.; Xing, G. Surface passivation using 2D perovskites toward efficient and stable perovskite solar cells. *Adv. Mater.* **2022**, *34*, 2105635. [CrossRef]

11. Ge, M.; Cao, C.; Huang, J.; Li, S.; Chen, Z.; Zhang, K.-Q.; Al-Deyab, S.; Lai, Y. A review of one-dimensional TiO$_2$ nanostructured materials for environmental and energy applications. *J. Mater. Chem. A* **2016**, *4*, 6772–6801. [CrossRef]
12. Wang, Y.; Liu, Z.; Li, Y.; Yang, X.; Zhao, L.; Peng, J. Boosting Photocatalytic Performance of ZnO Nanowires via Building Heterojunction with g-C$_3$N$_4$. *Molecules* **2023**, *28*, 5563. [CrossRef] [PubMed]
13. Zhang, S.; Yan, Y.; Hu, W.; Fan, Y. Mesoporous CuO Prepared in a Natural Deep Eutectic Solvent Medium for Effective Photodegradation of Rhodamine B. *Molecules* **2023**, *28*, 5554. [CrossRef] [PubMed]
14. Jatoi, A.W.; Khatri, Z.; Ahmed, F.; Memon, M.H. Effect of silicone nano, nano/micro and nano/macro-emulsion softeners on color yield and physical characteristics of dyed cotton fabric. *J. Surfactants Deterg.* **2015**, *18*, 205–211. [CrossRef]
15. Wang, X.; Zhao, Y.; Li, F.; Dou, L.; Li, Y.; Zhao, J.; Hao, Y. A chelation strategy for in-situ constructing surface oxygen vacancy on {001} facets exposed BiOBr nanosheets. *Sci. Rep.* **2016**, *6*, 24918. [CrossRef]
16. Wang, M.; Ge, R.; Zhao, P.; Williams, G.R.; Yu, D.; Bligh, S.A. Exploring wettability difference-driven wetting by utilizing electrospun chimeric Janus microfiber comprising cellulose acetate and polyvinylpyrrolidone. *Mater. Des.* **2023**, *226*, 111652. [CrossRef]
17. Fu, F.; Li, L.; Liu, L.; Cai, J.; Zhang, Y.; Zhou, J.; Zhang, L. Construction of cellulose based ZnO nanocomposite films with antibacterial properties through one-step coagulation. *ACS Appl. Mater. Interfaces* **2015**, *7*, 2597–2606. [CrossRef]
18. Abad, S.N.K.; Mozammel, M.; Moghaddam, J.; Mostafaei, A.; Chmielus, M. Highly porous, flexible and robust cellulose acetate/Au/ZnO as a hybrid photocatalyst. *Appl. Surf. Sci.* **2020**, *526*, 146237. [CrossRef]
19. Mahapatra, A.D.; Basak, D. Enhanced ultraviolet photosensing properties in Bi$_2$S$_3$ nanoparticles decorated ZnO nanorods' heterostructure. *J. Alloys Compd.* **2019**, *797*, 766–774. [CrossRef]
20. Luo, W.; Li, F.; Li, Q.; Wang, X.; Yang, W.; Zhou, L.; Mai, L. Heterostructured Bi$_2$S$_3$-Bi$_2$O$_3$ nanosheets with a built-in electric field for improved sodium storage. *ACS Appl. Mater. Interfaces* **2018**, *10*, 7201–7207. [CrossRef]
21. Ju, P.; Zhang, Y.; Hao, L.; Cao, J.; Zhai, X.; Dou, K.; Jiang, F.; Sun, C. 1D Bi$_2$S$_3$ nanorods modified 2D BiOI nanoplates for highly efficient photocatalytic activity: Pivotal roles of oxygen vacancies and Z-scheme heterojunction. *J. Mater. Sci. Technol.* **2023**, *142*, 45–59. [CrossRef]
22. Huang, W.; Xing, C.; Wang, Y.; Li, Z.; Wu, L.; Ma, D.; Dai, X.; Xiang, Y.; Li, J.; Fan, D. Facile fabrication and characterization of two-dimensional bismuth (III) sulfide nanosheets for high-performance photodetector applications under ambient conditions. *Nanoscale* **2018**, *10*, 2404–2412. [CrossRef]
23. Fenelon, E.; Bui, D.; Tran, H.H.; You, S.; Wang, Y.; Cao, T.; Van Pham, V. Straightforward synthesis of SnO$_2$/Bi$_2$S$_3$/BiOCl-Bi$_{24}$O$_{31}$C$_{l10}$ composites for drastically enhancing rhodamine B photocatalytic degradation under visible light. *ACS Omega* **2020**, *5*, 20438–20449. [CrossRef] [PubMed]
24. Sang, Y.; Cao, X.; Dai, G.; Wang, L.; Peng, Y.; Geng, B. Facile one-pot synthesis of novel hierarchical Bi$_2$O$_3$/Bi$_2$S$_3$ nanoflower photocatalyst with intrinsic pn junction for efficient photocatalytic removals of RhB and Cr (VI). *J. Hazard. Mater.* **2020**, *381*, 120942. [CrossRef]
25. Lu, J.; Han, Q.; Wang, Z. Synthesis of TiO$_2$/Bi$_2$S$_3$ heterojunction with a nuclear-shell structure and its high photocatalytic activity. *Mater. Res. Bull.* **2012**, *47*, 1621–1624. [CrossRef]
26. Ouyang, W.; Teng, F.; Jiang, M.; Fang, X. ZnO film UV photodetector with enhanced performance: Heterojunction with CdMoO$_4$ microplates and the hot electron injection effect of Au nanoparticles. *Small* **2017**, *13*, 1702177. [CrossRef]
27. Tian, C.; Zhang, Q.; Wu, A.; Jiang, M.; Liang, Z.; Jiang, B.; Fu, H. Cost-effective large-scale synthesis of ZnO photocatalyst with excellent performance for dye photodegradation. *Chem. Commun.* **2012**, *48*, 2858–2860. [CrossRef]
28. Bai, Z.; Fu, M.; Zhang, Y. Vertically aligned and ordered ZnO/CdS nanowire arrays for self-powered UV-visible photosensing. *J. Mater. Sci.* **2017**, *52*, 1308–1317. [CrossRef]
29. Yi, S.; Zhao, F.; Yue, X.; Wang, D.; Lin, Y. Enhanced solar light-driven photocatalytic activity of BiOBr-ZnO heterojunctions with effective separation and transfer properties of photo-generated chargers. *New J. Chem.* **2015**, *39*, 6659–6666. [CrossRef]
30. Yuan, X.; Wu, X.; Feng, Z.; Jia, W.; Zheng, X.; Li, C. Facile synthesis of heterojunctioned ZnO/Bi$_2$S$_3$ nanocomposites for enhanced photocatalytic reduction of aqueous Cr (VI) under visible-light irradiation. *Catalysts* **2019**, *9*, 624. [CrossRef]
31. Zhou, Z.; Peng, X.; Zhong, L.; Wu, L.; Cao, X.; Sun, R.C. Electrospun cellulose acetate supported Ag@AgCl composites with facet-dependent photocatalytic properties on degradation of organic dyes under visible-light irradiation. *Carbohydr. Polym.* **2016**, *136*, 322–328. [CrossRef] [PubMed]
32. Ai, Z.; Ho, W.; Lee, S. Efficient visible light photocatalytic removal of NO with BiOBr-graphene nanocomposites. *J. Phys. Chem. C* **2011**, *115*, 25330–25337. [CrossRef]
33. Qaiser, A.A.; Hyland, M.M.; Patterson, D.A. Surface and charge transport characterization of polyaniline-cellulose acetate composite membranes. *J. Phys. Chem. B* **2011**, *115*, 1652–1661. [CrossRef] [PubMed]
34. Naeem, H.; Tofil, H.M.; Soliman, M.; Hai, A.; Zaidi, S.H.H.; Kizilbash, N.; Alruwaili, D.; Ajmal, M.; Siddiq, M. Reduced graphene oxide-zinc sulfide nanocomposite decorated with silver nanoparticles for wastewater treatment by adsorption, photocatalysis and antimicrobial action. *Molecules* **2023**, *28*, 926. [CrossRef]
35. Jia, Y.; Liu, P.; Wang, Q.; Wu, Y.; Cao, D.; Qiao, Q.A. Construction of Bi$_2$S$_3$-BiOBr nanosheets on TiO$_2$ NTA as the effective photocatalysts: Pollutant removal, photoelectric conversion and hydrogen generation. *J. Colloid Inter. Sci.* **2021**, *585*, 459–469. [CrossRef]

36. Pan, L.; Yao, L.; Mei, H.; Liu, H.; Jin, Z.; Zhou, S.; Zhang, M.; Zhu, G.; Cheng, L.; Zhang, L. Structurally designable Bi_2S_3/P-doped ZnO S-scheme photothermal metamaterial enhanced CO_2 reduction. *Sep. Purif. Technol.* **2023**, *312*, 123365. [CrossRef]
37. Fang, L.; Zhang, B.; Li, W.; Li, X.; Xin, T.; Zhang, Q. Controllable synthesis of ZnO hierarchical architectures and their photocatalytic property. *Superlattices Microstruct.* **2014**, *75*, 324–333. [CrossRef]
38. Zeng, L.; Zhao, H.; Zhu, Y.; Chen, S.; Zhang, Y.; Wei, D.; Sun, J.; Fan, H. A one-pot synthesis of multifunctional Bi_2S_3 nanoparticles and the construction of core–shell Bi_2S_3@ Ce_6-CeO_2 nanocomposites for NIR-triggered phototherapy. *J. Mater. Chem. B* **2020**, *8*, 4093–4105. [CrossRef]
39. Wang, X.; Lv, R.; Wang, K. Synthesis of ZnO@ZnS-Bi_2S_3 core-shell nanorod grown on reduced graphene oxide sheets and its enhanced photocatalytic performance. *J. Mater. Chem. A* **2014**, *2*, 8304–8313.
40. Xiao, S.; Shen, Z.; Song, S.; Han, S.; Du, Y.; Wang, H. Enhanced sulfadiazine degradation in a multi-electrode paralleling DBD plasma system coupled with ZnO/cellulose acetate films. *J. Environ. Chem. Eng.* **2023**, *11*, 109063. [CrossRef]
41. Wang, Y.; Dai, L.; Qu, K.; Qin, L.; Zhuang, L.; Yang, H.; Xu, Z. Novel Ag-AgBr decorated composite membrane for dye rejection and photodegradation under visible light. *Front. Chem.* **2021**, *15*, 892–901. [CrossRef]
42. Jian, J.; Kuang, D.; Wang, X.; Zhou, H.; Gao, H.; Sun, W.; Yuan, Z.; Zeng, J.; You, K.; Luo, H.A. Highly dispersed Co/SBA-15 mesoporous materials as efficient and stable catalyst for partial oxidation of cyclohexane with molecular oxygen. *Mater. Chem. Phys.* **2020**, *246*, 122814. [CrossRef]
43. Jian, J.; Yang, D.; Liu, P.; You, K.; Sun, W.; Zhou, H.; Yuan, Z.; Ai, Q.; Luo, H. Solvent-free partial oxidation of cyclohexane to KA oil over hydrotalcite-derived Cu-MgAlO mixed metal oxides. *Chin. J. Chem. Eng.* **2022**, *42*, 269–276. [CrossRef]
44. Son, W.K.; Youk, J.H.; Lee, T.S.; Park, W.H. Preparation of antimicrobial ultrafine cellulose acetate fibers with silver nanoparticles. *Macromol. Rapid Commun.* **2004**, *25*, 1632–1637. [CrossRef]
45. El-Sheikh, S.M.; Azzam, A.B.; Geioushy, R.A.; Farida, M.; Salah, B.A. Visible-light-driven 3D hierarchical Bi_2S_3/BiOBr hybrid structure for superior photocatalytic Cr(VI) reduction. *J. Alloys Compd.* **2021**, *857*, 157513. [CrossRef]
46. Jatoi, A.W.; Kim, I.S.; Ni, Q. Cellulose acetate nanofibers embedded with AgNPs anchored TiO_2 nanoparticles for long term excellent antibacterial applications. *Carbohydr. Polym.* **2019**, *207*, 640–649. [CrossRef] [PubMed]
47. Ahmad, I.; Shukrullah, S.; Naz, M.Y.; Bhatti, H.N. Dual S-scheme ZnO-gC_3N_4-CuO heterosystem: A potential photocatalyst for H_2 evolution and wastewater treatment. *React. Chem. Eng.* **2023**, *8*, 1159–1175. [CrossRef]
48. Sivaranjini, B.; Mangaiyarkarasi, R.; Ganesh, V.; Umadevi, S. Vertical alignment of liquid crystals over a functionalized flexible substrate. *Sci. Rep.* **2018**, *8*, 8891. [CrossRef]
49. Xu, T.; Zhang, L.; Cheng, H.; Zhu, Y. Significantly enhanced photocatalytic performance of ZnO via graphene hybridization and the mechanism study. *Appl. Catal. B* **2011**, *101*, 382–387. [CrossRef]
50. Kumar, S.; Sharma, S.; Umar, A.; Kansal, S.K. Bismuth sulphide (Bi_2S_3) nanotubes as an efficient photocatalyst for methylene blue dye degradation. *Nanosci. Nanotechnol. Lett.* **2016**, *8*, 266–272. [CrossRef]
51. Wang, X.; Sui, Y.; Jian, J.; Yuan, Z.; Zeng, J.; Zhang, L.; Wang, T.; Zhou, H. Ag@AgCl nanoparticles in-situ deposited cellulose acetate/silk fibroin composite film for photocatalytic and antibacterial applications. *Cellulose* **2020**, *27*, 7721–7737. [CrossRef]
52. Ji, X.; Li, C.; Liu, J.; Zhang, T.; Yang, Y.; Yu, R.; Luo, X. Controlled Synthesis and Visible-Light-Driven Photocatalytic Activity of BiOBr Particles for Ultrafast Degradation of Pollutants. *Molecules* **2023**, *28*, 5558. [CrossRef]
53. Xu, J.; Jian, J.; Dan, Y.; Song, J.; Meng, L.; Deng, P.; Sun, W.; Zhang, Y.; Xiong, J.; Yuan, Z.; et al. Durable and recyclable BiOBr/silk fibroin-cellulose acetate composite film for efficient photodegradation of dyes under visible light irradiation. *Front. Chem. Sci. Eng.* **2023**, 1–11. [CrossRef]
54. Li, Y.; Sun, X.; Tang, Y.; Ng, Y.H.; Li, L.; Jiang, F.; Wang, J.; Chen, W.; Li, L. Understanding photoelectrocatalytic degradation of tetracycline over three-dimensional coral-like ZnO/$BiVO_4$ nanocomposite. *Mater. Chem. Phys.* **2021**, *271*, 124871. [CrossRef]
55. Murugadoss, G.; Salla, S.; Kumar, M.R.; Kandhasamy, N.; Al Garalleh, H.; Garaleh, M.; Brindhadevi, K.; Pugazhendhi, A. Decoration of ZnO surface with tiny sulfide-based nanoparticles for improve photocatalytic degradation efficiency. *Environ. Res.* **2023**, *220*, 115171. [CrossRef] [PubMed]
56. Zou, M.; Tan, C.; Yang, H.; Kuang, D.; Nie, Z.; Zhou, H. Facile preparation of recyclable and flexible BiOBr@TiO_2/PU-SF composite porous membrane for efficient photocatalytic degradation of mineral flotation wastewater. *J. Water Process Eng.* **2022**, *50*, 103127. [CrossRef]

Disclaimer/Publisher's Note: The statements, opinions and data contained in all publications are solely those of the individual author(s) and contributor(s) and not of MDPI and/or the editor(s). MDPI and/or the editor(s) disclaim responsibility for any injury to people or property resulting from any ideas, methods, instructions or products referred to in the content.

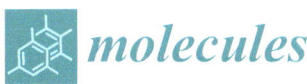

Article

The Fabrication of Halogen-Doped FeWO$_4$ Heterostructure Anchored over Graphene Oxide Nanosheets for the Sunlight-Driven Photocatalytic Degradation of Methylene Blue Dye

Muhammad Irfan [1], Noor Tahir [1], Muhammad Zahid [1,*], Saima Noreen [1], Muhammad Yaseen [2], Muhammad Shahbaz [3], Ghulam Mustafa [4], Rana Abdul Shakoor [5] and Imran Shahid [6,*]

[1] Department of Chemistry, University of Agriculture, Faisalabad 38040, Pakistan; mirfanjbd786@gmail.com (M.I.); noortahir17@yahoo.com (N.T.); saima_bashir03@yahoo.com (S.N.)
[2] Department of Physics, University of Agriculture, Faisalabad 38040, Pakistan
[3] Punjab Institute of Nuclear Medicine, Faisalabad 38800, Pakistan
[4] Department of Chemistry, University of Okara, Okara 56300, Pakistan
[5] Center for Advanced Materials (CAM), Qatar University, Doha P.O. Box 2713, Qatar
[6] Environmental Science Center, Qatar University, Doha P.O. Box 2713, Qatar
* Correspondence: rmzahid@uaf.edu.pk (M.Z.); ishahid@qu.edu.qa (I.S.)

Abstract: Rapid industrialization and urbanization are the two significant issues causing environmental pollution. The polluted water from various industries contains refractory organic materials such as dyes. Heterogeneous photocatalysis using semiconductor metal oxides is an effective remediation technique for wastewater treatment. In this research, we used a co-precipitation-assisted hydrothermal method to synthesize a novel I-FeWO$_4$/GO sunlight-active nanocomposite. Introducing dopant reductive iodine species improved the catalytic activity of FeWO$_4$/GO. I$^-$ ions improved the catalytic performance of H$_2$O$_2$ by doping into FeWO$_4$/GO composite. Due to I$^-$ doping and the introduction of graphene as a support medium, enhanced charge separation and transfer were observed, which is crucial for efficient heterogeneous surface reactions. Various techniques, like FTIR, SEM-EDX, XRD, and UV–Vis spectroscopy, were used to characterize composites. The Tauc plot method was used to calculate pristine and iodine-doped FeWO$_4$/GO bandgap. Iodine doping reduced the bandgap from 2.8 eV to 2.6 eV. The degradation of methylene blue (MB) was evaluated by optimizing various parameters like catalyst concentration, oxidant dose, pH, and time. The optimum conditions for photocatalysts where maximum degradation occurred were pH = 7 for both FeWO$_4$/GO and I-FeWO$_4$/GO; oxidant dose = 9 mM and 7 mM for FeWO$_4$/GO and I-FeWO$_4$/GO; and catalyst concentration = 30 mg and 35 mg/100 mL for FeWO$_4$/GO and I-FeWO$_4$/GO; the optimum time was 120 min. Under these optimum conditions, FeWO$_4$/GO and I-FeWO$_4$/GO showed 92.0% and 97.0% degradation of MB dye.

Keywords: iodine doping; halogenation; methylene blue degradation; photo-Fenton; heterogeneous catalysis; wastewater treatment

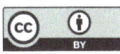

1. Introduction

Water contamination continuously increases due to the nonbiodegradability of industrial and agricultural wastes, resulting in severe diseases in humans and aquatic organisms [1]. Drinking and the utilization of polluted water cause approximately 1.4 thousand human deaths worldwide [2]. Nowadays, dyes are used in the pharmaceutical, textile, leather, and bleaching industries and for coloring purposes [3]. Textile processing loses almost half the amount in water bodies. Due to solubility and photoresistance stability, dyes contaminate water and cause various diseases such as jaundice, nausea, and cyanosis. Water resources become detrimental due to the release of dyes into the drinking water [4].

Such hazardous pollutants require extraordinary efforts [5]. Various techniques have been used to remove wastewater contaminants, such as filtration, chlorination, adsorption, reverse osmosis, precipitation, coagulation, and ion exchange [6]. These techniques have various limitations, including by-product formation [7], as well as being time-consuming and inefficient [8,9].

Advanced oxidation technologies have received great attention due to their role in water disinfection and dye degradation. The advanced oxidation process is the most crucial method for degrading many inorganic and organic pollutants released from industrial waste [10]. Different types of AOPs are used for water remediation, such as heterogeneous photocatalysis, Fenton, sono-Fenton, and photo-Fenton [11]. Advanced oxidation processes (AOPs) for wastewater treatment and the elimination of obstinate sustainable particulates have also been rapidly developed. Under ambient conditions, green technology AOPs utilize solar energy and help to remove hazardous materials from water.

In AOPs, reactive oxygen species (ROS) are generated, which degrade organic pollutants more effectively. AOPs have advantages owing to the formation of free radicals resulting from chemical reactions. During degradation, oxidizing agents such as charge carriers, superoxide radicals, and hydroxyl radicals effectively turn pollutants into harmless compounds. Various photocatalysts, such as metal ferrites, metal halides, and metal tungstates, have advantages in heterogeneous photocatalysis. Various limitations such as fast recombination of charge carriers, a lack of cost-effectiveness, and low surface area can hinder the degradation process [12]. The efficiency is improved using adsorbents that provide a surface for photocatalyst immobilization.

Among AOPs, the heterogeneous Fenton process is the most efficient and renewable. Due to its ability to degrade organic pollutants, the heterogeneous Fenton reaction, which uses Cu and Fe compounds and H_2O_2, has been intensively developed [13,14]. The consumption of H_2O_2 increases due to the low efficiency of the heterogeneous Fenton process. To overcome these limitations, composites of reductive metals like Fe, Mn, Cu, Ni, and Zn are used to activate H_2O_2, which improves the degradation of contaminants [15,16]. Reductive species such as I^- have good reducibility and therefore are used for improving the heterogeneous Fenton process. I^- is a more potent catalyst than a Fenton catalyst like Fe^{2+}.

Metal tungstates are ternary compounds that show excellent photocatalytic activity due to narrow bandgap and crystalline structure, resulting in the efficient utilization of sunlight and thus enhanced photoresponse [17]. The recombination time of photoexcited species is mainly reduced due to the narrow bandgap of ternary compounds. Some modifications are needed to improve the catalytic activity of metal tungstates. In the past decade, the photocatalytic activity of semiconductors was enhanced through several modification methods [18]. The coupling of metal tungstate with semiconductors with narrow bandgaps or transition metal doping enhances the photocatalytic activity of metal tungstate. The recombination time of charge carrier species is increased by providing a new energy level for charge carriers at which the trapping of e^- occurs through heterojunction formation. Photoexcited electrons are trapped at this new energy level, and doping enhances ternary compounds' activity responsiveness toward the visible region of ternary compounds, by introducing foreign ions, changing nanocomposite morphologies and changing the bandgap. The new energy band is formed above the valence band of the host due to the empty "d" orbitals of nonmetals. Due to this energy level, the photocatalyst shows degradation activity in the visible region through redshift in the bandgap [19].

The supporting material, graphene oxide (GO), increases the surface area due to sp^2 hybridization. The recombination time of holes and electrons increases by electrons shuttling between active co-catalyst sites and the photocatalyst, enhancing catalytic activity. Additionally, the photoresponse is enhanced through the adsorption of pollutants on the surface of GO. Tungstate composite with GO enhances the catalytic activity. P-type $FeWO_4$, with a bandgap of 2.0 eV, belongs to the wolframite family, which shows excellent photocatalytic activity due to various optical, electronic, and ferromagnetic properties [20].

In the present work, a novel I-FeWO$_4$/GO (I-FWGO) photocatalyst was synthesized and effectively used for methylene blue (MB) degradation under sunlight. The iodine doping of FeWO$_4$ enhanced the degradation efficiency. The iodine-doped FeWO$_4$ was hydrothermally treated with GO to form the doped hybrid composite. The novel I-doped FeWO$_4$/GO was characterized using FTIR, XRD, and SEM-EDX. Dye concentration and bandgap were monitored using UV–Vis spectroscopy. The dye degradation was assessed and optimized using activity parameters like time, oxidant dose, pH, and catalyst concentration. Iodine doping enhanced the photocatalytic activity of the composite in the visible region.

2. Results and Discussion

2.1. FTIR Analysis

The most important approach for finding composite functional groups is FTIR. FTIR provides information about the bonding that is present in composite materials. The characteristic peaks of undoped and iodine-doped iron tungstate/GO are shown in Figure 1. The broad absorption peaks around 3614 cm^{-1} and 3007 cm^{-1} are attributed to small -OH groups that were hydrothermally bonded to composites, indicating the presence of H$_2$O on the surface [21]. The typical elongated band at 567 cm^{-1} is related to bending vibrations due to Fe-O. The characteristic peaks of GO are shown around 1410 cm^{-1}, 1581 cm^{-1}, and 1711 cm^{-1}, which are attributed to COO$^-$, C=C, and C=O stretching vibrations, respectively [22]. In both composites, two characteristic peaks correspond to W-O stretching and O-W-O stretching peaks at 832 cm^{-1} and 1034 cm^{-1} [23]. In I-FWGO, the stretching peaks of O-W-O and F-O-W shifted due to the iodine doping into the Fe-O lattice [24,25]. The peak intensity in the iodine-doped composite was lower than in the undoped counterpart and pristine FeWO$_4$, confirming the successful insertion of dopant species in the host material [23].

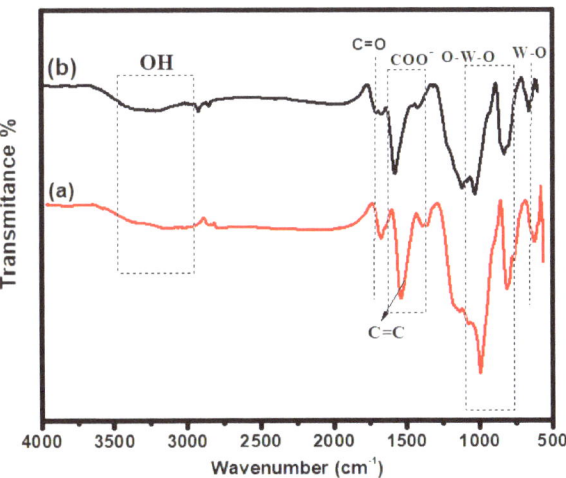

Figure 1. FTIR spectra: (**a**) FeWO$_4$/GO; (**b**) I-FeWO$_4$/GO.

2.2. XRD Analysis

XRD may be used to determine the crystalline size of nanocrystals. Figure 2 depicts the XRD pattern of I-FWGO and FeWO4/GO. In XRD spectra, diffraction peaks were observed at 2θ = 24.7°, 25.5°, 31.4°, 32.5°, 37.3°, 39.3°, 42.2°, 49.6°, 51.3°, 52.8°, 54.7°, 62.4°, and 66.0°, which were indexed to (011), (110), (020), (021), (200), (121), (022), (220), (122), (202), (032) and (312) crystal planes of I-doped FeWO$_4$/GO and FeWO$_4$/GO, respectively (JCPDS No. 46-1446) [26].

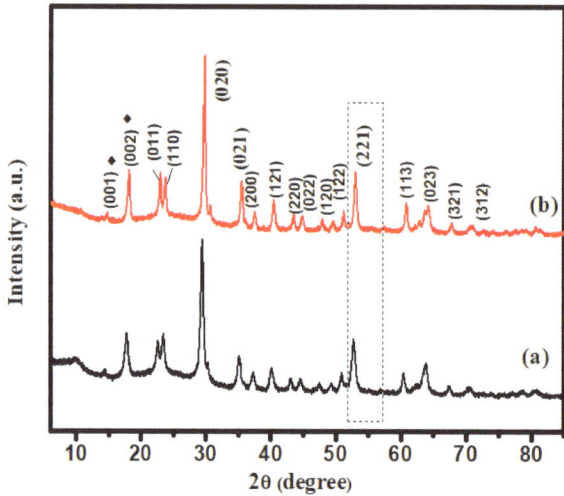

Figure 2. XRD spectra: (**a**) FeWO$_4$/GO; (**b**) I-FeWO$_4$/GO.

The high intensities of the I-FWGO peak demonstrated the influence of iodine doping on the crystal structure. Iodine doping led to a shift in the peak toward a higher 2θ value, indicating that I$^-$ substituted O^{2-} and increased the interlayer distance [27]. Crystal growth was restricted by the insertion of iodine, which blocked the grain boundary. Furthurmore, a slight shift in peak (221) was observed due to iodine doping [27]. The prominent peaks at 2θ = 13.6°, with d-spacings of 0.38 nm and 2θ = 17.1° in XRD patterns of both composites, are attributed to the (001) and (002) planes of graphene oxide, thus confirming its synthesis. The sharp peak at 2θ = 18.1°, corresponding to the (002) plane, might be attributed to restacked graphene sheets in the short-range order [28].

The Scherrer equation was used for crystalline size calculation, which is expressed in Equation (1).

$$D = \frac{0.9\lambda}{\beta \cos\theta} \tag{1}$$

where the crystal's crystalline size is "D", the Scherrer constant "K" value is "0.94", the wavelength "λ" of the X-ray source is 0.154 nm, the diffraction angle is "θ", and the entire width of the half maximum is "β." The crystalline sizes of I-FeWO$_4$/GO and FeWO$_4$/GO were 16.79 nm and 23.9 nm, respectively.

2.3. SEM-EDX

SEM characterizes the morphology and morphological changes at various resolutions, as shown in Figure 3. It can be clearly seen that the spherical nanoflake-like structure of FeWO$_4$ is well dispersed over small sheets of graphene oxide. Nanoparticle aggregation occurs due to the irregular edges of FeWO$_4$/GO. The SEM shows spherical-shaped particles of I-FeWO$_4$/GO with less agglomeration and uniformity of particles over small scattered sheets of GO. This uniformity and less aggregation result from surface area enhancement due to iodine doping [24]. The interaction of nonmetal ion species with metal tungstate forms interstitial spaces in metal oxide lattice. This ultimately leads to a faster nucleation rate and controlled growth kinetics, enhancing surface area [29]. The negatively charged iodide adsorbed on the composite surface, and as a result, the dispersion of nanoparticles increased in I-FeWO$_4$/GO compared with FeWO$_4$/GO. The iodine doping can be easily observed in SEM images of doped nanocomposite as compared to its undoped counterpart. The particle size of nanoparticles was computed using ImageJ v.1 software. The average particle size of FeWO$_4$/GO and I-FeWO$_4$/GO were 33 nm and 28.5 nm, respectively.

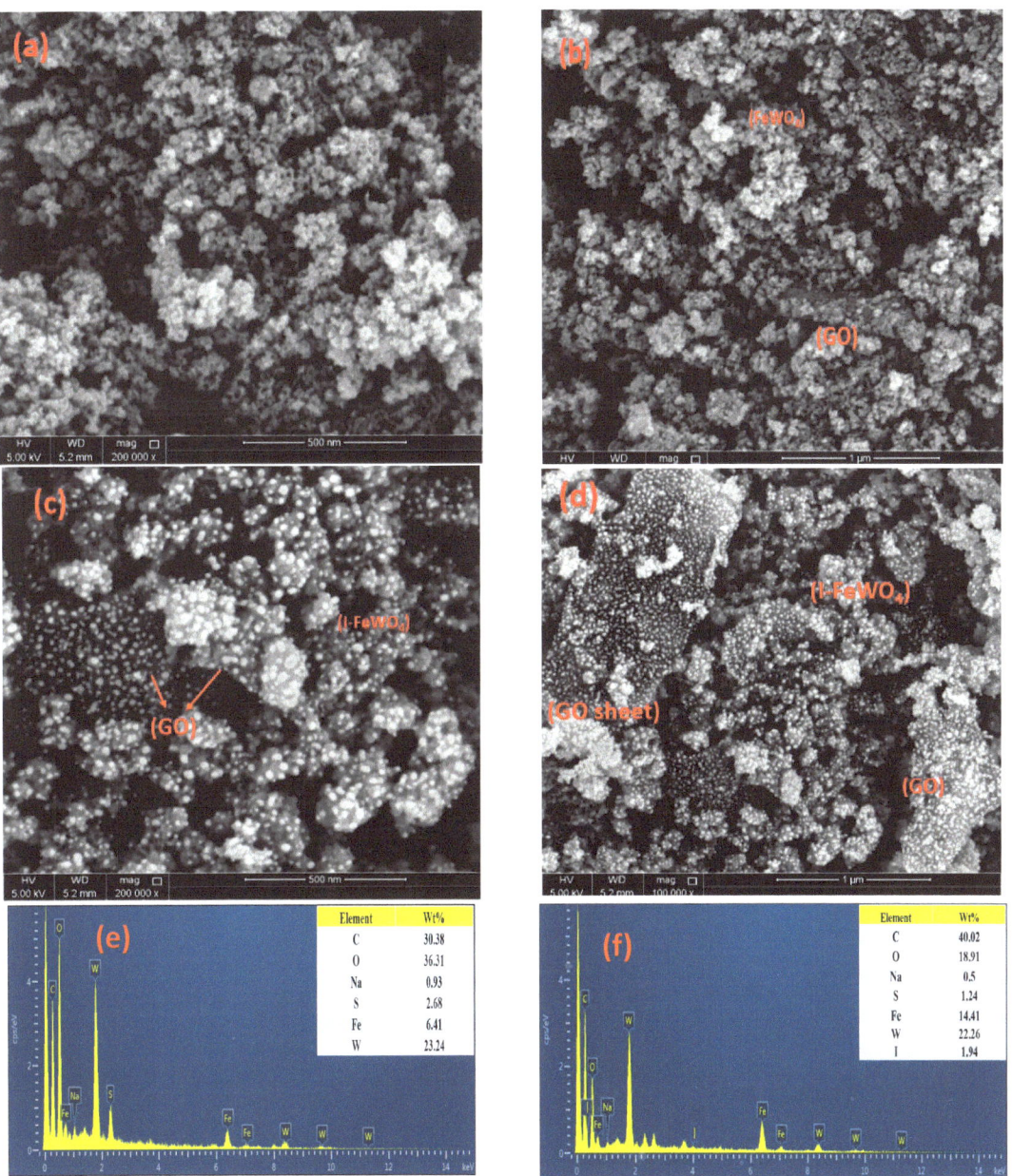

Figure 3. SEM images of FeWO$_4$-GO (**a**,**b**) and I-FeWO$_4$/GO (**c**,**d**) and EDX images of (**e**) FeWO$_4$−GO and (**f**) I-FeWO$_4$/GO.

The elemental analysis of the prepared FeWO$_4$/GO and I-FWGO was carried out through EDX, and the results are shown in Figure 3. Fe, W, O, and C show evidence of composite preparation with respective weight percentages in the inset. The iodine-doped FeWO$_4$/GO nanocomposite shows the presence of iodine and the successful incorporation of iodine in the host lattice [30].

2.4. Optical Study of FeWO₄/GO and I-FeWO₄/GO

The bandgap and optical properties of novel I-FeWO₄ and FeWO₄ were measured by observing UV–Vis spectra ranging from 200 to 800 nm. The Tauc plot method was used to determine the absorption edges of I-FeWO₄ and FeWO₄ in the visible region. The formation of heterojunction with GO and iodine doping improved the absorption ability of I-doped FeWO₄/GO. It enhanced the degradation activity by introducing new energy levels where electrons were quickly excited, and recombination was inhibited. The bandgap of the catalyst was calculated using Equation (2) as shown below:

$$(\alpha h v)^2 = B(h v - Eg) \qquad (2)$$

where α, Eg, v, and h represent the absorption coefficient, energy gap, light frequency, and proportionality constant. The plot between $(\alpha h v)^2$ and $h v$ was used for determining the bandgap.

In this composite, the bandgap of FeWO₄/GO was 2.8 eV, which is larger than the bandgap of I-FWGO (2.6 eV), as shown in Figure 4. Iodine was present at the interstice spaces of the FeWO₄/GO composite. The doped composite's bandgap was reduced due to reactive iodine species in the interstitial matrix of FeWO₄/GO, thereby enhancing the surface area. The photocatalytic activity of I-FWGO was more significant than FeWO₄/GO due to the easy excitation of electrons in the conduction band and the suppression of the charge carrier's recombination.

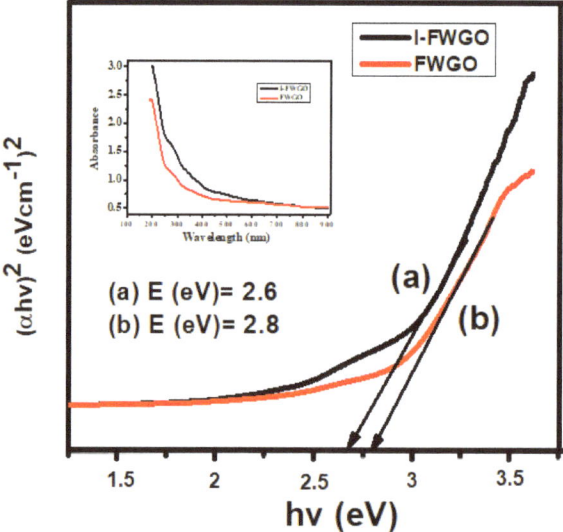

Figure 4. Bandgap of (**a**) I-FeWO₄/GO and (**b**) FeWO₄/GO.

3. Operating Parameters

Photocatalytic activities of composites were studied using several parameters, including catalyst concentration, pH, amount of H_2O_2, and irradiation time.

3.1. pH Effect

The pH value generally has an explicit influence on the photocatalytic degradation of hazardous dyes, and the breakdown performance is usually connected to the number of hydroxyl radicals (OH•) present in the medium, which significantly boosts the photodegradation efficiency in high-pH solutions. Additionally, the surface properties of photocatalysts play an essential role in the photodegradation of MB dye, which depends upon the pH of solutions. The influence of pH on the photocatalytic degradation of MB catalyzed by FWGO and I-FWGO nanocomposites is shown in Figure 5a. The degradation activity of the photocatalyst was changed under a broad range of pH (3–9) while preserving other variables unaltered (25 mg catalyst dosage and visible irradiation). The lowest decomposition performance was observed at the lowest pH value (pH = 3), with 58.0% and 68.0% of MB degraded using FWGO and I-FWGO after 100 min, respectively. However, increasing the pH to 7 resulted in the degradation of 94.3% and 95.3% of the MB dye in under 80 min using FWGO and I-FWGO respectively, due to the formation of many hydroxyl radicals [31]. Furthermore, dye adsorption on the catalytic surface increased with pH as MB dye has a positive charge and therefore is strongly adsorbed on negatively charged photocatalysts [29].

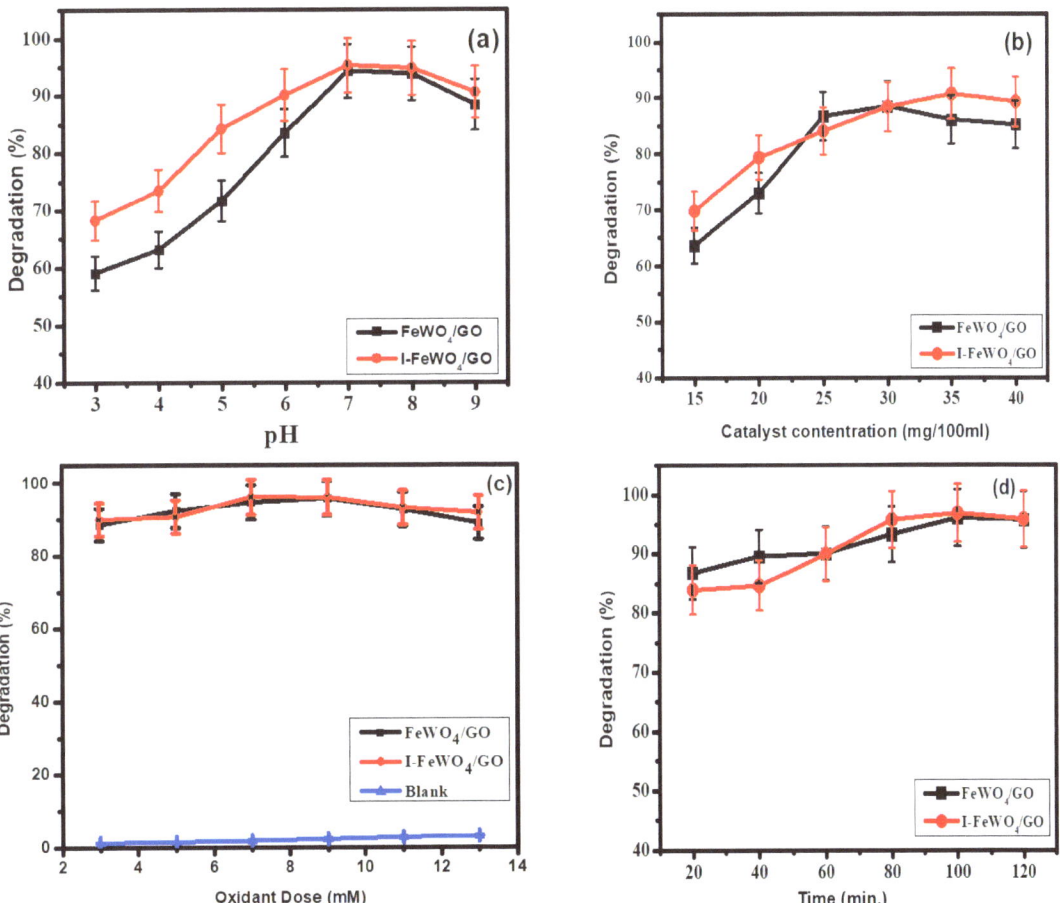

Figure 5. Optimized parameters: (**a**) pH; (**b**) catalyst load; (**c**) oxidant dose (H_2O_2); (**d**) time.

The pH is also depend on the point of zero charge, which is the threshold at which the surface of the photocatalyst has no charge. The photocatalyst has a negative charge on its surface if the pH is more than the point of zero charge. In the present study, the point of zero charge was 6.22 MB, and a cationic dye became readily adsorbed on the catalyst surface. Following thet, a reduction in photocatalytic activity was observed [32].

3.2. Influence of Catalyst Concentration on Photodegradation

The most critical parameter for the determination of photocatalytic activity is catalyst dose. The adsorption of dyes on catalyst surfaces plays an essential role in degradation. In this study, we used various catalyst concentrations (15–40 mg/100 mL dye solution) to determine the photocatalytic activity. The optimum concentrations for FWGO and I-FWGO were 30 mg and 35 mg respectively, at which maximum degradation rates of about 88.5% and 90.7% occurred under sunlight. $FeWO_4$ showed about 96.8% methyl blue degradation under UV light after 120 min (Figure 5b).

Initially, the degradation of MB increased sequentially with catalyst dose as the surface area of the catalyst was enhanced. More significant adsorption led to a higher rate of degradation. When the catalyst dose exceeded the optimum value, agglomeration occurred, and as a result, the surface area was reduced, and hence, the degradation of the dye decreased [21].

In this work, the heterojunction formation of $FeWO_4$ with graphene oxide and iodine doping improved the recombination rate of photogenerated e^- and h^+ by prolonging their suppression. Photoexcited electrons transfer from the conduction band (CB) of $FeWO_4$ toward the CB of GO. In contrast, h^+ transfers from the valence band (VB) of GO toward the VB of $FeWO_4$, and hence, the chance of recombination decreases, and degradation activity is enhanced. Iodine doping also enhanced the catalytic activity by improving the surface area of the catalyst. Iodide oxide converts into iodine and then into iodate at low pH. Due to these ions, the surface of the catalyst becomes negatively charged. IO^{3-} is a potent oxidizing agent like peroxide [33].

3.3. Oxidant Dose

Under the following conditions, the oxidant (H_2O_2) amount was optimized: MB solution (30 ppm); pH = 7; and catalyst dose = 30 mg/100 mL for $FeWO_4$/GO and 35 mg/100 mL for I-FWGO. The degradation of MB increased successively with oxidant dose (Figure 5c). The optimum oxidant value was 7 mM for I-doped $FeWO_4$/GO and 9 mM for $FeWO_4$/GO. The reduction of H_2O_2 to $OH^\bullet$ occurs by accepting electrons [34]. In photodegradation, the MB dye is effectively degraded by using $OH^\bullet$ radicals. Furthermore, $OH^\bullet$ radicals capture photoexcited electrons from the conduction band, and as a result, the recombination time increases.

$$H_2O_2 + e^-_{CB} \rightarrow HO^- + HO^\bullet$$

$$H_2O_2 + O_2^{\bullet -} \rightarrow HO^- + HO^\bullet + O_2$$

Increasing the amount of H_2O_2 over the optimum value limits the degradation efficiency because an oxidant quenches the $OH^\bullet$ radical [35–37]. In some cases, the large amount of hydrogen peroxide generates hydrogen peroxide that is less reactive than hydroxyl radicals [21].

$$H_2O_2 + HO^\bullet \rightarrow H_2O + HO_2^\bullet$$

$$HO_2^\bullet + HO^\bullet \rightarrow H_2O + O_2$$

Moreover, a reaction occurs between photogenerated holes and an excess amount of the oxidant, producing oxygen and proton. As a result, fewer $HO^\bullet$ radicals are generated, resulting in less degradation. Moreover, in the absence of the oxidant, the catalyst does not exhibit any significant photocatalytic activity.

$$H_2O_2 + 2h^+_{VB} \rightarrow O_2 + 2H^+$$

3.4. Irradiation Time

The irradiation time is the most crucial parameter for analyzing the degradation activities of the photocatalyst. All three optimized parameters were constant for time optimization. Degradation was retarded at the start of the reaction due to the formation of intermediate species that required enough time for degradation. However, it climbed over time until it reached 120 min (Figure 5d). The FWGO and I-FWGO photocatalysts exhibited 92.1% and 97% degradation after 120 min. The UV–Vis scans of dye degradation over time are demonstrated in Figure 6, showing the degradation of MB dye by both doped and undoped nanocomposites over time.

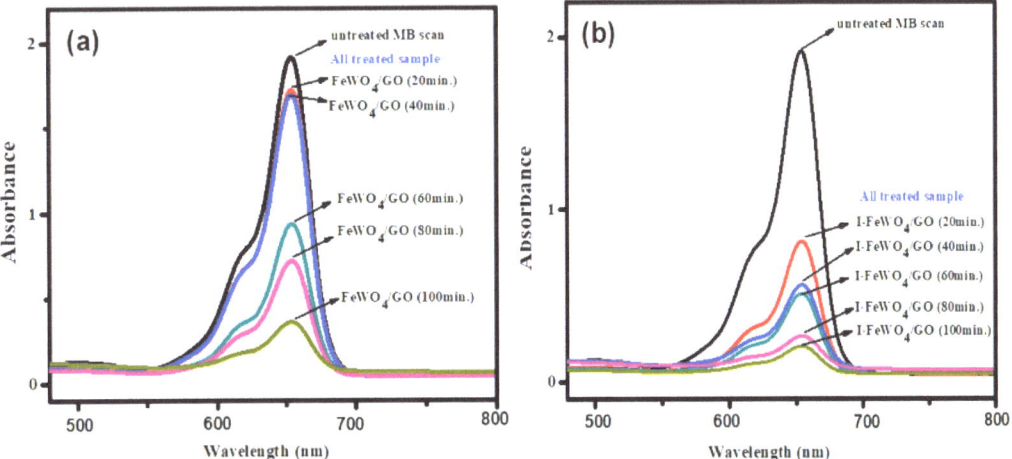

Figure 6. MB UV–Vis spectral changes during degradation over time using (**a**) FeWO$_4$/GO and (**b**) I-FeWO$_4$/GO.

3.5. Reaction Kinetics

For the quantitative study of MB, the pseudo-first- and pseudo-second-order kinetic models were used. When the pollutant concentration is in the millimolar (mM) range, Equations (3) and (4) are used for catalytic experiments. The equations for first- and second-order kinetic models are as follows:

$$\ln \frac{C_t}{C_o} = -K_1 t \quad (3)$$

$$\frac{1}{C_t} - \frac{1}{C_o} = K_2 t \quad (4)$$

where C_o is the initial dye concentration and C_t is the cncentration of MB at a time "t". For first- and second-order reaction kinetics, a linear response was observed from the plot of time (T) versus "ln (C_t/C_o)" and "$1/C_t - 1/C_o$". The "R^2" and "k" values are shown in Table 1. The values of "R^2" and "k" were more significant for I-I-FeWO$_4$/GO, indicating that iodine doping improved the catalytic activity (Figure 7).

Table 1. Reaction kinetics of FeWO$_4$/GO and I-FeWO$_4$/GO.

Photocatalyst	First-Order Kinetics		Second-Order Kinetics	
	R^2	K_1 (min^{-1})	R^2	K_2 (min^{-1})
FeWO$_4$/GO	0.9848	0.016	0.8603	0.0019
I-FeWO$_4$/GO	0.9903	0.0168	0.776	0.0026

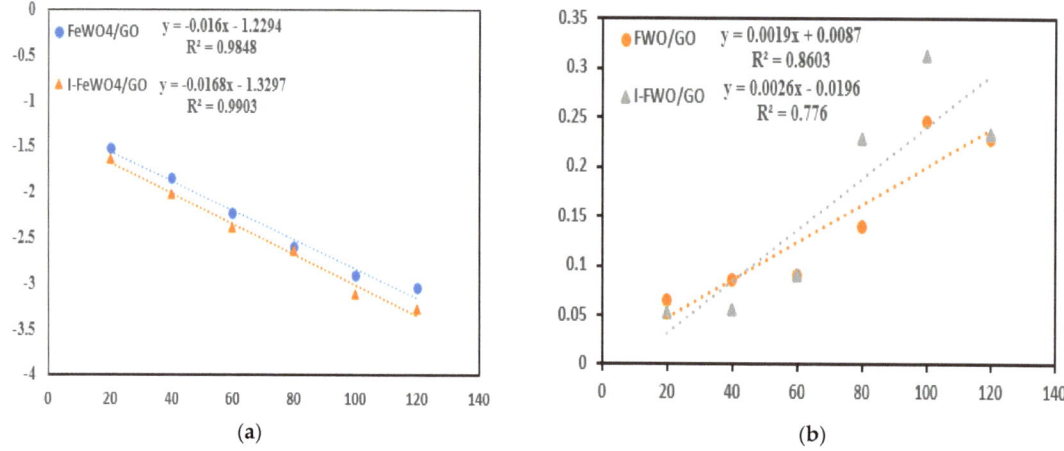

Figure 7. Reaction kinetics: (**a**) first-order kinetics; (**b**) second-order kinetics of FeWO$_4$/GO and I-FeWO$_4$/GO.

3.6. Degradation Using UV Irradiation

The photocatalytic activity of the prepared composite was also investigated under ultraviolet light, keeping the experimental conditions obtained from batch studies constant. Using UV light, the catalytic activity of novel I-FeWO$_4$/GO was analyzed by measuring absorbance using a spectrophotometer. Under optimized conditions, I-FeWO$_4$/GO exhibited 70.8% degradation after 2 h, which shows that iodine composites are adequate sunlight-activated catalysts for the degradation of pollutants.

3.7. Reusability

The reusability experiment is significant for evaluating the economic feasibility of catalysts under various conditions. The composite's stability was tested using a reusability trial test under optimized settings for up to five consecutive runs. All the optimized conditions from batch studies for the degradation of MB were kept constant. The sample was washed and dried five times and used for catalyst degradation. After five consecutive runs, the efficiency decreased from 97% to 75% using I-FeWO$_4$/GO, as shown in Figure 8.

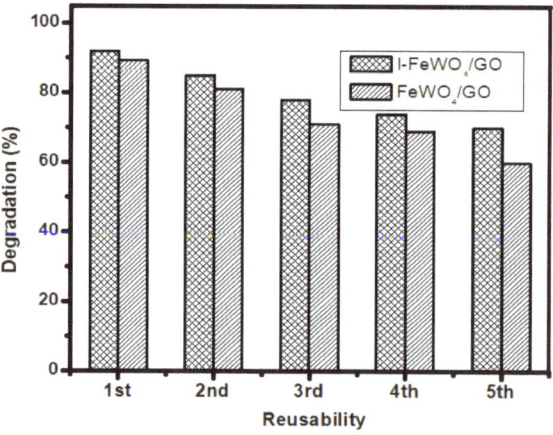

Figure 8. The reusability study using I-FeWO$_4$/GO and FeWO$_4$/GO.

3.8. Radical Scavenging Experiments and the Proposed Mechanism

Reactive species such as electron (e^-), hole (h^+), and hydroxyl radicals ($HO^\bullet$) play a key role in the photocatalytic activity. The efficiency of the radicals involved in the degradation process can be investigated by using radical scavenging species. For this purpose, 5 mM radical scavengers were used. The radical scavenger $K_2Cr_2O_7$ (potassium dichromate) was used for e^-, EDTA (ethylenediaminetetraacetate) was used for h^+, and DMSO (dimethyl sulfoxide) was used for $HO^\bullet$ as shown in Figure 9. After adding a precise number of these scavengers under optimal working conditions, the dye solution with the catalyst was exposed to sunlight. The results show a drastic reduction in dye solution degradation using DMSO. The degradation was decreased from 97% to 37% by using DMSO for I-I-FeWO$_4$/GO. Similarly, the contribution of electrons and hole scavengers also reduced the degradation.

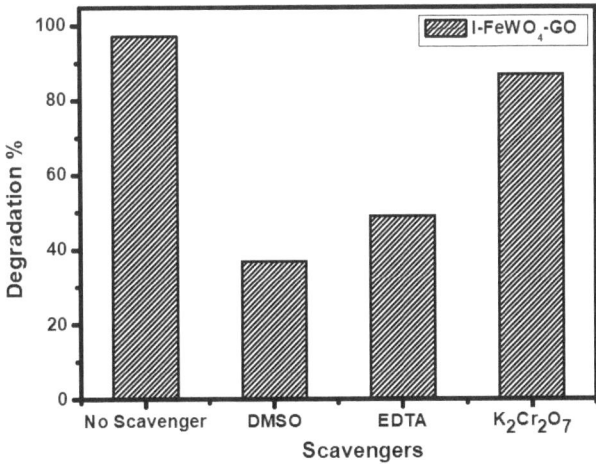

Figure 9. Radical scavenger effect of radical trapping scavengers.

The Proposed Mechanism of Degradation

Electrons and holes are the reactive oxygen species that initiate the degradation process. When sunlight falls on the I-FeWO$_4$/GO surface, the electrons are rapidly excited from the VB toward the CB due to iodine doping, which reduces the bandgap of FeWO$_4$. These photoexcited electrons move toward the CB of graphene oxide, and holes (h^+) remain in the VB of FeWO$_4$. In graphene oxide, h^+ moves toward the VB of FeWO$_4$. Fe^{2+} ions react with H_2O_2 and thus generate hydroxyl radicals and change into Fe^{3+} ions. The recombination time of the charge carrier is enhanced by receiving electrons from the conduction band by Fe^{3+}. Therefore, the generation of photo-Fenton reagents leads to a high degradation rate at neutral pH. This photogenerated h^+ reacts with H_2O_2, thus producing hydroxyl radicals. Additionally, many protons are present, which can react with $O^\bullet$ and generate OH°, which is used for degradation. The electron (e^-) in the CB oxidizes H_2O_2 to generate $OH^\bullet$ as swn in Figure 10. The mechanism is as follows:

$$I - FeWO_4(h^+ + e^-)/GO(e^- + h^+) \xrightarrow{h\nu} I - FeWO_4(h^+) + GO(e^-)$$

$$I - FeWO_4(h^+) + H_2O_2 \rightarrow I - FeWO_4 + H^+ + OH^\bullet$$

$$GO(e^-) + O_2 \rightarrow GO + O_2^{\bullet-}$$

$$OH^\bullet + OH^\bullet \rightarrow H_2O + O^\bullet$$

$$H^+ + O^\bullet \rightarrow OH^\bullet$$

$$H_2O_2 + O^\bullet \rightarrow OH^\bullet + OH^- + O_2$$

$$Fe^{2+} + H_2O_2 \rightarrow Fe^{3+} + OH^- + OH^\bullet$$

$$Fe^{3+} + H_2O_2 \rightarrow Fe^{2+} + HOO^\bullet + H^+$$

$$Fe^{3+} + H_2O \xrightarrow{h\nu} Fe^{2+} + OH^\bullet + H^+$$

$$OH^\bullet + MB \rightarrow Intermediate \rightarrow Degraded\ Products$$

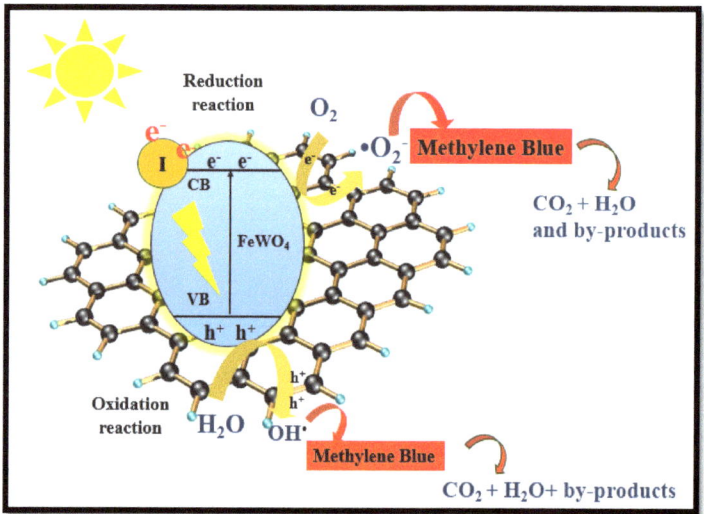

Figure 10. The proposed mechanism for the catalytic degradation of MB using I-FeWO$_4$/GO.

3.9. The Optimization of Interacting Parameters Using Response Surface Methodology (RSM)

The RSM method was used to determine the effects of the variables on the methylene blue degradation. The response was predicted using the second-order polynomials given below.

$$Y = \beta_0 + \sum_{i=1}^{k}\beta_i x_i + \sum_{i=1}^{k}\beta_{ii} x_i^2 + \sum_{i=1}^{k}\sum_{i \neq j=1}^{k}\beta_{ij} x_i x_j + \in \quad (5)$$

where the linear factor coefficient is "β_i"; the % degradation of MB is indicated by "Y"; the variables of "j" and "i" are "xj" and "xi"; the intercept term is "β_0"; the quadratic factor and the interaction factor are indicated by "β_{ii}" and "β_{ij}"; and "k" and "ε" represent the number of factors and the random error.

In Table 2, the results obtained using the Design-Expert v.1 software are shown. A regression model was developed as follows:

$$\begin{aligned}Y = &+95.20 - 0.47 * A - 0.78 * B + 0.058 * C + 3.30 * D - 7.92 * A * B + 1.55 * A * C - 1.42 * A * D - \\ &6.50 * B * C - 0.20 * B * D - 3.40 * C * D - 13.49 * A^2 - 13.58 * B^2 - 3.50 * C^2 - 3.12 * D^2\end{aligned} \quad (6)$$

where the MB degradation is represented by "Y', and pH, oxidant dose (mM), catalyst load (mg/100 mL), and time (mint.) are represented by "A", "C", "B", and "D", respectively. The final Equation (6) shows the "linear" (A, B, C, and D), "interaction" (AB, AD, AC, BD, BC, and CD), and "quadratic" (A^2, B^2, C^2, and D^2) effects.

Table 2. ANOVA table for I-FeWO$_4$/GO.

Source	Sum of Squares	df	Mean Square	F Value	p-Value Prob > F	Remarks
Model	11,015.3	14	786.8	14,219.36	<0.0001	significant
A—pH	5.23	1	5.23	94.46	<0.0001	
B—Catalyst	14.42	1	14.42	260.51	<0.0001	
C—Oxidant	0.082	1	0.082	1.48	0.2432	
D—Time	261.36	1	261.36	4723.37	<0.0001	
AB	1004.89	1	1004.89	18,160.66	<0.0001	
AC	38.44	1	38.44	694.7	<0.0001	
AD	32.49	1	32.49	587.17	<0.0001	
BC	676	1	676	12,216.87	<0.0001	
BD	0.64	1	0.64	11.57	0.004	
CD	184.96	1	184.96	3342.65	<0.0001	
A2	4992.69	1	4992.69	90,229.29	<0.0001	
B2	5057.66	1	5057.66	91,403.45	<0.0001	
C2	336.8	1	336.8	6086.76	<0.0001	
D2	266.43	1	266.43	4815.01	<0.0001	
Residual	0.83	15	0.055			
Lack of Fit	0.53	10	0.053	0.88	0.5961	not significant
Pure Error	0.3	5	0.06			
Cor Total	11016.1	29				
SD.	0.24		R^2		0.9998	
Mean	68.25		Adj. R^2		0.9998	
C.V.	0.34		Pred. R^2		0.9996	
PRESS	3.48		Adeq. Precision		335.872	

By using ANOVA, the validation of the model was investigated. The significance of the model was assessed by using the "F" value. The interaction of independent and dependent variables was investigated by using the R^2 value.

Optimization through Response Surface Methodology for Iodine-Doped Iron Tungstate/Graphene Oxide (I-FeWO$_4$/GO)

The antagonistic effects of pH and dye degradation are shown by negative signs. When the pH of the solution increased, the degradation % increased. At the same time, "B," "C," and "D" have +ve-signs, which show a synergistic effect on degradation. The dye degradation increased by increasing the oxidant dose, catalyst load, and time.

The ionic form and surface charge were immediately affected by changing the pH of the solution. At pH 6.22, I-FeWO$_4$/GO had zero charge on the surface. The mutual interaction between the catalyst concentration and pH is illustrated in Figure 11a. The catalyst concentration was set at 20–30 mg/100 mL, and pH was adjusted to 2–4. The degradation increased by increasing the pH of the solution to 7 due to the more significant interaction of MB with the catalyst. The degradation increased by increasing the catalyst concentration up to 25 mg/100 mL. The aggregation of the catalyst occurred when a high amount of catalyst was used; hence, a reduction in dye degradation was observed.

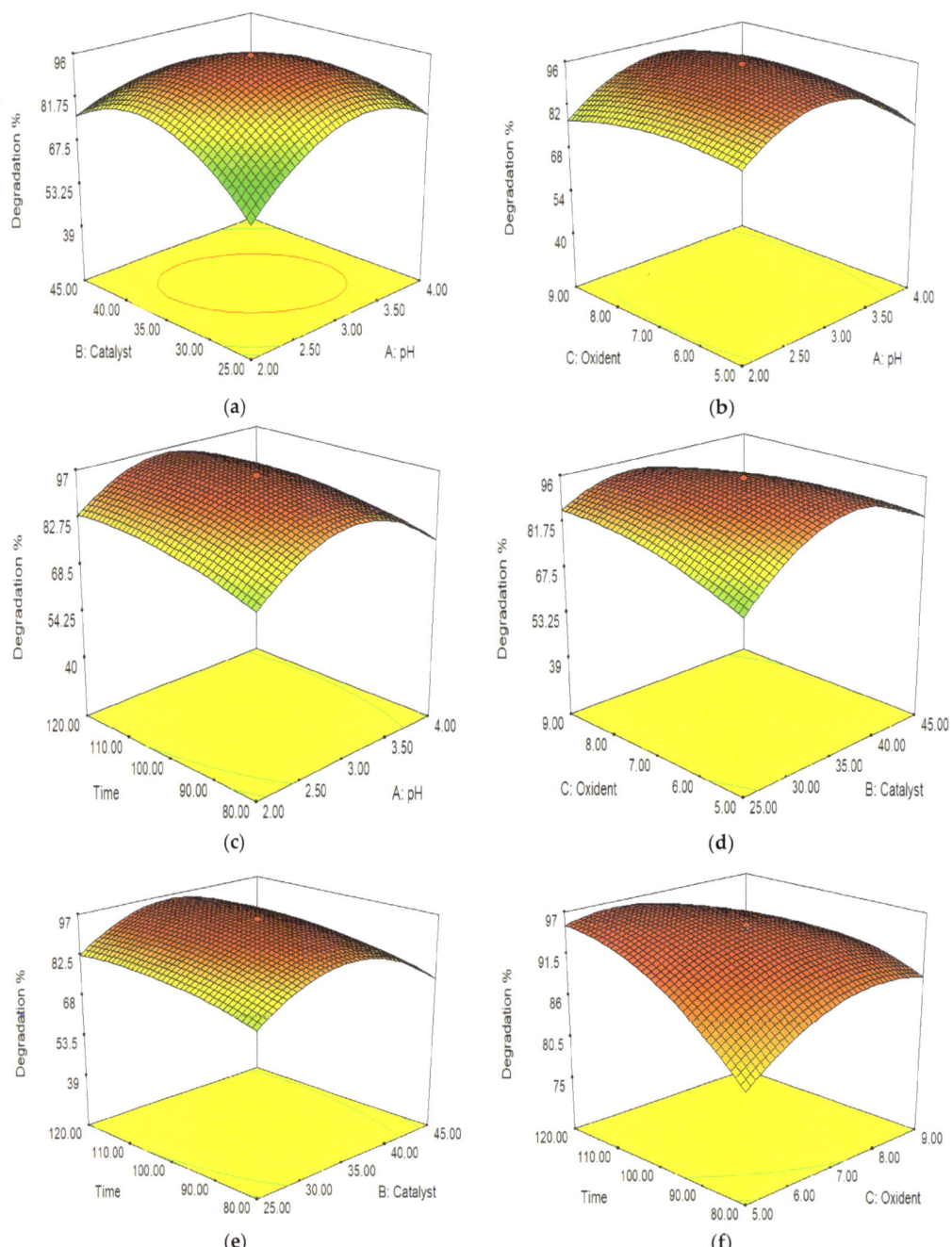

Figure 11. Interactions of (**a**) pH and catalyst load; (**b**) pH and oxidant dose; (**c**) pH and time; (**d**) oxidant dose and catalyst load; (**e**) time and catalyst load; and (**f**) time and oxidant dose.

The pH level and time play an important role in the catalytic activity. Initially, the intermediate products formed require enough time for complete mineralization. Hence, the degradation of dye increases with time. The interaction between the oxidant dose and pH is depicted in Figure 11b. The oxidant dose (H_2O_2) plays a significant role in degradation. The oxidant dose ranged from 5 to 9 mM. At 7 mM, maximum degradation occurred due to the formation and interaction of $OH°$ with dye; a further increase would reduce the catalytic activity due to the reduction in $OH°$ [38].

The combined effect of the catalyst concentration and oxidant dose is shown in Figure 11d. Increasing the oxidant dose to 7 mM enhanced the photocatalytic activity for I-FeWO$_4$/GO. The degradation of the dye remains constant if the amount of catalyst is increased, while the H_2O_2 concentration is low [39].

The interaction of the time parameter and the catalyst load is shown in Figure 11e. The catalytic activity was enhanced by increasing the concentration of the catalyst due to many active sites. If the catalyst concentration increased too much, degradation would decrease due to the agglomeration of the catalyst; hence, the surface area would be reduced. Initially, the degradation rate was low due to the production of resistant species. These intermediate products radially degraded with time [40].

4. Experimental Procedures

4.1. Materials and Reagents

In this study, an iodine-doped nanocomposite coupled with GO was prepared through a simple co-precipitation-assisted hydrothermal method. Analytical-grade reagents and chemicals were used for the synthesis of materials. Ammonium iron (II) sulfate (($NH_4)_2SO_4 \cdot FeSO_4 \cdot 6H_2O$) (99%), sodium tungstate dihydrate ($Na_2WO_4 \cdot 2H_2O$) (97%), ethanol (95.6%), and potassium iodide (KI) were obtained from UNI-CHEM. Sodium nitrate ($NaNO_3$), potassium permanganate ($KMnO_4$), sulfuric acid (H_2SO_4) (97%), and hydrogen peroxide (H_2O_2) (30% w/w) were purchased from Sigma-Aldrich (Hoboken, NJ, USA). The graphitic powder was acquired from Sharlau. The Fischer Scientific (Berlin, Germany) company provided the MB dye (purity 98%). Distilled water was obtained from the local water purification system used during the experiments.

4.2. Synthesis of Graphene Oxide (GO) and FeWO$_4$

Graphene oxide was prepared using the modified Hummer method, as reported in our previous work [23].

4.3. Synthesis of Iron Tungstate/Graphene Oxide (FeWO$_4$/GO)

For the synthesis of the FeWO$_4$/GO (FWGO) composite, the co-precipitation-assisted hydrothermal method was used. The sonication method was used to dissolve nearly 0.09 g of iron tungstate into 240 mL of deionized water. Sonication was accomplished by dissolving roughly 0.18 g of graphene oxide in 50 mL of deionized water (DI). The solutions were then vigorously magnetically stirred at room temperature for 30 min. The mixture was placed in an autoclave and heated at 160 °C for six hours. The final solution was cooled at room temperature (25 °C) and washed with water and ethanol. The samples were dried at 80 °C for 12 h in an oven.

4.4. Synthesis of Iodine-Doped Iron Tungstate (I-FeWO$_4$)

I-FeWO$_4$ was synthesized using a process described in our prior study. First, 1.176 g of Mohr's salt was dissolved in 30 mL of deionized water. In this Mohr's salt solution, we dissolved 0.99 g of sodium tungstate dihydrate and 1% potassium iodide in 30 mL of deionized water. For 30 min, magnetic stirring was employed to mix the precursors homogeneously. A 100 mL autoclave was filled to the top with the prepared solution and placed in the oven for 12 h at 200 °C. The autoclave was allowed to cool down to room temperature (25 °C), and the final solution was washed with distilled H_2O and ethanol to remove contaminants before drying for 12 h at 80 °C [24].

4.5. Synthesis of Iodine-Doped Iron Tungstate/Graphene Oxide (I-FeWO$_4$/GO)

A co-precipitation-assisted hydrothermal method was used to synthesize the novel I-FeWO$_4$/GO (I-FWGO). For sonication, 0.09 g of iodine-doped iron tungstate was dissolved into 240 mL of deionized water. Similarly, about 0.18 g of graphene oxide was dispersed into 50 mL of deionized water, and the solutions were mixed using sonication at room temperature for 30 min. The solutions were poured into a 500 mL autoclave and placed into an oven at 160 °C for 6 h. Later, it was cooled down to room temperature and then washed with water and ethanol. Finally, the samples at 80 °C were dried for 12 h in the oven. The visual explanation of the synthesis process is shown in Figure 12.

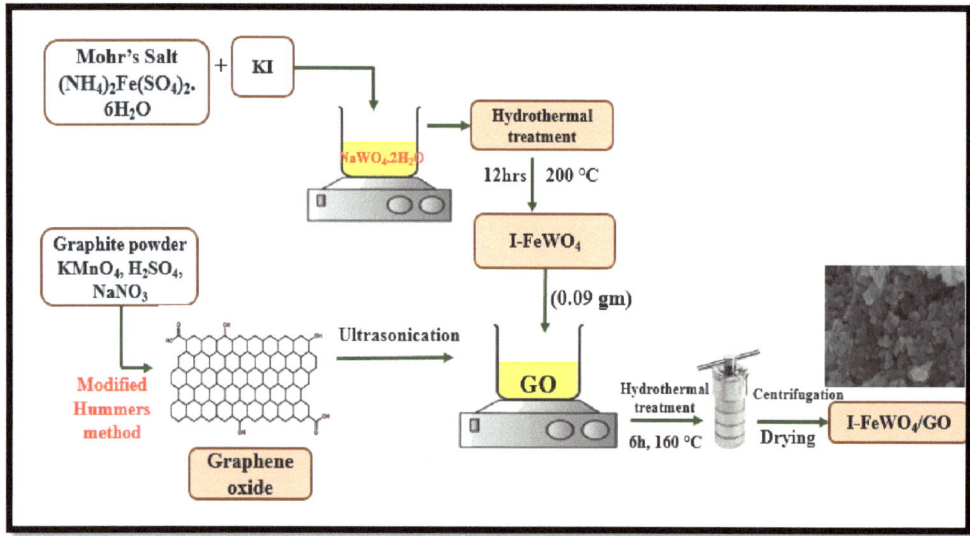

Figure 12. The schematic representation of I-FeWO$_4$/GO.

4.6. Characterization and Equipment Details

The prepared novel composites FeWO$_4$/GO and I-FeWO$_4$/GO were characterized using X-ray diffraction (Philips PANalytical Xpert pro-DY 3805 powder XRD, Amsterdam, The Netherlands) for the phase analysis of the composites. Scanning electron microscopy equipped with energy-dispersive X-ray (SEM-EDX; FEI NOVA 450 NANOSEM, Austin, TX, USA) was used for the determination of surface morphologies and the elemental analysis of the samples. The functional groups were identified using FTIR (Agilent Technologies Cary 360 FTIR spectrophotometer, Santa Clara, CA, USA). The dye absorption was analyzed using a "CECIL CE-7200 UV–Vis spectrophotometer" (Hanover, Germany).

4.7. Photocatalytic Degradation Experiment

The photocatalytic degradation of MB under sunlight was observed to investigate the catalytic capacity of the novel I-FeWO$_4$/GO catalyst generated. The support material has various applications in photocatalytic degradation due to its electrical and optical properties. Therefore, catalytic degradation is achieved by using materials similar to GO. To achieve adsorption–desorption equilibrium, the dye solution was put in the dark for half an hour. Following that, the dye solution with the catalyst was placed in sunlight for 120 min while using different oxidant dosages, catalyst concentrations, and pH levels. NaOH and HCl were used to maintain the pH of the solution. After each experiment, the catalyst was separated using a centrifuge machine, and the absorbance was assessed using a UV–Vis spectrophotometer at 665 nm. The percentage degradation of dye can be studied by using the following formula:

$$\% \text{ Degradation} = \left(1 - \frac{Co}{Ct}\right) \times 100 \tag{7}$$

where Ct is the final absorbance after sunlight irradiation, and Co is the initial absorbance of the dyes. A solar power meter was used to determine the intensity of sun, and a light meter was utilized to measure brightness.

5. Conclusions

A co-precipitation-assisted hydrothermal approach was used to synthesize undoped and doped $FeWO_4/GO$. Properties like morphology and band structure were used for evaluating the photocatalytic performance of the novel $I-FeWO_4/GO$ and $FeWO_4/GO$. After the optimization of the various parameters, $I-FeWO_4/GO$ showed greater degradation efficiency than $FeWO_4/GO$. Iodine doping restricts the grain boundary, increases the number of active sites for the adsorption of MB dye, and inhibits the recombination of holes and electrons. The crystalline sizes of $FeWO_4/GO$ and $I-FeWO_4/GO$ were 23.97 nm and 16.79 nm, respectively. $I-FeWO_4/GO$ and $FeWO_4/GO$ exhibited 97% and 92% of MB degradation after 120 min. The interaction and effects of the various parameters on degradation were studied by evaluating the results of RSM. Additionally, the novel $I-FeWO_4/GO$ also showed photocatalytic activity under UV. This research reveals that the electronic configuration of materials also improves the photocatalytic activity.

Author Contributions: Methodology, M.I., N.T. and S.N.; Software, M.S.; Validation, M.Z., M.S., R.A.S. and I.S.; Formal analysis, M.I., N.T., S.N., M.Y. and M.S.; Investigation, N.T., S.N., M.Y. and G.M.; Data curation, M.Z., G.M. and R.A.S.; Writing—original draft, M.I. and G.M.; Writing—review & editing, M.Z. and I.S.; Visualization, G.M. and R.A.S.; Supervision, M.Z. and I.S.; Project administration, I.S.; Funding acquisition, I.S. All authors have read and agreed to the published version of the manuscript.

Funding: Open Access funding provided by the Qatar National Library, Doha Qatar.

Institutional Review Board Statement: Not applicable.

Informed Consent Statement: Not applicable.

Data Availability Statement: Data is available on reasonable request.

Acknowledgments: Open Access funding provided by the Qatar National Library, Doha Qatar.

Conflicts of Interest: The authors declare no conflict of interest.

Sample Availability: Samples of the compounds are available from the authors.

References

1. Mitra, M.; Ghosh, A.; Mondal, A.; Kargupta, K.; Ganguly, S.; Banerjee, D. Facile synthesis of aluminium doped zinc oxide-polyaniline hybrids for photoluminescence and enhanced visible-light assisted photo-degradation of organic contaminants. *Appl. Surf. Sci.* **2017**, *402*, 418–428. [CrossRef]
2. Singh, P.; Sonu; Raizada, P.; Sudhaik, A.; Shandilya, P.; Thakur, P.; Agarwal, S.; Gupta, V.K. Enhanced photocatalytic activity and stability of AgBr/BiOBr/graphene heterojunction for phenol degradation under visible light. *J. Saudi Chem. Soc.* **2019**, *23*, 586–599. [CrossRef]
3. Lee, K.M.; Lai, C.W.; Ngai, K.S.; Juan, J.C. Recent developments of zinc oxide based photocatalyst in water treatment technology: A review. *Water Res.* **2016**, *88*, 428–448. [CrossRef]
4. Singh, P.; Sudhaik, A.; Raizada, P.; Shandilya, P.; Sharma, R. Hosseini-Bandegharaei, Photocatalytic performance and quick recovery of $BiOI/Fe_3O_4@$ graphene oxide ternary photocatalyst for photodegradation of 2, 4-dintirophenol under visible light. *Mater. Today Chem.* **2019**, *12*, 85–95. [CrossRef]
5. Sonu; Dutta, V.; Sharma, S.; Raizada, P.; Hosseini-Bandegharaei, A.; Gupta, V.K.; Singh, P. Review on augmentation in photocatalytic activity of $CoFe_2O_4$ via heterojunction formation for photocatalysis of organic pollutants in water. *J. Saudi Chem. Soc.* **2019**, *23*, 1119–1136. [CrossRef]

6. Raizada, P.; Sudhaik, A.; Singh, P.; Hosseini-Bandegharaei, A.; Thakur, P. Converting type II AgBr/VO into ternary Z scheme photocatalyst via coupling with phosphorus doped g-C_3N_4 for enhanced photocatalytic activity. *Sep. Purif. Technol.* **2019**, *227*, 115692. [CrossRef]
7. Zhang, L.; Qi, H.; Yan, Z.; Gu, Y.; Sun, W.; Zewde, A.A. Sonophotocatalytic inactivation of *E. coli* using ZnO nanofluids and its mechanism. *Ultrason. Sonochem.* **2017**, *34*, 232–238. [CrossRef] [PubMed]
8. Chandel, N.; Sharma, K.; Sudhaik, A.; Raizada, P.; Hosseini-Bandegharaei, A.; Thakur, V.K.; Singh, P. Magnetically separable ZnO/$ZnFe_2O_4$ and ZnO/$CoFe_2O_4$ photocatalysts supported onto nitrogen doped graphene for photocatalytic degradation of toxic dyes. *Arab. J. Chem.* **2020**, *13*, 4324–4340. [CrossRef]
9. Hasija, V.; Sudhaik, A.; Raizada, P.; Hosseini-Bandegharaei, A. Carbon quantum dots supported AgI/ZnO/phosphorus doped graphitic carbon nitride as Z-scheme photocatalyst for efficient photodegradation of 2, 4-dinitrophenol. *J. Environ. Chem. Eng.* **2019**, *7*, 103272. [CrossRef]
10. Raizada, P.; Sudhaik, A.; Singh, P.; Shandilya, P.; Saini, A.K.; Gupta, V.K.; Lim, J.-H.; Jung, H.; Hosseini-Bandegharaei, A. Fabrication of Ag_3VO_4 decorated phosphorus and sulphur co-doped graphitic carbon nitride as a high-dispersed photocatalyst for phenol mineralization and *E. coli* disinfection. *Sep. Purif. Technol.* **2019**, *212*, 887–900. [CrossRef]
11. Sharma, K.; Dutta, V.; Sharma, S.; Raizada, P.; Hosseini-Bandegharaei, A.; Thakur, P.; Singh, P. Recent advances in enhanced photocatalytic activity of bismuth oxyhalides for efficient photocatalysis of organic pollutants in water: A review. *J. Ind. Eng. Chem.* **2019**, *78*, 1–20. [CrossRef]
12. Iervolino, G.; Zammit, I.; Vaiano, V.; Rizzo, L. Limitations and Prospects for Wastewater Treatment by UV and Visible-Light-Active Heterogeneous Photocatalysis: A Critical Review. *Heterog. Photocatal.* **2020**, *26*, 225–264. [CrossRef]
13. Lyu, L.; Yan, D.; Yu, G.; Cao, W.; Hu, O. Efficient destruction of pollutants in water by a dual-reaction-center fenton-like process over carbon nitride compounds-complexed Cu (II)-$CuAlO_2$. *Environ. Sci. Technol.* **2018**, *52*, 4294–4304. [CrossRef] [PubMed]
14. Jiang, N.; Lyu, L.; Yu, G.; Zhang, L.; Hu, C. Dual-reaction-center Fenton-like process on–C(II) N–Cu linkage between copper oxides and defect-containing g-C_3N_4 for efficient removal of organic pollutants. *J. Mater. Chem.* **2018**, *36*, 17819–17828. [CrossRef]
15. Zhu, Y.; Zhu, R.; Xi, Y.; Zhu, J.; Zhu, G.; He, H. Strategies for enhancing the heterogeneous Fenton catalytic reactivity: A review. *Appl. Catal. B Environ.* **2019**, *255*, 117739. [CrossRef]
16. Diao, Y.; Yan, Z.; Guo, M.; Wang, X. Magnetic multi-metal co-doped magnesium ferrite nanoparticles: An efficient visible light-assisted heterogeneous Fenton-like catalyst synthesized from saprolite laterite ore. *J. Hazard. Mater.* **2018**, *344*, 829–838. [CrossRef]
17. Singh, P.; Shandilya, P.; Raizada, P.; Sudhaik, A.; Rahmani-Sani, A.; Hosseini-Bandegharaei, A. Review on various strategies for enhancing photocatalytic activity of graphene based nanocomposites for water purification. *Arab. J. Chem.* **2020**, *13*, 3498–3520. [CrossRef]
18. Li, B.; Lai, C.; Zeng, G.; Qin, L.; Yi, H.; Huang, D.; Zhou, C.; Liu, X.; Cheng, M.; Xu, P. Facile hydrothermal synthesis of Z-scheme $Bi_2Fe_4O_9$/Bi_2WO_6 heterojunction photocatalyst with enhanced visible light photocatalytic activity. *ACS Appl. Mater. Interfaces* **2018**, *10*, 18824–18836. [CrossRef] [PubMed]
19. Ahmad, I. Inexpensive and quick photocatalytic activity of rare earth (Er, Yb) co-doped ZnO nanoparticles for degradation of methyl orange dye. *Sep. Purif. Technol.* **2019**, *227*, 115726. [CrossRef]
20. Zhou, Y.-X.; Yao, H.-B.; Zhang, Q.; Gong, J.-Y.; Liu, S.-J.; Yu, S.-H. Hierarchical $FeWO_4$ Microcrystals: Solvothermal Synthesis and Their Photocatalytic and Magnetic Properties. *Inorg. Chem.* **2009**, *48*, 1082–1090. [CrossRef] [PubMed]
21. Rahman, M.U.; Qazi, U.Y.; Hussain, T.; Nadeem, N.; Zahid, M.; Bhatti, H.N.; Shahid, I. Solar driven photocatalytic degradation potential of novel graphitic carbon nitride based nano zero-valent iron doped bismuth ferrite ternary composite. *Opt. Mater.* **2021**, *120*, 111408. [CrossRef]
22. Marinoiu, A.; Raceanu, M.; Carcadea, E.; Varlam, M. Iodine-doped graphene–Catalyst layer in PEM fuel cells. *Appl. Surf. Sci.* **2018**, *456*, 238–245. [CrossRef]
23. Tahir, N.; Zahid, M.; Bhatti, I.A.; Jamil, Y. Fabrication of visible light active Mn-doped Bi_2WO_6-GO/MoS_2 heterostructure for enhanced photocatalytic degradation of methylene blue. *Environ. Sci. Pollut. Res.* **2021**, *29*, 6552–6567. [CrossRef] [PubMed]
24. Irfan, M.; Zahid, M.; Tahir, N.; Yaseen, M.; Qazi, U.Y.; Javaid, R.; Shahid, I. Enhanced photo-Fenton degradation of Rhodamine B using iodine-doped iron tungstate nanocomposite under sunlight. *Int. J. Environ. Sci. Technol.* **2023**, *20*, 3645–3660. [CrossRef]
25. Raja, K.; Ramesh, P.; Geetha, D. Structural, FTIR and photoluminescence studies of Fe doped ZnO nanopowder by co-precipitation method. *Spectrochim. Acta Part A Mol. Biomol. Spectrosc.* **2014**, *131*, 183–188. [CrossRef]
26. Wu, X.; Bao, C.; Niu, Q.; Lu, W. A novel method to construct a 3D $FeWO_4$ microsphere-array electrode as a non-enzymatic glucose sensor. *Nanotechnology* **2019**, *30*, 165501. [CrossRef]
27. Zhang, Y.; Zhao, Y.; Xiong, Z.; Gao, T.; Gong, B.; Liu, P.; Liu, J.; Zhang, J. Elemental mercury removal by I--doped Bi_2WO_6 with remarkable visible-light-driven photocatalytic oxidation. *Appl. Catal. B Environ.* **2021**, *282*, 119534. [CrossRef]
28. Zhang, B.; Shi, H.; Hu, X.; Wang, Y.; Liu, E.; Fan, J. A novel S-scheme MoS_2/$CdIn_2S_4$ flower-like heterojunctions with enhanced photocatalytic degradation and H_2 evolution activity. *J. Phys. D Appl. Phys.* **2020**, *53*, 205101. [CrossRef]
29. Nadeem, N.; Yaseen, M.; Rehan, Z.A.; Zahid, M.; Shakoor, R.A.; Jilani, A.; Iqbal, J.; Rasul, S.; Shahid, I. Coal fly ash supported $CoFe_2O_4$ nanocomposites: Synergetic Fenton-like and photocatalytic degradation of methylene blue. *Environ. Res.* **2022**, *206*, 112280. [CrossRef]

30. Zhang, J.; Huang, Z.-H.; Xu, Y.; Kang, F. Hydrothermal Synthesis of Iodine-Doped Nanoplates with Enhanced Visible and Ultraviolet-Induced Photocatalytic Activities. *Int. J. Photoenergy* **2012**, *2012*, 915386. [CrossRef]
31. Yang, S.; Huang, Y.; Wang, Y.; Yang, Y.; Xu, M.; Wang, G. Photocatalytic degradation of Rhodamine B with $H_3PW_{12}O_{40}/SiO_2$ sensitized by H_2O_2. *Int. J. Photoenergy* **2012**, *2012*, 927132. [CrossRef]
32. Mudhoo, A.; Paliya, S.; Goswami, P.; Singh, M.; Lofrano, G.; Carotenuto, M.; Carraturo, F.; Libralato, G.; Guida, M.; Usman, M.; et al. Fabrication, functionalization and performance of doped photocatalysts for dye degradation and mineralization: A review. *Environ. Chem. Lett.* **2020**, *18*, 1825–1903. [CrossRef]
33. Fox, P.M.; Davis, J.A.; Luther, G.W. The kinetics of iodide oxidation by the manganese oxide mineral birnessite. *Geochim. Cosmochim. Acta* **2009**, *73*, 2850–2861. [CrossRef]
34. Chu, W.; Choy, W.K.; So, T.Y. The effect of solution pH and peroxide in the TiO_2-induced photocatalysis of chlorinated aniline. *J. Hazard. Mater.* **2007**, *141*, 86–91. [CrossRef] [PubMed]
35. Soon, A.N.; Hameed, B. Heterogeneous catalytic treatment of synthetic dyes in aqueous media using Fenton and photo-assisted Fenton process. *Desalination* **2011**, *269*, 1–16. [CrossRef]
36. Enesca, A.; Isac, L.; Andronic, L.; Perniu, D.; Duta, A. Tuning SnO_2–TiO_2 tandem systems for dyes mineralization. *Appl. Catal. B Environ.* **2014**, *147*, 175–184. [CrossRef]
37. Visa, M.; Bogatu, C.; Duta, A. Tungsten oxide—Fly ash oxide composites in adsorption and photocatalysis. *J. Hazard. Mater.* **2015**, *289*, 244–256. [CrossRef]
38. Tabasum, A.; Zahid, M.; Bhatt, H.N.; Asghar, M. Fe_3O_4-GO composite as efficient heterogeneous photo-Fenton's catalyst to degrade pesticides. *Mater. Res. Express* **2018**, *6*, 015608. [CrossRef]
39. Yaqubzadeh, A.; Ahmadpour, A.; Bastami, T.R.; Hataminia, M. Low-cost preparation of silica aerogel for optimized adsorptive removal of naphthalene from aqueous solution with central composite design (CCD). *J. Non-Cryst. Solids* **2016**, *447*, 307–314. [CrossRef]
40. Daneshvar, N.; Aber, S.; Seyeddorraji, M.; Khataee, A.; Rasoulifard, M. Photocatalytic degradation of the insecticide diazinon in the presence of prepared nanocrystalline ZnO powders under irradiation of UV-C light. *Sep. Purif. Technol.* **2007**, *58*, 91–98. [CrossRef]

Disclaimer/Publisher's Note: The statements, opinions and data contained in all publications are solely those of the individual author(s) and contributor(s) and not of MDPI and/or the editor(s). MDPI and/or the editor(s) disclaim responsibility for any injury to people or property resulting from any ideas, methods, instructions or products referred to in the content.

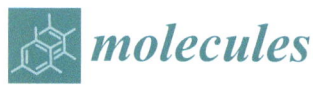

Article

Visible Light Motivated the Photocatalytic Degradation of P-Nitrophenol by Ca²⁺-Doped AgInS₂

Xuejiao Wang [1], Shuyuan Liu [1], Shu Lin [1], Kezhen Qi [1,*], Ya Yan [1,*] and Yuhua Ma [2,*]

[1] College of Pharmacy, Dali University, Dali 671000, China; 15187277683@163.com (X.W.)
[2] College of Chemistry and Chemical Engineering, Xinjiang Normal University, Urumqi 830054, China
* Correspondence: qkzh2003@aliyun.com (K.Q.); yanya@dali.edu.cn (Y.Y.); 15199141253@163.com (Y.M.)

Abstract: 4-Nitrophenol (4-NP) is considered a priority organic pollutant with high toxicity. Many authors have been committed to developing efficient, green, and environmentally friendly technological processes to treat wastewater containing 4-NP. Here, we investigated how the addition of Ca^{2+} affects the catalytic degradation of 4-NP with $AgInS_2$ when exposed to light. We synthesized $AgInS_2$ (AIS) and Ca^{2+}-doped $AgInS_2$ (Ca-AIS) with varying amounts of Ca^{2+} using a low-temperature liquid phase method. The SEM, XRD, XPS, HRTEM, BET, PL, and UV-Vis DRS characteristics were employed to analyze the structure, morphology, and optical properties of the materials. The effects of different amounts of Ca^{2+} on the photocatalytic degradation of 4-NP were investigated. Under visible light illumination for a duration of 120 min, a degradation rate of 63.2% for 4-Nitrophenol (4-NP) was achieved. The results showed that doping with an appropriate amount of Ca^{2+} could improve the visible light catalytic activity of AIS. This work provides an idea for finding suitable cheap alkaline earth metal doping agents to replace precious metals for the improvement of photocatalytic activities.

Keywords: $AgInS_2$; Ca^{2+}; doping; 4-Nitrophenol; visible photocatalytic degradation

Citation: Wang, X.; Liu, S.; Lin, S.; Qi, K.; Yan, Y.; Ma, Y. Visible Light Motivated the Photocatalytic Degradation of P-Nitrophenol by Ca^{2+}-Doped $AgInS_2$. *Molecules* **2024**, *29*, 361. https://doi.org/10.3390/molecules29020361

Academic Editor: Sugang Meng

Received: 2 December 2023
Revised: 25 December 2023
Accepted: 27 December 2023
Published: 11 January 2024
Corrected: 11 June 2024

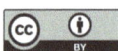

Copyright: © 2024 by the authors. Licensee MDPI, Basel, Switzerland. This article is an open access article distributed under the terms and conditions of the Creative Commons Attribution (CC BY) license (https:// creativecommons.org/licenses/by/ 4.0/).

1. Introduction

Environmental pollution has been intensified recently due to the increasing global population and frequent human activities. While people enjoy the benefits of chemical products and natural mineral resources, they have enforced the threat of toxic organic pollutants. Huge amounts of chemical wastes are discharged into the environment every year and cause great harm to the environment [1]. 4-Nitrophenol (4-NP) is a frequently used herbicide and fungicide that is widely used in medicine, dyes, and agricultural activities [2]. It is a highly toxic and insoluble organic pollutant in the environment, which has been detected in surface water and soil and even in beverages and food. It causes great harm to the human body and environment [3,4]. 4-NP is a member of 120 blacklisted priority pollutants by the U.S. Environmental Protection Agency. The delocalization of π electrons in the benzene ring makes 4-NP highly stable [5]. Therefore, finding a safe and efficient approach to degrade 4-NP is of utmost importance.

Common methods for the removal of 4-NP include photocatalytic oxidation [6], adsorption, and biological methods [7,8]. However, most of these technologies require further separation and purification steps to process substantial quantities of residual waste, potentially resulting in secondary pollution [9]. Photocatalytic oxidation has been proven to effectively degrade 4-NP into CO_2, H_2O, or other non-toxic compounds, with mild reaction conditions, low cost, and high efficiency [10,11]. During photocatalysis, the irradiation of the semiconductor produces excited electrons and holes, respectively, in the conduction and valance bands of the photocatalyst. These excited charges directly oxidize and reduce the target pollutant on the surface of the photocatalyst with the aid of highly reactive degrading species [12]. Amongst the various photocatalysts, TiO_2 is a widely used catalyst with many attractive characteristics. However, the band gap of TiO_2 is wide

(3.23 eV), limiting its ability to catalyze redox reactions under visible light irradiation [13]. By modifying TiO_2 or seeking new visible light-driven catalysts, there are several methods available for improving the catalytic performance of a catalyst: doping with metal or non-metallic ions, adjusting the morphology, loading precious metals, and utilizing composite semiconductors. Each of these approaches has been proven to enhance the efficiency and effectiveness of catalysts in various applications. By understanding and utilizing these methods, researchers can develop catalysts with improved performance for a wide range of chemical reactions [14,15].

As the I-III-VI ternary direct band gap semiconductor, $AgInS_2$ has attracted extensive attention due to its excellent light absorption characteristics, appropriate band gap width, high absorption coefficient, good radiation stability, and nonlinear optical properties [16]. There are two different polymorphs in $AgInS_2$ crystals: a tetragonal chalcopyrite structure at room temperature and an orthorhombic wurtzite structure at high temperature [17]. Furthermore, it is a non-toxic and environmentally friendly visible light sensitizer and has been used in fluorescence, solar cells, and photocatalysis, and it has garnered significant attention [18–20]. $AgInS_2$ has three phase structures: cubic, tetragonal, and orthogonal. Its wurtzite structure is composed of InS_4 and AgS_4 tetrahedrons in the orthorhombic system [21]. The unequal bonds between Ag-S and In-S can cause the tetrahedrons to twist, resulting in an internal electric field [22]. Under illumination, the electric field is conducive to the separation of charges and enhances photocatalytic activity. Its optical band gap (1.80~2.04 eV) is close to the optimal forbidden bandwidth (1.45 eV) of solar cell materials, making it an ideal choice as a photocatalytic material [23]. Although $AgInS_2$ has many advantages, its high charge recombination rate, low quantum efficiency, and strong photoetching badly limit its widespread application in the photocatalytic field. Therefore, it is essential to modify the $AgInS_2$ monomer and expand its application in the photocatalytic field. As a common cheap alkaline earth metal, calcium is used as a dopant in many semiconductors to reduce the band gap or interface resistance [24–26]. Based on the above analysis, it was speculated that AIS has certain degradation activity toward 4-NP under visible light. After introducing Ca^{2+}, the band gap and interface resistance of AIS could be reduced, thereby improving the photocatalytic activity of AIS. Given that the radius of Ca^{2+} (99 pm) is smaller than Ag^+ (115 pm) and larger than In^{3+} (80 pm) [27–29], it is speculated that after the introduction of Ca^{2+}, it replaces Ag^+ in entering the lattice of AIS. This modulation of the lattice is believed to adjust the band gap of AIS, thereby enhancing its degradation activity toward 4-NP under visible light.

The present study aims to explore the effect of introducing Ca^{2+} on the degradation of 4-NP by AIS under visible light, and the low-temperature liquid phase method was selected to synthesize AIS and Ca-AIS in different proportions. The influences of Ca doping on its morphology, band gap, and the electron hole recombination of AIS were also analyzed. The findings demonstrated that the presence of an appropriate amount of Ca^{2+} enhances the photocatalytic degradation performance of AIS. Herein, the potential mechanism for the photocatalytic degradation of 4-NP using Ca-doped AIS was proposed. We believe that this work will substitute precious metals as dopants to improve the performance of photocatalysts. Compared to noble metal elements, Ca is cheaper and can modify photocatalysts with less doping to improve its photocatalytic activity. Moreover, this method is easy to operate and requires lower cost.

2. Results and Discussion

2.1. Crystal Structure

To examine the crystal characteristics and phases of the samples, XRD analysis was conducted with AIS and 1%Ca-AIS samples. According to Figure 1a, the pure AIS sample exhibits distinct diffraction peaks at 26.5°, 28.4°, 44.5°, 48.0°, and 52.6°. These peaks correspond to crystal planes (002), (121), (320), (123), and (322), respectively, as indicated in the standard AIS spectrum with an orthogonal crystal structure (JCPD: 25-1328) [30]. Interestingly, no peaks related to impurities are detected, implying the successful synthesis of AIS. Upon the introduction of Ca^{2+}, there is no observable Ca-related peak in the XRD spectrum of the 1%Ca-AIS sample. The absence could be attributed to the low concentration of the Ca^{2+} dopant. Notably, the positions of all diffraction peaks remain unchanged, suggesting that Ca^{2+} does not significantly affect the crystal structure of AIS. However, the intensity of the characteristic diffraction peaks is slightly weakened, indicating that the introduction of Ca^{2+} can influence the crystallinity of AIS. These findings possibly suggest that Ca^{2+} is evenly distributed within the AIS matrix. Furthermore, the introduction of Ca^{2+} leads to the broadening of the characteristic diffraction peaks. This phenomenon is likely due to the smaller radius of Ca^{2+} (99 Å) compared to Ag^+ (115 Å) [28,31]. Based on the analysis mentioned above, it can be inferred that Ca^{2+} replaces Ag^+ within the AIS lattice upon introduction. Consequently, this substitution results in a reduction in the grain size of AIS [32].

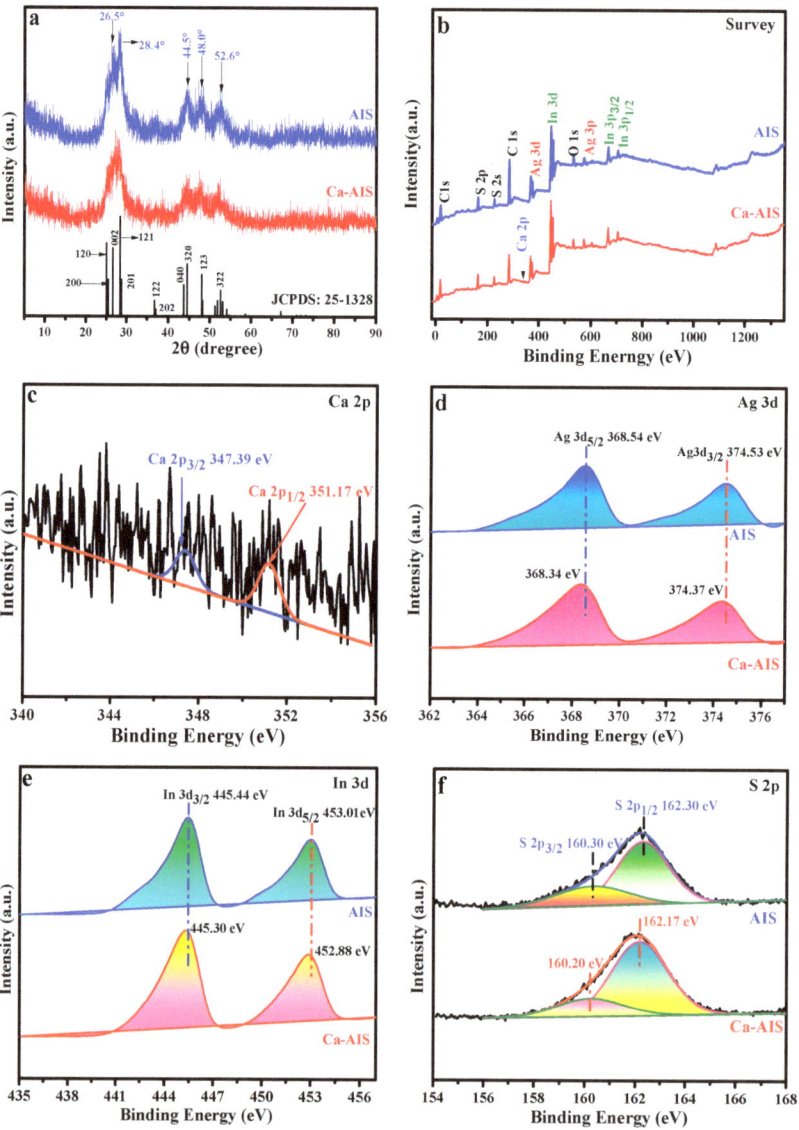

Figure 1. (**a**) XRD patterns of AIS and 1%Ca-AIS, (**b**) survey XPS spectrum and high-resolution XPS spectrum of AIS and 1%Ca-AIS: (**c**) Ca 2p; (**d**) Ag 3d; (**e**) In 3d; (**f**) S 2p.

The chemical composition and surface chemical state of AIS and 1%Ca-AIS samples were examined using XPS. As shown in Figure 1b, AIS contains not only Ag, In, and S but also O, C, and other elements. The C and O elements are produced in thioglycolic acid, the coating agent of the material, or the air. The obtained samples have no impurities, and the peak positions of Ag, In, and S are consistent with the previous report [33]. Figure 1c–f presents the high-resolution spectra of different elements in 1%Ca-AIS. Figure 1c reveals that the concentration of the doped Ca element is quite low, and a minimal amount of Ca is observed on the surface. The two main peaks of Ca 2p can be fitted, and a binding energy peak at 347.39 eV is ascribed to Ca $2p_{3/2}$, while another binding energy peak at 351.17 eV is associated with Ca $2p_{1/2}$. These findings indicate that Ca is present in the form of Ca^{2+} [34–36]. In Figure 1d, the two binding energy peaks at 374.53 eV and 368.54 eV are attributed to Ag $3d_{3/2}$ and Ag $3d_{5/2}$, respectively. This implies that the Ag in AIS has a valence state of +1 [37]. The Ca-AIS sample reveals distinguishable binding energy peaks of Ag $3d_{3/2}$ (374.37 eV) and Ag $3d_{5/2}$ (368.34 eV). The observed results propose that the presence of Ca^{2+} ions leads to a decrease in the binding capacity of Ag^+ ions toward the electrons existing in the crystal structure. The high-resolution spectrum of In 3d in Figure 1e exhibits two binding energy peaks at 445.44 eV and 453.01 eV, which correspond to In $3d_{3/2}$ and In $3d_{5/2}$, respectively [38]. After the incorporation of Ca^{2+}, a shift in the binding energy peaks can be observed, where the binding energy values for In $3d_{3/2}$ and In $3d_{5/2}$ undergo a change to 445.30 eV and 452.88 eV, respectively. This suggests that the presence of Ca reduces the binding strength of In^{3+} within the crystal lattice. These results demonstrate that Ca^{2+} replaces Ag^+ and enters the AIS lattice, resulting in the weakening of the binding ability of Ag^+ and In^{3+} to electrons. In Figure 1f, the peak corresponding to the binding energy of S $2p_{3/2}$ is detected at approximately 160.30 eV, while the peak for S $2p_{1/2}$ is observed at 162.30 eV. These results imply that the valence state of S in AIS is −2 [39–41]. Upon the introduction of Ca^{2+}, the binding energy peak of S $2p_{3/2}$ shifts to around 160.20 eV, and the binding energy of S $2p_{1/2}$ moves to 162.17 eV. This suggests a reduction in the binding affinity of S toward electrons after the introduction of Ca^{2+}. The XPS characterization results of the samples confirm that Ca^{2+} replaces Ag^+ in AIS. Although the oxidation states of the elements in AIS are unaffected by the introduction of Ca^{2+}, the binding ability of Ag, S, and In to electrons is reduced.

2.2. Morphology and Structure

SEM was used to examine the microscopic morphology of 1%Ca-AIS and AIS. Figure 2a indicates that the prepared AIS particles have rough surfaces, different shapes, uneven size, and serious agglomerations. AIS exhibits a particle size ranging from 361 to 630 nm. In Figure 2d, it is apparent that 1%Ca-AIS particles present smoother surfaces, improved sphericity, and a more uniform dispersion among the particles. The particle size distribution of Ca-AIS exhibits uniformity, with the average diameter ranging between 253 and 481 nm. According to SEM analysis, the doping of Ca^{2+} makes the surface of AIS smooth, the sphericity becomes better, the particle size becomes smaller, the size is more uniform, and the dispersion is better.

To further investigate the morphology and crystal lattice arrangement of both AIS and 1%Ca-AIS samples, a high-resolution TEM (HRTEM) analysis was conducted. The HRTEM analysis showcased in Figure 2b portrays the morphology of AIS, illustrating an aggregate structure with irregular particle sizes ranging from approximately 137 to 222 nm. As shown in Figure 2c, the measured interplanar spacings are 0.350 nm, 0.242 nm, 0.203 nm, and 0.174 nm, which corresponds to (200), (202), (320), and (322) crystal planes of AIS with an orthogonal crystal phase structure, respectively. According to the data displayed in Figure 2e, the addition of Ca^{2+} has a distinct impact on the characteristics of Ca-AIS particles. The Ca-AIS particles exhibit a smooth surface and possess a favorable sphericity, with an average size ranging from 106 to 166 nm. Figure 2f showcases clear lattice patterns on the surface of the particles, indicating the presence of well-defined crystal structures. The measured interplanar spacings of 0.189 nm and 0.335 nm that correspond to (123) and (002) crystal planes, respectively, are attributed to the orthogonal crystal phase of AIS. These findings are consistent with the obtained XRD results, affirming the accuracy and reliability of the HRTEM data.

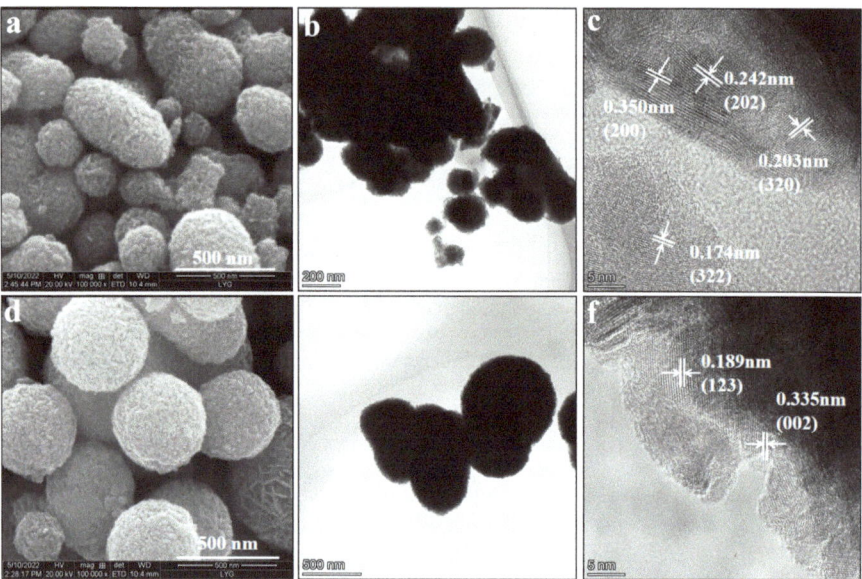

Figure 2. SEM, TEM, and HRTEM images of AIS (**a**–**c**) and 1%Ca-AIS (**d**–**f**).

2.3. BET

Nitrogen adsorption–desorption tests were employed to analyze the pore size and specific surface area of AIS and 1%Ca-AIS. The isotherms depicted in Figure 3a exhibit typical type IV characteristics with H3 hysteresis loops in the P/P_0 range of 0.4 to 1.0. These findings imply that both AIS and 1%Ca-AIS possess mesoporous structures [26,42]. The specific surface area of 1%Ca-AIS is slightly larger than AIS. A higher specific surface area is known to enhance photocatalytic activity and increase the number of active sites. Consequently, this suggests that 1%Ca-AIS may exhibit improved photocatalytic performance compared to AIS. Additionally, Figure 3b reveals that the introduction of Ca^{2+} increases the pore size, which, in turn, increases the effective contact area with pollutants and effectively enhances the adsorption performance of AIS.

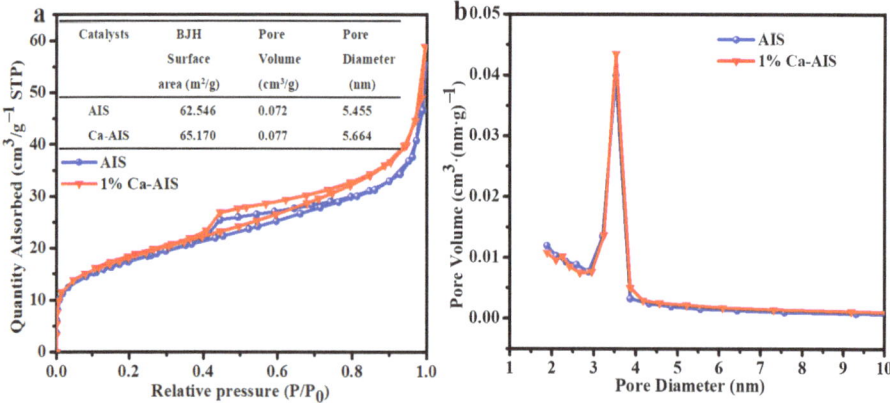

Figure 3. (**a**) N_2 adsorption–desorption isotherms and (**b**) corresponding pore size distributions of AIS and 1%Ca-AIS.

2.4. Electronic Structure

To evaluate the capacity of the samples to absorb visible light, UV-vis DRS characterizations of the samples were conducted. As depicted in Figure 4a, it is evident that Ca-AIS proportions demonstrate significant light absorption within the 400–700 nm range. Except for 3%Ca-AIS, which shows lower light absorption capacity compared to AIS, the other proportions of Ca-AIS demonstrate higher light absorption capacity than AIS, indicating that the introduction of the appropriate amount of Ca^{2+} is indeed conducive to the absorption of visible light. However, excessive Ca^{2+} will inhibit its optical utilization. The bandgap widths of AIS and 1%Ca-AIS were calculated according to Tauc's function by the Kubelka–Munk (KM) method: $\alpha h\nu = A(h\nu - E_g)^{n/2}$, where α is the absorbance coefficient of the substance, h is the Planck constant, A is the absorbance of the sample, E_g is the forbidden bandgap width of the substance, ν is the photon frequency [43,44], and n is equal to 1 or 4, and its value depends on the direct or indirect type conversion of the semiconductor. As we all know, $AgInS_2$ belongs to the direct transition semiconductor, and the value of n is 1 [45]. The relationship between $(\alpha h\nu)^2$ and $h\nu$ is illustrated in Figure 4b. By estimating and calculating the intercept of the tangent line with the curve, the band gap value (E_g) was determined as the point where the tangent intersects the x-axis, and it is obtained that the band gap energy (~1.68 eV) of 1%Ca-AIS is lower than AIS (~1.73 eV). Therefore, the enhanced photocatalytic efficiency of 1%Ca-AIS may be attributed to its strong light absorption.

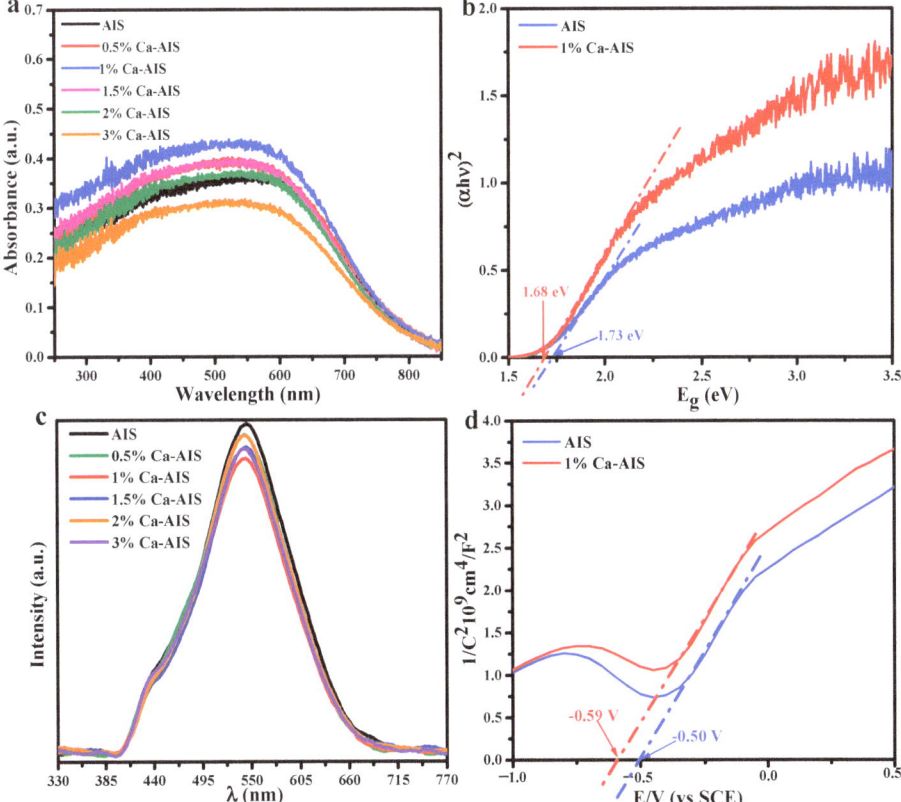

Figure 4. (**a**) UV–Vis DRS spectra, (**b**) band gap energy diagram, (**c**) fluorescence spectrum, (**d**) flat band potential diagrams of AIS and Ca-AIS.

The photoluminescence spectrum provides information about the separation effect of photogenerated electrons and holes. Figure 4c illustrates the fluorescence spectra of all samples, with the following measurement parameters: an excitation wavelength of 400 nm and a slit width of EX: 6HH and EM: 10. The results demonstrate that AgInS$_2$ exhibits the strongest emission peak at 544 nm. Upon the introduction of Ca^{2+}, the fluorescence intensity is weakened, as Ca^{2+} inhibits the recombination of e$^-$ and h$^+$. Notably, the fluorescence intensity of 1%Ca-AIS is the weakest, indicating better separation of electrons and holes, and the lifetime of photogenerated carriers is the longest, which indicates that the introduction of Ca^{2+} reduces the recombination rate of carriers facilitating the separation of photogenerated electrons and holes. This is beneficial for the photocatalytic degradation of pollutants. The PL spectrum further confirms that the separation rate of electron-hole pairs aligns with the corresponding efficiency of degradation, highlighting the enhanced ability of AIS to degrade organic pollutants upon the introduction of Ca^{2+}.

The impedance potential approach was employed to evaluate the flat band potential of the specimens. Specifically, AIS catalysts and 1%Ca-AIS catalysts were subjected to a series of experiments to determine their respective flat band potentials. The acquired data were reversed employing the Mott–Schottky theory, yielding Mott–Schottky curves for both AIS and 1%Ca-AIS catalysts. As depicted in Figure 4d, the patterns exhibit positive slopes, indicating that the specimens exhibit characteristics of n-type semiconductors. The point of intersection between the tangent lines of the Mott–Schottky curves and the x-axis yield values of -0.50 V and -0.59 V for AIS and 1%Ca-AIS catalysts, respectively, utilizing Formula (2) [29]:

$$E_0 = E_{fb} + \frac{RT}{F} \quad (1)$$

The point of intersection between the tangent of the Mott–Schottky curve and the x-axis is called intercept E_0. R represents the standard molar gas constant, the thermodynamic temperature is denoted as T, and the Faraday constant is represented by F. The flat band potentials (E_{fb}) for AIS and 1%Ca-AIS are determined as -0.53 V and -0.62 V (vs. SCE), respectively. The conduction band potentials of AIS and 1%Ca-AIS can be determined using a specific Formula (3):

$$E_{CB} = E_{fb} - kT \ln \frac{Nc}{N} \quad (2)$$

In this context, k denotes the Boltzmann constant, Nc indicates the effective state density of the conduction band, and N represents the doping concentration. Through calculations, the value of kTln(Nc/N) is approximately 0.1 eV. Consequently, the conduction band potentials (E_{CB}) for AIS and 1%Ca-AIS are found to be -0.63 V and -0.72 V, respectively. Furthermore, utilizing empirical Formula (4), the valence band potential (E_{VB}) of the semiconductor was calculated as follows [46]:

$$E_{CB} = E_{VB} - E_g \quad (3)$$

In this formula, E_{CB} represents the conduction band potential. The band gap energy is represented by Eg, and it determines the valence band potentials of AIS and 1%Ca-AIS. The calculated valence band potential values are 1.10 V for AIS and 0.96 V for 1%Ca-AIS.

2.5. Photoelectric Property and Photocatalytic Activity

The transient photocurrent response (I-t) curves and electrochemical impedance spectroscopy (EIS) provide a comprehensive understanding of the separation of electrons and holes in the sample. By analyzing the movement and behavior of charge carriers, we can identify limitations and opportunities for improvement in various applications, such as solar cells and photocatalysis. Figure 5a shows the diagrams of transient photocurrent response for AIS and 1%Ca-AIS. When the lamp is turned on for the first time, both AIS and 1%Ca-AIS exhibit good photocurrent response in the test, and the photocurrent intensity of 1%Ca-AIS (~2.920 μA/cm^2) is stronger than AIS (~2.56 μA/cm^2). Upon turning off the light, the current intensity of AIS and 1%Ca-AIS decreases rapidly. After performing the switch on and off for 10 consecutive operations, it becomes evident that both AIS and 1%Ca-AIS maintain excellent reproducibility in terms of photocurrent response. This observation implies the swift segregation of electrons and holes within the material. However, the photocurrent response of AIS and 1%Ca-AIS gradually decreases, which may be due to the partial loss of electrons in the closed circuit under current excitation. Nevertheless, the response intensity of 1%Ca-AIS remains higher than AIS, suggesting a better separation efficiency of electrons and holes in 1%Ca-AIS. This implies that there are more electrons in 1%Ca-AIS to participate in the catalytic reaction process, which proves that the introduction of Ca^{2+} can enhance the photocatalytic effect.

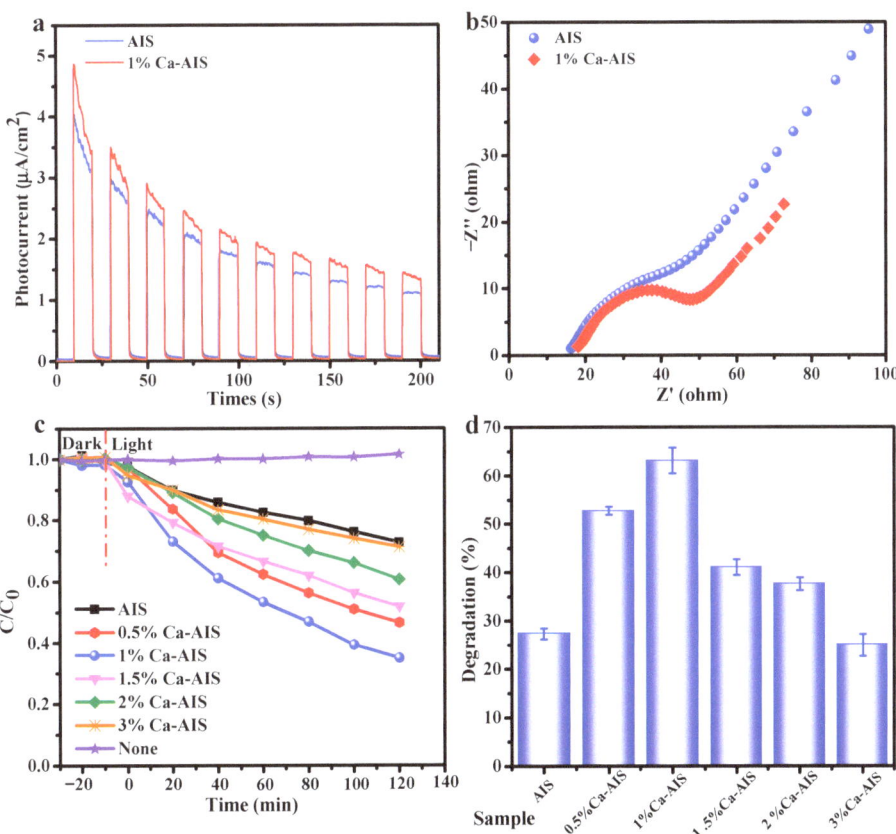

Figure 5. (**a**) Photocurrent response, (**b**) electrochemical impedance spectrum of AIS and 1%Ca-AIS, (**c**) photocatalytic removal curves, and (**d**) degradation rates of 4-NP by AIS and Ca-AIS under visible light irradiation over 120 min.

An examination of electrochemical impedance through the utilization of the "AC impedance" approach was conducted. The open circuit potential served as the primary voltage, maintaining stability throughout the testing process. For this particular experiment, a solution of 0.1 mol/L KCl incorporating 5 mm $K_3[Fe(CN)_6]$ and $K_4[Fe(CN)_6]$ was selected as the electrolyte solution. Figure 5b shows the EIS Nyquist curve obtained from this test. The charge transfer process occurring at the interface between the electrode and the electrolyte can be depicted by the arc observed in the EIS Nyquist curve. Typically, a decrease in the radius of the arc indicates a lower transfer resistance for carriers, thereby leading to enhanced separation and transmission efficiency of photogenerated electrons and holes [43]. The EIS Nyquist diagram reveals that the arc radius of 1%Ca-AIS is smaller compared to AIS. This signifies that the addition of Ca^{2+} improves electronic conductivity. It achieves this by efficiently segregating photogenerated carriers and promoting the swift transfer of interface charges to enhance the overall conductivity. Consequently, 1%Ca-AIS exhibits higher electronic conductivity and realizes the rapid transfer of interface charges, thus showing better photocatalytic activity.

Figure 5c depicts dark adsorption and photocatalytic degradation curves for both Ca-AIS and AIS under visible light. In the absence of light, the concentration of the 4-NP solution remains relatively constant with minimal changes. In Figure 5d, it is evident that the degradation rate of 4-NP under visible light without Ca^{2+} doping is 27.4% for AIS. However, upon the introduction of Ca^{2+}, the degradation rates of 4-NP under visible light for Ca-AIS increase significantly, with doping contents of 0.5% (52.7%), 1% (63.2%), 1.5% (41.1%), and 2% (37.6%). All these degradation rates are higher than pure AIS. Remarkably, the degradation rate of 4-NP with a doping content of 3% is slightly lower than AIS, measuring at 24.9%. Importantly, all the samples exhibit remarkable reproducibility in photocatalytic degradation. These experimental findings support the notion that pure AIS has the capability to harness visible light and generate active species that effectively degrade organic pollutants. Ca-AIS exhibits a consistent improvement in visible light photocatalytic performance for 4-NP upon the appropriate doping of Ca^{2+}. Nevertheless, it is crucial to exercise caution, as an excessive Ca^{2+} concentration impedes the visible light photocatalytic activity of Ca-AIS toward 4-NP. This suggests that the surplus Ca^{2+} functions as a center for recombination, leading to the recombination of charges and thereby impeding photocatalytic activity.

2.6. Photocatalytic Mechanism

Generally, during the process of a catalytic reaction, certain active species such as e^-, $\cdot O_2^-$, h^+, and $\cdot OH$ are produced [47,48]. To determine the active species that play the main role of oxidation and reduction in the catalytic reaction process and thereby speculate the mechanism of the catalytic process, we conducted active species capturing experiments for AIS and 1%Ca-AIS. It is well known that potassium persulfate (KPS), p-benzoquinone (BQ), potassium iodide (KI), n-butanol (N-BA), or isopropanol (IPA) are commonly used as capturing agents for e^-, $\cdot O_2^-$, h^+, and $\cdot OH$, respectively [49–51]. Figure 6a represents capturing experiments performed over a period of 120 min. Among the species, h^+ and $\cdot OH$ play a significant role in the photodegradation process of AIS, followed by e^-. Figure 6b displays the captured results of active species in 1%Ca-AIS. It is clear that the inclusion of the capturing agent significantly hinders the activity of 1%Ca-AIS in comparison to the photocatalytic degradation of 4- without a capturing agent, indicating that e^-, $\cdot O_2^-$, $\cdot OH$, and h^+ all play a role in the degradation of 4-NP by 1%Ca-AIS. The dominant active species in the degradation process of 1%Ca-AIS are $\cdot OH$ and h^+, followed by $\cdot O_2^-$. Based on the analysis, we propose a potential photocatalytic mechanism to elucidate the pathways of charge generation and transfer in Ca-AIS nanomaterials during the photocatalytic degradation of 4-NP. The overview of this mechanism is illustrated in Figure 6c. When AIS and Ca-AIS nanomaterials are exposed to visible light with energy that exceeds the band gap energy, the photon's energy is absorbed by electrons in the valence band, and they are sent to the conduction band. As a result, electrons (e^-) are generated in the conduction band, and holes (h^+) in the valence band are due to the photogenerated process. The production of $\cdot O_2^-$ can be ascribed to the observation that the CB potential of AIS (−0.63 V vs. SCE) and Ca-AIS (−0.72 V vs. SCE) exhibits a more unfavorable value compared to the redox potential of $O_2/\cdot O_2^-$ (−0.56 V vs. SCE) [52]. The generation of $\cdot O_2^-$ occurs when photogenerated electrons are present through a specialized pathway [44]. Since the VB potential of AIS and Ca-AIS is lower than $\cdot OH/H_2O$ (OH^-) (1.75 V vs. SCE),

·OH cannot be generated through the oxidation of H_2O or OH^- by photogenerated holes. Akira Fujishima proposed alternative pathways for the production of ·OH [53]:

$$O_2 + 2e^- + 2H^+ \rightarrow H_2O_2 \quad 0.44\ V(vs.\ SCE)$$
$$H_2O_2 + e^- \rightarrow ·OH + OH^- \quad 0.63\ V(vs.\ SCE) \quad (4)$$
$$H_2O_2 + ·O_2^- \rightarrow ·OH + OH^- + O_2 \quad 0.76\ V(vs.\ SCE)$$

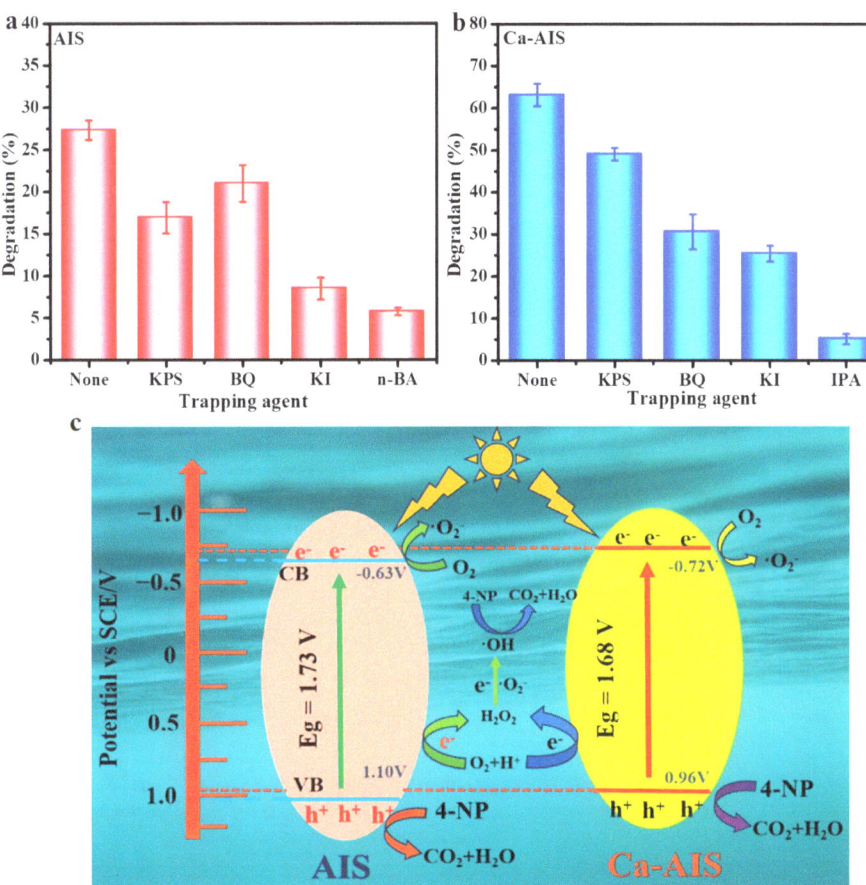

Figure 6. Photodegradation rates of 4-NP by (**a**) AIS and (**b**) 1%Ca-AIS with different active trapping agents and a photocatalysis mechanism diagram under visible light irradiation (**c**).

The VB potential of AIS (1.10 V vs. SCE) and Ca-AIS (0.96 V vs. SCE) are larger than the potential in the reaction formula, so ·OH may be generated through the above pathways in this reaction system. Due to ·OH, h^+, and $·O_2^-$ having strong oxidation, they react with 4-NP on the surface of the catalyst to generate CO_2 and H_2O and realize the degradation of 4-NP. By employing the inclusion of Ca^{2+}, we are able to resolve the instability and compound tendency of h^+ and e^- that are generated by AIS when exposed to light. The inclusion of Ca^{2+} aids in diminishing the resistance encountered during the transfer of electrons at the interface, thereby enhancing the separation and transfer of h^+ and e^-. As a result, the recombination of h^+ and e^- is effectively prevented. Moreover, the introduction of Ca^{2+} causes the CB potential of Ca-AIS to undergo a negative shift, resulting in a more reactive and vigilant e^-. This heightened e^- activity participates in the given reaction, actively leading to an increased production of H_2O_2, ·OH, and $·O_2^-$. Furthermore, the consumption of photogenerated electrons frees photogenerated holes for the oxidation reaction, allowing the involvement of more active species in the degradation of 4-NP [54]. Additionally, the narrow band gap of Ca-AIS suggests that it can effectively harness a broader range of light wavelengths, making it suitable for photocatalysis in a wider spectrum of conditions. Such characteristics of Ca-AIS make it a promising candidate for further exploration and development in the field of photocatalysis.

3. Materials and Methods

3.1. Materials

The experiment utilized analytically pure chemical reagents. $AgNO_3$ was procured from Guangdong Guangcai Technology Co., Ltd. (Shenzhen, China)., indium nitrate hydrate was obtained from Shanghai McLean Biochemical Technology Co., Ltd. (Shanghai, China), and thioglycolic acid (TGA) and thioacetamide (TAA) were purchased from Sinopharm Chemical Reagents Co., Ltd. (Beijing, China). $Ca(NO_3)_2 \cdot 4H_2O$ and isopropanol were acquired from Xilong Science Co., Ltd. (Shantou, China). P-benzoquinone (BQ) and potassium persulfate (KPS) were obtained from Sinopharm Chemical Reagent Co., Ltd. (Beijing, China), and KI was purchased from Tianjin Fengchuan Chemical Reagent Technology Co., Ltd. (Tianjin, China). Ultrapure water with a resistance of 18.25 MΩ cm was utilized in the whole experimental work.

3.2. Preparation of AIS and Ca-AIS

AIS: The catalyst was prepared using the low-temperature liquid phase method, with TGA serving as a stabilizer and TAA as the sulfur source [55]. $AgNO_3$ (0.2038 g), $In(NO_3)_3 \cdot xH_2O$ (1.023 g), and CH_3CSNH_2 [TAA (4.5078 g)] solutions were separately prepared in 50 mL of water. A total of 10 mL $AgNO_3$, 10 mL $In(NO_3)_3 \cdot xH_2O$, and 0.51 mL $C_2H_4O_2S$ (TGA) were transferred to a round bottom flask and mixed with 370 mL ultrapure water. Subsequently, after intense stirring for 15 min, a 10 mL TAA solution was precisely added to the above mixture under stirring. The mixture was promptly placed in a water bath at a constant temperature of 70 °C. The mixture was allowed to react for 5 h. The reaction system was then removed, cooled, and aged for 24 h to obtain the precipitate of AIS. To ensure the purity of the precipitate, filtration was carried out followed by washing with deionized water until the conductivity of the filtrate matched the deionized water. The desired AIS nanomaterial was obtained by vacuum drying at room temperature for 12 h.

Ca-AIS: For the preparation of Ca-doped AIS, the same procedure was followed, except $Ca(NO_3)_2 \cdot 4H_2O$ was added to form a mixed solution of $AgNO_3$, $In(NO_3)_3 \cdot xH_2O$ and $Ca(NO_3)_2 \cdot 4H_2O$ with different mass ratios (m ($Ca(NO_3)_2 \cdot 4H_2O$):m ($AgNO_3$ + In $(NO_3)_3 \cdot xH_2O$) = x%). The addition of $Ca(NO_3)_2 \cdot 4H_2O$ was just before the addition of TAA to obtain Ca-AIS with mass ratios of 0.5%, 1%, 1.5%, 2%, and 3%. The synthesis roadmap of Ca-AIS is shown in Figure 7.

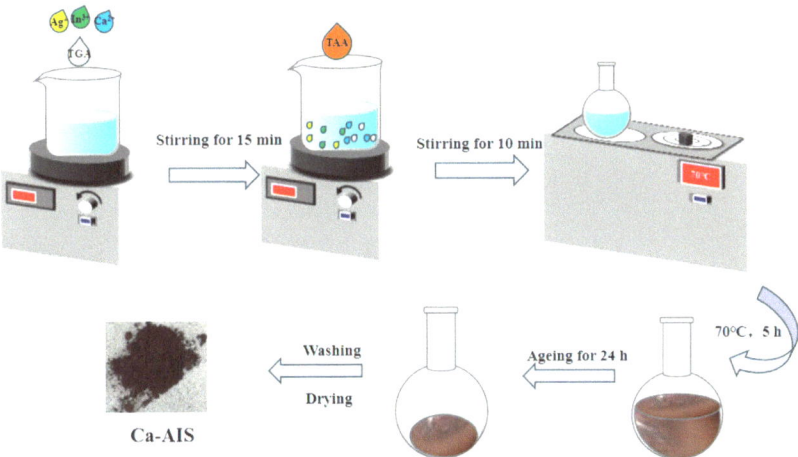

Figure 7. The synthesis roadmap of Ca-AIS.

3.3. Characterization

The crystallinity of the samples was analyzed using an X-ray diffractometer. The experiment employed a Cu-Kα as the light source, with the tube voltage set at 40 kV and current at 30 mA. The scanning range spanned from 5° to 90°. Binding energies were measured utilizing an X-ray photoelectron spectrometer, known as Escalab 250Xi (Thermo Fisher Scientific Shier Science & Technology Company, Waltham, MA, USA), and the radiation source employed was Al Ka. This allowed the determination of the type and valence state of the elements. The interface and surface morphology of the samples were examined using a Talos F200X (Thermo Fisher Scientific Shier Science & Technology Company, USA) high-resolution transmission electron microscope (HRTEM), as well as a JSM-7500F (Hitachi, Japan) scanning electron microscope (SEM). To obtain a UV-Vis absorption study of the samples, a TU-1901 UV-Vis (Beijing General Instrument Company, Beijing, China) spectrophotometer was utilized with a measurement range from 200 to 900 nm. $BaSO_4$ served as the test background. In our study, we utilized an RF-5301 (Shimadzu, Japan) fluorescence spectrophotometer to acquire the photoluminescence spectrum. The excitation wavelength employed was 400 nm, and the slit widths were set at EX: 6HH and EM: 10. Furthermore, the determination of Brunauer–Emmett–Teller (BET) surface areas was performed using a BSD-660M A3M. Before conducting the analysis, the samples underwent a 2 h degassing procedure at 120 °C.

3.4. Photocatalytic Activity

To assess the effectiveness of AIS and Ca-AIS as photocatalysts, a series of experiments were performed utilizing a photocatalytic apparatus. The light source utilized was an iodine tungsten lamp with a power of 1000 W. To eliminate light below 420 nm, a cutoff filter was applied. About 30 mg of the photocatalyst and 80 mL of the 4-NP solution (15 mg/L) were added to a quartz beaker. Before initiating the photocatalytic degradation process, the system was subjected to ultrasonic dispersion for 5 min. Subsequently, it was placed in the photocatalytic reaction device. The distance between the iodine tungsten lamp and the quartz beaker was adjusted to 10 cm. To ensure that the 4-NP diluent attained a state of dark adsorption–desorption equilibrium, the system was stirred in the dark for 30 min. Following this, the light source was turned on to initiate the photocatalytic reaction. The solution was continuously exposed to light for two hours. During this period, 8 mL of solution was taken out after every 20 min. After separation, the optical absorbance of the

supernatant was conducted at a wavelength of 317 nm, and the amount of 4-NP degraded was calculated as:
$$D(\%) = \frac{A_0 - A}{A_0} = \frac{C_0 - C}{C_0} \times 100\% \tag{5}$$

In this case, D represents the efficiency of degradation, A_0 and C_0 represent the absorbance and concentration of 4-NP prior to being measured after the dark adsorption–desorption equilibrium, and A and C denote the absorbance and concentration of 4-NP during the photocatalytic degradation over a given duration.

3.5. Active Species Capture

To investigate the active entities participating in the catalytic process, isopropyl alcohol (IPA) and n-butanol (n-BA) were employed to capture ·OH, while potassium persulfate (KPS), potassium iodide (KI), and p-benzoquinone (BQ) were utilized to capture e^-, h^+, and ·O_2^- separately. The same procedure was followed, as described for the measurement of the photocatalytic activities, except a small amount of the capturing agent was added in each case.

3.6. Flat Band Potential Test

To conduct the test for the flat charge potential of the catalyst, an electrochemical method with a three-electrode setup was employed. The experimental arrangement comprised three electrodes, namely the working electrode, reference electrode, and counter electrode. The working electrode consisted of a conductive glass of indium tin oxide (ITO) coated with a catalyst, the reference electrode was a saturated calomel electrode (SCE), and the counter electrode comprised platinum in a 0.1 mol/L Na_2SO_4 solution. The ITO glass (measuring 1 cm × 2 cm) was cleaned completely using distilled water, acetone, and ethanol. The first step in the preparation of the working electrode involved dispersing a 30 mg catalyst in 10 mL of ethanol. The mixture was ultrasonically treated for 30 min. Subsequently, 10 mL of ethylene glycol was added, followed by another 30 min ultrasonic treatment. The resulting mixture was magnetically stirred for 5 h, resulting in a viscous dispersion containing the catalyst. A droplet of the dispersion measuring 20 µL was then carefully placed on the ITO conductive glass. The glass was left undisturbed for 1 h and was subsequently dried using an infrared lamp to obtain the working electrode. To remove any traces of O_2 in the electrolyte, the solution underwent N_2 bubbling for 30 min. We conducted an analysis of the voltage stability using the "open circuit potential-time" method. A scanning voltage range of −1 V to 1 V we selected utilizing the "impedance-potential" method. The flat band potentials of the samples were determined by analyzing the information obtained from this curve to measure the Mott–Schottky (M-S) curve.

3.7. Photoelectric Chemical Test

Photocurrent tests were used to detect the response strength of the catalyst to light and the carrier separation efficiency. We utilized the CHI-66D model of the electrochemical workstation to assess the homeopathic photocurrent response (I-t) of the functioning electrode. Moreover, we designated the initial voltage as the stable voltage of the open circuit potential. Electrochemical impedance spectroscopy was used to detect the charge transfer rate. In this work, the electrochemical impedance model was CHI-66D, the test amplitude was 5 mV, and the frequency was $1-10^5$ Hz under open circuit voltage.

4. Conclusions

The main objective of this investigation was to fabricate pristine AIS and Ca^{2+}-doped AIS utilizing the liquid phase method at low temperatures. The structural arrangement of AIS crystals remained unaltered, even after the addition of Ca^{2+}. The detectable photocatalytic performance of Ca-AIS exhibited an escalation within a specific scope as the concentration of Ca^{2+} dopants increased. When the Ca^{2+} concentration was maintained at 1%, Ca-AIS was subjected to visible light for a duration of 120 min, and the degradation efficiency of P-Nitrophenol reached an impressive 63.2%. Despite the potential benefits of incorporating Ca^{2+} for improving the visible photocatalytic activity of AIS, it was observed that excessive Ca^{2+} content had a detrimental effect on the activity. Furthermore, Ca-AIS exhibited superior sphericity, smaller particle size, more uniformity in size, better dispersibility, and more active sites. Capturing experiments confirmed that the active species engaged in the degradation of 4-NP were ·OH and h^+. The introduction of Ca effectively suppressed the recombination of h^+ and e^- and generated more $·O_2^-$, resulting in improved photocatalytic activity of AIS. The target pollutant in this work was organic pollutant (4-NP) wastewater simulated under laboratory conditions. The complex actual wastewater situation in which multiple pollutants coexist has not been further explored. Therefore, it is necessary to explore the application of this system to composite pollutants and actual wastewater. Follow-up research can broaden its application areas to photocatalytic water splitting for hydrogen production and even try to treat some real industrial wastewater.

Furthermore, Ca-AIS can also be doped with different extraneous elements in an attempt to modify its energy band structure and electronic state, and then it can be compounded with magnetic semiconductors to find better combinations for achieving higher photocatalytic performance. Subsequently, these optimized combinations can be used in photocatalytic hydrogen production or acoustic catalysis experiments.

Author Contributions: X.W. conducted catalysts synthesis, characterization, and the activity test. S.L. (Shuyuan Liu) contributed to data analysis. S.L. (Shu Lin) discussed the photocatalytic mechanism. K.Q., Y.M. and Y.Y. conceived the project and wrote the manuscript. All authors have read and agreed to the published version of the manuscript.

Funding: This work was financially supported by the National Natural Science Foundation of China (Ggants 22362002, 22268003, 52272287) and a project from Yunnan Province (grants 202301AT070027, 202305AF150116).

Institutional Review Board Statement: Not applicable.

Informed Consent Statement: Not applicable.

Data Availability Statement: Data are contained within the article.

Conflicts of Interest: The authors declare no conflict of interest.

References

1. Tkaczyk, A.; Mitrowska, K.; Posyniak, A. Synthetic organic dyes as contaminants of the aquatic environment and their implications for ecosystems: A review. *Sci. Total Environ.* **2020**, *717*, 137222. [CrossRef] [PubMed]
2. Cushing, S.K.; Li, J.; Meng, F.; Senty, T.R.; Suri, S.; Zhi, M.; Li, M.; Bristow, A.D.; Wu, N. Photocatalytic activity enhanced by plasmonic resonant energy transfer from metal to semiconductor. *J. Am. Chem. Soc.* **2012**, *134*, 15033–15041. [CrossRef] [PubMed]
3. Shukla, S.S.; Dorris, K.L.; Chikkaveeraiah, B.V. Photocatalytic degradation of 2,4-dinitrophenol. *J. Hazard. Mater.* **2009**, *164*, 310–314. [CrossRef] [PubMed]
4. Watson, C.; Bahadur, K.; Briess, L.; Dussling, M.; Kohler, F.; Weinsheimer, S.; Wichern, F. Mitigating Negative Microbial Effects of p-Nitrophenol, Phenol, Copper and Cadmium in a Sandy Loam Soil Using Biochar. *Water Air Soil Pollut.* **2017**, *228*, 74. [CrossRef]
5. Balakrishnan, A.; Gaware, G.J.; Chinthala, M. Heterojunction photocatalysts for the removal of nitrophenol: A systematic review. *Chemosphere* **2023**, *310*, 136853. [CrossRef] [PubMed]
6. Nemiwal, M.; Zhang, T.C.; Kumar, D. Recent progress in g-C_3N_4, TiO_2 and ZnO based photocatalysts for dye degradation: Strategies to improve photocatalytic activity. *Sci. Total Environ.* **2021**, *767*, 144896. [CrossRef]
7. Kulkarni, M.; Chaudhari, A. Biodegradation of p-nitrophenol by P. putida. *Bioresour. Technol.* **2006**, *97*, 982–988. [CrossRef]
8. Chen, Q.; Ma, C.; Duan, W.; Lang, D.; Pan, B. Coupling adsorption and degradation in p-nitrophenol removal by biochars. *J. Clean. Prod.* **2020**, *271*, 122550. [CrossRef]
9. Fatima, R.; Afridi, M.N.; Kumar, V.; Lee, J.; Ali, I.; Kim, K.H.; Kim, J.O. Photocatalytic degradation performance of various types of modified TiO_2 against nitrophenols in aqueous systems. *J. Clean. Prod.* **2019**, *231*, 899–912. [CrossRef]
10. Mohan, B.S.; Ravi, K.; Anjaneyulu, R.B.; Sree, G.S.; Basavaiah, K. Fe_2O_3/RGO nanocomposite photocatalyst: Effective degradation of 4-Nitrophenol. *Phys. B* **2019**, *553*, 190–194. [CrossRef]
11. Kawase, Y.; Tokumura, M.; Salehi, Z.; Sugiyama, M. Photocatalytic degradation of p-nitrophenol by zinc oxide particles. *Water Sci. Technol.* **2012**, *65*, 1882–1886.

12. Koe, W.S.; Lee, J.W.; Chong, W.C.; Pang, Y.L.; Sim, L.C. An overview of photocatalytic degradation: Photocatalysts, mechanisms, and development of photocatalytic membrane. *Environ. Sci. Pollut. Res.* **2020**, *27*, 2522–2565. [CrossRef]
13. Zhang, J.J.; Gu, X.Y.; Zhao, Y.; Zhang, K.; Yan, Y.; Qi, K.Z. Photocatalytic Hydrogen Production and Tetracycline Degradation Using ZnIn$_2$S$_4$ Quantum Dots Modified g-C$_3$N$_4$ Composites. *Nanomaterials* **2023**, *13*, 305. [CrossRef] [PubMed]
14. Wang, L.Z.; Zhang, J.H.; Liu, H.M.; Huang, J. Design, modification and application of semiconductor photocatalysts. *J. Taiwan Inst. Chem. Eng.* **2018**, *93*, 590–602. [CrossRef]
15. Xia, Y.; Tian, Z.H.; Heil, T.; Meng, A.; Cheng, B.; Cao, S.W.; Yu, J.G.; Antonietti, M. Highly Selective CO$_2$ Capture and Its Direct Photochemical Conversion on Ordered 2D/1D Heterojunctions. *Joule* **2019**, *3*, 2792–2805. [CrossRef]
16. Song, J.H.; Zhang, J.J.; Qi, K.Z.; Imparato, C.; Liu, S.-Y. Exploration of the g-C$_3$N$_4$ Heterostructure with Ag–In Sulfide Quantum Dots for Enhanced Photocatalytic Activity. *ACS Appl. Electron. Mater.* **2023**, *5*, 4134–4144. [CrossRef]
17. Parbin, A.R. Bifunctional WO$_3$-AgInS$_2$ nanocomposite material: Enhanced electrical property and photocatalytic activity for degradation of methylene blue dye under visible-light irradiation. *Mater. Today Commun.* **2023**, *35*, 106447. [CrossRef]
18. Lei, Y.Q.; Xing, Y.; Fan, W.Q.; Song, S.Y.; Zhang, H.J. Synthesis, characterization and optical property of flower-like indium tin sulfide nanostructures. *Dalton Trans.* **2009**, 1620–1623. [CrossRef] [PubMed]
19. Lei, Y.Q.; Wang, G.H.; Zhou, L.; Hu, W.; Song, S.Y.; Fan, W.Q.; Zhang, H.J. Cubic spinel In$_4$SnS$_8$: Electrical transport properties and electrochemical hydrogen storage properties. *Dalton Trans.* **2010**, *39*, 7021–7024. [CrossRef]
20. Rengaraj, S.; Venkataraj, S.; Tai, C.-W.; Kim, Y.; Repo, E.; Sillanpaa, M. Self-Assembled Mesoporous Hierarchical-like In$_2$S$_3$ Hollow Microspheres Composed of Nanofibers and Nanosheets and Their Photocatalytic Activity. *Langmuir* **2011**, *27*, 5534–5541. [CrossRef]
21. Liu, B.J.; Li, X.Y.; Zhao, Q.D.; Ke, J.; Tadé, M.; Liu, S.M. Preparation of AgInS$_2$/TiO$_2$ Composites for Enhanced Photocatalytic Degradation of Gaseous o-dichlorobenzene under Visible Light. *Appl. Catal. B* **2016**, *185*, 1–10. [CrossRef]
22. Sun, L.J.; Wang, Y.; He, L.X.; Guo, J.; Deng, Q.W.; Zhao, X.; Yan, Y.; Qi, K.Z. Effect of cobalt doping on the photocatalytic performance of AgInS$_2$ for organic pollutant degradation and hydrogen production. *J. Alloys Compd.* **2022**, *926*, 166859. [CrossRef]
23. Yang, F.J.; Yang, B.Y.; Gu, X.Y.; Li, M.H.; Qi, K.Z.; Yan, Y. Detection of enrofloxacin residues in dairy products based on their fluorescence quenching effect on AgInS$_2$ QDs. *Spectrochim. Acta Part A* **2023**, *301*, 122985. [CrossRef]
24. Wu, F.F.; Liu, G.; Xu, X.X. Efficient photocatalytic oxygen production over Ca-modified LaTiO$_2$N. *J. Catal.* **2017**, *346*, 10–20. [CrossRef]
25. Ahmad, I.; Ahmed, E.; Ahmad, M.; Akhtar, M.S.; Basharat, M.A.; Khan, W.Q.; Ghauri, M.I.; Ali, A.; Manzoor, M.F. The investigation of hydrogen evolution using Ca doped ZnO catalysts under visible light illumination. *Mater. Sci. Semicond. Process.* **2020**, *105*, 104748. [CrossRef]
26. Chen, Y.F.; Duan, X.; Li, J.L.; Liu, W.Z.; Ren, S.; Yang, J.; Liu, Q.C. Hydrothermal synthesis of Ca doped β-In$_2$S$_3$ for effective dyes degradation. *Adv. Powder Technol.* **2021**, *32*, 1881–1890. [CrossRef]
27. Yao, L.; Wu, X.H.; Yang, S.H.; Zhang, Y.L. Structural and optical properties of Ca doped BiFeO$_3$ thin films prepared by a sol-gel method. *Ceram. Int.* **2017**, *43*, S470–S473. [CrossRef]
28. Yao, W.; Chen, Y.F.; Li, J.L.; Yang, J.; Ren, S.; Liu, W.Z.; Liu, Q.C. Photocatalytic degradation of methyl orange by Ca doped β-In$_2$S$_3$ with varying Ca concentration. *Res. Chem. Intermed.* **2022**, *48*, 1813–1829. [CrossRef]
29. Gu, X.Y.; Tan, C.; He, L.X.; Guo, J.; Zhao, X.; Qi, K.Z.; Yan, Y. Mn^{2+} doped AgInS$_2$ photocatalyst for formaldehyde degradation and hydrogen production from water splitting by carbon tube enhancement. *Chemosphere* **2022**, *304*, 135292. [CrossRef] [PubMed]
30. Kowalik, P.; Mucha, S.G.; Matczyszyn, K.; Bujak, P.; Mazur, L.M.; Ostrowski, A.; Kmita, A.; Gajewska, M.; Pron, A. Heterogeneity induced dual luminescence properties of AgInS$_2$ and AgInS$_2$–ZnS alloyed nanocrystals. *Inorg. Chem. Front.* **2021**, *8*, 3450–3462. [CrossRef]
31. Aazam, E.S. Photocatalytic oxidation of cyanide under visible light by Pt doped AgInS$_2$ nanoparticles. *J. Ind. Eng. Chem.* **2014**, *20*, 4008–4013. [CrossRef]
32. Yin, D.W.; Pei, L.; Liu, Z.; Yang, X.Y.; Xiang, W.D.; Zhang, X.Y. Synthesis, Characterization, and Photoluminescence on the Glass Doped with AgInS$_2$ Nanocrystals. *Adv. Condens. Matter Phys.* **2015**, *2015*, 141056.
33. Wang, H.J.; Li, J.Z.; Wan, Y.; Nazir, A.; Song, X.H.; Huo, P.W.; Wang, H.Q. Synthesis of AgInS$_2$ QDs-MoS$_2$/GO composite with enhanced interfacial charge separation for efficient photocatalytic degradation of tetracycline and CO$_2$ reduction. *J. Alloys Compd.* **2023**, *954*, 170159. [CrossRef]
34. Anand, P.; Jaihindh, D.P.; Chang, W.K.; Fu, Y.P. Tailoring the Ca-doped bismuth ferrite for electrochemical oxygen evolution reaction and photocatalytic activity. *Appl. Surf. Sci.* **2021**, *540*, 148387. [CrossRef]
35. E, T.; Ma, Z.; Cai, D.; Yang, S.; Li, Y. Enhancement of Interfacial Charge Transfer of TiO$_2$/Graphene with Doped Ca^{2+} for Improving Electrical Conductivity. *ACS Appl. Mater. Interfaces* **2021**, *13*, 41875–41885. [CrossRef] [PubMed]
36. Saumya; Dasauni, K.; Nailwal, T.K.; Voddumalla, S.; Nenavathu, B.P. Facile synthesis of Ca doped CuO nanoparticles and their investigation in antibacterial efficacy. *Biologia* **2023**, *78*, 903–911. [CrossRef]
37. Pham, X.N.; Vu, V.T.; Nguyen, H.V.T.; Nguyen, T.T.; Doan, H.V. Designing a novel heterostructure AgInS$_2$@MIL-101(Cr) photocatalyst from PET plastic waste for tetracycline degradation. *Nanoscale Adv.* **2022**, *4*, 3600–3608. [CrossRef]
38. Deng, F.; Zhong, F.; Hu, P.; Pei, X.L.; Luo, X.B.; Luo, S.L. Fabrication of In-rich AgInS$_2$ nanoplates and nanotubes by a facile low-temperature co-precipitation strategy and their excellent visible-light photocatalytic mineralization performance. *J. Nanopart. Res.* **2017**, *19*, 14. [CrossRef]

39. Chen, J.; Liu, W.X.; Gao, W.W. Tuning photocatalytic activity of In_2S_3 broadband spectrum photocatalyst based on morphology. *Appl. Surf. Sci.* **2016**, *368*, 288–297. [CrossRef]
40. Zhang, Z.W.; Xiao, A.; Yan, K.; Liu, Y.H.; Yan, Z.Y.; Chen, J.Q. $CuInS_2$/ZnS/TGA Nanocomposite Photocatalysts: Synthesis, Characterization and Photocatalytic Activity. *Catal. Lett.* **2017**, *147*, 1631–1639. [CrossRef]
41. Wang, L.; Cheng, B.; Zhang, L.; Yu, J. In situ Irradiated XPS Investigation on S-Scheme TiO_2@$ZnIn_2S_4$ Photocatalyst for Efficient Photocatalytic CO_2 Reduction. *Small* **2021**, *17*, 2103447. [CrossRef]
42. Cychosz, K.A.; Thommes, M. Progress in the Physisorption Characterization of Nanoporous Gas Storage Materials. *Engineering* **2018**, *4*, 559–566. [CrossRef]
43. Du, J.G.; Ma, S.L.; Liu, H.P.; Fu, H.C.; Li, L.; Li, Z.Q.; Li, Y.; Zhou, J.G. Uncovering the mechanism of novel $AgInS_2$ nanosheets/TiO_2 nanobelts composites for photocatalytic remediation of combined pollution. *Appl. Catal. B* **2019**, *259*, 118062. [CrossRef]
44. Zhao, Y.Y.; Fan, X.; Zheng, H.X.; Liu, E.Z.; Fan, J.; Wang, X.J. Bi_2WO_6/$AgInS_2$ S-scheme heterojunction: Efficient photodegradation of organic pollutant and toxicity evaluation. *J. Mater. Sci. Technol.* **2024**, *170*, 200–211. [CrossRef]
45. Li, Y.H.; Liu, Y.; Gao, G.; Zhu, Y.; Wang, D.; Ding, M.; Yao, T.T.; Liu, M.Y.; You, W.S. L-cysteine and urea synergistically-mediated one-pot one-step self-transformed hydrothermal synthesis of p-Ag_2S/n-$AgInS_2$ core-shell heteronanoflowers for photocatalytic MO degradation. *Appl. Surf. Sci.* **2021**, *548*, 149279. [CrossRef]
46. Zhang, J.J.; Zhao, Y.; Qi, K.Z.; Liu, S.-Y. $CuInS_2$ quantum-dot-modified g-C_3N_4 S-scheme heterojunction photocatalyst for hydrogen production and tetracycline degradation. *J. Mater. Sci. Technol.* **2024**, *172*, 145–155. [CrossRef]
47. Ran, X.Q.; Duan, L.; Chen, X.Y.; Yang, X. Photocatalytic degradation of organic dyes by the conjugated polymer poly(1,3,4-oxadiazole)s and its photocatalytic mechanism. *J. Mater. Sci.* **2018**, *53*, 7048–7059. [CrossRef]
48. Khairy, M.; Naguib, E.M.; Mohamed, M.M. Enhancement of Photocatalytic and Sonophotocatalytic Degradation of 4-nitrophenol by ZnO/Graphene Oxide and ZnO/Carbon Nanotube Nanocomposites. *J. Photochem. Photobiol. A* **2020**, *396*, 112507. [CrossRef]
49. Ryu, J.; Choi, W. Substrate-Specific Photocatalytic Activities of TiO_2 and Multiactivity Test for Water Treatment Application. *Environ. Sci. Technol.* **2008**, *42*, 294–300. [CrossRef]
50. Feng, C.; Chen, Z.Y.; Jing, J.P.; Hou, J. The photocatalytic phenol degradation mechanism of Ag-modified ZnO nanorods. *J. Mater. Chem. C* **2020**, *8*, 3000–3009. [CrossRef]
51. Luo, T.; Li, L.; Chen, Y.; An, J.; Liu, C.; Yan, Z.; Carter, J.H.; Han, X.; Sheveleva, A.M.; Tuna, F.; et al. Construction of C-C bonds via photoreductive coupling of ketones and aldehydes in the metal-organic-framework MFM-300(Cr). *Nat. Commun.* **2021**, *12*, 3583. [CrossRef] [PubMed]
52. Liu, B.W.; Bie, C.B.; Zhang, Y.; Wang, L.X.; Li, Y.J.; Yu, J.G. Hierarchically Porous ZnO/g-C_3N_4 S-Scheme Heterojunction Photocatalyst for Efficient H_2O_2 Production. *Langmuir* **2021**, *37*, 14114–14124. [CrossRef] [PubMed]
53. Cui, Q.F.; Gu, X.Y.; Zhao, Y.; Qi, K.Z.; Yan, Y. S-scheme $CuInS_2$/ZnS heterojunctions for the visible light-driven photocatalytic degradation of tetracycline antibiotic drugs. *J. Taiwan Inst. Chem. Eng.* **2023**, *142*, 104679. [CrossRef]
54. Liu, Y.; Hu, Z.F.; Jimmy, C. Photocatalytic degradation of ibuprofen on S-doped BiOBr. *Chemosphere* **2021**, *278*, 130376. [CrossRef] [PubMed]
55. Lv, X.H.; Lan, H.; Guo, J.; Guo, M.X.; Yan, Y. Synthesis of Au-loaded $AgInS_2$ nanoparticles with highly enhanced visible light photocatalytic performances. *J. Mater. Sci. Mater. Electron.* **2020**, *31*, 22284–22296. [CrossRef]

Disclaimer/Publisher's Note: The statements, opinions and data contained in all publications are solely those of the individual author(s) and contributor(s) and not of MDPI and/or the editor(s). MDPI and/or the editor(s) disclaim responsibility for any injury to people or property resulting from any ideas, methods, instructions or products referred to in the content.

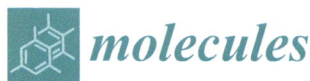

Article

Boosting the Activation of Molecular Oxygen and the Degradation of Rhodamine B in Polar-Functional-Group-Modified g-C₃N₄

Jing Chen [1,2,*], Minghua Yang [2], Hongjiao Zhang [2], Yuxin Chen [3], Yujie Ji [3], Ruohan Yu [3] and Zhenguo Liu [1,4,*]

[1] Key Laboratory of Flexible Electronics of Zhejiang Province, Ningbo Institute of Northwestern Polytechnical University, Ningbo 315103, China
[2] Department of Chemical and Material Engineering, Quzhou College of Technology, Quzhou 324002, China; yangmh@qzct.edu.cn (M.Y.); zhanghongjiao@qzct.edu.cn (H.Z.)
[3] Department of Chemistry, Lishui University, 1 Xueyuan Road, Lishui 323000, China; chenyuxin@lsu.edu.cn (Y.C.); jiyujie@lsu.edu.cn (Y.J.); yuruohan@lsu.edu.cn (R.Y.)
[4] School of Flexible Electronics and Henan Institute of Flexible Electronics, Henan University, Zhengzhou 450046, China
* Correspondence: chenjing@qzct.edu.cn (J.C.); iamzgliu@nwpu.edu.cn (Z.L.)

Abstract: Molecular oxygen activation often suffers from high energy consumption and low efficiency. Developing eco-friendly and effective photocatalysts remains a key challenge for advancing green molecular oxygen activation. Herein, graphitic carbon nitride (g-C₃N₄) with abundant hydroxyl groups (HCN) was synthesized to investigate the relationship between these polar groups and molecular oxygen activation. The advantage of the hydroxyl group modification of g-C₃N₄ included narrower interlayer distances, a larger specific surface area and improved hydrophilicity. Various photoelectronic measurements revealed that the introduced hydroxyl groups reduced the charge transfer resistance of HCN, resulting in accelerated charge separation and migration kinetics. Therefore, the optimal HCN-90 showed the highest activity for Rhodamine B photodegradation with a reaction time of 30 min and an apparent rate constant of 0.125 min^{-1}, surpassing most other g-C₃N₄ composites. This enhanced activity was attributed to the adjusted band structure achieved through polar functional group modification. The modification of polar functional groups could alter the energy band structure of photocatalysts, narrow band gap, enhance visible-light absorption, and improve photogenerated carrier separation efficiency. This work highlights the significant potential of polar functional groups in tuning the structure of g-C₃N₄ to enhance efficient molecular oxygen activation.

Keywords: polar functional group; g-C₃N₄; degradation; visible-light photocatalysis

1. Introduction

Synthetic dyes are common organic pollutants found in wastewater from industries, such as cosmetics, textiles, paints, and leather processing. Rhodamine B (RhB) is a water-soluble organic dye known for its industrial advantages, including its low cost and high color fastness [1]. Unfortunately, RhB exhibits potential neurotoxicity, genotoxicity, and carcinogenicity. Even trace amounts (approximately 1.0 mg/L) of RhB can have significant colorimetric effects on water, posing threats to both the environment and human health [2]. Several traditional methods have been developed to remove RhB from water, such as adsorption, membrane filtration, degradation, and coagulation [3]. Advanced oxidation processes (AOPs) are effective methods for removing difficult-to-degrade and non-biodegradable compounds, which makes them promising for RhB removal. Various advanced oxidation processes have been studied for RhB degradation, including ozone oxidation [4], Fenton and Fenton-like reactions [5–7], and photocatalysts [8,9]. These processes focus on generating reactive oxygen species (ROS) for degrading pollutants.

Molecular oxygen, as an environmentally friendly oxidant, is widely used in the field of environmental remediation [10]. By converting into reactive oxygen species (ROS), such as superoxide ($\cdot O_2^-$), hydrogen peroxide (H_2O_2), hydroxyl radical ($\cdot OH$), and singlet oxygen ($^1O_2$), molecular oxygen can exhibit excellent performances in pollutant degradation and clean energy conversion [11]. Therefore, promoting the activation of molecular oxygen into ROS has garnered significant research interest in recent years. Nevertheless, the direct oxidation of molecular oxygen is limited due to spin-forbidden reactions [12]. Traditional physical and chemical methods for activating molecular oxygen tend to have high energy consumption and low efficiency. This is mainly attributed to the high energy of the O=O bond (494 kJ/mol) [13]. Interestingly, photocatalysis presents a viable approach for molecular oxygen activation. Photogenerated electrons in the excited state can overcome the spin-forbidden barrier, transforming molecular oxygen into ROS [14]. Thus, developing high-performance photocatalysts through rational design emerges as a promising strategy to enhance activation efficiency [15,16].

Due to its abundant active edge sites and hierarchical nanostructures [17], g-C_3N_4 has emerged as a highly effective visible light-driven catalyst. It exhibits versatile applications in many fields, such as pollutant degradation [18], hydrogen evolution [19], CO_2 reduction [20], and organic matter conversion [21]. However, the slow kinetic processes and the rapid recombination rate of photo-generated charges have significantly limited the application efficacy. Various modification strategies including doping, texture engineering, and semiconductor coupling have been pioneered [22,23]. Notably, functional group modification is a molecular doping process that optimizes the intrinsic conjugation system, optoelectronic properties, and energy band structure of g-C_3N_4. Novel functional groups, including hydroxyl, amino, carboxyl, cyano, urea, and carbon rings, have been continuously introduced to g-C_3N_4 to improve its photocatalytic performance [24].

Polar functional groups may induce local charge redistribution when introduced to the g-C_3N_4 matrix and surface. This results in effective local spatial charge separation, interfacial charge transfer, and a significant increase in carrier densities [25]. Li et al. developed surface-alkalized g-C_3N_4 (CN-KCl/NH_4Cl), achieving a 3.2-times boost in photocatalytic H_2 evolution. The addition of hydroxyl groups increased the conduction band potential, resulting in more reducing electrons and accelerating the rate of photoexcited electrons transferred to reactants [26]. Yu et al. enhanced the generation rate of H_2 11-fold through the surface hydroxylation of g-C_3N_4 using post-hydrothermal and plasmonic treatment [27]. Furthermore, polar functional group modifications can improve the interaction between the catalyst and the target. Nan et al. demonstrated that grafting hydroxyl groups to g-C_3N_4 might increase the affinity of the catalyst surface, allowing it to adsorb more CO_2 and H_2O molecules and effectively enhancing the photocatalytic process [28]. Polar functional groups can also improve the hydrophilicity of g-C_3N_4, facilitating a more effective dispersion of the catalyst in water and ensuring its proper utilization. Special procedures for preparing hydroxylation oxygen plasma [29,30], chemical oxidization [31], and hydrothermalization [32–34] have also been attempted. Nevertheless, the current processes would probably introduce unnecessary recombination centers for electron-hole pairs, which may cause a decrease in photocatalytic efficiency and chemical pollution. Furthermore, the complexity and high expense of the operation processes and unpredictable risks in the action process hinder the further development of these technologies. Therefore, a simple and environmentally friendly method to modify g-C_3N_4 with hydroxyl groups is highly desired.

Herein, we developed a novel hydroxyl-group-modified g-C_3N_4 (HCN) with ultrasonic-assisted hydrogen peroxide (H_2O_2). The introduction of hydroxyl groups into g-C_3N_4 promoted the interaction between photo-excited electrons and protons in water and enhanced the proton exchange process. The band gap energy of optimal samples was reduced, and the separation efficiency of photoexcited electrons and holes improved, resulting in a more favorable environment for the generation of reactive oxygen species. A significant improvement was observed in the photocatalytic performance of HCN. Specifically, the photocatalytic degradation constants of RhB for HCN-90 were 3.5 times higher than those for g-C_3N_4. This improvement was primarily attributed to the hydroxyl groups, which facilitated the mass transfer and interfacial charge transfer processes.

2. Results and Discussion

2.1. Characterization of g-C_3N_4 and HCN

TEM images of the g-C_3N_4 and HCN-90 are shown in Figure 1a,b, respectively. Notably, HCN-90 and g-C_3N_4 exhibited similar morphology. HCN-90 exhibited a darker color to g-C_3N_4. This difference could be attributed to the presence of more polar functional groups on the surface of HCN-90, altering its electronic arrangement and the conjugation system. Next, XRD analysis was performed to investigate changes in crystal phase structures and crystallinity (Figure 1c). Both g-C_3N_4 and HCN-90 showed two characteristic diffraction peaks of g-C_3N_4 (JCPDS No. 87-1526) at 2θ = 27.5° (002) and 13.0° (100) [35]. These peaks corresponded to the tri-s-triazine ring in-plane compression and interlayer stacking structure of the conjugated aromatic system, respectively [36]. The significant decrease in the (001) diffraction peak of HCN-90 indicated disruption in the orderly stacking structure within the tri-s-triazine planes. Compared to g-C_3N_4, the diffraction peak at (002) for HCN-90 showed a slight rightward shift from 27.5° to 27.6°, indicating a reduction in the interlayer spacing [37]. Furthermore, the intensity of the (002) plane in HCN-90 decreased, supporting the conclusion of a shortened interlayer distance. Narrower interlayer distances were beneficial for faster charge transfer [38].

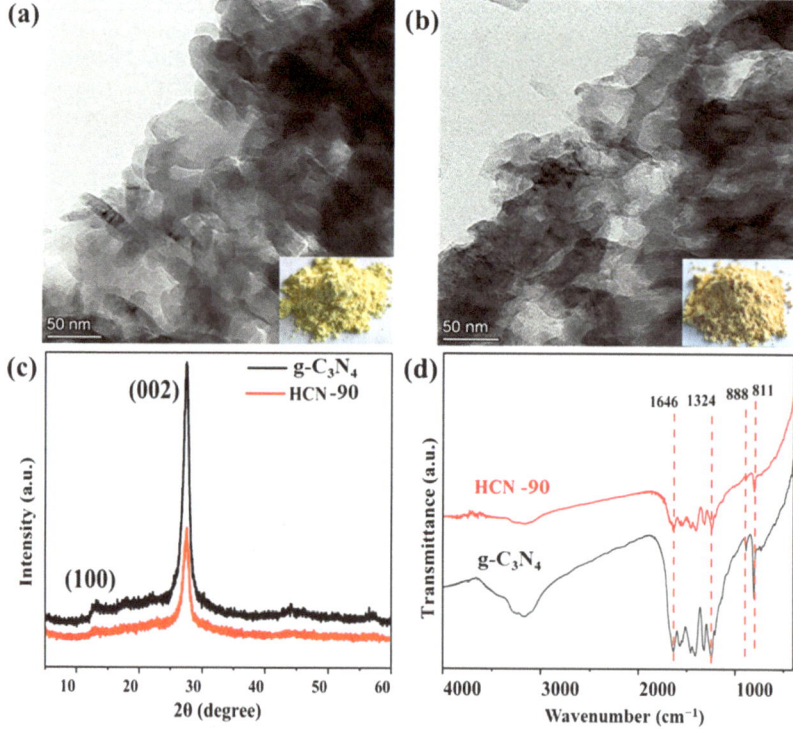

Figure 1. (**a**) TEM images of g-C_3N_4; (**b**) TEM images of HCN-90; (**c**) XRD patterns of g-C_3N_4 and HCN-90; (**d**) FT-IR spectra of g-C_3N_4 and HCN-90.

FT-IR spectroscopy was employed to assess the structure of g-C_3N_4 and HCN-90 (Figure 1d). HCN-90 exhibited a significant increase in broadband intensity in the 3000–3500 cm^{-1} region compared to g-C_3N_4. These broad peaks could be attributed to N-H and O-H stretching vibrational modes [39]. The increased broadband strength in HCN-90 indicated the formation of abundant surface hydroxyl groups. In the region of 1200–1650 cm^{-1}, these bands corresponded to the typical stretching mode of C-N heterocycles [40]. Specifically, the peaks at 1324 cm^{-1} reflected the out-of-plane bending vibration characteristic of the heptazine ring [41]. The absorption band at 888 cm^{-1} was attributed to an N-H deformation mode [42], indicating an incomplete condensation of the amino groups. The sharp absorption peak around 811 cm^{-1} was associated with the typical breathing mode of the tri-s-triazine unit [43]. A similar structure indicated that the structure of HCN-90 remained unchanged.

XPS analysis was conducted to examine the surface composition and chemical states of g-C$_3$N$_4$ and HCN-90. In the XPS survey spectra (Figure 2a), O 1s, N 1s, and C 1s peaks were observed. Elemental analysis further revealed that the O-atom contents of g-C$_3$N$_4$ and HCN-90 were 3.06% and 6.36%. These results suggested the introduction of oxygen-containing functional groups in the samples following treatment with H$_2$O$_2$. The high-resolution C 1s spectrum (Figure 2b) of g-C$_3$N$_4$ exhibited three distinct peaks. The peak at 284.8 eV corresponded to the indeterminate carbon (sp3 C-C), whereas those at 286.3 eV and 288.7 eV arose from the C-N and N=C-N in the heptazine heterocycles [44]. The high-resolution N 1s spectra (Figure 2c) displayed peaks at 398.5 eV, 400.1 eV, and 401.0 eV, corresponding to C-N=C, C-N(-C)-C, and C-NH$_2$, respectively [45]. The high-resolution O 1s spectra (Figure 2d) revealed two O species in g-C$_3$N$_4$ and HCN-90, with binding energies of 531.3 eV (O-H) and 533.8 eV (O-N). The former corresponded to surface hydroxyl groups, while the latter originated from intermediate products of melamine thermal polymerization [46]. Notably, the calculated atomic percentages of the O-H of g-C$_3$N$_4$ and HCN-90 were 19.81% and 47.51%, respectively. This suggested that the oxygen species predominantly existed as hydroxyl groups with hydroxyl on the surface. The contact angle (CA) measurements further supported the results, as shown for HCN-90 and g-C$_3$N$_4$ (Figure 2e). The reduced CA could be attributed to the abundance of hydroxyl groups on the surface.

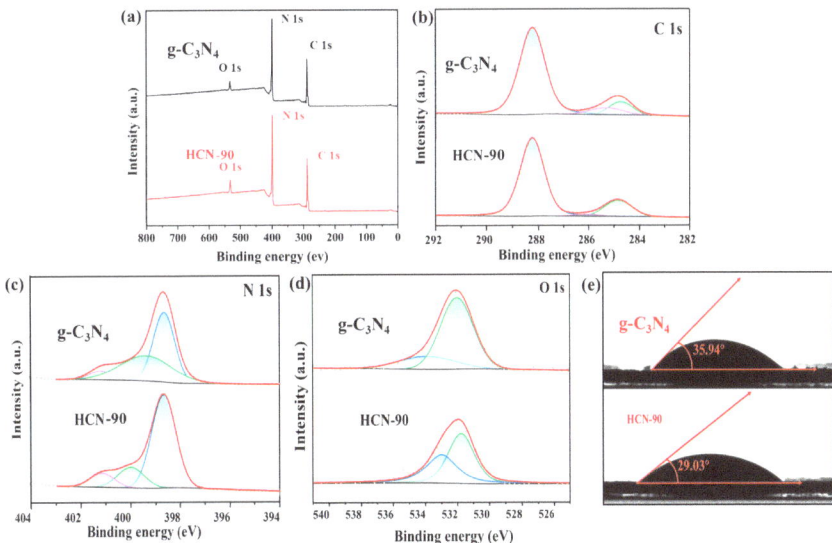

Figure 2. XPS spectra of g-C$_3$N$_4$ and HCN-90: (**a**) survey; (**b**) C 1s; (**c**) N 1s; (**d**) O 1s; (**e**) water contact angles.

Figure 3a shows the N$_2$ isothermal adsorption–desorption curves of g-C$_3$N$_4$ and HCN-90. Both curves exhibited typical IV adsorption patterns with H3-type hysteresis loops, indicating the presence of mesopores and macropores in both samples. The smaller hysteresis loop observed in g-C_3N_4 at high P/P_0 was ascribed to the aggregation of g-C_3N_4 particles. Importantly, the specific surface area of HCN-90 measured 27.3 m^2/g, surpassing the 11.5 m^2/g recorded for g-C_3N_4. This expanded the specific surface area and provided numerous active sites for adsorption and surface reactions, effectively enhancing the photocatalytic reaction.

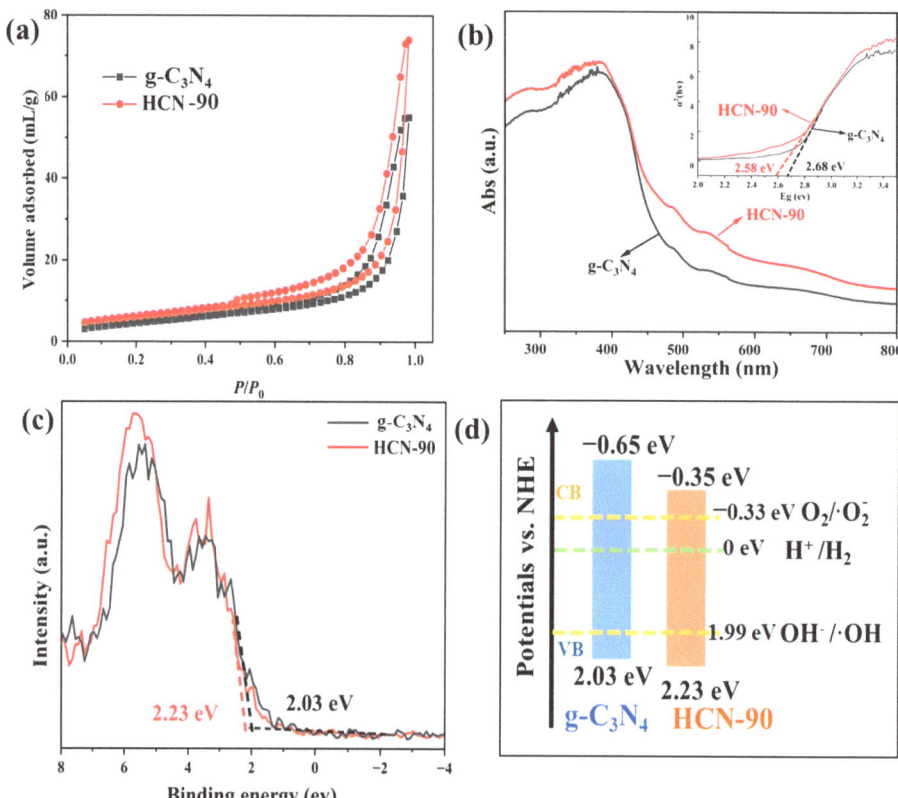

Figure 3. (**a**) Nitrogen adsorption–desorption isotherms; (**b**) UV–vis diffuse reflectance spectra; (**c**) XPS valence band spectra; (**d**) band alignments of g-C_3N_4 and HCN-90.

The photo-redox reaction is primarily governed by the potentials of valence bands (VBs) and conduction bands (CBs), as well as the bandgap energy of materials. Consequently, further investigation into the band structure and electronic conductivity was conducted. Diffuse reflectance spectroscopy (DRS) was used to characterize the light absorption properties. As shown in Figure 3b, the absorption edge of HCN-90 showed a red shift compared to that of g-C_3N_4. The red shift in the absorption edge correlated with a change in color from yellow in g-C_3N_4 to dark yellow in HCN-90. According to the Kubelka–Munk equation, the band gap of HCN-90 and g-C_3N_4 could be deduced [9]. The band gap of g-C_3N_4 was 2.70 eV, consistent with previously reported results [8]. For HCN-90, the value was approximately 2.58 eV.

The valence band X-ray photoelectron spectroscopy (VB XPS) spectrum in Figure 3c was used to estimate the band edge potentials of g-C_3N_4 and HCN-90. The VB potentials for g-C_3N_4 and HCN-90 were measured at 2.03 eV and 2.23 eV, respectively. The positive shift in the VB of HCN-90 enhanced the oxidizing capacity of holes and improved its photo-oxidation capability. In combination with the results of the DRS, the CB edge potentials of g-C$_3$N$_4$ and HCN-90 were estimated at −0.65 eV and −0.35 eV, respectively. The reduction in the CB facilitated the transfer of surface charge carriers and promoted the generation of reactive oxygen species.

Figure 3d illustrates the comprehensive influences of the polar functional group modifications on the band structure, including the potentials of key reactions. The potential of the CB remained more negative than the redox potentials of O$_2$/·O$_2^-$, suggesting that photogenerated electrons could potentially be trapped by adsorbed O$_2$. This trapping mechanism resulted in the production of reactive species, preventing light-induced carrier recombination [47]. The suitable band structure thermodynamically enabled boost-photo-induced charge separation and molecular oxygen activation.

2.2. Photoelectric Property

Energy transfer for the activation of molecular oxygen was greatly facilitated by improving intersystem crossover processes to reduce non-radiative attenuation [48]. Electrochemical impedance spectroscopy (EIS) was employed to study the interfacial charge transfer capability. Figure 4a displays the EIS Nyquist plots of g-C$_3$N$_4$ and HCN-90, with the inset showing the corresponding equivalent circuit model for analysis. In the equivalent circuit model, R_{ct}, C_d and R_s represented charge transfer resistance, double layer capacitance, and the electrolyte solution resistance, respectively. The smaller arc radius observed for HCN-90 compared to g-C$_3$N$_4$ indicated lower surface impedance and faster charge transfer in HCN-90. This observation supported the proposition that polar functional groups contribute to the enhanced separation of photogenerated electrons and holes, thereby improving photocatalytic activity [49].

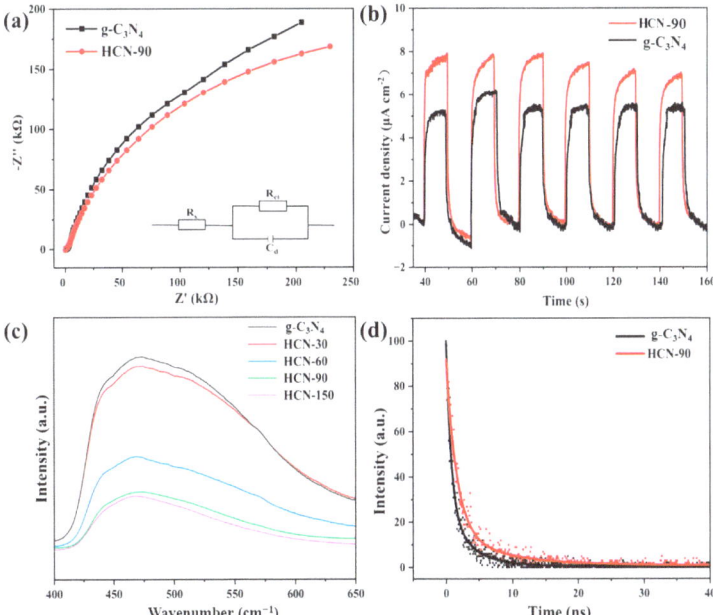

Figure 4. (**a**) EIS Nyquist plots; (**b**) transient state photocurrent spectra; (**c**) steady-state fluorescence spectra; (**d**) time-resolved fluorescence spectra.

The transient photocurrent response of the samples was measured and is shown in Figure 4b. All samples exhibited a rapid and reproducible photocurrent response during each illumination cycle. Notably, the photocurrent of HCN-90 was observed to be larger than that of g-C$_3$N$_4$, confirming the constructive role of polar functional groups in enhancing charge migration and separation. Fluorescence spectroscopy provided valuable insights into the separation and recombination of photogenerated electron-hole pairs. In Figure 4c, the photoluminescence intensity of g-C_3N_4 was stronger than that in HCN, and the fluorescence intensity of HCN gradually decreased with prolonged H_2O_2 treatment time. This phenomenon was likely attributed to the abundant polar functional groups, which enhanced charge trapping and effective charge transfer [50]. Consequently, this prolonged the charge carrier lifetime and contributed to the improvement in photocatalytic activity. The fluorescence decay curves were employed to explore the transfer efficiency of carriers. As illustrated in Figure 4d, the findings were fitted using the tri-exponential decay function. The average lifetime increased from 2.51 ns (g-C_3N_4) to 4.78 ns (HCN-90). The extended charge carrier lifetime of HCN-90 could be attributed to the electrical interaction between hydroxyl groups and graphitic carbonitride. These findings indicated that HCN-90 has better electron-hole pair separation.

2.3. Visible-Light Photocatalytic Activity Measurements

The photocatalytic activities were assessed by monitoring the photodegradation of RhB in visible light irradiation. As shown in Figure 5a, the degradation rate showed no significant changes without the photocatalyst, indicating that the RhB degradation was caused by photodegradation rather than self-decomposition. The degradation rate of pure g-C_3N_4 was only 59.4%, whereas HCN consistently achieved degradation rates above 96%. The photocatalytic activities of HCN gradually increased with ultrasonic-assisted hydrogen peroxide treatment time. The results demonstrated that modification with hydroxyl groups significantly improved the photocatalytic activity, likely due to enhanced separation of photogenerated carriers and a narrowed band gap, thereby boosting the activation of molecular oxygen.

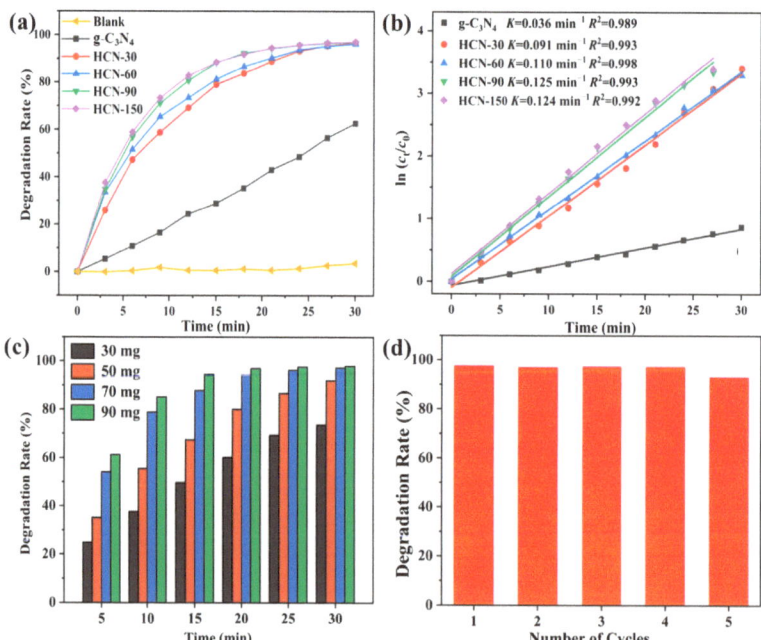

Figure 5. (**a**) Photocatalytic degradation of RhB; (**b**) first-order kinetics plot; (**c**) effect of dosage on degradation rate; (**d**) reusability of HCN-90.

The kinetics of the photocatalytic degradation of RhB were further investigated. A first-order linear relationship was observed in the plots of ln (c_t/c_0) versus irradiation time (Figure 5b). The calculated reaction rate constants (K) were 0.036, 0.091, 0.110, 0.125, and 0.124 min^{-1} for g-C$_3$N$_4$, HCN-30, HCN-60, HCN-90, and HCN-150, respectively. Apparently, HCN-90 demonstrated the highest kinetic parameters, approximately 3.5 times that of g-C$_3$N$_4$. The enhanced photocatalytic performance of HCN-90 could be attributed to its larger specific surface area and improved charge carrier separation. The higher specific surface area increased chemisorption and mass transfer. The enhanced charge separation improved the photo responsiveness, contributing to the overall improved catalytic activity. Notably, HCN-90 was selected for further studies due to cost and time constraints, even though HCN-150 showed comparable photocatalytic performance.

Further investigation was conducted into the usage conditions of HCN-90. Figure 5c depicted the effect of HCN-90 dosage on the photodegradation of RhB. With increased HCN-90 dosage, the degradation rate of RhB also increased. At dosages of 30 mg, 50 mg, 70 mg, and 90 mg, the degradation rates of RhB within 30 min were 72.9%, 92.07%, 96.9%, and 97.7%, respectively. Higher catalyst dosages resulted in increased active substances, thereby enhancing the photodegradation rate within a specific range. However, excessive photocatalysts could only lead to the increased adsorption of pollutants. Moreover, a high concentration of suspension in the solution might hinder incident light penetration, thereby reducing photodegradation efficiency [51]. Ultimately, the optimal dosage of HCN-90 was found to be 70 mg.

Additionally, the reusability of HCN-90 was evaluated through five consecutive reaction cycles (Figure 5d). Over the five cycles, the photodegradation rates of RhB by HCN-90 were 98.8%, 97.4%, 96.8%, 97.0%, and 92.8% within 30 min, respectively. This indicated that HCN-90 exhibited negligible deactivation, underscoring its commendable cycle stability.

The photocatalytic performance was strongly influenced by the solvent pH (Figure 6a). HCN-90 exhibited an optimal photocatalytic efficiency at pH = 1, achieving 99% degradation within 30 min. While there was a slight decrease in performance with an increasing pH within the range of 3–9, degradation rates remained above 85% within the same timeframe. However, at pH = 11, the degradation efficiency significantly declined to 55% after 30 min. This decline could be attributed to the pH-dependent structural characteristics of RhB, where protonation of the carboxyl group occurred when the solution pH was below the pKa of RhB (3.70) [51,52]. Figure 6b illustrates the effect of temperature on the photocatalytic rate of HCN-90. At 278 K, 288 K, 308 K, and 318 K, RhB degradation rates were 84.6%, 92.1%, 97.0%, and 97.2% (within 30 min), respectively. The increase in the catalytic rate was mainly due to the accelerated molecular thermal motion, facilitating the activation process of pollutants on the catalyst surface.

To elucidate the photocatalytic mechanism, experiments were conducted using various radical scavengers to degrade RhB. As shown in Figure 6c, photocatalytic activities remained unaffected after adding IPA, L-his, and K$_2$Cr$_2$O$_7$ as quenchers for ·OH, ^{1}O$_2$, and e$^-$, respectively. The results suggested that ·OH, ^{1}O$_2$, and e$^-$ were not responsible for the degradation of RhB. However, introducing p-BQ and KI resulted in the RhB degradation rate decreasing from 96.9% to 6.9% and 64.9%, respectively. These findings indicated that ·O$_2^-$ radicals were the primary active component and h$^+$ was also involved in the photodegradation of RhB. Furthermore, replacing O$_2$ with N$_2$ hindered the photocatalytic reaction, suggesting that O$_2$ was essential.

The absorption spectra of RhB degradation with HCN-90 under visible light were shown in Figure 6d. Upon visible light irradiation, the characteristic peak of RhB at 554 nm gradually decreased and exhibited a blue-shift. Over the first 10 min, the peaks shifted from 552 nm to 497 nm, indicating the decomposition of RhB into N,N,N'-triethyl-rhodamine (539 nm); N,N'-diethyl-rhodamine (528 nm); N-ethyl-rhodamine (502 nm); and Rhodamine (497 nm) [53]. In the final 5 min, the maximum peak declined without an obvious peak, suggesting the further degradation of RhB into small molecules such as CO$_2$ and H$_2$O [54]. Thus, RhB photodegradation involved de-ethylation and the destruction of the conjugated structure [52]. RhB degradation was further confirmed by LC–MS, and the results are shown in Figure S1. Based on the mass spectra and molecular weight analysis, the catalysis process led to the degradation of RhB.

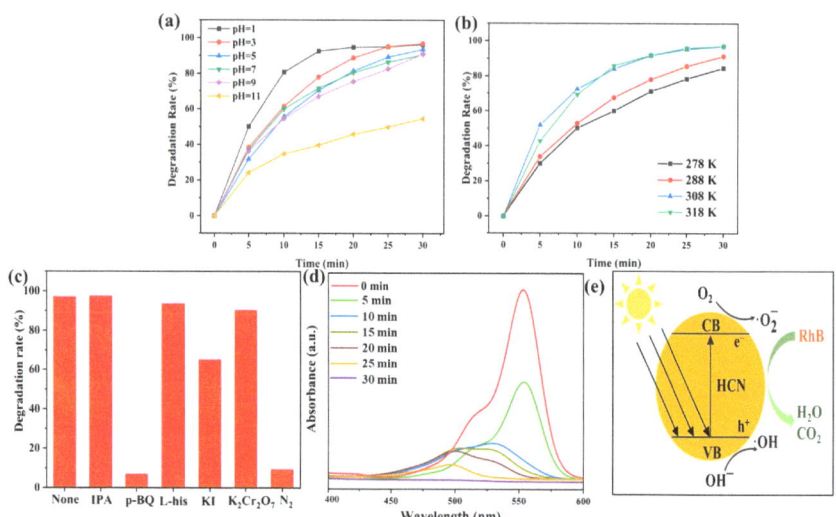

Figure 6. (**a**) Effect of pH on degradation rate; (**b**) effect of temperature on degradation rate; (**c**) effect of scavengers on degradation rate; (**d**) absorption spectra of RhB during the photocatalytic process by HCN-90; (**e**) possible mechanism schematic for RhB degradation under visible light irradiation.

Based on these results, a proposed mechanism for the enhanced photoactivity of HCN is illustrated in Figure 6e. HCN was excited by photon energy, generating electrons and holes to form electron-hole pairs. The electron acceptor adsorbed on the surface of HCN induced photogenerated electrons in the CB and reacted with O_2 to produce $\cdot O_2^-$. The $\cdot O_2^-$ exhibited strong reducibility and participated in the degradation of RhB. Additionally, holes in the VB could react with OH^- to produce highly oxidizing $\cdot OH$. However, due to the high potential of $OH^-/\cdot OH$, only a small amount of $\cdot OH$ was produced in the photocatalytic process. Therefore, $\cdot O_2^-$ and h^+ as the main active substances were responsible partially or completely for redox RhB to achieve a degradation effect. The comparison of this study with recently published results on the photocatalytic degradation of RhB is presented in Table 1. HCN-90 exhibited the efficient catalysis of RhB degradation under visible-light irradiation (420 nm), showcasing excellent reusability and rapid degradation rates. These findings demonstrated its practical applicability in wastewater remediation.

Table 1. The photocatalytic performance of different g-C_3N_4 composites for RhB photodegradation.

Catalyst	Irradiation Source	Irradiation Time (min)	Degradation Rate (%)	RhB Concentration (mg/L)	Catalyst Dosage (g/L)	Reusability	K (min^{-1})	Ref.
HCN-90	50 W LED	30	98.8	5	0.47	After five cycles: 93%	0.125	This work
g-C$_3$N$_4$/SmVO$_4$	500 W Xe arc lamp	120	>90	10	1	After ten cycles: 93%	0.0345	[8]
TiO$_2$@g-C$_3$N$_4$	300 W Xe arc lamp	100	93.3	4.79	1.33	After five cycles: 90%	0.021	[55]
40-OCN	30 W LED lamp	140	>90	30	1	After five cycles: >80%	0.0193	[56]
g-C$_3$N$_4$/CNTs	300 W xenon lamp	60	98.1	10	0.2	After five cycles: 90%	0.051	[53]
g-C$_3$N$_4$/AgI	500 W Xe lamp	100	73.86	20	0.67	After four cycles: >70%	0.0723	[57]
FeCN-7	300 W xenon lamp	60	-	20	2	After three cycles: 95%	0.117	[58]
CoFe$_2$O$_4$/g-C$_3$N$_4$	500 W Halogen lamp	120	57	-	0.6	After five cycles: 55%	-	[59]
CN-UM/Mt	300 W Xe lamp	60	almost 99	10	0.5	-	0.053	[60]
g-C$_3$N$_4$/5-rGO/SnO$_2$	100 W halogen lamp	120	83.2	7.2	0.15	-	0.0285	[61]
Zn$_2$Ti$_3$O$_8$/g-C$_3$N$_4$	400 W visible lamp	90	89.0	10	0.5	After five cycles: 83%	0.0211	[62]

3. Materials and Methods

3.1. Materials

Melamine ($C_3H_6N_6$, >99.0%), hydrogen peroxide (H_2O_2, ≥30%), p-benzoquinone (p-BQ, $C_6H_4O_2$, >99%), potassium iodide (KI, ≥99%), and potassium dichromate ($K_2Cr_2O_7$, ≥99.8%) were supplied by Adamas Chemical Reagent Co., Ltd., Shanghai, China. Rhodamine B (RhB, $C_{28}H_{31}ClN_2O_3$, >98.0%), isopropyl alcohol (IPA, C_3H_8O, >99.5%), and L-histidine (L-his, $C_6H_9N_3O_2$, >99.0%) were supplied by Tokyo Chemical Industry Co., Ltd., Tokyo, Japan.

3.2. Preparation of HCN

Pure g-C_3N_4 was synthesized via thermal polycondensation. In detail, 5 g of melamine was placed into an alumina crucible (Titan Technology Co., Shanghai, China) and heated in a muffle furnace (Yiheng Scientific Instrument Co., Shanghai, China) at 550 °C for 4 h, with a heating rate of 5 °C/min. Subsequently, the product was further heated at 550 °C for another 4 h to obtain the g-C_3N_4. HCN was synthesized through ultrasound-assisted oxidation with hydrogen peroxide. Typically, 0.5 g of g-C_3N_4 was mixed with a 7.5 mL H_2O_2 solution (30 wt%) and subjected to ultrasonicated using bath sonication (Dekang Cleaning Electronic Appliance Co., Shenzhen, China, power 60 W, frequency 40 kHz) for 30–150 min. Finally, the products were washed with deionized water three times and collected through centrifugation. The final products were obtained by drying at 60 °C overnight, while the corresponding solids were named HCN-x (x is the time of ultrasonication).

3.3. Characterization

X-ray diffraction (XRD) measurements were conducted by using a Bruker D8 Advance X-ray powder diffractometer (Bruker Co., Billerica, MA, USA) equipped with Cu Kα radiation (λ = 1.5406 Å) and a scanning speed of 10°/min. The accelerating voltage and emission current were set at 40 mV and 40 mA, respectively, with a scanning range from 5° to 60°. Transmission electron microscopy (TEM) imaging was performed using a JEOL-2010 transmission electron microscope (JEOL Ltd., Akishima, Japan). Fourier Transform Infrared Spectra (FT-IR) were collected with a Nicolet iS50 Spectrometer (Thermo Fisher Scientific Inc., Waltham, MA, USA) using KBr as diluents. The surface chemical state was analyzed by X-ray Photoelectron Spectroscopy (XPS) using a Thermo Fisher Escalab 250Xi apparatus (Thermo Fisher Scientific Inc., Waltham, MA, USA) with an Al-Kα source. The water contact angle was recorded by sessile drop analysis Dataphysics OCA20 (DataPhysics Instruments, Filderstadt, Germany). Specific surface areas were determined by Brunauer–Emmett–Teller (BET) analysis using a Micromeritics automatic surface area analyzer Gemini 2360 (Shimadzu Co., Kyoto, Japan) with nitrogen adsorption at 77 K. Ultraviolet-Visible Diffuse Reflectance Spectra (UV–vis DRS) were recorded with a Model Shimadzu UV 2550 spectrophotometer (Shimadzu Co., Kyoto, Japan) in the range of 250 nm to 800 nm. Time-resolved fluorescence spectra were obtained using an Edinburgh FLS 900 (Edinburgh Instruments Ltd., Edinburgh, England). A Waters SQD2 (Waters Co., Milford, CT, USA) Liquid Chromatography mass spectrometer (LC–MS) was used to identify the degradation intermediates of RhB. The mobile phase was methanol and a 0.2% methane acid solution. The gradient elution was programmed as follows: methanol was obtained at 70% and kept for 1 min, then linearly decreased to 10% over 8 min.

The electrochemical station employed was CHI 660D (Shanghai Chenhua Instrument Co., Shanghai, China), and the test system constituted a three-electrode system with a working electrode prepared by the drop-coating method, Ag/AgCl as the reference electrode, and Pt as the counter electrode. The electrolyte solution was 0.1 M Na_2SO_4. The working electrode was prepared by weighing 2.5 mg of catalyst and 50 μL of Nafion solution, followed by dispersion through ultrasonication with the addition of 0.45 mL of a water and ethanol mixture (1:9 volume ratio). A 20 μL drop of the dispersion was pipetted onto a square (1 × 1 cm^2) of conductive glass and dried in a natural environment.

Electrochemical impedance spectroscopy was performed in the frequency range of 0.05 Hz to 100 kHz at 0.7 V under irradiation.

3.4. Evaluation of Photocatalytic Activity

The photocatalytic degradation performances of samples were evaluated by using Rhodamine B (RhB) as the probe pollutant under visible light. Briefly, photocatalysts (70 mg) were weighed into an RhB solution (150 mL, 5 mg/L). After mixing, the reaction system was placed in the dark for 30 min to achieve adsorption equilibrium. Photodegradation was initiated by 420 nm LED (50 W) at room temperature, and the monitor wavelength was 554 nm. After the reaction, 5 mL of solvent was extracted from the reaction suspension to determine the RhB concentration. The degradation rate was calculated by using the following formula:

$$\text{Degradation rate (\%)} = \frac{c_0 - c_t}{c_0} \times 100\% \tag{1}$$

where c_0 is the concentration of the reactant before illumination (mg/L), and c_t is the concentration of the reactant after a certain illumination period (mg/L). The initial pH (1, 3, 5, 7, 9, and 11), temperature (278 K, 288 K, 303 K, and 318 K), and dosage (30 mg, 50 mg, 70 mg, and 90 mg) on the degradation effect of Rh B (5 mg/L, 150 mL) were examined by changing the test conditions, respectively.

4. Conclusions

In summary, g-C_3N_4 modified with hydroxyl groups was prepared, characterized, and evaluated for its effectiveness in the photodegradation of RhB under visible light irradiation. By optimizing the duration of ultrasound-assisted oxidation with hydrogen peroxide, HCN-90 was synthesized, exhibiting a higher specific surface area, improved hydrophilia, and narrower interlayer distances. The hydroxyl groups on the surface acted as charge trapping centers, accelerating carrier separation efficiency. With a lower conduction band energy and narrower bandgap, HCN-90 facilitated molecular oxygen activation. Compared to pristine g-C_3N_4, HCN-90 demonstrated a 3.5-fold increase in the photodegradation rate of RhB (0.115 min^{-1}). Even after five cycles, the photocatalytic efficacy of RhB degradation remained at 93%. Additionally, the RhB solutions were effectively degraded by HCN-90 under visible light irradiation within 30 min, resulting in a colorless solution. This bonding strategy presents a promising model for developing high-performance and eco-friendly photocatalysts for green molecular oxygen activation. The straightforward synthesis method, along with excellent recycling capabilities and rapid kinetics, positions HCN-90 as a viable candidate for industrial application.

Supplementary Materials: The following supporting information can be downloaded at: https://www.mdpi.com/article/10.3390/molecules29163836/s1, Figure S1: (**a**) Total ion chromatogram and MS spectra of RhB intermediates at different retention times: (**b**) 0.99 min; (**c**) 0.48 min; (**d**) 0.32 min.

Author Contributions: Conceptualization, J.C. and Z.L.; investigation, Y.J. and R.Y.; methodology, M.Y. and H.Z.; validation, Y.C.; writing—original draft, J.C. All authors have read and agreed to the published version of the manuscript.

Funding: This research was funded by the Fundamental Research Funds of Lishui (Grant No. 2023GYX46), "Pioneer" and "Leading Goose" R&D programs of Zhejiang (Grant No. 2024C01251(SD2)), Key Research and Development Projects of Quzhou (Grant No. 2023K259), Key R&D Special Project of He'nan (Grant No. 231111232500), MIIT Dedicated Program (Grant No. TC220A04A-206).

Institutional Review Board Statement: Not applicable.

Informed Consent Statement: Not applicable.

Data Availability Statement: Data are contained within the article; further inquiries can be directed to the corresponding author.

Acknowledgments: We would like to thank the researchers in the Shiyanjia Lab (https://www.shiyanjia.com/order-2496416.html, accessed on 6 August 2024) for their help with the XPS analysis.

Conflicts of Interest: The authors declare no conflicts of interest.

References

1. Mohod, A.V.; Momotko, M.; Shah, N.S.; Marchel, M.; Imran, M.; Kong, L.; Boczkaj, G. Degradation of Rhodamine dyes by Advanced Oxidation Processes (AOPs)—Focus on cavitation and photocatalysis—A critical review. *Water Resour. Ind.* **2023**, *30*, 100220. [CrossRef]
2. Teo, S.H.; Ng, C.H.; Islam, A.; Abdulkareem-Alsultan, G.; Joseph, C.G.; Janaun, J.; Taufiq-Yap, Y.H.; Khandaker, S.; Islam, G.J.; Znad, H.; et al. Sustainable toxic dyes removal with advanced materials for clean water production: A comprehensive review. *J. Clean. Prod.* **2022**, *332*, 130039. [CrossRef]
3. Ajiboye, T.O.; Oyewo, O.A.; Onwudiwe, D.C. Adsorption and photocatalytic removal of Rhodamine B from wastewater using carbon-based materials. *FlatChem* **2021**, *29*, 100277. [CrossRef]
4. Lara-Ramos, J.A.; Diaz-Angulo, J.; Machuca-Martinez, F. Use of modified flotation cell as ozonation reactor to minimize mass transfer limitations. *Chem. Eng. J.* **2021**, *405*, 126978. [CrossRef]
5. Sharmoukh, W.; Abdelhamid, H.N. Fenton-like Cerium Metal—Organic Frameworks (Ce-MOFs) for Catalytic Oxidation of Olefins, Alcohol, and Dyes Degradation. *J. Clust. Sci.* **2023**, *34*, 2509–2519. [CrossRef]
6. Wang, C.; Shi, P.; Guo, C.; Guo, R.; Qiu, J. $CuCO_2O_4$/CF cathode with bifunctional and dual reaction centers exhibits high RhB degradation in electro-Fenton systems. *J. Electroanal. Chem.* **2024**, *956*, 118072. [CrossRef]
7. Zanaty, M.; Zaki, A.H.; El-Dek, S.I.; Abdelhamid, H.N. Zeolitic imidazolate framework@hydrogen titanate nanotubes for efficient adsorption and catalytic oxidation of organic dyes and microplastics. *J. Environ. Chem. Eng.* **2024**, *12*, 112547. [CrossRef]
8. Li, T.; Zhao, L.; He, Y.; Cai, J.; Luo, M.; Lin, J. Synthesis of $g-C_3N_4$/$SmVO_4$ composite photocatalyst with improved visible light photocatalytic activities in RhB degradation. *Appl. Catal. B Environ.* **2013**, *129*, 255–263. [CrossRef]
9. Yu, J.; Bao, P.; Liu, J.; Jin, Y.; Li, J.; Lv, Y. Cu and Ni dual-doped ZnO nanostructures templated by cellulose nanofibrils for the boosted visible-light photocatalytic degradation of wastewater pollutants. *Green Chem.* **2023**, *25*, 10530–10537. [CrossRef]
10. Tang, C.; Qiu, X.; Cheng, Z.; Jiao, N. Molecular oxygen-mediated oxygenation reactions involving radicals. *Chem. Soc. Rev.* **2021**, *50*, 8067–8101. [CrossRef]
11. Zhan, H.; Zhou, Q.; Li, M.; Zhou, R.; Mao, Y.; Wang, P. Photocatalytic O_2 activation and reactive oxygen species evolution by surface B-N bond for organic pollutants degradation. *Appl. Catal. B Environ.* **2022**, *310*, 121329. [CrossRef]
12. Zhao, K.; Zhang, L.; Wang, J.; Li, Q.; He, W.; Yin, J.J. Surface Structure-Dependent Molecular Oxygen Activation of BiOCl Single-Crystalline Nanosheets. *J. Am. Chem. Soc.* **2013**, *135*, 15750–15753. [CrossRef] [PubMed]
13. Anglada, J.M.; Martins-Costa, M.; Francisco, J.S.; Ruiz-Lopez, M.F. Interconnection of reactive oxygen species chemistry across the interfaces of atmospheric, environmental, and biological processes. *Acc. Chem. Res.* **2015**, *48*, 575–583. [CrossRef] [PubMed]
14. Ben, H.; Liu, Y.; Liu, X.; Liu, X.; Ling, C.; Liang, C.; Zhang, L. Diffusion-Controlled Z-Scheme-Steered Charge Separation across PDI/BiOI Heterointerface for Ultraviolet, Visible, and Infrared Light-Driven Photocatalysis. *Adv. Funct. Mater.* **2021**, *31*, 202102315. [CrossRef]
15. Li, Q.; Li, F.T. Recent advances in molecular oxygen activation via photocatalysis and its application in oxidation reactions. *Chem. Eng. J.* **2021**, *421*, 129915. [CrossRef]
16. Zhang, J.; Wang, X.; Dai, J.; Songsiriritthigul, P.; Oo, T.Z.; Zaw, M.; Lwin, N.W.; Aung, S.H.; Chen, F. Defect engineering in 0D/2D TiO_2/$g-C_3N_4$ heterojunction for boosting photocatalytic degradation of tetracycline in a tetracycline/Cu^{2+} combined system. *Colloids Surf. A Physicochem. Eng. Asp.* **2024**, *680*, 132624. [CrossRef]
17. Kumar, A.; Thakur, P.R.; Sharma, G.; Naushad, M.; Rana, A.; Mola, G.T.; Stadler, F.J. Carbon nitride, metal nitrides, phosphides, chalcogenides, perovskites and carbides nanophotocatalysts for environmental applications. *Environ. Chem. Lett.* **2018**, *17*, 655–682. [CrossRef]
18. Che, H.; Wang, P.; Chen, J.; Gao, X.; Liu, B.; Ao, Y. Rational design of donor-acceptor conjugated polymers with high performance on peroxydisulfate activation for pollutants degradation. *Appl. Catal. B Environ.* **2022**, *316*, 121611. [CrossRef]
19. Li, G.; Xie, Z.; Chai, S.; Chen, X.; Wang, X. A facile one-step fabrication of holey carbon nitride nanosheets for visible-light-driven hydrogen evolution. *Appl. Catal. B Environ.* **2021**, *283*, 119637. [CrossRef]
20. Sun, S.; Peng, B.; Song, Y.; Wang, R.; Song, H.; Lin, W. Engineering Z-Scheme FeOOH/PCN with Fast Photoelectron Transfer and Surface Redox Kinetics for Efficient Solar-Driven CO_2 Reduction. *ACS Appl. Mater. Interfaces* **2023**, *15*, 12957–12966. [CrossRef]
21. Wang, X.; Tang, W.; Jiang, L.; Feng, J.; Yang, J.; Zhou, S.; Li, W.; Yuan, X.; Wang, H.; Wang, J.; et al. Mechanism insights into visible light-induced crystalline carbon nitride activating periodate for highly efficient ciprofloxacin removal. *Chem. Eng. J.* **2023**, *471*, 144521. [CrossRef]
22. Tan, J.; Li, Z.; Li, J.; Wu, J.; Yao, X.; Zhang, T. Graphitic carbon nitride-based materials in activating persulfate for aqueous organic pollutants degradation: A review on materials design and mechanisms. *Chemosphere* **2021**, *262*, 127675. [CrossRef] [PubMed]
23. Huang, C.; Wen, Y.; Ma, J.; Dong, D.; Shen, Y.; Liu, S.; Ma, H.; Zhang, Y. Unraveling fundamental active units in carbon nitride for photocatalytic oxidation reactions. *Nat. Commun.* **2021**, *12*, 320. [CrossRef] [PubMed]

24. Wang, N.; Cheng, L.; Liao, Y.; Xiang, Q. Effect of Functional Group Modifications on the Photocatalytic Performance of g-C_3N_4. *Small* **2023**, *19*, e2300109. [CrossRef] [PubMed]
25. Che, H.; Gao, X.; Chen, J.; Hou, J.; Ao, Y.; Wang, P. Iodide-Induced Fragmentation of Polymerized Hydrophilic Carbon Nitride for High-Performance Quasi-Homogeneous Photocatalytic H_2O_2 Production. *Angew. Chem. Int. Ed.* **2021**, *60*, 25546–25550. [CrossRef] [PubMed]
26. Li, Y.; Xu, H.; Ouyang, S.; Lu, D.; Wang, X.; Wang, D.; Ye, J. In situ surface alkalinized g-C_3N_4 toward enhancement of photocatalytic H_2 evolution under visible-light irradiation. *J. Mater. Chem. A* **2016**, *4*, 2943–2950. [CrossRef]
27. Yu, S.; Li, J.; Zhang, Y.; Li, M.; Dong, F.; Zhang, T.; Huang, H. Local spatial charge separation and proton activation induced by surface hydroxylation promoting photocatalytic hydrogen evolution of polymeric carbon nitride. *Nano Energy* **2018**, *50*, 383–392. [CrossRef]
28. Li, J.; He, C.; Xu, N.; Wu, K.; Huang, Z.; Zhao, X.; Nan, J.; Xiao, X. Interfacial bonding of hydroxyl-modified g-C_3N_4 and $Bi_2O_2CO_3$ toward boosted CO_2 photoreduction: Insights into the key role of OH groups. *Chem. Eng. J.* **2023**, *452*, 139191. [CrossRef]
29. She, X.; Zhu, X.; Yang, J.; Song, Y.; She, Y.; Liu, D.; Wu, J.; Yu, Q.; Li, H.; Liu, Z.; et al. Grain-boundary surface terminations incorporating oxygen vacancies for selectively boosting CO_2 photoreduction activity. *Nano Energy* **2021**, *84*, 105869. [CrossRef]
30. Bu, X.; Li, J.; Yang, S.; Sun, J.; Deng, Y.; Yang, Y.; Wang, G.; Peng, Z.; He, P.; Wang, X.; et al. Surface Modification of C_3N_4 through Oxygen-Plasma Treatment: A Simple Way toward Excellent Hydrophilicity. *ACS Appl. Mater. Interfaces* **2016**, *8*, 31419–31425. [CrossRef]
31. Li, H.J.; Sun, B.W.; Sui, L.; Qian, D.J.; Chen, M. Preparation of water-dispersible porous g-C_3N_4 with improved photocatalytic activity by chemical oxidation. *Phys. Chem. Chem. Phys.* **2015**, *17*, 3309–3315. [CrossRef] [PubMed]
32. Li, X.; Zhang, X.; Ma, H.; Wu, D.; Zhang, Y.; Du, B.; Wei, Q. Cathodic electrochemiluminescence immunosensor based on nanocomposites of semiconductor carboxylated g-C_3N_4 and graphene for the ultrasensitive detection of squamous cell carcinoma antigen. *Biosens. Bioelectron.* **2014**, *55*, 330–336. [CrossRef] [PubMed]
33. Wang, B.; Zhong, X.; Chai, Y.; Yuan, R. Ultrasensitive electrochemiluminescence biosensor for organophosphate pesticides detection based on carboxylated graphitic carbon nitride-poly(ethylenimine) and acetylcholinesterase. *Electrochim. Acta* **2017**, *224*, 194–200. [CrossRef]
34. Ming, L.; Yue, H.; Xu, L.; Chen, F. Hydrothermal synthesis of oxidized g-C_3N_4 and its regulation of photocatalytic activity. *J. Mater. Chem. A* **2014**, *2*, 19145–19149. [CrossRef]
35. Moon, G.-h.; Fujitsuka, M.; Kim, S.; Majima, T.; Wang, X.; Choi, W. Eco-Friendly Photochemical Production of H_2O_2 through O_2 Reduction over Carbon Nitride Frameworks Incorporated with Multiple Heteroelements. *ACS Catal.* **2017**, *7*, 2886–2895. [CrossRef]
36. You, Q.; Zhang, Q.; Gu, M.; Du, R.; Chen, P.; Huang, J.; Wang, Y.; Deng, S.; Yu, G. Self-assembled graphitic carbon nitride regulated by carbon quantum dots with optimized electronic band structure for enhanced photocatalytic degradation of diclofenac. *Chem. Eng. J.* **2022**, *431*, 133927. [CrossRef]
37. Luo, L.; Gong, Z.; Ma, J.; Wang, K.; Zhu, H.; Li, K.; Xiong, L.; Guo, X.; Tang, J. Ultrathin sulfur-doped holey carbon nitride nanosheets with superior photocatalytic hydrogen production from water. *Appl. Catal. B Environ.* **2021**, *284*, 119742. [CrossRef]
38. Merschjann, C.; Tschierlei, S.; Tyborski, T.; Kailasam, K.; Orthmann, S.; Hollmann, D.; Schedel-Niedrig, T.; Thomas, A.; Lochbrunner, S. Complementing Graphenes: 1D Interplanar Charge Transport in Polymeric Graphitic Carbon Nitrides. *Adv. Mater.* **2015**, *27*, 7993–7999. [CrossRef] [PubMed]
39. Zhu, B.; Xia, P.; Ho, W.; Yu, J. Isoelectric point and adsorption activity of porous g-C_3N_4. *Appl. Surf. Sci.* **2015**, *344*, 188–195. [CrossRef]
40. Yan, S.C.; Li, Z.S.; Zou, Z.G. Photodegradation Performance of g-C_3N_4 Fabricated by Directly Heating Melamine. *Langmuir* **2009**, *25*, 10397–10401. [CrossRef]
41. Liu, J.; Zhang, T.; Wang, Z.; Dawson, G.; Chen, W. Simple pyrolysis of urea into graphitic carbon nitride with recyclable adsorption and photocatalytic activity. *J. Mater. Chem.* **2011**, *21*, 14398–14401. [CrossRef]
42. Dong, F.; Wang, Z.; Sun, Y.; Ho, W.-K.; Zhang, H. Engineering the nanoarchitecture and texture of polymeric carbon nitride semiconductor for enhanced visible light photocatalytic activity. *J. Colloid Interface Sci.* **2013**, *401*, 70–79. [CrossRef] [PubMed]
43. Xiang, Q.; Yu, J.; Jaroniec, M. Preparation and Enhanced Visible-Light Photocatalytic H_2-Production Activity of Graphene/C_3N_4 Composites. *J. Phys. Chem. C* **2011**, *115*, 7355–7363. [CrossRef]
44. Feng, J.; Li, M. Large-Scale Synthesis of a New Polymeric Carbon Nitride—C_3N_3 with Good Photoelectrochemical Performance. *Adv. Funct. Mater.* **2020**, *30*, 2001502. [CrossRef]
45. Xie, Y.; Li, Y.; Huang, Z.; Zhang, J.; Jia, X.; Wang, X.-S.; Ye, J. Two types of cooperative nitrogen vacancies in polymeric carbon nitride for efficient solar-driven H_2O_2 evolution. *Appl. Catal. B Environ.* **2020**, *265*, 118581. [CrossRef]
46. Fu, J.; Zhu, B.; Jiang, C.; Cheng, B.; You, W.; Yu, J. Hierarchical Porous O-Doped g-C_3N_4 with Enhanced Photocatalytic CO_2 Reduction Activity. *Small* **2017**, *13*, 1603938. [CrossRef] [PubMed]
47. Liang, Q.; Li, Z.; Huang, Z.H.; Kang, F.; Yang, Q.H. Holey Graphitic Carbon Nitride Nanosheets with Carbon Vacancies for Highly Improved Photocatalytic Hydrogen Production. *Adv. Funct. Mater.* **2015**, *25*, 6885–6892. [CrossRef]
48. Zhang, L.; Zhang, J.; Yu, H.; Yu, J. Emerging S-Scheme Photocatalyst. *Adv. Mater.* **2022**, *34*, e2107668. [CrossRef]
49. Yang, H.; Xu, B.; Yuan, S.; Zhang, Q.; Zhang, M.; Ohno, T. Synthesis of Y-doped CeO_2/PCN nanocomposited photocatalyst with promoted photoredox performance. *Appl. Catal. B Environ.* **2019**, *243*, 513–521. [CrossRef]

50. Huang, J.; Li, D.; Li, R.; Zhang, Q.; Chen, T.; Liu, H.; Liu, Y.; Lv, W.; Liu, G. An efficient metal-free phosphorus and oxygen co-doped g-C$_3$N$_4$ photocatalyst with enhanced visible light photocatalytic activity for the degradation of fluoroquinolone antibiotics. *Chem. Eng. J.* **2019**, *374*, 242–253. [CrossRef]
51. Yi-Zhu, P.; Wan-Hong, M.; Man-Ke, J.; Xiao-Rong, Z.; Johnson, D.M.; Ying-Ping, H. Comparing the degradation of acetochlor to RhB using BiOBr under visible light: A significantly different rate-catalyst dose relationship. *Appl. Catal. B Environ.* **2016**, *181*, 517–523. [CrossRef]
52. Shi, W.; Fang, W.X.; Wang, J.C.; Qiao, X.; Wang, B.; Guo, X. pH-controlled mechanism of photocatalytic RhB degradation over g-C$_3$N$_4$ under sunlight irradiation. *Photochem. Photobiol. Sci.* **2021**, *20*, 303–313. [CrossRef] [PubMed]
53. Liu, G.; Liao, M.; Zhang, Z.; Wang, H.; Chen, D.; Feng, Y. Enhanced photodegradation performance of Rhodamine B with g-C3N4 modified by carbon nanotubes. *Sep. Purif. Technol.* **2020**, *244*, 116618. [CrossRef]
54. Meng, X.; Li, Z.; Zeng, H.; Chen, J.; Zhang, Z. MoS$_2$ quantum dots-interspersed Bi$_2$WO$_6$ heterostructures for visible light-induced detoxification and disinfection. *Appl. Catal. B Environ.* **2017**, *210*, 160–172. [CrossRef]
55. Ma, L.; Wang, G.; Jiang, C.; Bao, H.; Xu, Q. Synthesis of core-shell TiO$_2$@g-C$_3$N$_4$ hollow microspheres for efficient photocatalytic degradation of rhodamine B under visible light. *Appl. Surf. Sci.* **2018**, *430*, 263–272. [CrossRef]
56. Tran, D.A.; Nguyen Pham, C.T.; Nguyen Ngoc, T.; Nguyen Phi, H.; Hoai Ta, Q.T.; Truong, D.H.; Nguyen, V.T.; Luc, H.H.; Nguyen, L.T.; Dao, N.N.; et al. One-step synthesis of oxygen doped g-C3N4 for enhanced visible-light photodegradation of Rhodamine B. *J. Phys. Chem. Solids* **2021**, *151*, 109900. [CrossRef]
57. Huang, H.; Li, Y.-X.; Wang, H.-L.; Jiang, W.-F. In situ fabrication of ultrathin-g-C$_3$N$_4$/AgI heterojunctions with improved catalytic performance for photodegrading rhodamine B solution. *Appl. Surf. Sci.* **2021**, *538*, 148132. [CrossRef]
58. Nguyen Van, M.; Mai, O.L.T.; Pham Do, C.; Lam Thi, H.; Pham Manh, C.; Nguyen Manh, H.; Pham Thi, D.; Do Danh, B. Fe-Doped g-C$_3$N$_4$: High-Performance Photocatalysts in Rhodamine B Decomposition. *Polymers* **2020**, *12*, 1963. [CrossRef]
59. Dharani, S.; Gnanasekaran, L.; Arunachalam, S.; Zielinska-Jure, A.; Almoallim, H.S.; Soto-Moscoso, M. Photodegrading rhodamine B dye with cobalt ferrite-graphitic carbon nitride (CoFe$_2$O$_4$/g-C$_3$N$_4$) composite. *Environ. Res.* **2024**, *258*, 119484. [CrossRef]
60. Chen, Y.; Yu, Y.; Yan, Z.; Li, T.; Jing, Q.; Liu, P. Montmorillonite induced assembly of multi-element doped g-C$_3$N$_4$ nanosheets with enhanced activity for Rhodamine B photodegradation. *Appl. Clay Sci.* **2022**, *218*, 106432. [CrossRef]
61. Ali, G.; Jazib Abbas Zaidi, S.; Abdul Basit, M.; Park, T.J. Synergetic performance of systematically designed g-C$_3$N$_4$/rGO/SnO$_2$ nanocomposite for photodegradation of Rhodamine-B dye. *Appl. Surf. Sci.* **2021**, *570*, 151140. [CrossRef]
62. Reza Saadati-Gullojeh, M.; Ghanbari, M.; Salavati-Niasari, M. Facile preparation and characterization of Zn$_2$Ti$_3$O$_8$/g-C$_3$N$_4$ nanocomposites for degradation of rhodamine B under simulated sunlight. *Sol. Energy* **2024**, *268*, 112316. [CrossRef]

Disclaimer/Publisher's Note: The statements, opinions and data contained in all publications are solely those of the individual author(s) and contributor(s) and not of MDPI and/or the editor(s). MDPI and/or the editor(s) disclaim responsibility for any injury to people or property resulting from any ideas, methods, instructions or products referred to in the content.

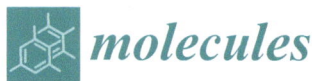

Article

MgO Nanoparticles as a Promising Photocatalyst towards Rhodamine B and Rhodamine 6G Degradation

Maria-Anna Gatou [1,*,†], Natalia Bovali [1,†], Nefeli Lagopati [2,3] and Evangelia A. Pavlatou [1,*]

1. Laboratory of General Chemistry, School of Chemical Engineering, National Technical University of Athens, Zografou Campus, 15772 Athens, Greece; natalia.bovali@gmail.com
2. Laboratory of Biology, Department of Basic Medical Sciences, Medical School, National and Kapodistrian University of Athens, 11527 Athens, Greece; nlagopati@med.uoa.gr
3. Biomedical Research Foundation, Academy of Athens, 11527 Athens, Greece
* Correspondence: mgatou2@mail.ntua.gr (M.-A.G.); pavlatou@chemeng.ntua.gr (E.A.P.)
† These authors contributed equally to this work.

Abstract: The increasing global requirement for clean and safe drinking water has necessitated the development of efficient methods for the elimination of organic contaminants, especially dyes, from wastewater. This study reports the synthesis of magnesium oxide (MgO) nanoparticles via a simple precipitation approach and their thorough characterization using various techniques, including XRD, FT-IR, XPS, TGA, DLS, and FESEM. Synthesized MgO nanoparticles' photocatalytic effectiveness was evaluated towards rhodamine B and rhodamine 6G degradation under both UV and visible light irradiation. The results indicated that the MgO nanoparticles possess a face-centered cubic structure with enhanced crystallinity and purity, as well as an average crystallite size of approximately 3.20 nm. The nanoparticles demonstrated a significant BET surface area (52 m^2/g) and a bandgap value equal to 5.27 eV. Photocatalytic experiments indicated complete degradation of rhodamine B dye under UV light within 180 min and 83.23% degradation under visible light. For rhodamine 6G, the degradation efficiency was 92.62% under UV light and 38.71% under visible light, thus verifying the MgO catalyst's selectivity towards degradation of rhodamine B dye. Also, reusability of MgO was investigated for five experimental photocatalytic trials with very promising results, mainly against rhodamine B. Scavenging experiments confirmed that •OH radicals were the major reactive oxygen species involved in the photodegradation procedure, unraveling the molecular mechanism of the photocatalytic efficiency of MgO.

Keywords: MgO; precipitation approach; photocatalysis; organic dyes; rhodamine B; rhodamine 6G; photocatalysis mechanism; photocatalyst selectivity; scavengers; reusability

Citation: Gatou, M.-A.; Bovali, N.; Lagopati, N.; Pavlatou, E.A. MgO Nanoparticles as a Promising Photocatalyst towards Rhodamine B and Rhodamine 6G Degradation. *Molecules* **2024**, *29*, 4299. https://doi.org/10.3390/molecules29184299

Academic Editor: Sugang Meng

Received: 27 June 2024
Revised: 6 September 2024
Accepted: 10 September 2024
Published: 11 September 2024

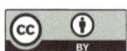

Copyright: © 2024 by the authors. Licensee MDPI, Basel, Switzerland. This article is an open access article distributed under the terms and conditions of the Creative Commons Attribution (CC BY) license (https://creativecommons.org/licenses/by/4.0/).

1. Introduction

The rising global need for clean and safe drinking water is a direct consequence of water pollution, which also leads to epidemics in various countries [1]. Contaminated water is a major cause of widespread waterborne diseases [2]. Organic pollutants, including dyes, contribute to health problems such as cancer in both humans and animals. Additionally, water pollution has been linked to higher mortality rates [3].

Even though organic water pollution occurs through various industrial sources, including textile, pharmaceutical, papermaking, leather, printing, cosmetics, and food processing, the textile industry constitutes a significant factor as it contributes to the generation of a vast quantity of dye-containing wastewater, since it is estimated that annually ≈700,000 tons of dyes are produced, while due to inefficiencies in the dyeing process, around 200,000 tons of dyes are released into water bodies during dyeing and finishing operations. Dyes possess an aromatic molecular structure attributed to hydrocarbons, such as C_6H_6, $C_6H_5CH_3$, $C_{14}H_{10}$, C_8H_{10}, $C_{10}H_8$, etc. [4,5]. In addition, they contain auxochromes (-NH_2, -Cl, -OH, -COOH, etc.), as well as chromophores (carbonyl, azo, nitroso, nitro, sulfur functional groups, etc.). Chromophores, which receive electrons, provide color, while auxochromes, which donate electrons, enhance the adhesion and solubility of color on substrates. Many dyes dissolve in water, and even at concentrations below 1 ppm, these dyes color industrial wastewater, which reduces sunlight penetration into water bodies. This affects oxygen levels, hinders photosynthesis, and disrupts the balance of eutrophication processes [6,7].

Among numerous dyes, rhodamine B (RhB) and rhodamine 6G (R6G), which are being extensively used, pose a pivotal threat to aquatic ecosystems and human health. Rhodamine B is an aminoxanthene anionic dye, and it is acknowledged for its mutagenic, noxious, chemically inert, and non-biodegradable properties, making it particularly hazardous. In particular, it causes acute and chronic toxicity, while its accumulation within the body may potentially induce harm to the liver, kidneys, reproductive system, and nervous system, as well as promote carcinogenesis. Moreover, it can lead to allergies or skin irritation upon contact and, when inhaled, may cause coughing, shortness of breath, and chest pain [8]. Rhodamine 6G, also called rhodamine 590, is part of the xanthenes family and is commonly used in drug synthesis and in producing dyes like fluorescein and eosin. This dye constitutes a cationic polar compound with a stable heterocyclic structure, notable for its enhanced visible light absorption and intense fluorescence [9]. Rhodamine 6G is extensively utilized in dyeing materials such as acrylic, nylon, silk, and wool, while it constitutes the preferred dye towards dye laser applications and hydraulic flow pattern visualization, where it is utilized as a fluorescent tracer [10]. Additionally, R6G frequently serves as a sensitizer [11]. Recently, there has been an increasing focus on integrating R6G into both inorganic and organic matrices for use in areas like solid-state laser technology, optoelectronics, and optical filters [12–14]. Previous studies of our research group focusing on the degradation of various pollutants and dyes, such as methylene blue, methyl orange, brilliant green, etc., have shown that rhodamine is a very stable pollutant and is considered a very reliable system for a photocatalytic study; thus, it is selected also for this study, in parallel with the use of rhodamine 6G [15].

Currently, a range of standard treatment approaches is utilized, involving chemical precipitation, separation, adsorption, coagulation, reverse osmosis, ion exchange, flocculation, activated carbon adsorption, incineration, filtration, biopolymeric hybrid membrane technology, and electrochemical oxidation [16,17]. Nonetheless, these techniques frequently lead to incomplete dye degradation, generating secondary pollutants that require additional treatment and potentially exacerbating pollution [18,19]. To address these issues, there is rising interest in advanced oxidation processes (AOPs), which use semiconducting materials as an alternative to conventional approaches [20], offering various benefits, such as lower equipment demands, non-selective oxidation, straightforward control, cost-efficiency, and organic dyes' complete conversion into harmless byproducts like CO_2, H_2O, other inorganic compounds, and/or less toxic organic compounds that are environmentally safe [21,22]. A distinguishing aspect of AOPs is their ability to produce reactive agents such as •OH, which enable the rapid and non-selective oxidation of organic pollutants. Particularly interesting is the use of heterogeneous photocatalysis with oxide-based nanomaterials, which effectively removes water-soluble organic contaminants from water/wastewater upon exposure to light [23].

Overall, in photocatalytic degradation, suspended particles in a water solution act as photocatalysts when exposed to light. In this process, the photocatalyst, which is typically composed of semiconductors with distinct electronic band structures characterized by a band gap (E_g) separating the valence band (VB) and the conduction band (CB), plays a crucial role. The absorbance of photons, characterized by sufficient energy, leads to the generation of electron–hole (e^--h^+) pairs within the semiconductor particles. Subsequently, these carriers undergo charge separation, promoting reactive species' production such as H_2O, •OH, and $^1O_2$. It is important to note that the recombination of e^- and h^+ does not require their participation in chemical reactions. The oxidative agents catalyze organic pollutants' decomposition on or near the catalysts' surface, eventually converting them into harmless substances [24].

Metal oxide semiconductors such as TiO_2, ZnO, CuO, Fe_2O_3, Mn_2O_3, ZrO_2, Co_3O_4, and WO_3 exhibit outstanding adsorption properties and serve as effective catalysts because of their high reactivity, enhanced sensitivity to light, large surface area per unit mass, cost-effectiveness, non-toxicity, and enhanced catalytic performance in dye degradation through photodegradation [25].

Magnesium oxide (MgO) nanoparticles have attracted significant interest among metal oxide nanoparticles due to their excellent biocompatibility, non-toxicity, and strong stability under various conditions [26]. Additionally, the FDA considers MgO safe for human consumption [27]. MgO nanoparticles exhibit beneficial physicochemical properties, including increased ionic character, a significant specific surface area, unique crystal structures, and oxygen vacancies [28,29]. Nano-MgO particles can be fabricated utilizing a plethora of physicochemical techniques, such as sol–gel [30], microwave-assisted [31], solvothermal/hydrothermal [32], combustion [33], precipitation [34], environmentally friendly green synthesis [35], vapor deposition method [36], plasma irradiation [37], ultrasonic irradiation [38], etc. A variety of approaches have been employed to synthesize nano-MgO particles possessing decreased crystallite size and enhanced surface area, features that are acknowledged for augmenting photocatalytic performance towards organic dyes' degradation upon irradiation [39,40] (Table 1). Among the utilized approaches, the precipitation method finds widespread application in synthesizing nanoparticles, as it is facile, cost-efficient, and useful for large-scale production [41].

Table 1. Comparison of various synthetic approaches towards MgO nanoparticles' fabrication, regarding the average crystallite size and specific surface area.

Synthetic Approach	Average Crystallite Size (nm)	Specific Surface Area (m²/g)	Reference
Sol–gel	12–13	-	[42]
Microwave-assisted sol–gel	9.5–10.5	243.2	[43]
Ultrasonic-assisted sol–gel	19.2	-	[44]
Modified thermal/sol–gel	23.6	257.3	[45]
Solid-state chemical	10.5	213	[40]
Microwave irradiation	16	70	[46]
Precipitation	25	216.9	[47]

In this study, MgO nanopowder was synthesized using a simple precipitation approach using $Mg(NO_3)_2$ (precursor) and NaOH as the precipitant. The physical characteristics of the nanopowder were comprehensively examined using techniques such as FESEM, XRD, FTIR, BET, DLS, and DRS. Following this, the photocatalytic efficiency of the material in degrading rhodamine B and rhodamine 6G was assessed under both UV and visible light, with a focus on its potential selectivity towards specific organic dyes. Additionally, the study aimed to elucidate the photocatalytic degradation mechanisms of the dyes under different light conditions, using scavengers during the experimental procedure to evaluate the oxidative potential of MgO nanoparticles that mediate the photocatalytic efficiency of this material.

2. Results

2.1. Characterization of MgO Powder

2.1.1. XRD Analysis

XRD was utilized in order to evaluate MgO powder's crystallinity. The indexed peaks in the acquired pattern (Figure 1) are fully consistent with that of bulk MgO ((JCPDS) card no. 00-004-0829), certifying their monocrystallinity as well as face-centered cubic structure [48]. No additional impurity-related peak was spotted in the spectrum, within the detection limit of XRD, verifying the produced sample's enhanced purity [49]. The formed peaks at two-theta (2θ) values, 36.85°, 42.83°, 61.20°, 74.58°, and 78.51°, are attributed to the (111), (200), (220), (311), and (222) (Miller indices) planes, respectively [50].

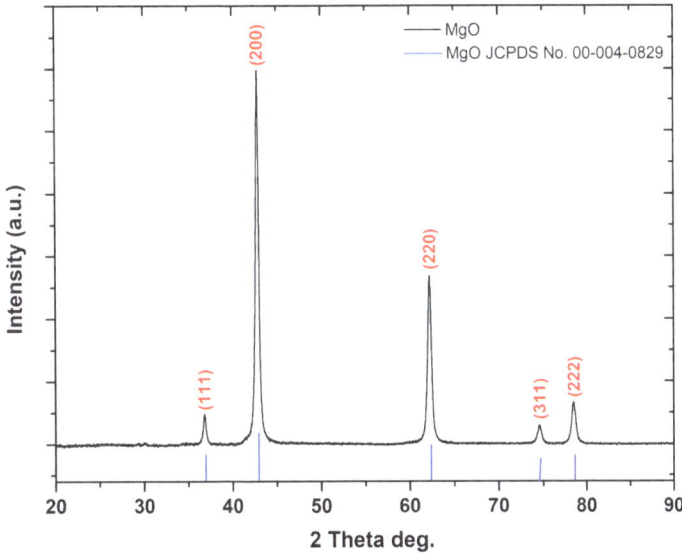

Figure 1. XRD diffractogram of the as-prepared MgO powder.

The as-produced MgO powder's average crystallite size was determined through the Debye–Scherrer equation, its interplanar d-spacing according to Bragg's Law Equation, and the crystallinity index (CI%), as previous studies have already analytically presented (Tables 2 and 3) [51–53]. Bragg peak broadening (β) constitutes the composition of both the instrumental and sample-dependent effects. The instrumental peak width was corrected according to each diffraction peak of MgO material using the following equation (Equation (1)) [54]:

$$\beta^2 = \beta^2_{measured} - \beta^2_{instrumental} \quad (1)$$

Table 2. Crystal lattice indices, average crystallite size, FWHM (Full Width at Half Maximum), and crystallinity index of the synthesized MgO powder.

Sample ID	Crystal Lattice Index ($a = b = c$)			Average Crystallite Size (D, nm) *	FWHM	CI (%)
	a	b	c			
MgO	4.2194	4.2194	4.2194	3.23	0.4562	80.49

* The (200) plane's peak was used to estimate the crystallite size.

Table 3. d-Spacing calculations for MgO powder.

Bragg's Angle		d_{hkl} (Å)	d_{hkl} (nm)	hkl
2θ	θ			
36.85	18.43	2.4372	0.2437	111
42.83	21.42	2.1097	0.2110	200
61.20	30.60	1.5132	0.1513	220
74.58	37.29	1.2714	0.1271	311
78.51	39.26	1.2173	0.1217	222

The usual procedure towards instrumental broadening correction is determining the diffraction line breadth of a "coarse" material, such that broadening due to small crystallite size and lattice distortion is minimal. Thus, the "coarse" material chosen for reference was pure MgO (44–53 μm) and measured ten times in order to obtain statistical validity [55].

The value of the lattice constant was calculated using the following equation (Equation (2)), considering a cubic structure ($a = b = c$) (Table 2):

$$d = \frac{a}{\sqrt{h^2 + k^2 + l^2}} \qquad (2)$$

Additionally, the Nelson–Riley function (Equation (3)) was utilized for estimating the lattice constant due to its more enhanced precision in estimating lattice parameters after eradicating 2θ systematic errors for high angle reflections.

$$F(\theta) = \frac{1}{2}\left(\frac{cos^2\theta}{sin\theta}\right) + \left(\frac{cos^2\theta}{\theta}\right) \qquad (3)$$

By extrapolating the lattice parameter's straight line against an extrapolation function of θ to the value of 0 (Figure S1), the average lattice parameter (a) is determined. The acquired value aligns closely with the one reported in similar studies [56].

Thus, the lattice parameter (a) is measured equal to 4.2170 Å, which is marginally increased than the previously documented 4.2113 Å, according to the reference CIF (Crystallographic Information File) file [57]. Such a minor discrepancy in the lattice parameter is anticipated for nanoparticles possessing crystallite sizes in the tens of nanometers range.

In general, crystal imperfections and distortions lead to strain-induced broadening, which is expressed as $\varepsilon \approx \beta_s/\tan\theta$. A key aspect of Scherrer's equation is its dependence on the diffraction angle θ. Unlike the Scherrer equation, which involves a $1/\cos\theta$ relationship, the Williamson–Hall approach shows variation with $\tan\theta$. This distinction is crucial because it enables the differentiation of reflection broadening when both small crystallite size and micro-strain co-exist. The following approaches consider that size and strain broadening are additive components of the total integral breadth of a Bragg peak [58]. The differing θ dependencies form the foundation for separating size and strain broadening in the W-H analysis. By combining the Scherrer equation with $\varepsilon \approx \beta_s/\tan\theta$, the following equations are obtained (Equations (4) and (5)):

$$\beta_{hkl} = \beta_s + \beta_D \qquad (4)$$

$$\beta_{hkl} = \left(\frac{k\lambda}{D\cos\theta}\right) + (4\varepsilon \tan\theta) \qquad (5)$$

where β_s refers to the broadening due to small crystallite size and β_D represents the broadening due to lattice distortions or micro-strain. The rearrangement of Equation (5) leads to the following equation (Equation (6)):

$$\beta_{hkl}\cos\theta = \left(\frac{k\lambda}{D}\right) + (4\varepsilon \sin\theta) \qquad (6)$$

where β_{hkl} constitutes the FWHM measured in radians, k equals to 0.9, λ corresponds to the wavelength of the X-rays (λ = 1.5406 Å), θ stands for the diffraction angle, D denotes the particle size, and ε constitutes the micro-strain [59]. Additionally, Equation (6) assumes that strain is uniform across all crystallographic directions, reflecting the isotropic nature of the crystal, where material properties do not vary based on the direction of measurement. A plot of βcos θ versus 4sin θ was made for the preferred orientation peaks of nano-MgO (Figure S2). In this plot, the slope corresponds to the strain, while the y-intercept indicates particle size. Typically, a negative slope indicates the presence of compressive micro-strain [60], whereas a positive slope suggests the possible presence of tensile micro-strain [59].

Based on the obtained results, the MgO powder presents a positive slope, thus affirming the existence of tensile micro-strain. In particular, the micro-strain within the sample was determined to be 2.16×10^{-3}, indicating a small but noteworthy value, possibly attributed to the extremely small crystallite size of MgO, which was determined to be equal to 3.42 nm through the Williamson–Hall approach and equal to 3.23 nm applying the Scherrer approach. This small crystallite size prevents the relaxation of strain within the lattice [61]. Both for Scherrer and W-H calculations, zero shifts were accounted for by correcting 2θ.

2.1.2. FT-IR Analysis

In the FT-IR spectrum of the studied MgO powder (Figure 2), bands at 468.62, 863.95, 1432.85, and 3421.10 cm^{-1} are illustrated.

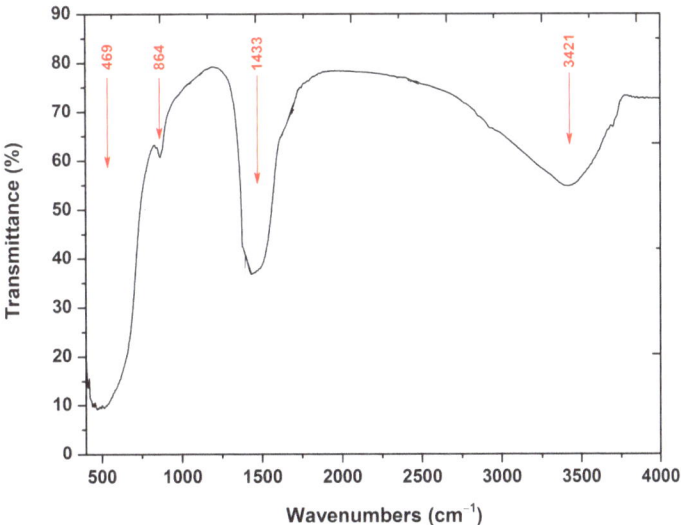

Figure 2. FT-IR spectrum of the synthesized MgO powder.

In particular, the major band observed at ≈469 cm^{-1} is attributed to Mg-O vibrations [62]. The bands observed at approximately 864 and 1433 cm^{-1} are associated with carbonate species that are chemisorbed surficially on MgO [63], while the broad band depicted at 3421 cm^{-1} corresponds to the O-H stretching, as well as bending vibrations of H_2O molecules [62,63], possibly due to atmospheric humidity during the conduction of the powder's measurement [64].

2.1.3. N_2-Sorption Analysis

The N_2-sorption isotherm of the MgO powder is depicted in Figure 3.

Based on the acquired data, the as-synthesized powder displays a type IV isotherm, characterized by a narrow hysteresis loop and the absence of a saturation plateau, suggesting mesopores and macropores existence. The pore size distribution as obtained from the desorption curve via the BJH approach is depicted in the inset in Figure 3. This distribution is broad, covering both the mesopore range (2–50 nm) and the macropore range (>50 nm), consistent with the N_2-sorption isotherm findings [65–67]. The physical parameters are summarized in Table 4, including the BET surface area, micropore surface area, cumulative volume, as well as average pore diameter. The prepared MgO powder exhibits an increased BET surface area, correlating with the small crystallite size, as observed through the XRD analysis (Table 2).

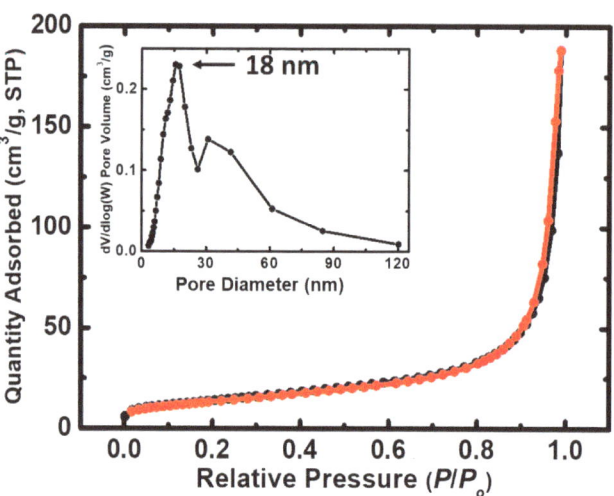

Figure 3. N$_2$-sorption diagram of the prepared MgO powder (sorption: black line; desorption: red line). The pore size distribution utilizing the BJH approach is indicated in the inset.

Table 4. Data obtained via the BET approach. (a) Specific surface area estimated utilizing Brunauer–Emmett–Teller theory, (b) micropore surface area through t-plot analysis, based on the Harkins and Jura model, (c) cumulative volume of pores in the range 1.7 and 300 nm from N$_2$-sorption data and the BJH desorption approach, and (d) average pore diameter, evaluated by the 4 V/σ approach (V was equated to the maximum volume of N$_2$ adsorbed along the isotherm as P/P$_o$ → 1.0).

Sample ID	BET Surface Area (m^2/g)	Micropore Surface Area (m^2/g)	Cumulative Pore Volume (cm^3/g)	Average Pore Diameter (nm)
MgO	52	2	0.3	21

2.1.4. XPS Analysis

XPS analysis was conducted to examine the prepared MgO powder's surficial chemical composition. Figure 4 shows the wide survey spectrum of the as-synthesized powder. All peaks were expected due to the specific synthetic procedure that was employed. Figure S3a,b illustrates the detailed Mg2p XPS peak and the MgKLL X-ray-induced Auger spectrum (XAES). By adding the binding energy of Mg2p and the kinetic energy of MgKL$_{23}$L$_{23}$, the modified Auger parameter, which is an accurate method for chemical species characterization, is derived. The Mg2p binding energy was equal to 49.5 eV, and the modified Auger parameter was estimated as 1231.1 eV, both assigned to MgO [68]. Figure 5 indicates the deconvoluted O1s peak, which is a peak consisting of two components corresponding to oxides Mg-O (529.8 eV) and hydroxides Mg-OH (531.8 eV) [69]. The atomic percentage of Mg and O was calculated from the intensity (peak area) of the XPS peaks weighted with the corresponding relative sensitivity factors (RSF), taking into account the analyzer's transmission characteristics, and was equal to 49.9% at. Mg and 50.1% at. O.

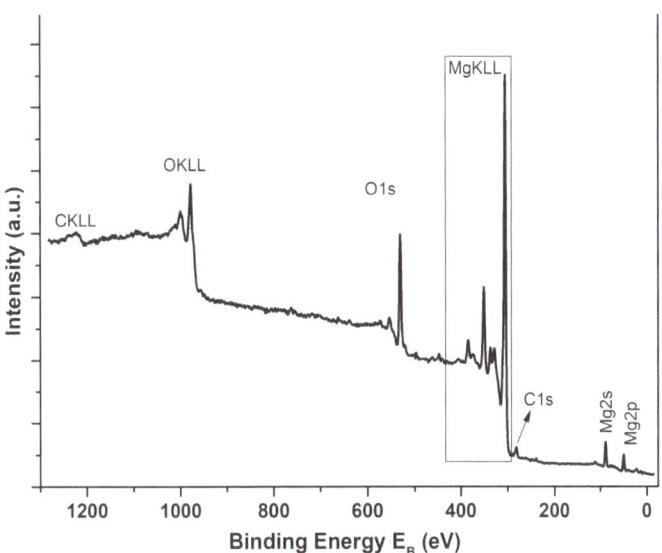

Figure 4. Wide survey XPS spectrum of the studied MgO powder.

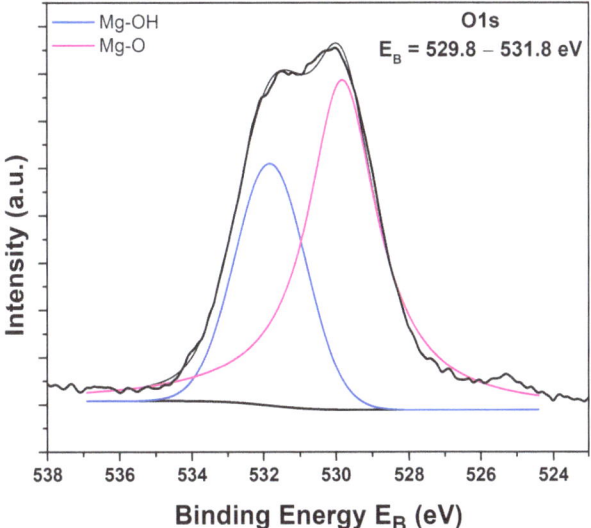

Figure 5. Deconvoluted O1s peak of the synthesized MgO powder.

2.1.5. TGA Analysis

The thermal stability of the developed MgO powder was investigated through thermogravimetric analysis by assessing weight loss, as depicted in Figure 6. Thermal decomposition occurred across three stages within the temperature range of 30–692 °C. The first stage, from 30 to 160 °C, resulted in 3.59% weight loss due to the evaporation of H_2O and a minor amount of adsorbed CO_2, probably due to prolonged storage [70]. During the second stage, between 165 and 345 °C, a 6.55% weight loss was noted, attributed to the decomposition of traces of $Mg(OH)_2$ that have not been converted to MgO during calcination and organic residues' oxidation, yielding carbon dioxide and water vapor. The third stage, ranging from 525 to 692 °C, led to a 3.92% weight loss due to carbonate decomposition and oxidation of remaining organic compounds. Above 692 °C, there was negligible weight loss, implying stabilization of the crystalline solid phases (magnesium hydroxide), as well as the enhanced thermal robustness of the synthesized MgO powder [71].

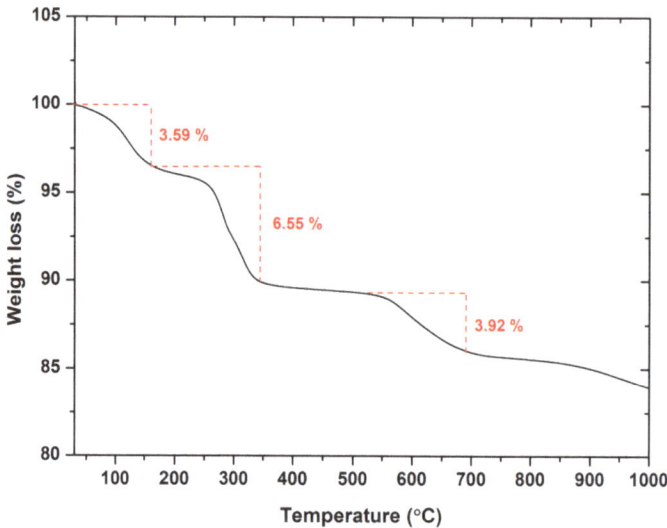

Figure 6. TGA spectrum of the as-prepared MgO powder.

2.1.6. Dynamic Light Scattering (DLS) Analysis

A crucial approach for characterizing nanoparticles is dynamic light scattering (DLS), which provides critical information about the size distribution of colloidal samples. It offers the ability to distinguish whether the studied nanoparticles are polydispersed (variation in size) or monodispersed (uniformity in size). Additionally, DLS analysis is instrumental in detecting aggregation or agglomeration that directly influences stability, reactivity, as well as efficacy of the examined nanostructure [72].

In the present study, the dynamic light scattering measurements were performed at a pH equal to 6.81 ± 0.01. Figure S4a depicts the distribution of hydrodynamic radius as a function of scattered light intensity of the studied MgO powder. Based on the acquired results, the as-utilized synthetic procedure yielded MgO possessing particle sizes within the range 10–100 nm and possessing an average particle size equal to ≈27 nm. The acquired value indicated the successful production of relatively small nanoparticles that are advantageous for photocatalytic applications. In general, smaller nanoparticles tend to exhibit enhanced stability in suspension and reduced aggregation or settling over time [73]. Moreover, decreased particle sizes offer increased surface area-to-volume ratios, potentially enhancing photocatalytic effectiveness [74]. In addition, the PDI (polydispersity index) value of the as-prepared MgO was equal to 0.197, confirming the uniform distribution of particle sizes as well as a monodisperse nature (PDI in the range 0–0.4) [75] (Table 5).

Table 5. Size distribution and zeta potential data acquired from DLS measurements utilizing an aqueous dispersion solution of the examined MgO powder.

Sample ID	Hydrodynamic Diameter (D_h) (nm)	Zeta Potential (mV)	PDI
MgO	27.11 ± 0.93	−50.8 ± 0.6	0.197 ± 0.093

Furthermore, the zeta potential unveils important aspects of nanoparticles' stability and behavior within a colloidal system [76]. Typically, dispersion systems characterized by zeta potential values ranging from ±0 to ±10 mV are considered highly unstable, while those between ±10 and ±20 mV are deemed stable. Furthermore, zeta potential values from ±20 to ±30 mV indicate moderately stable dispersions, and values exceeding ±30 mV indicate extremely stable dispersions [77]. The zeta potential of the as-synthesized MgO nanoparticles was measured equal to −50.8 mV (Figure S4b, Table 5), indicating their stability within the colloidal system. An enhanced absolute zeta potential value, particularly negative as observed from the obtained data, promotes strong repulsion among particles, thereby preventing agglomeration or precipitation over time.

2.1.7. Diffuse Reflectance UV–Vis Spectroscopy (DRS) Analysis

Determining the energy band gap (E_g) is essential for studies involving photocatalysis. Figure S5a presents the diffuse reflectance spectra (DRS) of the synthesized MgO powder.

To evaluate the powder's reflectance, the Kubelka–Munk approach was utilized, as depicted in Figure S5a, following Equation (7) [78]:

$$F(R) = \frac{(1-R)^2}{2R} \qquad (7)$$

where R constitutes the reflectance.

As illustrated in Figure S5a, the absorption edge of the as-studied powder is located at ≈213 nm. Figure S5b depicts the direct energy band gap of the studied powder using the Kubelka–Munk model against energy through the extrapolation of the linear part of the spectra $(F(R)h\nu)^{1/2}$ vs. $h\nu$. The E_g was determined utilizing Tauc's equation (Equation (8)):

$$\alpha h\nu = A(h\nu - E_g)^n \qquad (8)$$

where h constitutes the Planck's constant, ν stands for the frequency, α corresponds to the absorption coefficient, and $n = \frac{1}{2}$ [53].

The studied MgO powder exhibited a band gap value equal to 5.27 eV. This finding is consistent with previous research, where E_g values for nano-MgO ranging from 5.0 to 6.2 eV were reported [79]. Additionally, the obtained energy band gap value is decreased, compared to the 7.8 eV reported for bulk MgO [80]. The reduced E_g value of the examined MgO powder could be attributed to its small crystallite size, as energy band gap narrowing may occur in the nano-scale region due to the high surface area to volume ratio of the crystallites [79]. This aspect is regarded as beneficial for enhancing the overall photocatalytic effectiveness of the as-prepared MgO powder [81].

2.1.8. FESEM Analysis

The primary morphological characteristics of the synthesized MgO powder were assessed through FESEM observation, as illustrated in Figure 7.

Based on the obtained data, the observed nanoparticles display a combination of nearly spherical and hexagonal shapes, while they are also interconnected. This agglomeration might be attributed to electrostatic attraction, as well as polarity [82].

2.2. Photocatalytic Study of MgO Powder

2.2.1. Study of the Photocatalytic Effectiveness towards Rhodamine B (RhB) Degradation

The photocatalytic capability of the as-developed MgO powder was primarily assessed by evaluating its efficiency towards RhB degradation within an aqueous solution under both visible and UV light illumination. The trials were carried out at room temperature and pH = 6.71 ± 0.01. Figure 8a,b illustrates the photocatalytic performance of MgO powder upon UV and visible light irradiation, respectively. Control experiments included photolysis (RhB photolysis) and adsorption–desorption equilibrium (RhB dark) in the absence of irradiation but with constant stirring for the same duration as the photocatalytic trials. The findings revealed that ≈3% of RhB degraded under both visible and UV light exposure, indicating an extremely low degradation rate of RhB in the absence of the examined powder. Moreover, consistent results from the trials implemented under dark conditions confirmed the dye's robustness [83].

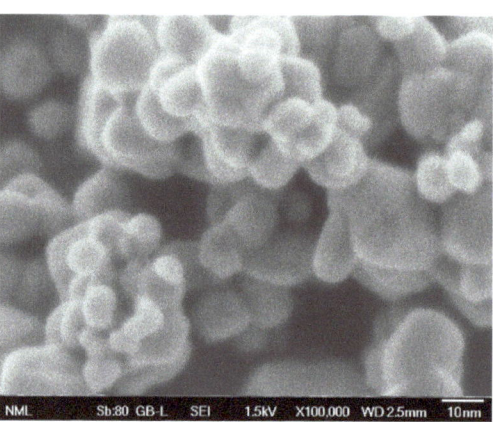

Figure 7. Representative FESEM image of the examined MgO powder at ×100,000 magnification.

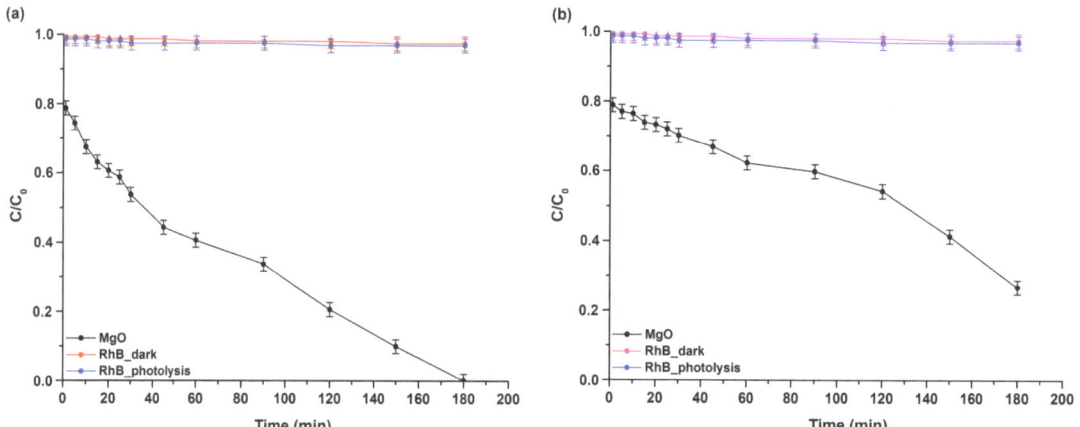

Figure 8. RhB's degradation curve for the studied MgO powder vs. time upon (**a**) UV light exposure and (**b**) visible-light exposure. RhB's photolysis and degradation under dark conditions are also included.

According to the received data, during the photocatalytic experiments, the examined powder exhibited high efficiency, as it led to RhB's complete degradation (100%) within 180 min upon UV light illumination, as well as 83.23 ± 0.83% under visible light exposure within the same 180 min timeframe. Additionally, Figure S6a,b illustrates the UV–visible spectra documented throughout the photocatalytic trials, which were used to track the dye's degradation progress over time, analyze the underlying degradation mechanisms, and evaluate the photocatalytic performance of the powder. Generally, RhB degradation proceeds through two known pathways: (a) N-de-ethylation and (b) disruption of its conjugated structure. Pathway (a) is characterized by a blue shift in the absorption maximum, while the pathway (b) shows a gradual decrease in absorption without a significant blue shift [84]. The real-time UV–visible spectra obtained during the photocatalytic trials of the

MgO powder under UV (Figure S6a) and visible light (Figure S6b) clearly demonstrate the involvement of the second pathway during RhB's degradation.

For the confirmation of the results obtained from RhB's photocatalytic degradation, further analysis was conducted via TOC measurements so as to determine the percentage of mineralization of the examined dye attained during the photocatalytic process. RhB's mineralization percentage was estimated via Equation (9):

$$Mineralization\ (\%) = \left(1 - \frac{TOC_{final}}{TOC_{initial}}\right) \times 100 \quad (9)$$

where $TOC_{initial}$ refers to the medium's initial total organic carbon concentration prior to photocatalytic trials, while TOC_{final} denotes the medium's total organic carbon concentration upon the completion of the photocatalytic procedure [85]. According to the TOC analysis, the MgO powder demonstrated almost total mineralization (98.83 ± 0.97%) of RhB dye upon UV light exposure, as well as an increased mineralization rate (80.04 ± 1.13%) under visible light illumination, thus validating the data acquired from RhB's degradation study.

Study of RhB's Photocatalytic Degradation Kinetics

Figure 9 indicates the outcomes derived from the investigation utilizing the pseudo-first-order kinetic model upon UV and visible light exposure, presenting a plot of $-\ln(C/C_0)$ against time, as described by Equation (10) [86]:

$$-\ln\left(\frac{C}{C_0}\right) = k_1 t \quad (10)$$

where C_0 and C are ascribed to the initial and reaction-time RhB concentrations, respectively, k_1 constitutes the photocatalytic oxidation's apparent rate constant (min^{-1}), while t stands for the irradiation time. The apparent rate constants of the as-prepared MgO powder under both types of irradiation derive from the linearly fitted plot's slope.

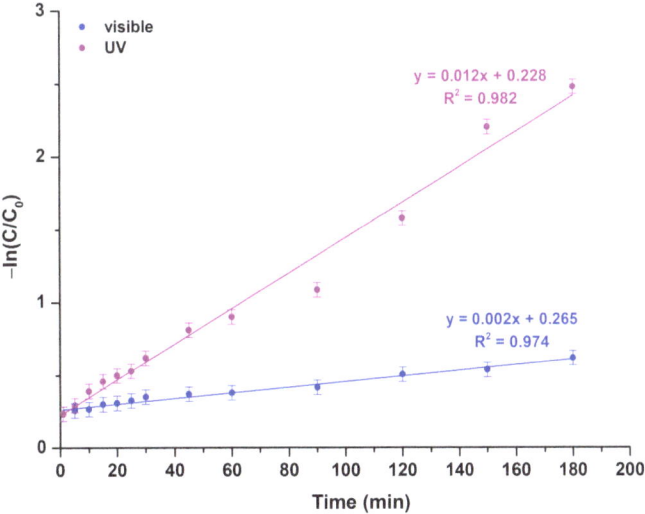

Figure 9. Photocatalytic kinetic model studies for the studied MgO powder, based on a pseudo-first-order model upon UV and visible light illumination.

However, the photocatalytic kinetics can alternatively be described by the pseudo-second-order equation (Equation (11)) [53]:

$$\frac{t}{q_t} = \frac{1}{k_2 q_e^2} + \frac{1}{q_e} t \tag{11}$$

where q_t and q_e constitute the amount of the pollutant adsorbed at time t and equilibrium, respectively (mg/g), and k_2 corresponds to the rate constant (g/mg·min).

In contrast to the results observed with the pseudo-first-order kinetics (Figure 9), the R^2 values acquired from the pseudo-second-order kinetic model (Figure S7) indicate a considerably decreased goodness of fit [53]. Table 6 details the kinetic parameters for the examined MgO powder.

Table 6. Kinetic parameters of the studied powder upon UV and visible light photocatalytic trials.

Sample ID	Pseudo-First-Order Kinetic Model		Pseudo-Second-Order Kinetic Model	
	k_1 (min^{-1})	R^2	k_2 (g/mg·min)	R^2
MgO (visible)	0.002	0.974	10.747	0.778
MgO (UV)	0.012	0.982	5.545	0.906

In photocatalytic systems, rate constants are strongly influenced by crystallite size and specific surface area, both of which play critical roles in determining photocatalytic efficiency. A smaller crystallite size generally leads to a higher surface-to-volume ratio, which increases the number of active sites available for catalytic reactions, thereby enhancing overall performance [87]. However, this variability in surface area complicates direct comparisons between different photocatalysts, as larger specific surface areas may artificially boost rate constants by providing more reaction sites without necessarily improving the material's intrinsic photocatalytic ability [88]. For instance, studies have shown that photocatalysts with larger surface areas often exhibit higher degradation efficiencies, due to increased dye adsorption (dye sensitization) rather than enhanced photocatalytic mechanisms [89]. As such, comparing photocatalysts with different specific surface areas may result in misleading conclusions about their relative efficiencies. In this study, the MgO nanoparticles demonstrated a surface area of 52 m^2/g, which likely contributes to their observed photocatalytic performance.

Mechanism Study

During the photocatalytic oxidation procedure, several key oxidative species play a crucial role, including superoxide radicals (•O$_2^-$), singlet oxygen (^{1}O$_2$), electrons (e$^-$), holes (h$^+$), as well as hydroxyl radicals (•OH). In order to better understand the underlying photocatalytic mechanism, extensive studies were carried out to specify the active species. This involved a series of scavenging experiments in order to identify these specific species. In particular, p-benzoquinone (p-BQ, C$_6$H$_4$(=O)$_2$, ≥98%, Sigma-Aldrich, Darmstadt, Germany), sodium azide (NaN$_3$, ≥99.5%, Sigma-Aldrich, Darmstadt, Germany), silver nitrate (AgNO$_3$, >99%, Sigma-Aldrich, Darmstadt, Germany), disodium ethylenediaminetetraacetate (EDTA-2Na, C$_{10}$H$_{14}$N$_2$Na$_2$O$_8$•2H$_2$O, ≥97%, Sigma-Aldrich, Darmstadt, Germany), and t-butanol (t-BuOH, (CH$_3$)$_3$COH, ≥99.5%, Sigma-Aldrich, Darmstadt, Germany) were added to the RhB dye's solution, in order to selectively capture the •O$_2^-$, ^{1}O$_2$, e$^-$, h$^+$, and •OH, respectively [90,91].

Derived from the outcomes depicted in Figure 10a,b, rhodamine B's degradation effectiveness on the surface of the MgO powder endured a prominent reduction to 14.69 ± 1.03% and 13.23 ± 1.11% under UV and visible light illumination, respectively, upon adding t-BuOH into the photocatalytic reaction solution, thus confirming that the •OH radicals had a major effect on RhB's photocatalytic degradation in both irradiation conditions. On the contrary, $\bullet O_2^-$, $^1O_2$, as well as photogenerated e^- and h^+, were not the principal reactive species participating in the process.

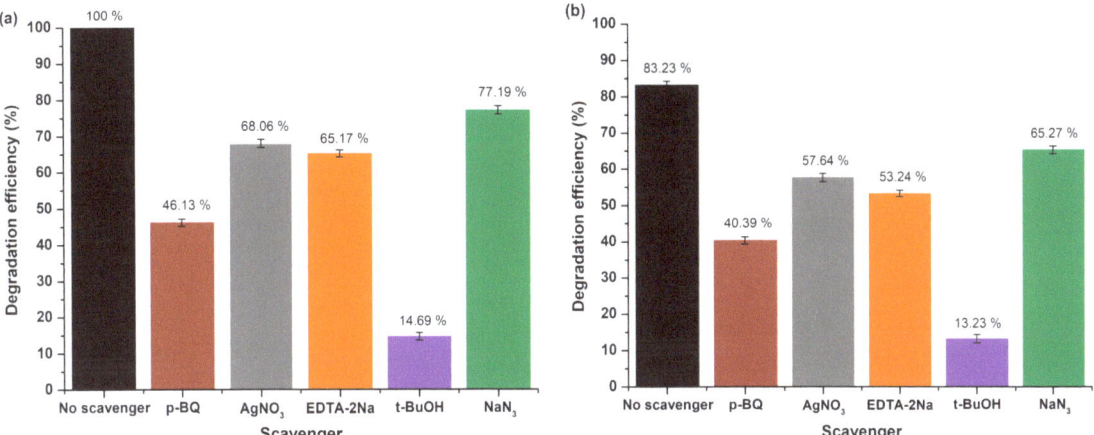

Figure 10. Scavenging trials for RhB's degradation over MgO powder under (**a**) UV and (**b**) visible light exposure.

In accordance with the results of the scavenging experiments, a feasible mechanism is outlined (Figure 11). When MgO nanoparticles are exposed to light (UV or visible) in the VB and CB, electrons and holes are produced within the reaction medium. Then, these photogenerated e^- interact surficially with the photocatalyst, leading to the oxidation of O_2 to $\bullet O_2^-$, while the photogenerated h^+ tend to reduce -OH groups deriving from H_2O molecules to $\bullet OH$ radicals. Subsequently, a reaction among $\bullet O_2^-$ and H_2O leads to the generation of -OH and HOO$\bullet$ radicals, which in turn produce $\bullet OH$ radicals. These free radicals facilitate the decomposition of RhB dye into both gaseous and liquid oxidation byproducts such as CO_2 and H_2O. The following equations illustrate the procedure of radical generation and demonstrate that $\bullet OH$ radicals are predominantly in charge of RhB's degradation (Equations (12)–(18)):

$$MgO + h\nu \rightarrow h_{VB}^+ + e_{CB}^- \tag{12}$$

$$H_2O \rightarrow H^+ + -OH \tag{13}$$

$$h_{VB}^+ + -OH \rightarrow \bullet OH \tag{14}$$

$$e_{CB}^- + O_2 \rightarrow \bullet O_2^- \tag{15}$$

$$\bullet O_2^- + H_2O \rightarrow HOO\bullet + -OH \tag{16}$$

$$HOO\bullet + -OH \rightarrow 2\bullet OH + O_2 \tag{17}$$

$$\bullet OH + RhB \rightarrow oxidation\ byproducts + CO_2 + H_2O \tag{18}$$

Reusability Study

Figure 12a,b demonstrates the reusability of the MgO nanopowder under both UV and visible light exposure across five successive photocatalytic cycles (catalyst loading = 5 mg, pH = 6.71 ± 0.01, initial concentration of RhB = 10 mg/L). After each degradation cycle, the photocatalyst underwent centrifugation and multiple washes with distilled H_2O, followed by drying in a vacuum oven (70 °C, 24 h) in preparation for the next trial, with no further treatment [92]. The photocatalyst showed significant photostability under both light sources, as an approximate 5% (5.46 ± 0.83%) (Figure 12a) and a ≈7% (7.32 ± 1.01%) (Figure 12b) decrease in its photocatalytic efficiency was observed in the case of UV and visible light irradiation, respectively, after five consecutive cycles. These results verify the robustness of the examined photocatalyst throughout repeated photocatalytic trials.

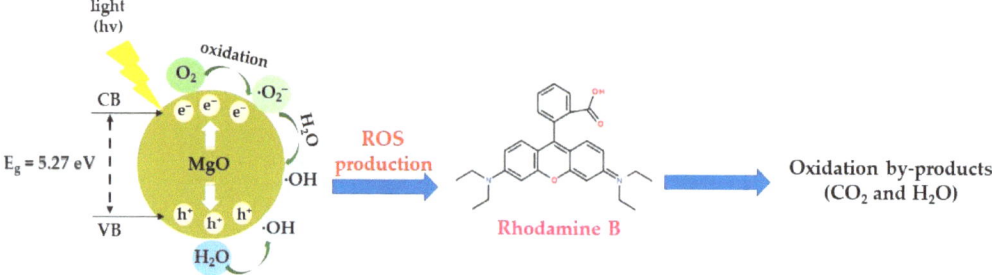

Figure 11. Proposed photocatalytic mechanism of MgO powder towards RhB degradation under both UV and visible light exposure.

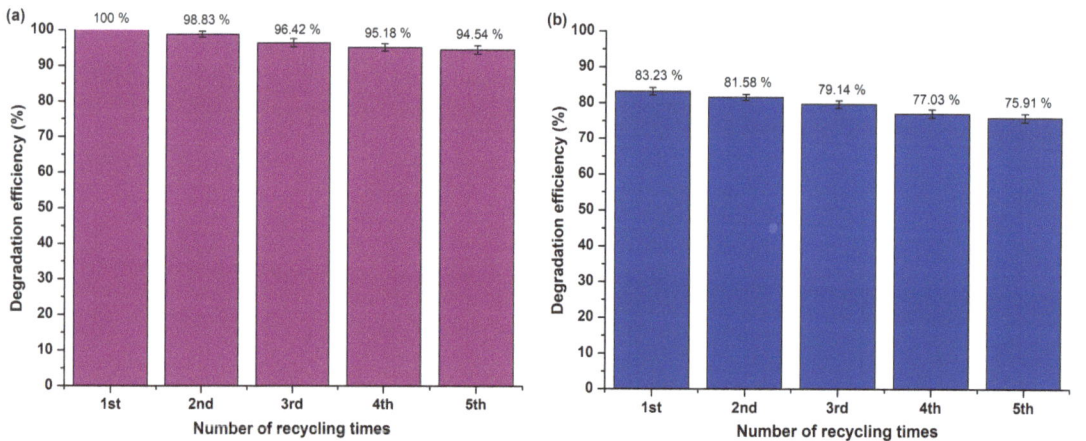

Figure 12. Reusability effectiveness of MgO powder after five experimental photocatalytic trials towards RhB degradation upon (**a**) UV and (**b**) visible light illumination.

Additionally, the studied powder was examined for its stability after five experimental cycles under the as-mentioned conditions through XRD (Figure S8). The analysis revealed that the MgO powder indicated insignificant changes in their crystalline phases, with only a slight increase in peaks' intensity, proving that the examined photocatalyst maintained its structure after RhB's degradation trials and exposure to air, presenting enhanced photochemical robustness. Moreover, the modest augmentation in peaks' intensity may be attributed to crystallite size's growth, because of the photoirradiation activation procedure [93].

2.2.2. Study of the Photocatalytic Effectiveness towards Rhodamine 6G (R6G) Degradation

MgO's capability was also evaluated towards R6G's (aqueous solution) photocatalytic degradation under the same irradiation conditions as the ones described in the case of rhodamine B. During R6G's photocatalytic trials, temperature and pH conditions were set at 25 °C and 7.48 ± 0.01. Control trials were also conducted, including photolysis (R6G photolysis) and adsorption–desorption equilibrium (R6G dark) in the absence of light illumination upon continual stirring for the same duration as the photocatalysis procedure. The data acquired from these trials and for both irradiation types, verified the dye's robustness, as ≈2% of R6G was degraded [86] (Figure 13).

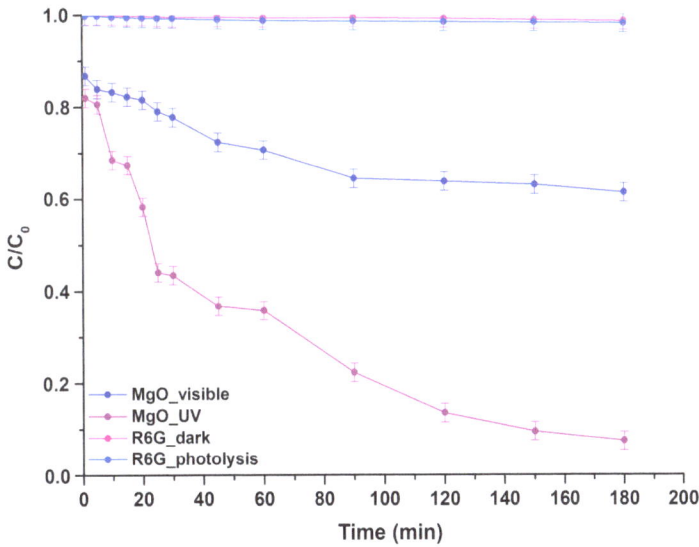

Figure 13. Degradation curves of R6G for the studied MgO powder vs. time upon UV and visible light exposure. R6G's photolysis and degradation under dark conditions are also included.

Throughout the photocatalytic trials, the studied powder demonstrated enhanced effectiveness towards R6G degradation under UV light illumination, achieving a degradation rate equal to 92.62 ± 0.84% over 180 min, whereas a rate of the order of 38.71 ± 1.43% was attained upon visible light irradiation within the same period.

Based on the data derived from the photocatalytic effectiveness studies for RhB, as well as R6G, the MgO powder achieved 100% and 83.23 ± 0.83% RhB degradation upon UV and visible light irradiation within 180 min, respectively, while 92.62 ± 0.84% and 38.71 ± 1.43% of R6G was degraded in the same timeframe upon UV and visible light illumination, respectively. Consequently, the as-mentioned photocatalyst exhibits selective activity favoring RhB's photocatalytic degradation, primarily in the case of visible light irradiation (Figure 14). This phenomenon might be attributed to the pH that was prevalent during the experimental procedure. According to other studies, rhodamine B can be effectively degraded in generally acidic conditions, while rhodamine 6G requires highly basic conditions [94]. In these series of experiments, pH was approximately 7 (in the case of rhodamine B, pH was 6.71, and for rhodamine 6G, pH was 7.48). It might be possible to obtain even more promising results for rhodamine 6G for a pH of around 10.

Figure S9a,b represents the real-time UV–visible spectra as received during the photocatalytic trials. In general, R6G dye contains a chromophore made up of benzene and xanthene rings, connected by ethylamine ($CH_3CH_2NH_2$) as the auxochrome. The chromophore determines the dye's color, while the auxochrome influences the color's intensity. The photocatalytic degradation of R6G typically follows two main pathways: breaking the conjugated chromophores or N-deethylation of the auxochromes. Previous research has outlined that a shift to a shorter absorption wavelength (blue shift) indicates a degradation pathway via N-deethylation [95]. Based on the emerged spectra, the peak at 526 nm (absorption maximum), which is attributed to a xanthene compound [96], remains constant, presenting no significant blue or red shift, thus rendering the *N*-deethylation pathway less probable in R6G's degradation.

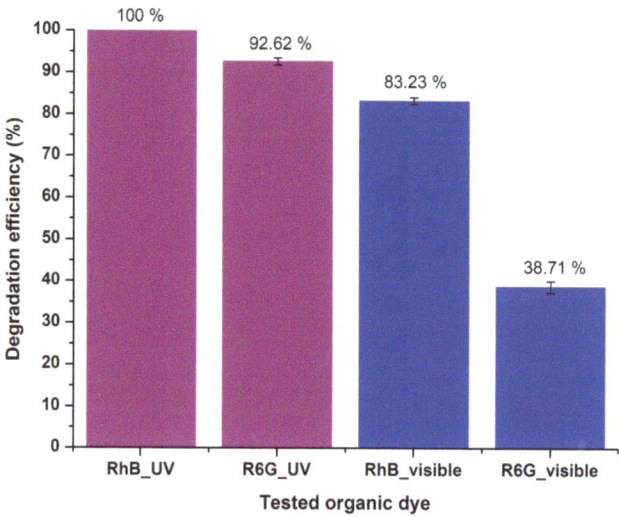

Figure 14. Selectivity of MgO photocatalyst.

TOC analysis was similarly conducted to assess the extent of R6G's mineralization (Equation (9)) during photocatalysis, so as to affirm the validity of degradation experiments. The as-mentioned analysis indicated that the MgO powder achieved a more increased mineralization rate of R6G upon UV light illumination (90.03 ± 1.31% instead of 36.49 ± 1.14% in the case of visible light irradiation), thus validating the results obtained from the photocatalytic degradation study.

Study of R6G's Photocatalytic Degradation Kinetics

Kinetic model studies upon UV and visible light illumination were conducted based on the pseudo-first-order (Equation (10) and Figure 15) and pseudo-second-order (Equation (11) and Figure S10) models.

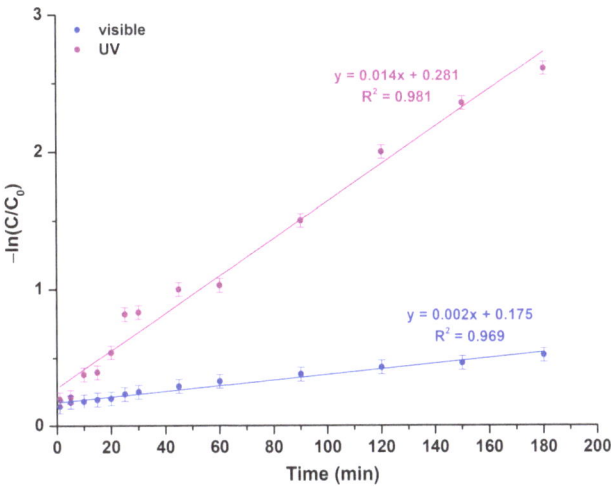

Figure 15. Photocatalytic kinetic model studies for the examined MgO powder, based on a pseudo-first-order model upon UV and visible light illumination.

In opposition to the pseudo-first-order model, the pseudo-second-order is characterized by inferior R^2 values (Table 7). Consequently, it can be inferred that the photocatalytic degradation of R6G in the presence of the as-synthesized MgO powder upon both UV and visible light illumination is best elucidated by a pseudo-first-order reaction kinetic model.

Table 7. Kinetic parameters of the studied powder upon UV and visible light photocatalysis towards degradation of R6G dye.

Sample ID	Pseudo-First-Order Kinetic Model		Pseudo-Second-Order Kinetic Model	
	k_1 (min^{-1})	R^2	k_2 (g/mg·min)	R^2
MgO (visible)	0.002	0.969	1.772	0.911
MgO (UV)	0.014	0.981	0.756	0.907

Mechanism Study

Comprehensive studies were conducted to determine the active species involved by emphasizing validating R6G's photocatalytic degradation mechanism. Similar to the approach outlined in the case of RhB dye, experimental trials were performed to scavenge and capture the entagled active species. Consequently, AgNO$_3$, EDTA-2Na, p-BQ, NaN$_3$, and t-BuOH were added to R6G's aqueous solution to selectively trap, as well as specify e$^-$, h$^+$, •O$_2^-$ radicals, ^{1}O$_2$, and •OH radicals, respectively (Figure 16a,b).

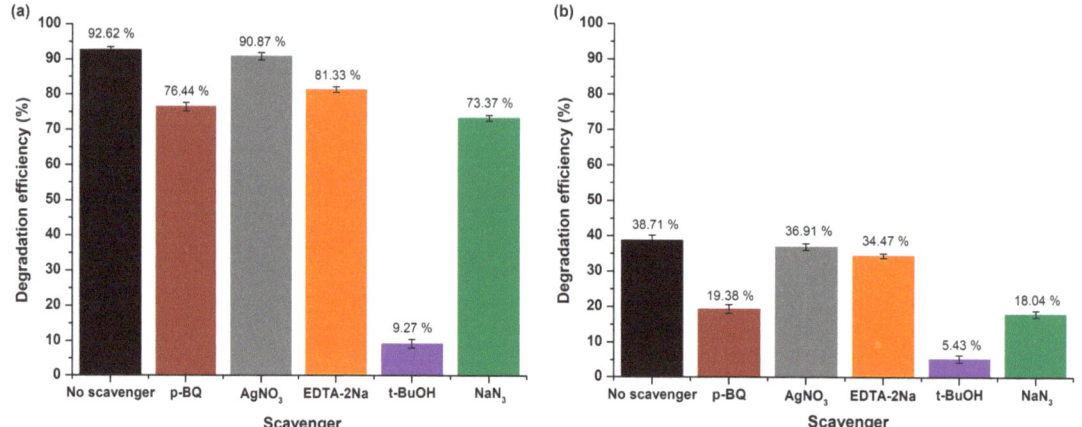

Figure 16. Scavenging trials for R6G's degradation over MgO powder under (**a**) UV and (**b**) visible light exposure.

According to the received data, R6G's capability presented a notable reduction to 9.27 ± 1.23% and 5.43 ± 1.01% under UV and visible light photocatalysis, respectively, after introducing t-BuOH into the photocatalytic reaction solution, thus justifying that •OH radicals played a crucial role on R6G's degradation in both irradiation conditions. However, when visible light was utilized as the source of irradiation, less oxidative species like $•O_2^-$ radicals and $^1O_2$ indicated a slightly enhanced contribution to the degradation of R6G, possibly because under visible light the mechanism of self-sensitization was involved in the dye's degradation [92]. Additionally, in both irradiation conditions, h^+ had a minor effect on the degradation procedure, while the role of photogenerated e^- was negligible, proving the efficient e^- transfer from MgO's surface towards the adsorbed molecules for the generation of reactive species [97].

As a result, taking also into account the as-received real-time UV–visible data, the suggested mechanism involves the cleavage of conjugated chromophores, where the predominant •OH radicals fragment R6G chromophore's structural ring, leading to the effective dye's degradation into mineralized by-products (CO_2 and H_2O).

Reusability Study

The reusability of the studied nano-MgO powder upon both UV and visible light illumination across five sequential photocatalytic cycles (catalyst loading = 5 mg, pH = 7.48 ± 0.01, R6G's initial concentration equal to 10 mg/L) was assessed (Figure 17a,b) through the perpetual process as in the case of RhB. The examined photocatalyst presented notable photostability under both utilized light sources, achieving a ≈6% decrease in its photocatalytic efficiency upon UV (5.98 ± 0.54%) and visible (6.27 ± 0.71%) light irradiation after the completion of the reusability experimental trials.

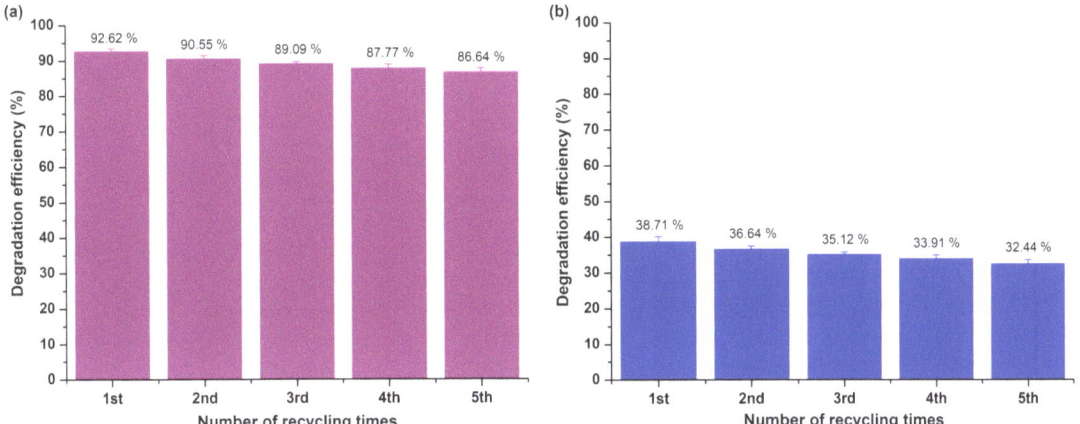

Figure 17. Reusability effectiveness of MgO powder after five experimental photocatalytic trials towards R6G degradation upon (**a**) UV and (**b**) visible light illumination.

3. Discussion

This study successfully synthesized MgO nanoparticles using a simple precipitation method and evaluated their photocatalytic efficiency in degrading rhodamine B (RhB) and rhodamine 6G (R6G) upon UV and visible light illumination. The characterization of MgO nanoparticles confirmed their crystallinity, purity, and favorable surface properties, which are crucial for photocatalytic applications.

The XRD analysis revealed that the synthesized MgO nanoparticles possess a pure face-centered cubic structure with high crystallinity that is known to enhance photocatalytic activity towards degradation of organic dyes, indicating successful synthesis without significant impurities. The average crystallite size, determined using the Debye–Scherrer equation, was approximately 3.23 nm, which is beneficial for enhancing photocatalytic activity due to the increased surface area-to-volume ratio.

FT-IR analysis further confirmed the presence of characteristic Mg-O vibrations and minor surface-adsorbed carbonate species, while the N_2-sorption isotherms suggested a mesoporous and macroporous structure, which is advantageous for dye adsorption and subsequent degradation. The BET surface area of 52 m^2/g supports the observed high photocatalytic activity.

The photocatalytic studies demonstrated that MgO nanoparticles exhibit excellent degradation capabilities for both RhB and R6G dyes. Under UV light, MgO achieved complete degradation of RhB within 180 min, while under visible light, it achieved 83.23% degradation. For R6G, the degradation efficiency was 92.62% under UV light and 38.71% under visible light, indicating a higher photocatalytic activity towards RhB under visible light. These results highlight the potential of MgO nanoparticles as effective photocatalysts for the degradation of organic dyes in wastewater.

The results align well with previous studies that have highlighted the effectiveness of metal oxide nanoparticles in photocatalytic applications. For instance, TiO_2 and ZnO have been widely studied and reported to exhibit significant photocatalytic properties. However, MgO offers several advantages, including non-toxicity, biocompatibility, and a lower band gap, which enhances its activity under visible light.

The photocatalytic mechanism proposed in this study is consistent with the general principles observed in other semiconductor photocatalysts. Electron-hole pairs' generation upon light irradiation and the subsequent production of ROS like •OH radicals play a crucial role in dyes' degradation. The scavenging experiments confirmed that •OH radicals are the dominant species in the degradation process for both RhB and R6G, similar to findings in studies involving TiO_2 and ZnO photocatalysts.

The findings of this study have significant implications for wastewater treatment, particularly in industries that discharge dye-contaminated effluents. The high photocatalytic efficiency of MgO nanoparticles under both UV and visible light suggests their potential application in real-world scenarios, where visible light comprises a major portion of the solar spectrum. This could lead to more sustainable and cost-effective wastewater treatment processes. Comparing the results obtained from previous studies, that had focused on the use of well-established photocatalysts, such as pure TiO_2 and ZnO, it is clear that MgO powder could totally degrade rhodamine B upon a 3 h UV light irradiation, while ZnO [98] and TiO_2 nanoparticles [99] needed less than 3 h for the same effect. Under visible light irradiation, MgO powder led to 83.23% degradation of rhodamine B, while ZnO nanoparticles could totally degrade rhodamine B in the same timeframe [98]. TiO_2 is not so efficient under visible light irradiation (TiO_2 Evonik P25 can degrade rhodamine B by 48% after 240 min) [100], and this is why it is widely doped for the enhancement of its photocatalytic performance under visible light irradiation. Regarding rhodamine 6G, MgO achieved 92.62% and 38.71% degradation after 3 h of UV and visible light illumination, respectively. According to Pino et al., when UV or visible light is applied for 90 min to irradiate a solution of rhodamine 6G in the presence of TiO_2 Evonik P25, a degradation percentage of 22% is determined [14]. MgO led to a 35% degradation of rhodamine 6G after 90 min of visible light irradiation and ~70% under UV light irradiation, thus MgO is proven as an efficient photocatalyst of rhodamine 6G. ZnO degraded by 72% rhodamine 6G, under UV light irradiation for 120 min, according to Yudasari et al. [101]. In the same timeframe, MgO degraded by >85% rhodamine 6G. Also, according to Khoza et al., ZnO composites led to a 50% degradation of rhodamine 6G after 60 min of photoactivation with visible light, showing also excellent reusability after five cycles [102]. So, MgO seems to be a very promising photocatalyst against rhodamine B or rhodamine 6G, compared to TiO_2 and ZnO.

Furthermore, the study highlights the importance of nanoparticle size, surface area, and the presence of active sites in enhancing photocatalytic activity. These insights can guide the design and synthesis of more efficient photocatalysts in the future.

Future research could focus on optimizing the synthesis process to further reduce the particle size and increase the surface area of MgO nanoparticles, thereby enhancing their photocatalytic efficiency. Additionally, exploring the doping of MgO with other metal ions could improve visible light's absorption and enhance the generation of ROS.

Investigating the reusability and stability of MgO nanoparticles in long-term photocatalytic applications is also crucial. While this study demonstrated significant photostability over five cycles, extended research is required to grasp the mechanisms behind any noted deactivation and to develop strategies for regeneration.

Finally, extending the study to other types of organic pollutants and exploring the photocatalytic performance of MgO in real wastewater samples would provide a more comprehensive understanding of its potential applications in environmental remediation.

In conclusion, this study underscores the potential of MgO nanoparticles as efficient photocatalysts towards organic dye degradation, paving the way for their application in sustainable wastewater treatment technologies.

4. Materials and Methods

4.1. Synthesis of MgO Powder

The synthesis of MgO powder was conducted utilizing a facile precipitation approach, founded on the synthetic protocol of Karthikeyan and colleagues [103], upon some alterations. In particular, 6.4103 g of magnesium nitrate hexahydrate ($Mg(NO_3)_2 \bullet 6H_2O$, 99%, Sigma-Aldrich, Darmstadt, Germany) were added in 100 mL of lab-distilled water. Subsequently, 100 mL of a 0.25 M sodium hydroxide solution (NaOH, 99.5%, Panreac Quimica SA, Barcelona, Spain) were poured dropwise into the aforementioned aqueous solution. The acquired mixture underwent continuous magnetic stirring for 4 h at 25 °C until the emergence of a white-colored suspension. The completion of the reaction procedure was indicated by the formation of a white precipitate, which was acquired through centrifugation and was subsequently triturated and purified via rinsing with double-distilled (18.2 MΩ·cm) water and centrifugation for eliminating potential impurities. Then, the obtained precipitate underwent drying at 80 °C for 6 h and was further calcinated at 500 °C (4 h), finally resulting in a white powder's production (Figure 18). The reaction that took place during the synthetic procedure is outlined through the following equation (Equation (19)):

$$Mg(NO_3)_2 + NaOH \rightarrow Mg(OH)_2 \downarrow + NaNO_3 + H_2O \tag{19}$$

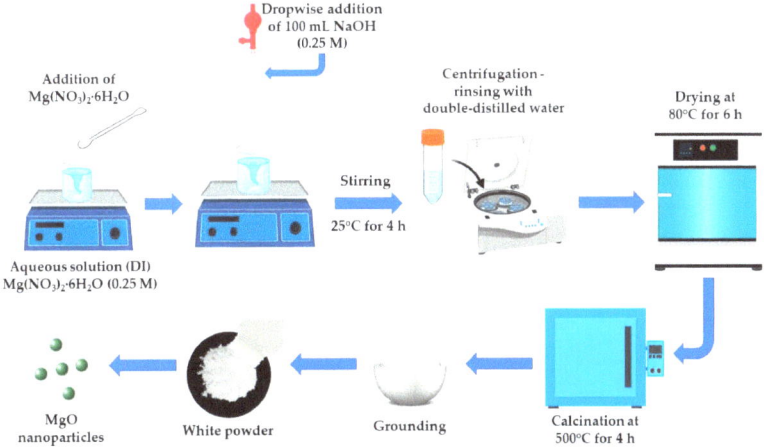

Figure 18. Schematic illustration for the synthetic procedure of MgO powder.

$Mg(OH)_2$ formed by the reaction of $Mg(NO_3)_2$ with NaOH when calcinated at 500 °C for 4 h results in the formation of MgO (Equation (20)) [104]:

$$Mg(OH)_2 \rightarrow MgO + H_2O \tag{20}$$

4.2. Characterization of MgO Nanopowder

FESEM analysis was utilized in order to assess the morphology of the MgO powder (FESEM, JSM-7401F, JEOL, Tokyo, Japan).

Regarding the XRD analysis, a Brucker D8 Advance (Brucker, Karlsruhe, Germany) X-ray diffractometer was utilized, implementing CuKα radiation (λ = 1.5406 Å) (40 kV, 40 mA). The measurements were conducted at a 2-theta angle ranging from 20° to 90° (0.01°/1.0 s).

FTIR measurements were also performed, and spectra were acquired at 25 °C in the range from 400 cm^{-1} to 4000 cm^{-1} (resolution: 4 cm^{-1}) through a FTIR JASCO4200 apparatus (Oklahoma City, OK, USA), possessing a Ge crystal.

The synthesized powder's N_2 adsorption was examined via a ChemBET 3000 instrument (Yumpu, Diepoldsau, Switzerland) to ascertain the BET specific area. Before each measurement, the MgO powder passed through a degassing process (80 °C, 24 h).

Thermogravimetric analysis was performed utilizing a Mettler Toledo TGA/DSC 1 HT apparatus (Mettler Toledo GmbH, Greifensee, Switzerland). Measurements were conducted under N_2 flow (10 mL/min) in the range 30–1000 °C and a heating rate equal to 10 °C/min.

XPS analysis (Leybold SPECS LHS/EA10, Leybold GmbH, Cologne, Germany) was implemented in order to assess the examined powder's surficial chemical states. An ultra-high vacuum chamber (P ≈ 5 × 10^{-10} mbar) equipped with a SPECS Phoibos

100 hemispherical electron analyzer (Berlin, Germany) with a delay line detector (DLD) and an unmonochromized dual-anode Mg/Al X-ray source were utilized for the measurements. A MgKα line at 1253.6 eV and an analyzer pass energy of 10 eV (giving a FWHM equal to 0.85 eV for the Ag $3d_{5/2}$ peak) were utilized. A fitting routine was used for analyzing the XPS core level spectra, leading to each spectrum's decomposition into individual mixed Gaussian–Lorentzian peaks upon a Shirley background subtraction. Errors regarding peak areas were found equal to ≈10%, and the accuracy for binding energies' assignments was approximately 0.1 eV. The samples, which were originally in powder form, were compressed into pellets for measurement. Analysis was conducted on a 3 mm diameter area, with the XPS spectra documented at 25 °C.

The hydrodynamic diameter, as well as the distribution of the powder's particles in an aqueous dispersion, was assessed through dynamic light scattering (DLS) (Malvern Zetasizer Nano ZS, Malvern Panalytical Ltd., Malvern, UK). The scattering intensity's recording was achieved using a 633 nm laser and a 173° scattering angle.

Diffuse reflectance measurements for obtaining the E_g values were evaluated via a UV–vis spectrometer (Jasco UV/Vis/NIR V-770, Interlab, Athens, Greece) possessing an integrating sphere.

RhB's and R6G's mineralization percentage was evaluated by TOC analysis (TOC-LCSH/CSN, Shimadzu Scientific Instruments, Columbia, MD, USA).

4.3. Photocatalytic Efficiency Study of MgO Nanopowder

The photocatalytic effectiveness of the as-prepared MgO powder upon both UV and visible light irradiation was initially evaluated towards the degradation of rhodamine B through the addition of 0.005 g of the powder in a 10 ppm aqueous solution (250 mL) of RhB ($C_{28}H_{31}ClN_2O_3$, ≥95%, Penta-Chemicals Unlimited, Prague, Czech Republic) at 25 °C and pH value equal to 6.71 ± 0.01. Before each photocatalytic experiment, the rhodamine B solution was saturated for 1 h via extra-pure O_2 (99.999%) flow.

In addition, the assessment of the MgO's photocatalytic activity was conducted under UV and visible light illumination towards rhodamine 6G ($C_{28}H_{31}N_2O_3Cl$, 99%, Sigma-Aldrich, Darmstadt, Germany) degradation, using the same conditions as described in the case of rhodamine B with the only difference that the pH value of the dye's solution was equal to 7.48 ± 0.01.

The photoreactor that was utilized for the photocatalytic experiments was equipped with four parallel lamps placed 10 cm above each sample's surface [78]. Blacklight lamps (368 nm, 830 lumens, incident light flux: 0.184 μmol quanta/s, Sylvania, Wilmington, NC, USA) were employed as the UV irradiation source, while 15 W visible light lamps (900 lumens, 400 nm cutoff filter, incident light flux: 0.371 μmol quanta/s, OSRAM GmbH, Munich, Germany) comprised the visible light irradiation source. All the experiments were conducted at 25 °C [53,78]

The derived absorbance of the studied MgO powder was estimated at 554 nm [53] and 525 nm [105] for RhB and R6G, respectively, utilizing a spectrometer (Thermo Fisher Scientific Evolution 200, Thermo Fisher Scientific, Waltham, MA, USA). The C/C_0 ratio, where C is ascribed to RhB's and R6G's concentration after a certain time of photocatalysis and C_0 corresponds to RhB and R6G initial concentration, was acquired indirectly by the evaluation of the measured absorption A (absorption at each time) to the initial absorption ($A_{initial}$) [78].

5. Conclusions

In this study, magnesium oxide (MgO) nanoparticles were synthesized using a simple precipitation method and characterized by various techniques, confirming their high purity, crystallinity, and appropriate physicochemical properties for photocatalytic applications. The MgO nanoparticles demonstrated significant photocatalytic efficiency in degrading rhodamine B (RhB) and rhodamine 6G (R6G) dyes under both UV and visible light irradiation. The nanoparticles exhibited complete degradation of RhB under UV light within 180 min and achieved notable degradation levels for R6G as well. The study's findings underscore the potential of MgO nanoparticles as a promising photocatalyst, particularly for the selective degradation of hazardous dyes such as RhB, thereby contributing to the development of more effective wastewater treatment technologies. Additionally, the reusability of MgO nanoparticles across multiple trials further emphasizes their practical applicability, making them a viable candidate for large-scale environmental remediation efforts. Future research could focus on optimizing the synthesis process to enhance the photocatalytic performance of MgO nanoparticles under visible light and exploring their efficacy in degrading other persistent organic pollutants.

Supplementary Materials: The following supporting information can be downloaded at: https://www.mdpi.com/article/10.3390/molecules29184299/s1: Figure S1: Nelson–Riley plot of the synthesized MgO powder; Figure S2: Williamsons-Hall (W-H) plot of the as-studied MgO powder; Figure S3: (a) Mg2p peak and (b) XAES detailed region of Mg KLL of the MgO powder; Figure S4: (a) Size distribution diagram and (b) zeta potential diagram of the as-synthesized MgO powder; Figure S5: (a) F(R) reflectance plotted against wavelength for the MgO powder under study and (b) the E_g of the same powder; Figure S6: Real-time UV–visible spectra obtained upon (a) UV and (b) visible light induced photocatalytic degradation of RhB utilizing the as-synthesized MgO powder; Figure S7: Photocatalytic kinetic model studies for the studied MgO powder, following a pseudo-second-order model upon UV and visible light illumination; Figure S8: XRD patterns of MgO photocatalyst after the reusability studies; Figure S9: Real-time UV–visible spectra obtained upon (a) UV and (b) visible light induced photocatalytic degradation of R6G utilizing the as-synthesized MgO powder; Figure S10: Photocatalytic kinetic model studies for the examined MgO powder, following a pseudo-second-order model upon UV and visible light illumination.

Author Contributions: Conceptualization, E.A.P.; methodology, E.A.P., M.-A.G. and N.B.; validation, E.A.P., M.-A.G. and N.B.; formal analysis, M.-A.G. and N.B.; investigation, M.-A.G. and N.B.; resources, E.A.P.; writing—original draft preparation, M.-A.G. and N.B.; writing—review and editing, M.-A.G., N.B., N.L. and E.A.P.; visualization, M.-A.G. and N.B.; supervision, E.A.P. All authors have read and agreed to the published version of the manuscript.

Funding: This research received no external funding.

Institutional Review Board Statement: Not applicable.

Informed Consent Statement: Not applicable.

Data Availability Statement: Data are contained within the article and Supplementary Materials.

Acknowledgments: The authors would like to thank Labrini Sygellou from Foundation of Research and Technology Hellas, Institute of Chemical Engineering Sciences (Patras, Greece) for XPS analysis, as well as Christos Zotiadis from Laboratory of Polymer Technology, School of Chemical Engineering, National Technical University of Athens (Greece) for TGA measurements.

Conflicts of Interest: The authors declare no conflicts of interest.

References

1. Jaspal, D.; Malviya, A. Composites for wastewater purification: A review. *Chemosphere* **2020**, *246*, 125788. [CrossRef] [PubMed]
2. Sharma, V.K.; Jinadatha, C.; Lichtfouse, E. Environmental chemistry is most relevant to study coronavirus pandemics. *Environ. Chem. Lett.* **2020**, *18*, 993–996. [CrossRef]
3. Sarkar, S.; Banerjee, A.; Halder, U.; Biswas, R.; Bandopadhyay, R. Degradation of Synthetic Azo Dyes of Textile Industry: A Sustainable Approach Using Microbial Enzymes. *Water Conserv. Sci. Eng.* **2017**, *2*, 121–131. [CrossRef]
4. Zare, E.N.; Motahari, A.; Sillanpää, M. Nanoadsorbents based on conducting polymer nanocomposites with main focus on polyaniline and its derivatives for removal of heavy metal ions/dyes: A review. *Environ. Res.* **2018**, *162*, 173–195. [CrossRef] [PubMed]
5. Tara, N.; Siddiqui, S.; Rathi, G.; Inamuddin, I.; Asiri, A.M. Nano-engineered adsorbent for removal of dyes from water: A review. *Curr. Anal. Chem.* **2019**, *16*, 14–40. [CrossRef]
6. Saeed, M.; Khan, I.; Adeel, M.; Akram, N.; Muneer, M. Synthesis of a CoO–ZnO photocatalyst for enhanced visible-light assisted photodegradation of methylene blue. *New J. Chem.* **2022**, *46*, 2224–2231. [CrossRef]
7. Kocijan, M.; Ćurković, L.; Vengust, D.; Radošević, T.; Shvalya, V.; Gonçalves, G.; Podlogar, M. Synergistic remediation of organic dye by titanium dioxide/reduced graphene oxide nanocomposite. *Molecules* **2023**, *28*, 7326. [CrossRef]

8. Ngoc, P.K.; Mac, T.K.; Nguyen, H.T.; Thanh, T.D.; Van Vinh, P.; Phan, B.T.; Duong, A.T.; Das, R. Superior organic dye removal by $CoCr_2O_4$ nanoparticles: Adsorption kinetics and isotherm. *J. Sci. Adv. Mater. Devices* **2022**, *7*, 100438. [CrossRef]
9. Zehentbauer, F.M.; Moretto, C.; Stephen, R.; Thevar, T.; Gilchrist, J.R.; Pokrajac, D.; Richard, K.L.; Kiefer, J. Fluorescence spectroscopy of Rhodamine 6G: Concentration and solvent effects. *Spectrochim. Acta Part A* **2014**, *121*, 147–151. [CrossRef]
10. Tarud, F.; Aybar, M.; Pizarro, G.; Cienfuegos, R.; Pastén, P. Integrating fluorescent dye flow-curve testing and acoustic Doppler velocimetry profiling for in situ hydraulic evaluation and improvement of clarifier performance. *Water Environ. Res.* **2010**, *82*, 675–685. [CrossRef]
11. Wu, T.; Liu, G.; Zhao, J.; Hidaka, H.; Serpone, N. Photoassisted degradation of dye pollutants. v. self-photosensitized oxidative transformation of rhodamine b under visible light irradiation in aqueous TiO_2 dispersions. *Phys. Chem. B* **1998**, *102*, 5845–5851. [CrossRef]
12. Vanamudan, A.; Pamidimukkala, P. Chitosan, nanoclay and chitosan-nanoclay composite as adsorbents for Rhodamine-6G and the resulting optical properties. *Int. J. Biol. Macromol.* **2015**, *74*, 127–135. [CrossRef] [PubMed]
13. Barranco, A.; Groening, P. Fluorescent plasma nanocomposite thin films containing nonaggregated rhodamine 6G laser dye molecules. *Langmuir* **2006**, *22*, 6719–6722. [CrossRef] [PubMed]
14. Pino, E.; Calderón, C.; Herrera, F.; Cifuentes, G.; Arteaga, G. Photocatalytic degradation of aqueous rhodamine 6G using supported TiO_2 catalysts. a model for the removal of organic contaminants from aqueous samples. *Front. Chem.* **2020**, *8*, 365. [CrossRef] [PubMed]
15. Kassalia, M.-E.; Nikolaou, Z.; Pavlatou, E.A. Photocatalytic testing protocol for N-Doped TiO_2 nanostructured particles under visible light irradiation using the statistical Taguchi experimental design. *Appl. Sci.* **2023**, *13*, 774. [CrossRef]
16. Sansenya, T.; Masri, N.; Chankhanittha, T.; Senasu, T.; Piriyanon, J.; Mukdasai, S.; Nanan, S. Hydrothermal synthesis of ZnO photocatalyst for detoxification of anionic azo dyes and antibiotic. *J. Phys. Chem. Solids* **2022**, *160*, 110353. [CrossRef]
17. Crini, G.; Lichtfouse, E. Advantages and disadvantages of techniques used for wastewater treatment. *Environ. Chem. Lett.* **2019**, *17*, 145–155. [CrossRef]
18. Vaez, Z.; Javanbakht, V. Synthesis, characterization and photocatalytic activity of ZSM-5/ZnO nanocomposite modified by Ag nanoparticles for methyl orange degradation. *J. Photochem. Photobiol. A* **2020**, *388*, 112064. [CrossRef]
19. Khataee, A.R.; Pons, M.N.; Zahraa, O. Photocatalytic degradation of three azo dyes using immobilized TiO_2 nanoparticles on glass plates activated by UV light irradiation: Influence of dye molecular structure. *J. Hazard. Mater.* **2009**, *168*, 451–457. [CrossRef]
20. John Peter, I.; Praveen, E.; Vignesh, G.; Nithiananthi, P. ZnO nanostructures with different morphology for enhanced photocatalytic activity. *Mater. Res. Express* **2017**, *4*, 124003. [CrossRef]
21. Ameen, S.; Akhtar, M.S.; Seo, H.K.; Shin, H.S. Mineralization of rhodamine 6G dye over rose flower-like ZnO nanomaterials. *Mater. Lett.* **2013**, *113*, 20–24. [CrossRef]
22. Zhang, D.E.; Ren, L.Z.; Hao, X.Y.; Pan, B.B.; Wang, M.Y.; Ma, J.J.; Li, F.; Li, S.A.; Tong, Z.W. Synthesis and photocatalytic property of multilayered Co_3O_4. *Appl. Surf. Sci.* **2015**, *355*, 547–552. [CrossRef]
23. Ani, I.J.; Akpan, U.G.; Olutoye, M.A.; Hameed, B.H. Photocatalytic degradation of pollutants in petroleum refinery wastewater by TiO_2- and ZnO-based photocatalysts: Recent development. *J. Clean. Prod.* **2018**, *205*, 930–954. [CrossRef]
24. Sinar Mashuri, S.I.; Ibrahim, M.L.; Kasim, M.F.; Mastuli, M.S.; Rashid, U.; Abdullah, A.H.; Islam, A.; Asikin Mijan, N.; Tan, Y.H.; Mansir, N.; et al. Photocatalysis for organic wastewater treatment: From the basis to current challenges for society. *Catalysts* **2020**, *10*, 1260. [CrossRef]
25. Kuruthukulangara, N.; Asharani, I.V. Photocatalytic degradation of Rhodamine B, a carcinogenic pollutant, by MgO nanoparticles. *Inorg. Chem. Commun.* **2024**, *160*, 111873. [CrossRef]
26. Abdel-Aziz, M.M.; Emam, T.M.; Elsherbiny, E.A. Bioactivity of magnesium oxide nanoparticles synthesized from cell filtrate of endobacterium *Burkholderia rinojensis* against *Fusarium oxysporum*. *Mater. Sci. Eng. C Mater. Biol. Appl.* **2020**, *109*, 110617. [CrossRef]
27. Aničić, N.; Vukomanović, M.; Koklič, T.; Suvorov, D. Fewer defects in the surface slows the hydrolysis rate, decreases the ROS generation potential, and improves the non-ROS antimicrobial activity of MgO. *Small* **2018**, *14*, 1800205. [CrossRef]
28. Anand, K.V.; Anugraga, A.R.; Kannan, M.; Singaravelu, G.; Govindaraju, K. Bio-engineered magnesium oxide nanoparticles as nano-priming agent for enhancing seed germination and seedling vigour of green gram (*Vigna radiata* L.). *Mater. Lett.* **2020**, *271*, 127792. [CrossRef]
29. Verma, S.K.; Nisha, K.; Panda, P.K.; Patel, P.; Kumari, P.; Mallick, M.A.; Sarkar, B.; Das, B. Green synthesized MgO nanoparticles infer biocompatibility by reducing in vivo molecular nanotoxicity in embryonic zebrafish through arginine interaction elicited apoptosis. *Sci. Total Environ.* **2020**, *713*, 136521. [CrossRef]
30. Baraket, L.; Ghorbel, A. Control preparation of aluminium chromium mixed oxides by sol-gel process. In *Studies in Surface Science and Catalysis*; Delmon, B., Jacobs, P.A., Maggi, R., Martens, J.A., Grange, P., Poncelet, G., Eds.; Preparation of Catalysts VII; Elsevier: Amsterdam, The Netherlands, 1998; Volume 118, pp. 657–667. [CrossRef]
31. Heo, Y.J.; Park, S.J. Facile synthesis of MgO-modified carbon adsorbents with microwave-assisted methods: Effect of MgO particles and porosities on CO_2 capture. *Sci. Rep.* **2017**, *7*, 5653. [CrossRef]
32. Feng, S.H.; Li, G.H. Chapter 4—Hydrothermal and Solvothermal Syntheses. In *Modern Inorganic Synthetic Chemistry*, 2nd ed.; Xu, R., Xu, Y., Eds.; Elsevier: Amsterdam, The Netherlands, 2017; pp. 73–104. [CrossRef]

33. Yeh, C.L. Combustion Synthesis: Principles and Applications. In *Reference Module in Materials Science and Materials Engineering*; Elsevier: Amsterdam, The Netherlands, 2016. [CrossRef]
34. Rane, A.V.; Kanny, K.; Abitha, V.K.; Thomas, S. Methods for Synthesis of Nanoparticles and Fabrication of Nanocomposites. In *Synthesis of Inorganic Nanomaterials*; Mohan Bhagyaraj, S., Oluwafemi, O.S., Kalarikkal, N., Thomas, S., Eds.; Micro and Nano Technologies; Woodhead Publishing: Cambridge, UK, 2018; pp. 121–139. [CrossRef]
35. Pal, G.; Rai, P.; Pandey, A. Green synthesis of nanoparticles: A greener approach for a cleaner future. In *Green Synthesis, Characterization and Applications of Nanoparticles*; Shukla, A.K., Iravani, S., Eds.; Micro and Nano Technologies; Elsevier: Amsterdam, The Netherlands, 2019; pp. 1–26. [CrossRef]
36. Lai, Y.F.; Chaudouët, P.; Charlot, F.; Matko, I.; Dubourdieu, C. Magnesium oxide nanowires synthesized by pulsed liquid-injection metal organic chemical vapor deposition. *Appl. Phys. Lett.* **2009**, *94*, 022904. [CrossRef]
37. Sirota, V.; Selemenev, V.; Kovaleva, M.; Pavlenko, I.; Mamunin, K.; Dokalov, V.; Prozorova, M. Synthesis of magnesium oxide nanopowder by thermal plasma using magnesium nitrate hexahydrate. *Phys. Res. Int.* **2016**, *4*, 6853405. [CrossRef]
38. Gandhi, S.; Abiramipriya, P.; Pooja, N.; Jeyakumari, J.J.L.; Arasi, A.Y.; Dhanalakshmi, V.; Gopinathan, M.R.; Anbarasan, R. Synthesis and characterizations of nano-sized MgO and its nano composite with poly(vinyl alcohol). *J. Non-Cryst. Solids* **2011**, *357*, 181–185. [CrossRef]
39. Bartley, J.K.; Xu, C.; Lloyd, R.; Enache, D.I.; Knight, D.W.; Hutchings, G.J. Simple method to synthesize high surface area magnesium oxide and its use as a heterogeneous base catalyst. *Appl. Catal. B* **2012**, *128*, 31–38. [CrossRef]
40. Zhang, H.; Hu, J.; Xie, J.; Wang, S.; Cao, Y. A solid-state chemical method for synthesizing MgO nanoparticles with superior adsorption properties. *RSC Adv.* **2019**, *9*, 2011–2017. [CrossRef]
41. Gatou, M.-A.; Skylla, E.; Dourou, P.; Pippa, N.; Gazouli, M.; Lagopati, N.; Pavlatou, E.A. Magnesium oxide (MgO) nanoparticles: Synthetic strategies and biomedical applications. *Crystals* **2024**, *14*, 215. [CrossRef]
42. Jeevanandam, J.; Chan, Y.S.; Danquah, M.K. Calcination-dependent morphology transformation of sol-gel-synthesized MgO nanoparticles. *ChemistrySelect* **2017**, *2*, 10393–10404. [CrossRef]
43. Mirzaei, H.; Davoodnia, A. Microwave assisted sol-gel synthesis of MgO nanoparticles and their catalytic activity in the synthesis of hantzsch 1,4-dihydropyridines. *Chin. J. Catal.* **2012**, *33*, 1502–1507. [CrossRef]
44. Wong, C.W.; Chan, Y.S.; Jeevanandam, J.; Pal, K.; Bechelany, M.; Abd Elkodous, M.; El-Sayyad, G.S. Response surface methodology optimization of mono-dispersed MgO nanoparticles fabricated by ultrasonic-assisted sol-gel method for outstanding antimicrobial and antibiofilm activities. *J. Clust. Sci.* **2020**, *31*, 367–389. [CrossRef]
45. Mashayekh-Salehi, A.; Moussavi, G.; Yaghmaeian, K. Preparation, characterization and catalytic activity of a novel mesoporous nanocrystalline MgO nanoparticle for ozonation of acetaminophen as an emerging water contaminant. *Chem. Eng. J.* **2017**, *310*, 157–169. [CrossRef]
46. Gajengi, A.L.; Sasaki, T.; Bhanage, B.M. Mechanistic aspects of formation of MgO nanoparticles under microwave irradiation and its catalytic application. *Adv. Powder Technol.* **2017**, *28*, 1185–1192. [CrossRef]
47. Najafi, A. A novel synthesis method of hierarchical mesoporous MgO nanoflakes employing carbon nanoparticles as the hard templates for photocatalytic degradation. *Ceram. Int.* **2017**, *43*, 5813–5818. [CrossRef]
48. John Sushma, N.; Prathyusha, D.; Swathi, G.; Madhavi, T.; Deva Prasad Raju, B.; Mallikarjuna, K.; Kim, H.S. Facile approach to synthesize magnesium oxide nanoparticles by using *Clitoria ternatea*-characterization and in vitro antioxidant studies. *Appl. Nanosci.* **2016**, *6*, 437–444. [CrossRef]
49. Aljabali, A.A.A.; Obeid, M.A.; Bakshi, H.A.; Alshaer, W.; Ennab, R.M.; Al-Trad, B.; Al Khateeb, W.; Al-Batayneh, K.M.; Al-Kadash, A.; Alsotari, S.; et al. Synthesis, characterization, and assessment of anti-cancer potential of ZnO nanoparticles in an in vitro model of breast cancer. *Molecules* **2022**, *27*, 1827. [CrossRef] [PubMed]
50. Almontasser, A.; Parveen, A.; Azam, A. Synthesis, Characterization and antibacterial activity of magnesium oxide (MgO) nanoparticles. *IOP Conf. Ser. Mater. Sci. Eng.* **2019**, *577*, 012051. [CrossRef]
51. Limón-Rocha, I.; Guzmán-González, C.A.; Anaya-Esparza, L.M.; Romero-Toledo, R.; Rico, J.L.; González-Vargas, O.A.; Pérez-Larios, A. Effect of the precursor on the synthesis of ZnO and its photocatalytic activity. *Inorganics* **2022**, *10*, 16. [CrossRef]
52. Levin, A.A.; Narykova, M.V.; Lihachev, A.I.; Kardashev, B.K.; Kadomtsev, A.G.; Brunkov, P.N.; Panfilov, A.G.; Prasolov, N.D.; Sultanov, M.M.; Kuryanov, V.N.; et al. Modification of the structural, microstructural, and elastoplastic properties of aluminum wires after operation. *Metals* **2021**, *11*, 1955. [CrossRef]
53. Gatou, M.-A.; Fiorentis, E.; Lagopati, N.; Pavlatou, E.A. Photodegradation of rhodamine B and phenol using TiO_2/SiO_2 composite nanoparticles: A comparative study. *Water* **2023**, *15*, 2773. [CrossRef]
54. Rani, N.; Chahal, S.; Chauhan, A.S.; Kumar, R.; Shukla, R.; Singh, S.K. X-ray analysis of MgO nanoparticles by modified Scherer's Williamson-Hall and size-strain method. *Mater. Today Proc.* **2019**, *12*, 543–548. [CrossRef]
55. Rosauer, E.A.; Handy, R.L. Crystallite-size determination of MgO by X-ray diffraction line broadening. *Proc. Iowa Acad. Sci.* **1961**, *68*, 357–371. Available online: https://scholarworks.uni.edu/pias/vol68/iss1/53 (accessed on 10 August 2024).
56. Savita, S.; Jain, M.; Manju, V.; Vij, A.; Thakur, A. Impact of annealing on the structural properties of MgO nanoparticles by XRD analysis and Rietveld refinement. *AIP Conf. Proc.* **2019**, *2093*, 020024. [CrossRef]
57. Boiocchi, M.; Caucia, F.; Merli, M.; Prella, D.; Ungaretti, L. Crystal-chemical reasons for the immiscibility of periclase and wüstite under lithospheric P, T conditions. *Eur. J. Mineral.* **2001**, *13*, 871–881. [CrossRef]

58. Zak, A.K.; Majid, W.A.; Abrishami, M.E.; Yousefi, R. X-ray analysis of ZnO nanoparticles by Williamson-Hall and size-strain plot methods. *Solid State Sci.* **2011**, *13*, 251–256. [CrossRef]
59. Tripathi, A.K.; Singh, M.K.; Mathpal, M.C.; Mishra, S.K.; Agarwal, A. Study of structural transformation in TiO_2 nanoparticles and its optical properties. *J. Alloys Compd.* **2013**, *549*, 114–120. [CrossRef]
60. Prabhu, R.R.; Abdul Khadar, M. Study of optical phonon modes of CdS nanoparticles using Raman spectroscopy. *Bull. Mater. Sci.* **2008**, *31*, 511–515. [CrossRef]
61. Kurian, M.; Kunjachan, C. Investigation of size dependency on lattice strain of nanoceria particles synthesised by wet chemical methods. *Int. Nano Lett.* **2014**, *4*, 73–80. [CrossRef]
62. Khaleel, W.A.; Sadeq, S.A.; Alani, I.A.M.; Ahmed, M.H.M. Magnesium oxide (MgO) thin film as saturable absorber for passively mode locked erbium-doped fiber laser. *Opt. Laser Technol.* **2019**, *115*, 331–336. [CrossRef]
63. Sutradhar, N.; Sinhamahapatra, A.; Pahari, S.K.; Pal, P.; Bajaj, H.C.; Mukhopadhyay, I.; Panda, A.B. Controlled synthesis of different morphologies of MgO and their use as solid base catalysts. *J. Phys. Chem. C* **2011**, *115*, 12308–12316. [CrossRef]
64. Kaningini, G.A.; Azizi, S.; Nyoni, H.; Mudau, F.N.; Mohale, K.C.; Maaza, M. Green synthesis and characterization of zinc oxide nanoparticles using bush tea (*Athrixia phylicoides* DC) natural extract: Assessment of the synthesis process. *F1000Research* **2021**, *10*, 1077. [CrossRef]
65. Al-Arjan, W.S. Zinc oxide nanoparticles and their application in adsorption of toxic dye from aqueous solution. *Polymers* **2022**, *14*, 3086. [CrossRef]
66. Thommes, M.; Kaneko, K.; Neimark, A.; Olivier, J.; Rodriguez-Reinoso, F.; Rouquerol, J.; Sing, K. Physisorption of gases, with special reference to the evaluation of surface area and pore size distribution (IUPAC Technical Report). *Pure Appl. Chem.* **2015**, *87*, 1051–1069. [CrossRef]
67. Turcu, E.; Coromelci, C.G.; Harabagiu, V.; Ignat, M. Enhancing the photocatalytic activity of TiO_2 for the degradation of Congo red dye by adjusting the ultrasonication regime applied in its synthesis procedure. *Catalysts* **2023**, *13*, 345. [CrossRef]
68. Khairallah, F.; Glisenti, A. XPS study of MgO nanopowders obtained by different preparation procedures. *Surf. Sci. Spectra* **2006**, *13*, 58–71. [CrossRef]
69. Ardizzone, S.; Bianchi, C.L.; Fadoni, M.; Vercelli, B. Magnesium salts and oxide: An XPS overview. *Appl. Surf. Sci.* **1997**, *119*, 253–259. [CrossRef]
70. Proniewicz, E.; Vijayan, A.M.; Surma, O.; Szkudlarek, A.; Molenda, M. Plant-assisted green synthesis of MgO nanoparticles as a sustainable material for bone regeneration: Spectroscopic properties. *Int. J. Mol. Sci.* **2024**, *25*, 4242. [CrossRef] [PubMed]
71. Srivastava, V.; Sharma, Y.C.; Sillanpää, M. Green synthesis of magnesium oxide nanoflower and its application for the removal of divalent metallic species from synthetic wastewater. *Ceram. Int.* **2015**, *41*, 6702–6709. [CrossRef]
72. Mourdikoudis, S.; Pallares, R.M.; Thanh, N.T. Characterization techniques for nanoparticles: Comparison and complementarity upon studying nanoparticle properties. *Nanoscale* **2018**, *10*, 12871–12934. [CrossRef]
73. Bélteky, P.; Rónavári, A.; Zakupszky, D.; Boka, E.; Igaz, N.; Szerencsés, B.; Pfeiffer, I.; Vágvölgyi, C.; Kiricsi, M.; Kónya, Z. Are smaller nanoparticles always better? Understanding the biological effect of size-dependent silver nanoparticle aggregation under biorelevant conditions. *Int. J. Nanomed.* **2021**, *16*, 3021–3040. [CrossRef]
74. Ramezani Farani, M.; Farsadrooh, M.; Zare, I.; Gholami, A.; Akhavan, O. Green synthesis of magnesium oxide nanoparticles and nanocomposites for photocatalytic antimicrobial, antibiofilm and antifungal applications. *Catalysts* **2023**, *13*, 642. [CrossRef]
75. Danaei, M.; Dehghankhold, M.; Ataei, S.; Hasanzadeh Davarani, F.; Javanmard, R.; Dokhani, A.; Khorasani, S.; Mozafari, M.R. Impact of particle size and polydispersity index on the clinical applications of lipidic nanocarrier systems. *Pharmaceutics* **2018**, *10*, 57. [CrossRef]
76. Yuan, T.; Gao, L.; Zhan, W.; Dini, D. Effect of particle size and surface charge on nanoparticles diffusion in the brain white matter. *Pharm. Res.* **2022**, *39*, 767–781. [CrossRef] [PubMed]
77. Sharma, S.K.; Gupta, S.M. Preparation and evaluation of stable nanofluids for heat transfer application: A review. *Exp. Therm Fluid Sci.* **2016**, *79*, 202–212. [CrossRef]
78. Gatou, M.-A.; Kontoliou, K.; Volla, E.; Karachalios, K.; Raptopoulos, G.; Paraskevopoulou, P.; Lagopati, N.; Pavlatou, E.A. Optimization of ZnO nanoparticles' synthesis via precipitation method applying Taguchi robust design. *Catalysts* **2023**, *13*, 1367. [CrossRef]
79. Kumar, A.; Kumar, J. On the synthesis and optical absorption studies of nano-size magnesium oxide powder. *J. Phys. Chem. Solids* **2008**, *69*, 2764–2772. [CrossRef]
80. Kurth, M.; Graat, P.C.J.; Mittemeijer, E.J. The oxidation kinetics of magnesium at low temperatures and low oxygen partial pressures. *Thin Solid Films* **2006**, *500*, 61–69. [CrossRef]
81. Sun, M.; Fang, Y.; Sun, S.; Wang, Y. Surface co-modification of TiO_2 with N doping and Ag loading for enhanced visible-light photoactivity. *RSC Adv.* **2016**, *6*, 12272–12279. [CrossRef]
82. Nagappa, B.; Chandrappa, G.T. Mesoporous nanocrystalline magnesium oxide for environmental remediation. *Microporous Mesoporous Mater.* **2007**, *106*, 212–218. [CrossRef]
83. Lagopati, N.; Kitsiou, P.; Kontos, A.; Venieratos, P.; Kotsopoulou, E.; Kontos, A.; Dionysiou, D.; Pispas, S.; Tsilibary, E.; Falaras, P. Photo-induced treatment of breast epithelial cancer cells using nanostructured titanium dioxide solution. *J. Photochem. Photobiol. A Chem.* **2010**, *214*, 215–223. [CrossRef]

84. Fu, H.; Pan, C.; Yao, W.; Zhu, Y. Visible-light-induced degradation of rhodamine B by nanosized Bi_2WO_6. *J. Phys. Chem. B* **2005**, *109*, 22432–22439. [CrossRef]
85. Uribe-López, M.C.; Hidalgo-López, M.C.; López-González, R.; Frías-Márquez, D.M.; Núñez-Nogueira, G.; Hernández-Castillo, D.; Alvarez-Lemus, M.A. Photocatalytic activity of ZnO nanoparticles and the role of the synthesis method on their physical and chemical properties. *J. Photochem. Photobiol. A* **2021**, *404*, 112866. [CrossRef]
86. Dodoo-Arhin, D.; Asiedu, T.; Agyei-Tuffour, B.; Nyankson, E.; Obada, D.; Mwabora, J.M. Photocatalytic degradation of Rhodamine dyes using zinc oxide nanoparticles. *Mater. Today Proc.* **2021**, *38*, 809–815. [CrossRef]
87. Hu, C.; Lu, T.; Chen, F.; Zhang, R.; Lian, C.; Zheng, S.; Hu, Q.; Duo, S. Enhancement of photocatalytic performance of TiO_2 produced by an alcohothermal approach through inclusion of water. *Mater. Res. Bull.* **2014**, *53*, 42–48. [CrossRef]
88. Bhatkhande, D.S.; Pangarkar, V.G.; Beenackers, A.A.C.M. Photocatalytic degradation for environmental applications-a review. *J. Chem. Technol. Biotechnol.* **2002**, *77*, 102–116. [CrossRef]
89. Kader, D.A.; Mohammed, S.J. Emerging developments in dye-sensitized metal oxide photocatalysis: Exploring the design, mechanisms, and organic synthesis applications. *RSC Adv.* **2023**, *13*, 26484–26508. [CrossRef] [PubMed]
90. Trenczek-Zajac, A.; Synowiec, M.; Zakrzewska, K.; Zazakowny, K.; Kowalski, K.; Dziedzic, A.; Radecka, M. Scavenger-supported photocatalytic evidence of an extended type I electronic structure of the $TiO_2@Fe_2O_3$ interface. *ACS Appl. Mater. Interfaces* **2022**, *14*, 38255–38269. [CrossRef] [PubMed]
91. Algethami, F.K.; Katouah, H.A.; Al-Omar, M.A.; Almehizia, A.A.; Amr, A.E.G.E.; Naglah, A.M.; Al-Shakliah, N.S.; Fetoh, M.E.; Youssef, H.M. Facile synthesis of magnesium oxide nanoparticles for studying their photocatalytic activities against orange G dye and biological activities against some bacterial and fungal strains. *J. Inorg. Organomet. Polym. Mater.* **2021**, *31*, 2150–2160. [CrossRef]
92. Farhadian, N.; Akbarzadeh, R.; Pirsaheb, M.; Jen, T.C.; Fakhri, Y.; Asadi, A. Chitosan modified N, S-doped TiO_2 and N, S-doped ZnO for visible light photocatalytic degradation of tetracycline. *Int. J. Biol. Macromol.* **2019**, *132*, 360–373. [CrossRef]
93. Iskandar, F.; Nandiyanto, A.; Yun, K.; Hogan, C., Jr.; Okuyama, K.; Biswas, P. Enhanced photocatalytic performance of brookite TiO_2 macroporous particles prepared by spray drying with colloidal templating. *Adv. Mater.* **2007**, *19*, 1408–1412. [CrossRef]
94. Mohod, A.V.; Momotko, M.; Shah, N.S.; Marchel, M.; Imran, M.; Kong, L.; Boczkaj, G. Degradation of Rhodamine dyes by Advanced Oxidation Processes (AOPs)-Focus on caviatation and photocatalysis—A critical review. *Water Resour. Ind.* **2023**, *30*, 100220. [CrossRef]
95. Chen, F.; Zhao, J.; Hidaka, H. Highly selective deethylation of rhodamine B: Adsorption and photooxidation pathways of the dye on the TiO_2/SiO_2 composite photocatalyst. *Int. J. Photoenergy* **2003**, *5*, 674957. [CrossRef]
96. Taniguchi, M.; Lindsey, J.S. Database of absorption and fluorescence spectra of> 300 common compounds for use in photochem CAD. *J. Photochem. Photobiol.* **2018**, *94*, 290–327. [CrossRef] [PubMed]
97. Sudrajat, H.; Babel, S. Comparison and mechanism of photocatalytic activities of N-ZnO and N-ZrO_2 for the degradation of rhodamine 6G. *Environ. Sci. Pollut. Res.* **2016**, *23*, 10177–10188. [CrossRef] [PubMed]
98. Gatou, M.-A.; Lagopati, N.; Vagena, I.-A.; Gazouli, M.; Pavlatou, E.A. ZnO nanoparticles from different precursors and their photocatalytic potential for biomedical use. *Nanomaterials* **2023**, *13*, 122. [CrossRef] [PubMed]
99. Ruíz-Santoyo, V.; Marañon-Ruiz, V.F.; Romero-Toledo, R.; González Vargas, O.A.; Pérez-Larios, A. Photocatalytic degradation of Rhodamine B and methylene orange using TiO_2-ZrO_2 as nanocomposite. *Catalysts* **2021**, *11*, 1035. [CrossRef]
100. Tsoukleris, D.S.; Gatou, M.-A.; Lagopati, N.; Sygellou, L.; Christodouleas, D.C.; Falaras, P.; Pavlatou, E.A. Chemically modified TiO_2 photocatalysts as an alternative disinfection approach for municipal wastewater treatment plant effluents. *Water* **2023**, *15*, 2052. [CrossRef]
101. Yudasari, N.; Anugrahwidya, R.; Tahir, D.; Suliyanti, M.M.; Herbani, Y.; Imawan, C.; Khalil, M.; Djuhana, D. Enhanced photocatalytic degradation of rhodamine 6G (R6G) using ZnO–Ag nanoparticles synthesized by pulsed laser ablation in liquid (PLAL). *J. Alloys Compd.* **2021**, *886*, 161291. [CrossRef]
102. Phindile Khoza, P.; Nyokong, T. Visible light transformation of Rhodamine 6G using tetracarbazole zinc phthalocyanine when embedded in electrospun fibers and in the presence of ZnO and Ag particles. *J. Coord. Chem.* **2015**, *68*, 1117–1131. [CrossRef]
103. Karthikeyan, V.; Dhanapandian, S.; Manoharan, C. Characterization and antibacterial behavior of MgO-PEG nanoparticles synthesized via co-precipitation method. *Int. Lett. Chem. Phys. Astron.* **2016**, *70*, 33–41. [CrossRef]
104. Mehta, M.; Mukhopadhyay, M.; Christian, R.; Mistry, N. Synthesis and characterization of MgO nanocrystals using strong and weak bases. *Powder Technol.* **2012**, *226*, 213–221. [CrossRef]
105. Sugiarto, I.T.; Putri, K.Y. Analysis of dual peak emission from Rhodamine 6G organic dyes using photoluminescence. *J. Phys. Conf. Ser.* **2017**, *817*, 012047. [CrossRef]

Disclaimer/Publisher's Note: The statements, opinions and data contained in all publications are solely those of the individual author(s) and contributor(s) and not of MDPI and/or the editor(s). MDPI and/or the editor(s) disclaim responsibility for any injury to people or property resulting from any ideas, methods, instructions or products referred to in the content.

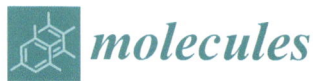

Article

Visible Light Photoactivity of g-C$_3$N$_4$/MoS$_2$ Nanocomposites for Water Remediation of Hexavalent Chromium

Chunmei Tian [1], Huijuan Yu [1], Ruiqi Zhai [1], Jing Zhang [1], Cuiping Gao [1], Kezhen Qi [2], Yingjie Zhang [1,3,*], Qiang Ma [4,*] and Mengxue Guo [5]

[1] College of Agriculture and Biological Science, Dali University, Dali 671000, China; tiancm1985@hotmail.com (C.T.); hjyu_yhj@163.com (H.Y.); zhairuiqi2023@163.com (R.Z.); zj2452488891@163.com (J.Z.); gaocp_dlu@163.com (C.G.)
[2] College of Pharmacy, Dali University, Dali 671000, China; qkzh2003@aliyun.com
[3] Key Laboratory of Ecological Microbial Remediation Technology of Yunnan Higher Education Institutes, Dali University, Dali 671000, China
[4] School of Architecture and Civil Engineering, Chengdu University, Chengdu 610106, China
[5] Resources and Environment Institute, Yunnan Land and Resources Vocational College, Kunming 652501, China; mxx921@163.com
* Correspondence: yjzhang_dlu@163.com (Y.Z.); maqiang@cdu.edu.cn (Q.M.)

Abstract: Water pollution has becoming an increasingly serious issue, and it has attracted a significant amount of attention from scholars. Here, in order remove heavy metal hexavalent chromium (Cr (VI)) from wastewater, graphitic carbon nitride (g-C$_3$N$_4$) was modified with molybdenum disulfide (MoS$_2$) at different mass ratios via an ultrasonic method to synthesize g-C$_3$N$_4$/MoS$_2$ (CNM) nanocomposites as photocatalysts. The nanocomposites displayed efficient photocatalytic removal of toxic hexavalent chromium (Cr (VI)) from water under UV, solar, and visible light irradiation. The CNM composite with a 1:2 g-C$_3$N$_4$ to MoS$_2$ ratio achieved optimal 91% Cr (VI) removal efficiency at an initial 20 mg/L Cr (VI) concentration and pH 3 after 120 min visible light irradiation. The results showed a high pH range and good recycling stability. The g-C$_3$N$_4$/MoS$_2$ nanocomposites exhibited higher performance compared to pure g-C$_3$N$_4$ due to the narrowed band gap of the Z-scheme heterojunction structure and effective separation of photo-generated electron–hole pairs, as evidenced by structural and optical characterization. Overall, the ultrasonic synthesis of g-C$_3$N$_4$/MoS$_2$ photocatalysts shows promise as an efficient technique for enhancing heavy metal wastewater remediation under solar and visible light.

Keywords: g-C$_3$N$_4$/MoS$_2$ composites; Z-scheme heterojunction; hexavalent chromium Cr (VI); photocatalyst

Citation: Tian, C.; Yu, H.; Zhai, R.; Zhang, J.; Gao, C.; Qi, K.; Zhang, Y.; Ma, Q.; Guo, M. Visible Light Photoactivity of g-C$_3$N$_4$/MoS$_2$ Nanocomposites for Water Remediation of Hexavalent Chromium. *Molecules* **2024**, *29*, 637. https://doi.org/10.3390/molecules29030637

Academic Editor: Sugang Meng

Received: 31 December 2023
Revised: 21 January 2024
Accepted: 26 January 2024
Published: 30 January 2024

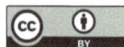

Copyright: © 2024 by the authors. Licensee MDPI, Basel, Switzerland. This article is an open access article distributed under the terms and conditions of the Creative Commons Attribution (CC BY) license (https://creativecommons.org/licenses/by/4.0/).

1. Introduction

Water scarcity and water pollution have long been major global concerns; in recent decades, the rapid development of the economy and industrialization led to increasingly serious environmental pollution problems. Water quality has decreased since a large amount of industrial wastewater, which contained heavy metals, was discharged into the water system [1,2]. Chromium is one of the common sources of heavy metal pollution and mainly exists in Cr (III) and Cr (VI) in water [3]. Cr (III) is one of the essential elements in the human body, which can participate in the metabolism of human fat and is widely used in the adjuvant therapy of diabetes [4]. Cr (VI) poses a lasting threat to the environment and human health and can enter the human body through skin-to-skin contact or breathing. In addition, Cr (VI) has strong oxidation and can oxidize human hemoglobin into methemoglobin, which may cause cancer risk after long-term or short-term exposure [5,6]. Therefore, it is highly important that we find a way to handle Cr (VI) in industrial wastewater economically and efficiently and make it meet the discharge standard.

At present, reducing Cr (VI) to Cr (III) in wastewater is an important way of alleviating chromium pollution in water [7,8], and common methods for treating chrome-containing heavy metal wastewater include the adsorption method [9,10], chemical reduction method [11,12], and biological method [13,14]. In the process of Cr (VI) removal, these methods consume a large amount of power and other resources, have high costs, and may cause other forms of pollution. However, existing treatment methods for the removal of pollutants in the process of treatment have complexity and high costs, and they are prone to secondary pollution and other shortcomings.

Photocatalytic technology is widely used [15–17], which has the advantages of no secondary contamination and strong redox capacity and is widely used in pollutant degradation [18,19], hydrogen generation [20,21] and CO_2 photoreduction [22]. It is one of the best ways to solve future pollution problems [23]. Bi-bridge S-scheme Bi_2S_3/BiOBr heterojunction (Bi_2S_3/Bi/BiOBr), produced by the one-pot solvothermal method, has shown high visible light photocatalytic reduction performance, and the removal efficiency of Cr (VI) was 97% [24]. Graphitic carbon nitride (g-C_3N_4)'s band gap is 2.7 eV; it is a common photocatalyst with high stability and environmental friendliness [25–27]. Currently, thermal polycondensation is commonly used in the preparatory work of g-C_3N_4, which makes the preparation of g-C_3N_4 simple [28–30]. However, due to the rapid recombination rate of photo-generated electrons and holes and the low light absorption range and surface range [31–33], the photocatalytic performance of g-C_3N_4 photocatalysts is low, which makes the use of g-C_3N_4 limited. Numerous researchers have found that the photocatalytic performance of g-C_3N_4 could be improved by conducting morphology regulation [34,35], ion doping [36–38], and heterojunction construction [39–41]. Li et al. [42] prepared ultra-thin tubular lateral heterostructures (LHSs) of graphitic carbon nitride and carbon dots (CN/C-Dots) by one-step thermal polymerization; they found that the CN/C-Dots LHSs exhibited excellent electrocatalysts for a hydrogen evolution reaction, due to which the charge carriers' transport was enhanced and the specific surface area was increased, meaning more active sites of CN. Renji Rajendran et al. [43] developed a g-C_3N_4/TiO_2/α-Fe_2O_3 ternary magnetic nanocomposite with a Z-scheme by facile calcination and a hydrothermal process. The g-C_3N_4/TiO_2/α-Fe_2O_3 ternary magnetic nanocomposite exhibited excellent photocatalytic performance for the degradation of Rhodamine B (RhB); under visible light exposure, the degradation rate was 95.7%, which was due to the formation of the Z-scheme enhancing the separation and migration of photoexcited electron and hole pairs and the light absorption range. Photocatalysts have been widely used for various purposes. However, photocatalysts still have the shortcomings of low utilization of visible light and high requirements for reaction conditions. MoS_2 has attracted attention as a transition metal dichalcogenide with good chemical stability and adjustable bandwidth [44].

In this work, g-C_3N_4/MoS_2 samples with different mass ratios were prepared by the ultrasonic method, and the photocatalytic removal efficiencies of Cr (VI) under different light irradiation sources (ultraviolet light, solar light and visible light) were investigated. g-C_3N_4/MoS_2 composites showed strong photocatalytic activity. When the pH value was 3, the initial concentration of Cr (VI) was 20 mg/L, and the photocatalyst demonstrated strong photocatalytic activity. Compared with pure g-C_3N_4, the doping of MoS_2 is beneficial for narrowing the band gap and reducing the recombination rate of photo-generated electrons and holes, and the photocatalytic performance of CNM (1:2) increased. The composite photocatalyst has a wide pH range and can still show a high removal rate after multiple reuses, overcoming the shortcomings of existing difficult-to-recover photocatalysts.

2. Results and Discussion

2.1. Characterization

2.1.1. XRD

The X-ray diffraction (XRD) pattern characterization of g-C_3N_4, MoS_2, and CNM (1:2) is shown in Figure 1. g-C_3N_4 had diffraction peaks at 13.1° and 27.6°, which corresponded to the (100) and (002) planes, respectively [45]. The characteristic diffraction peaks of

13.9°, 32.8° and 58.6° were attributed to the (002), (100), and (110) planes, respectively [46]. Compared with g-C$_3$N$_4$ and MoS$_2$, there is a shift in the peak position of the CNM (1:2) composites, which may be caused by the increased interlayer distance of the defect modified samples [47]. The diffraction peaks of the CNM (1:2) composites were 13.3°, 27.9°, 32.8° and 57.6°, respectively. These were attributed to (100), (002), (100), and (110). The CNM (1:2) composites showed diffraction peaks belonging to g-C$_3$N$_4$ and MoS$_2$, which indicated the MoS$_2$ had successfully combined with g-C$_3$N$_4$.

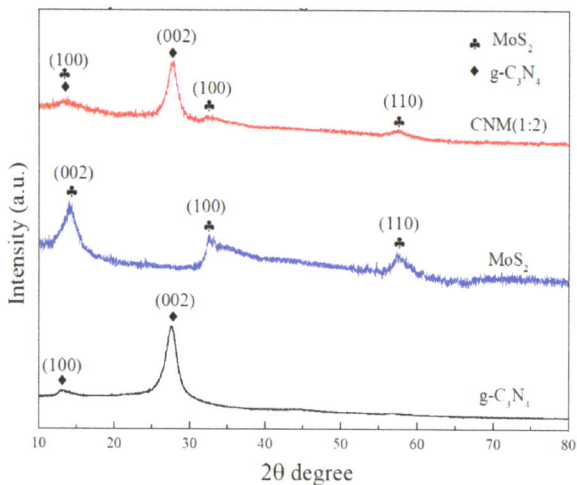

Figure 1. XRD patterns of g-C$_3$N$_4$, MoS$_2$, and CNM (1:2).

2.1.2. SEM

Scanning electron microscopy (SEM) images of g-C$_3$N$_4$ and g-C$_3$N$_4$/MoS$_2$ are shown in Figure 2. Figure 2a,b show SEM images of g-C$_3$N$_4$ and CNM (1:2), g-C$_3$N$_4$ had a massive structure, which was combined with a layered structure. CNM (1:2) had a porous structure, the reason for this result may be that during the ultrasonic treatment, the g-C$_3$N$_4$ was stripped and combined with MoS$_2$, and a large number of pore structures were formed in the process. Ultrasonic treatment can effectively promote g-C$_3$N$_4$ and MoS$_2$ recombination, effectively accelerate the separation of photo-generated carriers, and improve the photo-generated carrier migration rate, thus improving the photocatalytic activity of composite photocatalytic materials. The CNM (1:2) complex can accelerate the separation of photo-generated carriers and increase the migration rate of photo-generated carriers, thus improving the photocatalytic activity of the composite photocatalyst. Figure 2c–h reveal CNM (1:2) as well as corresponding elemental mapping of C, N, S, and Mo, and EDS of CNM (1:2). The mapping of SEM confirmed that the elements of C, N, S, and Mo exist in CNM (1:2), and it indicated that g-C$_3$N$_4$ and MoS$_2$ had been successfully combined. In the process of MoS$_2$ doping g-C$_3$N$_4$, a g-C$_3$N$_4$/MoS$_2$ photocatalyst with more voids was formed, which increased the area of the photocatalyst in contact with pollutants, and increased the number of active sites on its surface, thus increasing its photocatalytic activity.

2.1.3. XPS

The X-ray photoelectron spectroscopy (XPS) spectra of and CNM (1:2) and used CNM (1:2) are displayed in Figure 3, and the spectra of g-C$_3$N$_4$ were shown in previous articles [30]. The survey spectra of CNM (1:2) and used CNM (1:2) are shown in Figure 3a, the main elements are C, N, O, S and Mo, indicating g-C$_3$N$_4$ and MoS$_2$ were successfully combined. In Figure 3b, the C 1s spectrum of CNM (1:2) has three peaks at 288.2, 286.4, and 284.8 eV; the 288.2 eV is attributed to O-C-N, the 286.4 eV is attributed to C-O, and the 284.8 eV belongs to C-C [48]. In the C 1s spectrum of used CNM (1:2), the peaks shifted to 288.8, 286.4 and 284.8 eV, respectively [49]. The N 1s of CNM (1:2) has three peaks at 404.3, 400.3 and 398.5 eV, which are attributed to N-H bonds, N-(C)$_3$, and C = N-C [50]. Additionally, the N 1s peaks of the used CNM (1:2) were shifted to 404.5 eV (N-H), 401.3 eV (C-N-H), and 399.2 eV (N-(C)$_3$) [51], as shown in Figure 3c. The Mo 3d of CNM (1:2) had four peaks at 235.1, 231.5, 228.1 and 225.4 eV, with the peaks corresponding to Mo^{6+}, Mo 3d$_{3/2}$, Mo 3d$_{5/2}$ and S 2s, attributed to the 1T-phase MoS$_2$ [52,53]. In the Mo 3d spectrum of used CNM (1:2), the peaks shifted to 235.8, 232.3, 228.9, and 226.2 eV, respectively [45]. Figure 3e shows the S 2p spectra of CNM (1:2); it has three peaks at 168.2, 162.2, and 161 eV, which correspond to S_2^{2-}, S 2p$_{1/2}$, and S 2p$_{3/2}$ [53]. In the S 2p spectrum of used CNM (1:2), those peaks shifted to 169.1, 162.9, and 161.7 eV [45]. In Figure 3f, the presence of Cr was not detected on the surface of the reused photocatalysts, which ensures that the active sites on the surface of the photocatalyst were not covered. The XPS characterization results again confirm that both g-C$_3$N$_4$ and MoS$_2$ have been successfully compounded, and Cr was not detected in the reused CNM (1:2), thus ensuring the excellent reusable performance of the photocatalyst.

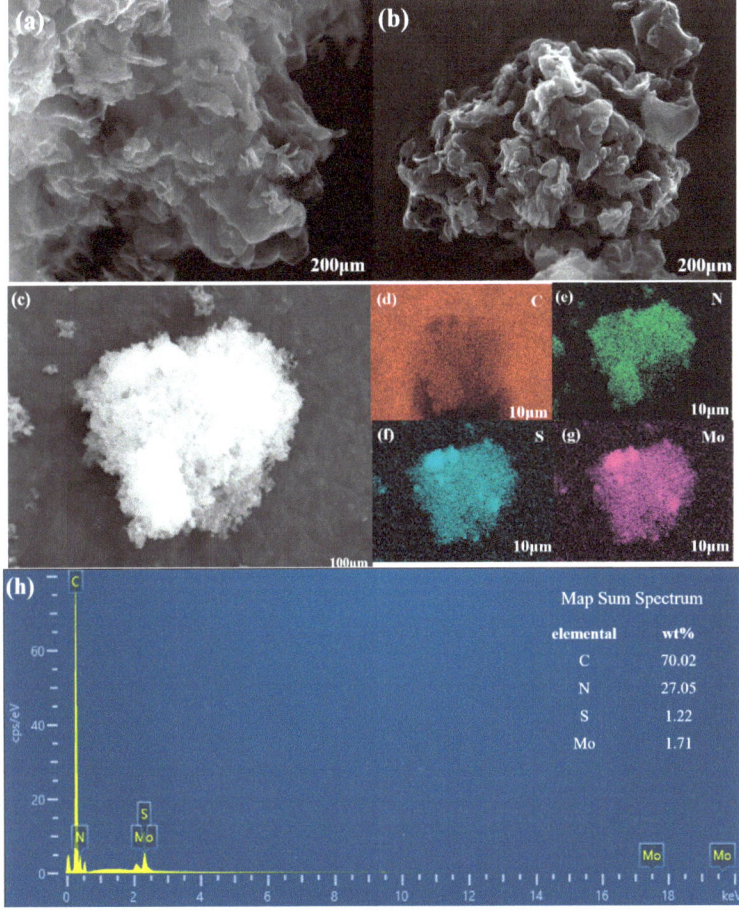

Figure 2. SEM images of samples: (**a**) g-C$_3$N$_4$, (**b**) CNM (1:2), (**c**) SEM image of CNM (1:2), and corresponding elemental mapping of (**d**) C, (**e**) N, (**f**) S, and (**g**) Mo. (**h**) EDS spectrum of CNM (1:2).

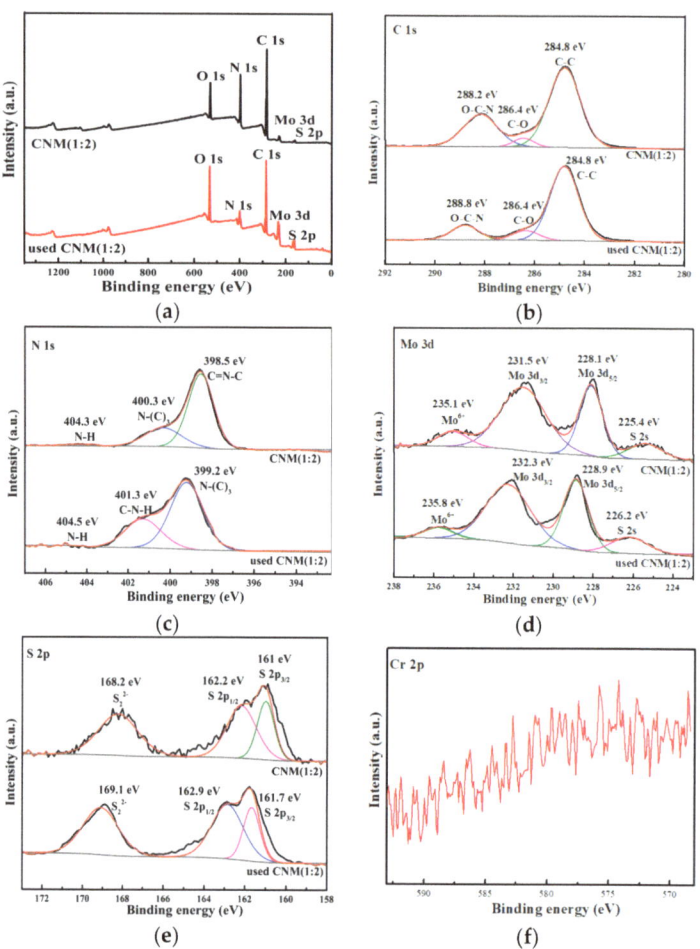

Figure 3. XPS spectra of CNM (1:2) and used CNM (1:2): (**a**) Survey spectra, (**b**) C 1s, (**c**) N 1s, (**d**) Mo 3d, (**e**) S 2p, (**f**) Cr 2p.

2.1.4. BET

The Brunauer–Emmett–Teller N_2 adsorption–desorption isotherms of g-C_3N_4, MoS_2 and CNM (1:2) are shown in Figure 4. The specific surface area and pore volumes of g-C_3N_4, MoS_2, and CNM (1:2) are listed in Table 1. The specific surface area of CNM (1:2) (30.7214 $m^2 \cdot g^{-1}$) is higher than that of g-C_3N_4 (27.3882 $m^2 \cdot g^{-1}$) and MoS_2 (10.5045 $m^2 \cdot g^{-1}$). In addition, we found that the pore volumes of g-C_3N_4 (0.2385 $cm^3 \cdot g^{-1}$) and MoS_2 (0.0332 $cm^3 \cdot g^{-1}$) are lower than that of CNM (1:2) (0.3498 $cm^3 \cdot g^{-1}$). The increase in specific surface area and pore volume is beneficial to providing more photocatalytic active sites and improving the activity of CNM (1:2).

Table 1. Specific surface area and pore volumes of g-C_3N_4, MoS_2, and CNM (1:2).

Samples	S_{BET} ($m^2 \cdot g^{-1}$)	V_{Pore} ($cm^3 \cdot g^{-1}$)
g-C_3N_4	27.3882	0.2385
MoS_2	10.5045	0.0332
CNM (1:2)	30.7214	0.3498

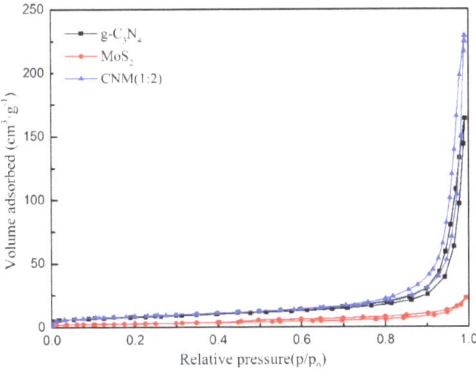

Figure 4. N$_2$ adsorption–desorption isotherms of g-C$_3$N$_4$, MoS$_2$ and CNM (1:2).

2.1.5. UV–Vis Diffuse Reflectance Spectra

UV–vis diffuse reflectance spectra images of g-C$_3$N$_4$ and CNM (1:2) are displayed in Figure 5a. g-C$_3$N$_4$ had an absorption edge at 450 nm, while the absorption edge of CNM (1:2) was redshifted, and the absorption range was 200–800 nm. This indicates that the doping of MoS$_2$ could effectively improve the utilization ratio of the photocatalyst in visible light, and the light absorption of the photocatalyst was enhanced, thus achieving the purpose of improving the photocatalytic activity of CNM (1:2). The plots of the transformed Kubelka–Munk function versus the photon energy of g-C$_3$N$_4$ and CNM (1:2) are shown in Figure 5b. The value of the band gap can be calculated according to the formula $(ah\nu)^{1/2} = A(h\nu - E_g)$, $h\nu = hc/\lambda$; the results show that the band gaps of g-C$_3$N$_4$ and CNM (1:2) are 2.72 and 2.31 eV, respectively. The doping of MoS$_2$ is beneficial to narrowing the band gap and reducing the recombination rate of photo-generated electrons and holes.

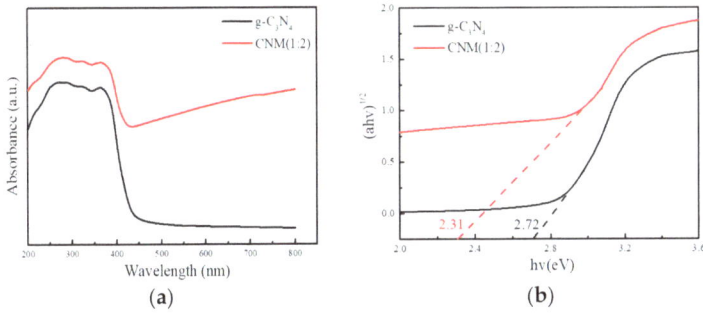

Figure 5. (**a**) UV–vis diffuse reflectance spectra. (**b**) Plots of the transformed Kubelka–Munk function versus the photon energy of g-C$_3$N$_4$ and CNM (1:2).

2.1.6. PL Spectra

The separation and transfer ability of photo-excited carriers in the g-C$_3$N$_4$, MoS$_2$ and CNM (1:2) are measured with PL spectra. As displayed in Figure 6, the g-C$_3$N$_4$ and CNM (1:2) exhibited broad peaks at 435 nm. g-C$_3$N$_4$ showed a stronger fluorescence emission peak intensity, which indicates the higher recombination efficiency of the electron–hole pairs. After adding MoS$_2$, the CNM (1:2) showed a low PL intensity, the carrier separation efficiency was enhanced, and the electron pairs' separation rate was reduced in the CNM (1:2) nanocomposite. Therefore, the results confirmed the photocatalytic performance of CNM (1:2) increased.

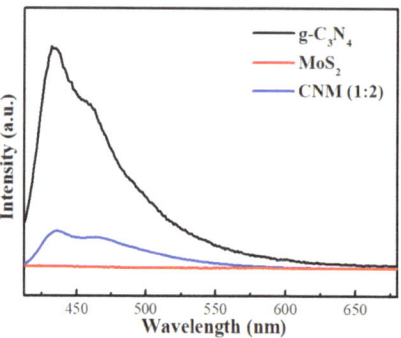

Figure 6. PL spectra of g-C$_3$N$_4$, MoS$_2$, and CNM (1:2).

2.1.7. Transient Photocurrent Responses

The separation and transfer of photo-excited carriers on g-C$_3$N$_4$ MoS$_2$ and CNM (1:2) were investigated. The transient photocurrent spectrum of the samples is shown in Figure 7. The CNM (1:2) showed the highest photocurrent density during the samples; it showed that the separation efficiency of the photogenerated electrons and holes is significantly improved after the doping MoS$_2$. This result confirms that CNM (1:2) can effectively reduce the recombination rate of electrons and holes, thereby increasing the photocatalytic activity of the photocatalysts.

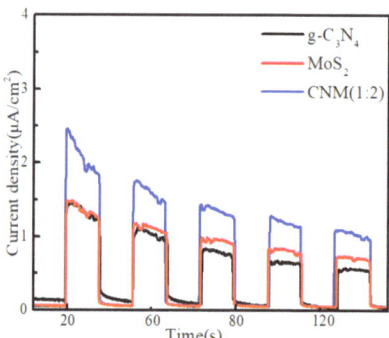

Figure 7. Transient photocurrent responses of g−C$_3$N$_4$ MoS$_2$ and CNM (1:2).

2.2. Photocatalysis

2.2.1. Photocatalytic Performance of Different Photocatalysts

The removal rates and the pseudo-first-order reaction kinetics of Cr (VI) by g-C$_3$N$_4$, MoS$_2$, CNM (1:1), CNM (1:2), CNM (1:4), CNM (2:1), and CNM (4:1) were shown in Figure 8a,b. In order to select the optimal ratio of g and m, we prepared photocatalysts with different mass ratios, as shown in Figure 8a, the results show that doping with different MoS$_2$ masses has a great influence on the photocatalytic activity of the photocatalysts. When the mass ratio of g-C$_3$N$_4$ to MoS$_2$ was 2:1 (CNM (1:2)), it had the best rate of removal of Cr (VI). At the same time, the pseudo-first-order reaction kinetics model shows that the reaction rates of g-C$_3$N$_4$, MoS$_2$, CNM (1:1), CNM (1:2), CNM (1:4), CNM (2:1) and CNM (4:1) are, respectively, 0.0006, 0.0010, 0.0028, 0.0102, 0.0052, 0.0022, and 0.0018 min^{-1}. It was found that when the content of MoS$_2$ was too high, the removal efficiency of Cr (VI) was decreased. Excessive MoS$_2$ made the charge transfer rate too fast, which increases the recombination probability of photo-generated electrons and holes; therefore, the photocatalytic activity decreased.

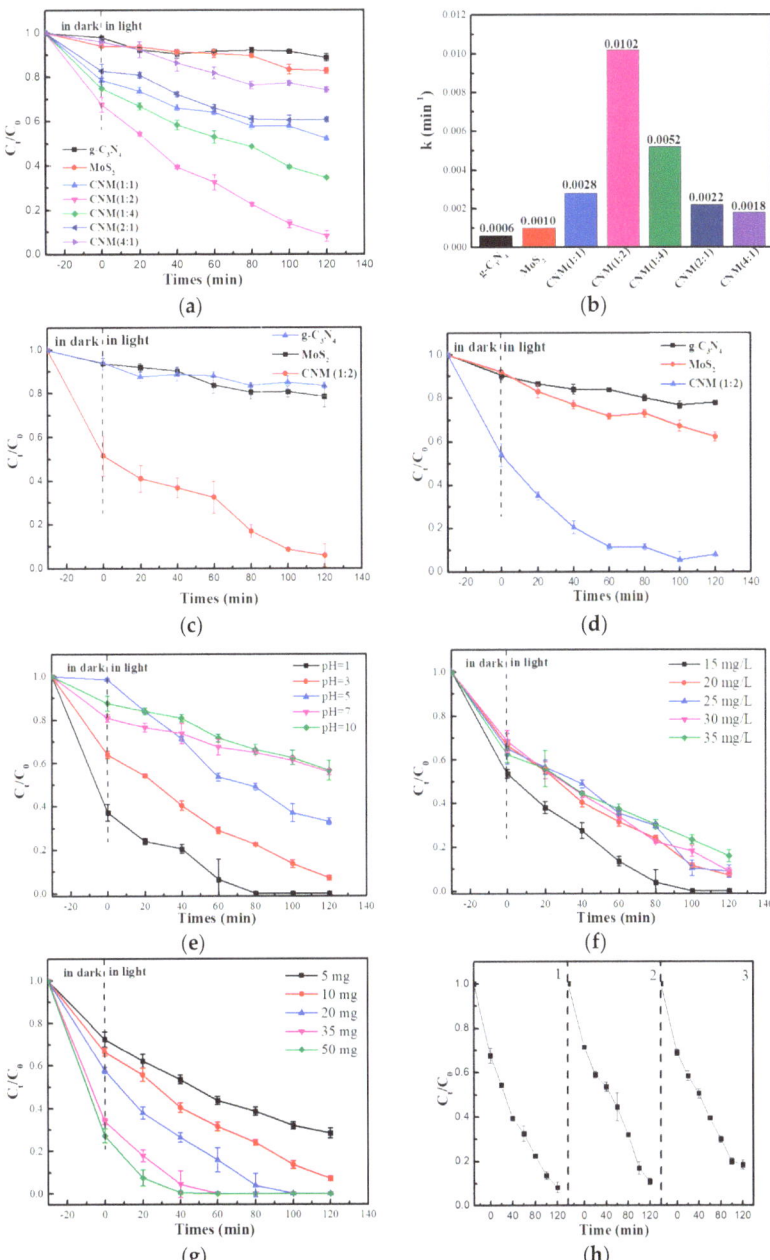

Figure 8. (**a**) The removal of Cr (VI) by different photocatalysts. (**b**) Pseudo−first−order reaction kinetics. (**c**) Photocatalytic removal of Cr (VI) under ultraviolet light. (**d**) Photocatalytic removal of Cr (VI) under solar light. (**e**) Effect of pH. (**f**) Effect of initial concentration. (**g**) Effect of photocatalytic dosage. (**h**) Recyclability of CNM (1:2).

In order to investigate the removal ability of photocatalysts, we explored the Cr (VI) removal rate of photocatalysts under different forms of light illumination (ultraviolet light, solar light, and visible light), and the results displayed in Figure 8c,d. The removal rate of Cr (VI) by CNM (1:2) was 91.6% under the illumination of ultraviolet light, and the removal rate of Cr (VI) was 91% and 86% under solar light and visible light, respectively. The results revealed that with the different forms of light irradiation, the photocatalytic removal performance of Cr (VI) had a weak effect. At the same time, we investigated the effects of pH value, initial concentration, and dosage on the removal rate (in Figure 8e–g), The experimental results show that with the increase in the pH value, the reducibility of the photocatalyst to Cr (VI) decreases gradually. When the solution is neutral or alkaline, the removal rate of Cr (VI) reduced to 40%, but the removal rate is as high as about 65% under weak acid conditions, which affirms that photocatalysts have a high application range. The stability of the photocatalysts was experimentally assessed three times under visible light (in Figure 8h), and the results showed that the CNM (1:2) photocatalysts still had strong photocatalytic activity after multiple cycles. This effectively solves the shortcomings of traditional photocatalysts that can only remove Cr (VI) under strong acid conditions and provides data support for the practical engineering application of photocatalysts in the future.

2.2.2. Scavenging Study

In order to investigate the main reactive radicals in the reactions, scavenger tests were performed and the results are displayed in Figure 9a. In this study, ethylenediaminetetraacetic acid disodium salt (EDTA−2Na), potassium persulfate ($K_2S_2O_8$), and ascorbic acid ($C_6H_8O_6$) were used as the scavenger for scavenge holes (h^+), electrons (e^-), and superoxide radicals ($\cdot O_2^-$), respectively. The test results showed that the removal of Cr (VI) by the CNM (1:2) photocatalyst was significantly decreased after the addition of $K_2S_2O_8$, which implied that the e^- played an important role in the removal of Cr (VI), and the results displayed that the addition of ascorbic acid and EDTA-2Na have a slight influence on the removal of Cr (VI), which shows that $\cdot O_2^-$ and h^+ do not play a key role in the reaction.

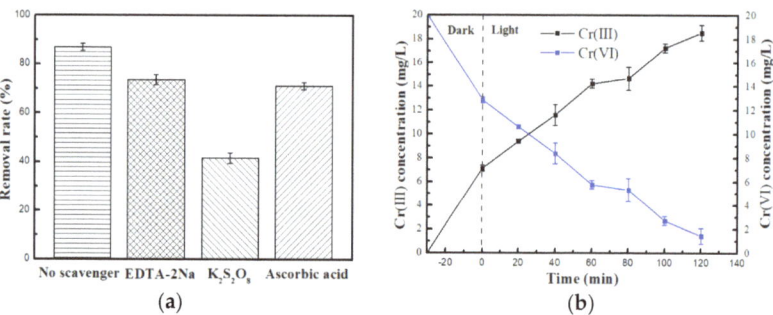

Figure 9. (**a**) The effect of reactive scavengers. (**b**) Variation in Cr valence at different reaction times.

To evaluate the reaction mechanism of CNM (1:2)'s photocatalytic reduction of Cr (VI), an inductively coupled plasma–mass spectrometer (ICP-MS) was used to analyze the concentration of chromium. Ultraviolet-visible spectrophotometry was performed to measure the concentration of Cr (VI), which can determine the valence state change of chromium during the reaction (Figure 9b). The results show that the content of total chromium did not change with the increase in reaction time, but the concentration of Cr (VI.) decreased with the increase in light time. The presence of chromium in aqueous solution mainly includes Cr (III) and Cr (VI), from which it can be inferred that with the increase in reaction time, Cr (VI) in water is reduced to Cr (III). The content of total chromium in the solution remains unchanged, which indicates that the Cr (VI) in the water is reduced to Cr (III) by photocatalysis during the reaction process. Chromium is mainly present in water in the form of minimally toxic Cr (III) instead of being adsorbed on the surface of the photocatalyst; this means it will not form a buildup on the surface of the material and affect the performance of the photocatalyst, which is beneficial for recycling of photocatalysts.

2.2.3. Mechanisms of Photocatalysis

A possible photocatalytic mechanism of CNM (1:2) removal Cr (VI) is shown in Figure 10. Additionally, the figure shows that under the excitation of light, a large number of electron and hole pairs are generated on the surface of photocatalysts, which greatly increases the activity of the photocatalyst for pollutant removal [54]. The band gap of CNM (1:2) was significantly narrower than that of the g-C_3N_4 and MoS_2, which is due to the photoexcited electrons' (e^-) transition from the conduction band (CB) of g-C_3N_4 to the CB of MoS_2, and the holes' (h^+) transition from the valence band (VB) of MoS_2 to the VB of g-C_3N_4, which is beneficial to the narrowing of the band gap and reduces the recombination rate of photo-generated electrons and holes. The photocatalyst can absorb more energy under the same light conditions and be excited to generate more photo-generated electron–hole pairs, thus improving the photocatalytic performance of CNM (1:2) and enhancing the removal rate of Cr (VI) by CNM (1:2). This is due to Z-scheme heterojunction formed between g-C_3N_4 and MoS_2 [44]. The reaction equation is shown in Equations (1)–(4).

$$\text{g-}C_3N_4 + h\nu \rightarrow \text{g-}C_3N_4\ (e^- + h^+) \quad (1)$$

$$\text{g-}C_3N_4 + MoS_2 \rightarrow \text{g-}C_3N_4 + MoS_2(e^-) \quad (2)$$

$$MoS_2\ (e^-) + O_2 \rightarrow MoS_2 + \cdot O_2^- \quad (3)$$

$$Cr\ (VI) + e^- \rightarrow Cr\ (III) \quad (4)$$

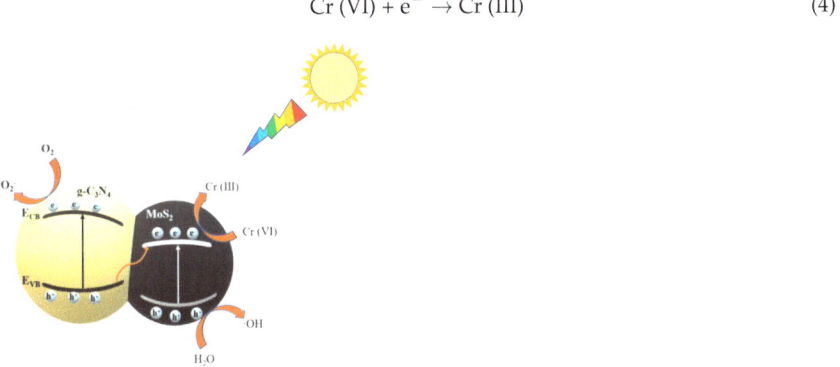

Figure 10. The mechanism for removal of Cr (VI) by CNM (1:2).

3. Materials and Methods

3.1. Materials

Thiourea (H_2NCSNH_2, AR) was purchased from Hengxing chemical preparation(Tianjin, China), ammonium molybdate ((NH_4)$_6Mo_7O_{24}\cdot 4H_2O$, AR) was acquired from Taishan Chemical Plant (Shandong, China), urea (H_2NCONH_2, AR) was obtained from Tianjin Zhiyuan chemical reagent co(Tianjin, China), ethylenediaminetetraacetic acid disodium salt (EDTA-2Na), potassium persulfate ($K_2S_2O_8$), ascorbic acid ($C_6H_8O_6$), hydrochloric acid (HCL), and sodium hydroxide (NaOH) were obtained from Xilong scientific (Guangzhou, China).

3.2. Preparation of Photocatalysts

3.2.1. Preparation of g-C_3N_4

g-C_3N_4 was prepared by the thermal polymerization method. Then, 20 g of urea were loaded into a crucible and wrapped in tin foil, with a 5 °C·min^{-1} heating rate, before being kept at 550 °C for 4 h. After cooling to room temperature, the yellow g-C_3N_4 was obtained, using an agate mortar grind to obtain the powdered g-C_3N_4.

3.2.2. Preparation of MoS_2

The MoS_2 was prepared by the hydrothermal method. Then, 0.4 g ammonium molybdate (($NH_4)_6Mo_7O_{24}·4H_2O$) and 0.8 g thiourea (H_2NCSNH_2) were added to 10 mL of deionized water, stirred for 30 min, and ultrasound-treated for 30 min. The solution was transferred to a hydrothermal reactor and heated for 10 h at 200 °C, after which the solution was cooled to room temperature and strained and washed with deionized water and anhydrous ethanol 3 times, aiming to remove any impurities. The samples were kept at 60 °C for 12 h; the black MoS_2 was obtained using an agate mortar to grind it into a powder (which was bagged for later use).

3.2.3. Preparation of $g-C_3N_4/MoS_2$ with Different Mass Ratios

$g-C_3N_4/MoS_2$ with different mass ratios was prepared by the ultrasonic method. The 0.2 g $g-C_3N_4$ and 0.4 g MoS_2 were added to 400 mL of deionized water and ultrasound-treated for 180 min. The $g-C_3N_4/MoS_2$ was obtained and denoted CNM (1:2); the CNM (1:4), CNM (2:1), CNM (4:1), and CNM (1:1) were obtained in the same way, and the different samples were obtained by changing the mass ratios of $g-C_3N_4$ and MoS_2, as shown in Figure 11.

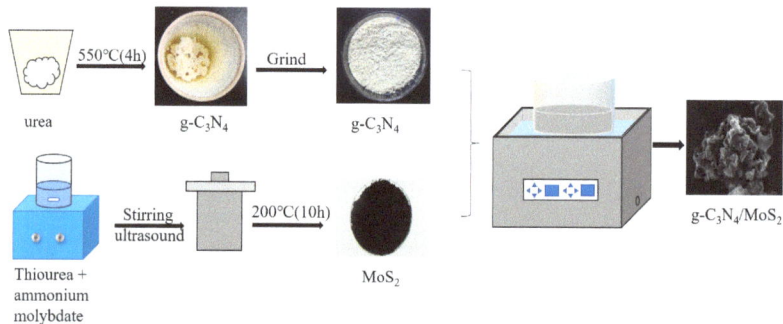

Figure 11. The preparation process of photocatalysts.

3.3. Characterization of Photocatalysts

The crystal structures of the photocatalysts were characterized by X-ray diffraction (XRD, Rigaku SmartLab SE, Rigaku Corp., Tokyo, Japan) with Cu-kα radiation. The morphology and structure of the photocatalysts were determined using scanning electron microscopy (SEM, TESCAN MIRA LMS, TESCAN CHINA, Ltd., Shanghai, China). X-ray photoelectron spectroscopy (XPS, Thermo Scientific k-Alpha, Thermo Fisher Scientific Co., Ltd., Shanghai, China) was used to characterize the elemental composition and valence state of the photocatalysts. The optical properties of photocatalysts were measured using a UV–visible spectrophotometer (UV–vis, UV-3600i plus, Shimadzu Corp., Kyoto, Japan). The surface area and pore size of photocatalysts were tested by the Brunauer–Emmett–Teller method (BET, Micromeritics ASAP2460, Micromeritics Corp., Norcross, GA, USA). The steady and transient photoluminescence spectra of photocatalysts were assessed using a fluorescence spectrometer (PL, FLS980, Edinburgh Instruments Ltd., Shanghai, China). The metal element content was tested using an inductively coupled plasma–mass spectrometer (ICP-MS, PerkinElmer NexION 2000, Perkinelmer, MS, USA).

3.4. Photocatalytic Tests

The photocatalytic performance of $g-C_3N_4$, CNM (1:2), CNM (1:4), CNM (2:1), CNM (4:1) and CNM (1:1) was tested in the photoreactor. A 300 W Xe lamp supported by CEL-LAM with a cutoff filter (λ > 420 nm) was used as the source of solar light and visible light. CEL-LAM 500 was the source of UV light, and the reaction took place at room temperature. A 10 mg photocatalyst was put into the 100 mL Cr (VI) solution (20 mg·L^{-1}), and the pH value was 3. The photocatalyst and the 20 mg·L^{-1} Cr (VI) solution were stirred in the dark for 30 min to achieve adsorption–desorption equilibrium, and 2 mL of solution was taken each time to analyze the concentration of Cr (VI). After turning on the light source, samples were taken at 20, 40, 60, 80, 100, and 120 min, respectively. The same 2 mL of solution was taken at a time and filtered using a biofilter membrane (0.45 μm) to obtain a filtrate without photocatalyst. We then determined the water quality and amount of chromium (VI)-1,5 dtphenylcarbohydrazide using a spectrophotometric method (GB 7467-87) [55] to analyze the concentration of hexavalent chromium. The removal rate (%) was calculated according to Equation (5):

$$\text{removal rate } (\%) = \frac{C_0 - C_t}{C_0} \times 100\% \quad (5)$$

C_0: the initial concentration of Cr (VI); C_t: the concentration of Cr (VI) at the corresponding time.

4. Conclusions

Z-scheme g-C_3N_4/MoS_2 nanocomposite heterojunctions were successfully synthesized using an ultrasonic method and demonstrated efficient photocatalytic removal of toxic Cr (VI) from water under UV, visible, and solar light irradiation. The nanocomposites, especially those with the optimized 1:2 g-C_3N_4/MoS_2 ratio, exhibited enhanced photoactivity compared to pure g-C_3N_4, with over 90% Cr (VI) removal achieved. The superior performance is attributed to the combined effects of the narrowed heterostructure band gap, which enables visible light response, and the effective separation of photo-generated electron–hole pairs at the interfaced junction between the two semiconductors. The results showed that the MoS_2 could be located at the g-C_3N_4, which was beneficial for the enhancement of photocatalytic activity, owing to the g-C_3N_4/MoS_2 nanocomposites having a broad range of light response and the separation and transfer efficiencies of photo-generated electron–hole pairs being improved. Overall, this work highlights the promise of ultrasonically synthesized g-C_3N_4/MoS_2 nanocomposites for tackling the pressing environmental challenge of heavy metal wastewater treatment using solar-driven photocatalysis. Further optimization to translate this efficient lab-scale Cr (VI) remediation to real-world applications should be pursued.

Author Contributions: Conceptualization, C.T. and H.Y.; methodology, C.T.; software, H.Y.; validation, R.Z., J.Z. and C.G.; formal analysis, Y.Z.; investigation, K.Q.; resources, H.Y.; data curation, Q.M.; writing—original draft preparation, C.T.; writing—review and editing, H.Y.; visualization, M.G.; supervision, Y.Z.; project administration, Q.M.; funding acquisition, Y.Z., H.Y., C.G. and K.Q. All authors have read and agreed to the published version of the manuscript.

Funding: This research was funded by the Yunnan Province Education Department Scientific Research Fund Project, grant number: 2024J0828; The Basic Research Project of the Yunnan Province Science and Technology Department, grant number: 202201AU070004; The Yunnan Province Education Department Scientific Research Fund Project, grant number: 2023J0959, 2023Y1049 and the National Natural Science Foundation of China, grant number 52272287, 22268003.

Institutional Review Board Statement: Not applicable.

Informed Consent Statement: Not applicable.

Data Availability Statement: The data presented in this study are available upon request from the corresponding author. The data are not publicly available due to ethical considerations.

Conflicts of Interest: The authors declare no conflicts of interest.

References

1. Chen, Z.; Kahn, M.E.; Liu, Y.; Wang, Z. The Consequences of Spatially Differentiated Water Pollution Regulation in China. *J. Environ. Econ. Manag.* **2018**, *88*, 468–485. [CrossRef]
2. Wang, Q.; Yang, Z. Industrial Water Pollution, Water Environment Treatment, and Health Risks in China. *Environ. Pollut.* **2016**, *218*, 358–365. [CrossRef]

3. Barrera-Díaz, C.E.; Lugo-Lugo, V.; Bilyeu, B. A Review of Chemical, Electrochemical and Biological Methods for Aqueous Cr(VI) Reduction. *J. Hazard. Mater.* **2012**, *223–224*, 1–12. [CrossRef]
4. Schroeder, H.A. The Ce: Role of Chromium in Mammalian Nutrition. *Am. J. Clin. Nutr.* **1968**, *21*, 230–244. [CrossRef]
5. Chen, Y.; Qian, Y.; Ma, J.; Mao, M.; Qian, L.; An, D. New Insights into the Cooperative Adsorption Behavior of Cr(VI) and Humic Acid in Water by Powdered Activated Carbon. *Sci. Total Environ.* **2022**, *817*, 153081. [CrossRef]
6. Hansen, M.B.; Johansen, J.D.; Menné, T. Chromium Allergy: Significance of Both Cr(III) and Cr(VI). *Contact Dermat.* **2003**, *49*, 206–212. [CrossRef]
7. Qi, Y.; Jiang, M.; Cui, Y.-L.; Zhao, L.; Liu, S. Novel Reduction of Cr(VI) from Wastewater Using a Naturally Derived Microcapsule Loaded with Rutin–Cr(III) Complex. *J. Hazard. Mater.* **2015**, *285*, 336–345. [CrossRef] [PubMed]
8. Zhou, L.; Liu, Y.; Liu, S.; Yin, Y.; Zeng, G.; Tan, X.; Hu, X.; Hu, X.; Jiang, L.; Ding, Y.; et al. Investigation of the Adsorption-Reduction Mechanisms of Hexavalent Chromium by Ramie Biochars of Different Pyrolytic Temperatures. *Bioresour. Technol.* **2016**, *218*, 351–359. [CrossRef] [PubMed]
9. Acharya, J.; Sahu, J.N.; Sahoo, B.K.; Mohanty, C.R.; Meikap, B.C. Removal of Chromium(VI) from Wastewater by Activated Carbon Developed from Tamarind Wood Activated with Zinc Chloride. *Chem. Eng. J.* **2009**, *150*, 25–39. [CrossRef]
10. Attia, A.A.; Khedr, S.A.; Elkholy, S.A. Adsorption of Chromium Ion (VI) by Acid Activated Carbon. *Braz. J. Chem. Eng.* **2010**, *27*, 183–193. [CrossRef]
11. Jiang, B.; Gong, Y.; Gao, J.; Sun, T.; Liu, Y.; Oturan, N.; Oturan, M.A. The Reduction of Cr(VI) to Cr(III) Mediated by Environmentally Relevant Carboxylic Acids: State-of-the-Art and Perspectives. *J. Hazard. Mater.* **2019**, *365*, 205–226. [CrossRef]
12. Liu, X.; Chu, G.; Du, Y.; Li, J.; Si, Y. The Role of Electron Shuttle Enhances Fe(III)-Mediated Reduction of Cr(VI) by Shewanella Oneidensis MR-1. *World J. Microbiol. Biotechnol.* **2019**, *35*, 64. [CrossRef]
13. Liu, F.; Hua, S.; Wang, C.; Qiu, M.; Jin, L.; Hu, B. Adsorption and Reduction of Cr(VI) from Aqueous Solution Using Cost-Effective Caffeic Acid Functionalized Corn Starch. *Chemosphere* **2021**, *279*, 130539. [CrossRef]
14. Yang, H.; Kim, N.; Park, D. Ecotoxicity Study of Reduced-Cr(III) Generated by Cr(VI) Biosorption. *Chemosphere* **2023**, *332*, 138825. [CrossRef]
15. Li, H.; Tu, W.; Zhou, Y.; Zou, Z. Z-Scheme Photocatalytic Systems for Promoting Photocatalytic Performance: Recent Progress and Future Challenges. *Adv. Sci.* **2016**, *3*, 1500389. [CrossRef]
16. Li, S.; Cai, M.; Wang, C.; Liu, Y. Ta_3N_5/CdS Core–Shell S-Scheme Heterojunction Nanofibers for Efficient Photocatalytic Removal of Antibiotic Tetracycline and Cr(VI): Performance and Mechanism Insights. *Adv. Fiber Mater.* **2023**, *5*, 994–1007. [CrossRef]
17. Wen, X.-J.; Shen, C.-H.; Fei, Z.-H.; Fang, D.; Liu, Z.-T.; Dai, J.-T.; Niu, C.-G. Recent Developments on AgI Based Heterojunction Photocatalytic Systems in Photocatalytic Application. *Chem. Eng. J.* **2020**, *383*, 123083. [CrossRef]
18. Li, S.; Cai, M.; Liu, Y.; Wang, C.; Yan, R.; Chen, X. Constructing $Cd_{0.5}Zn_{0.5}S/Bi_2WO_6$ S-Scheme Heterojunction for Boosted Photocatalytic Antibiotic Oxidation and Cr(VI) Reduction. *Adv. Powder Mater.* **2023**, *2*, 100073. [CrossRef]
19. Zhang, G.; Chen, D.; Li, N.; Xu, Q.; Li, H.; He, J.; Lu, J. Fabrication of Bi_2MoO_6/ZnO Hierarchical Heterostructures with Enhanced Visible-Light Photocatalytic Activity. *Appl. Catal. B Environ.* **2019**, *250*, 313–324. [CrossRef]
20. Meng, A.; Zhu, B.; Zhong, B.; Zhang, L.; Cheng, B. Direct Z-Scheme TiO_2/CdS Hierarchical Photocatalyst for Enhanced Photocatalytic H2-Production Activity. *Appl. Surf. Sci.* **2017**, *422*, 518–527. [CrossRef]
21. Zhang, J.; Hu, W.; Cao, S.; Piao, L. Recent Progress for Hydrogen Production by Photocatalytic Natural or Simulated Seawater Splitting. *Nano Res.* **2020**, *13*, 2313–2322. [CrossRef]
22. Liu, X.; Chen, T.; Xue, Y.; Fan, J.; Shen, S.; Hossain, M.S.A.; Amin, M.A.; Pan, L.; Xu, X.; Yamauchi, Y. Nanoarchitectonics of MXene/Semiconductor Heterojunctions toward Artificial Photosynthesis via Photocatalytic CO_2 Reduction. *Coord. Chem. Rev.* **2022**, *459*, 214440. [CrossRef]
23. Li, S.; Wang, C.; Liu, Y.; Liu, Y.; Cai, M.; Zhao, W.; Duan, X. S-Scheme MIL-101(Fe) Octahedrons Modified Bi_2WO_6 Microspheres for Photocatalytic Decontamination of Cr(VI) and Tetracycline Hydrochloride: Synergistic Insights, Reaction Pathways, and Toxicity Analysis. *Chem. Eng. J.* **2023**, *455*, 140943. [CrossRef]
24. He, R.; Wang, Z.; Deng, F.; Li, X.; Peng, Y.; Deng, Y.; Zou, J.; Luo, X.; Liu, X. Tunable Bi-Bridge S-Scheme Bi_2S_3/BiOBr Heterojunction with Oxygen Vacancy and SPR Effect for Efficient Photocatalytic Reduction of Cr(VI) and Industrial Electroplating Wastewater Treatment. *Sep. Purif. Technol.* **2023**, *311*, 123176. [CrossRef]
25. Chen, Y.; Huang, W.; He, D.; Situ, Y.; Huang, H. Construction of Heterostructured G-C_3N_4/Ag/TiO_2 Microspheres with Enhanced Photocatalysis Performance under Visible-Light Irradiation. *ACS Appl. Mater. Interfaces* **2014**, *6*, 14405–14414. [CrossRef]
26. Han, Q.; Hu, C.; Zhao, F.; Zhang, Z.; Chen, N.; Qu, L. One-Step Preparation of Iodine-Doped Graphitic Carbon Nitride Nanosheets as Efficient Photocatalysts for Visible Light Water Splitting. *J. Mater. Chem. A* **2015**, *3*, 4612–4619. [CrossRef]
27. Pasupuleti, K.S.; Chougule, S.S.; Vidyasagar, D.; Bak, N.; Jung, N.; Kim, Y.-H.; Lee, J.-H.; Kim, S.-G.; Kim, M.-D. UV Light Driven High-Performance Room Temperature Surface Acoustic Wave NH_3 Gas Sensor Using Sulfur-Doped g-C_3N_4 Quantum Dots. *Nano Res.* **2023**, *16*, 7682–7695. [CrossRef]
28. Cui, Y.; Ding, Z.; Liu, P.; Antonietti, M.; Fu, X.; Wang, X. Metal-Free Activation of H_2O_2 by g-C_3N_4 under Visible Light Irradiation for the Degradation of Organic Pollutants. *Phys. Chem. Chem. Phys.* **2012**, *14*, 1455–1462. [CrossRef]
29. Preeyanghaa, M.; Vinesh, V.; Sabarikirishwaran, P.; Rajkamal, A.; Ashokkumar, M.; Neppolian, B. Investigating the Role of Ultrasound in Improving the Photocatalytic Ability of CQD Decorated Boron-Doped g-C_3N_4 for Tetracycline Degradation and First-Principles Study of Nitrogen-Vacancy Formation. *Carbon* **2022**, *192*, 405–417. [CrossRef]

30. Yu, H.; Ma, Q.; Gao, C.; Liao, S.; Zhang, Y.; Quan, H.; Zhai, R. Petal-like g-C_3N_4 Enhances the Photocatalyst Removal of Hexavalent Chromium. *Catalysts* **2023**, *13*, 641. [CrossRef]
31. Mo, F.; Liu, Y.; Xu, Y.; He, Q.; Sun, P.; Dong, X. Photocatalytic Elimination of Moxifloxacin by Two-Dimensional Graphitic Carbon Nitride Nanosheets: Enhanced Activity, Degradation Mechanism and Potential Practical Application. *Sep. Purif. Technol.* **2022**, *292*, 121067. [CrossRef]
32. Sun, H.; Guo, F.; Pan, J.; Huang, W.; Wang, K.; Shi, W. One-Pot Thermal Polymerization Route to Prepare N-Deficient Modified g-C_3N_4 for the Degradation of Tetracycline by the Synergistic Effect of Photocatalysis and Persulfate-Based Advanced Oxidation Process. *Chem. Eng. J.* **2021**, *406*, 126844. [CrossRef]
33. Wang, J.; Wang, S. A Critical Review on Graphitic Carbon Nitride (g-C_3N_4)-Based Materials: Preparation, Modification and Environmental Application. *Coord. Chem. Rev.* **2022**, *453*, 214338. [CrossRef]
34. Cheng, C.; Dong, C.-L.; Shi, J.; Mao, L.; Huang, Y.-C.; Kang, X.; Zong, S.; Shen, S. Regulation on Polymerization Degree and Surface Feature in Graphitic Carbon Nitride towards Efficient Photocatalytic H_2 Evolution under Visible-Light Irradiation. *J. Mater. Sci. Technol.* **2022**, *98*, 160–168. [CrossRef]
35. Song, X.; Wang, M.; Liu, W.; Li, X.; Zhu, Z.; Huo, P.; Yan, Y. Thickness Regulation of Graphitic Carbon Nitride and Its Influence on the Photocatalytic Performance towards CO_2 Reduction. *Appl. Surf. Sci.* **2022**, *577*, 151810. [CrossRef]
36. Bu, Y.; Chen, Z. Effect of Oxygen-Doped C_3N_4 on the Separation Capability of the Photoinduced Electron-Hole Pairs Generated by O-C_3N_4@TiO_2 with Quasi-Shell-Core Nanostructure. *Electrochim. Acta* **2014**, *144*, 42–49. [CrossRef]
37. Cao, L.; Wang, R.; Wang, D. Synthesis and Characterization of Sulfur Self-Doped g-C_3N_4 with Efficient Visible-Light Photocatalytic Activity. *Mater. Lett.* **2015**, *149*, 50–53. [CrossRef]
38. Ranjbakhsh, E.; Izadyar, M.; Nakhaeipour, A.; Habibi-Yangjeh, A. Quantum Chemistry Calculations of S, P, and O-Doping Effect on the Photocatalytic Molecular Descriptors of g-C_3N_4 Quantum Dots. *J. Iran. Chem. Soc.* **2022**, *19*, 3513–3528. [CrossRef]
39. Li, K.; Huang, Z.; Zeng, X.; Huang, B.; Gao, S.; Lu, J. Synergetic Effect of Ti^{3+} and Oxygen Doping on Enhancing Photoelectrochemical and Photocatalytic Properties of TiO_2/g-C_3N_4 Heterojunctions. *ACS Appl. Mater. Interfaces* **2017**, *9*, 11577–11586. [CrossRef] [PubMed]
40. Sun, M.; Yan, Q.; Yan, T.; Li, M.; Wei, D.; Wang, Z.; Wei, Q.; Du, B. Facile Fabrication of 3D Flower-like Heterostructured g-C_3N_4/SnS_2 Composite with Efficient Photocatalytic Activity under Visible Light. *RSC Adv.* **2014**, *4*, 31019–31027. [CrossRef]
41. Wang, X.; Yang, W.; Li, F.; Xue, Y.; Liu, R.; Hao, Y. In Situ Microwave-Assisted Synthesis of Porous N-TiO_2/g-C_3N_4 Heterojunctions with Enhanced Visible-Light Photocatalytic Properties. *Ind. Eng. Chem. Res.* **2013**, *52*, 17140–17150. [CrossRef]
42. Li, B.; Fang, Q.; Si, Y.; Huang, T.; Huang, W.-Q.; Hu, W.; Pan, A.; Fan, X.; Huang, G.-F. Ultra-Thin Tubular Graphitic Carbon Nitride-Carbon Dot Lateral Heterostructures: One-Step Synthesis and Highly Efficient Catalytic Hydrogen Generation. *Chem. Eng. J.* **2020**, *397*, 125470. [CrossRef]
43. Rajendran, R.; Vignesh, S.; Raj, V.; Palanivel, B.; Ali, A.M.; Sayed, M.A.; Shkir, M. Designing of TiO_2/α-Fe_2O_3 Coupled g-C_3N_4 Magnetic Heterostructure Composite for Efficient Z-Scheme Photo-Degradation Process under Visible Light Exposures. *J. Alloys Compd.* **2022**, *894*, 162498. [CrossRef]
44. Sharma, G.; Naushad, M.; ALOthman, Z.A.; Iqbal, J.; Bathula, C. High Interfacial Charge Separation in Visible-Light Active Z-Scheme g-C_3N_4/MoS_2 Heterojunction: Mechanism and Degradation of Sulfasalazine. *Chemosphere* **2022**, *308*, 136162. [CrossRef] [PubMed]
45. Sivakumar, S.; Daniel Thangadurai, T.; Manjubaashini, N.; Nataraj, D. Two-Dimensional z-Type MoS_2/g-C_3N_4 Semiconductor Heterojunction Nanocomposites for Industrial Methylene Blue Dye Degradation under Daylight. *Colloids Surf. A Physicochem. Eng. Asp.* **2022**, *654*, 130090. [CrossRef]
46. Sima, L.; Li, D.; Dong, L.; Zhang, F. Facile Preparation of Porous G-C_3N_4/MoS_2 Heterojunction for Hydrogen Production under Simulated Sunlight. *Mater. Today Sustain.* **2022**, *20*, 100217. [CrossRef]
47. Lyu, H.; Zhu, W.; Chen, K.; Gao, J.; Xie, Z. 3D Flower-Shaped g-C_3N_4/MoS_2 Composite with Structure Defect for Synergistic Degradation of Dyes. *J. Water Process Eng.* **2024**, *57*, 104656. [CrossRef]
48. Zhao, L.; Guo, L.; Tang, Y.; Zhou, J.; Shi, B. Novel G-C_3N_4/C/Fe_2O_3 Composite for Efficient Photocatalytic Reduction of Aqueous Cr(VI) under Light Irradiation. *Ind. Eng. Chem. Res.* **2021**, *60*, 13594–13603. [CrossRef]
49. Zhang, B.; Hu, X.; Liu, E.; Fan, J. Novel S-Scheme 2D/2D BiOBr/g-C_3N_4 Heterojunctions with Enhanced Photocatalytic Activity. *Chin. J. Catal.* **2021**, *42*, 1519–1529. [CrossRef]
50. Wu, Z.; He, X.; Xue, Y.; Yang, X.; Li, Y.; Li, Q.; Yu, B. Cyclodextrins Grafted MoS_2/g-C_3N_4 as High-Performance Photocatalysts for the Removal of Glyphosate and Cr (VI) from Simulated Agricultural Runoff. *Chem. Eng. J.* **2020**, *399*, 125747. [CrossRef]
51. Xue, Y.; Ji, Y.; Wang, X.; Wang, H.; Chen, X.; Zhang, X.; Tian, J. Heterostructuring Noble-Metal-Free 1T' Phase MoS_2 with g-C_3N_4 Hollow Nanocages to Improve the Photocatalytic H_2 Evolution Activity. *Green Energy Environ.* **2023**, *8*, 864–873. [CrossRef]
52. Bashal, A.H.; Alkanad, K.; Al-Ghorbani, M.; Ben Aoun, S.; Bajiri, M.A. Synergistic Effect of Cocatalyst and S-Scheme Heterojunction over 2D/2D g-C_3N_4/MoS_2 Heterostructure Coupled Cu Nanoparticles for Selective Photocatalytic CO_2 Reduction to CO under Visible Light Irradiation. *J. Environ. Chem. Eng.* **2023**, *11*, 109545. [CrossRef]
53. Yuan, H.; Fang, F.; Dong, J.; Xia, W.; Zeng, X.; Shangguan, W. Enhanced Photocatalytic Hydrogen Production Based on Laminated MoS_2/g-C_3N_4 Photocatalysts. *Colloids Surf. A Physicochem. Eng. Asp.* **2022**, *641*, 128575. [CrossRef]

54. Pasupuleti, K.S.; Vidyasagar, D.; Ambadi, L.N.; Bak, N.; Kim, S.-G.; Kim, M.-D. UV Light Activated G-C$_3$N$_4$ Nanoribbons Coated Surface Acoustic Wave Sensor for High Performance Sub-Ppb Level NO$_2$ Detection at Room Temperature. *Sens. Actuators B Chem.* **2023**, *394*, 134471. [CrossRef]
55. *GB 7467-87*; Water Quality-Determination of Chromiun(VI)-1,5 Dtphenylcarbohydrazide Spectrophotometric Method. Ministry of Ecology and Environment of the People's Republic of China: Beijing, China, 1987.

Disclaimer/Publisher's Note: The statements, opinions and data contained in all publications are solely those of the individual author(s) and contributor(s) and not of MDPI and/or the editor(s). MDPI and/or the editor(s) disclaim responsibility for any injury to people or property resulting from any ideas, methods, instructions or products referred to in the content.

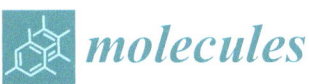

Article

Photoredox-Catalyzed Synthesis of 3-Sulfonylated Pyrrolin-2-ones via a Regioselective Tandem Sulfonylation Cyclization of 1,5-Dienes

Ran Ding [1,*], Liang Li [1], Ya-Ting Yu [1], Bing Zhang [1] and Pei-Long Wang [2,3,*]

[1] College of Chemistry and Materials Engineering, Anhui Science and Technology University, Bengbu 233100, China; ll15855863179@126.com (L.L.); yyt2747196669@126.com (Y.-T.Y.); zhangbing2168@126.com (B.Z.)
[2] Key Laboratory of Green and Precise Synthetic Chemistry and Applications, Ministry of Education, School of Chemistry and Materials Science, Huaibei Normal University, Huaibei 235000, China
[3] Information College, Huaibei Normal University, Huaibei 235000, China
* Correspondence: dingran@mail.ustc.edu.cn (R.D.); wangpl@chnu.edu.cn (P.-L.W.)

Abstract: A mild, visible-light-induced, regioselective cascade sulfonylation-cyclization of 1,5-dienes with sulfonyl chlorides through the intermolecular radical addition/cyclization of alkenes C(sp^2)-H was developed. This procedure proceeds well and affords a mild and efficient route to a range of monosulfonylated pyrrolin-2-ones at room temperatures.

Keywords: regioselective; dienes; radical; cyclization; pyrrolin-2-ones

1. Introduction

Pyrrolin-2-ones, which constitute one of the most prominent classes of skeletons exhibiting unique biological activities, are prevalent in a large number of biological pharmaceutical molecules [1,2] and natural products, like chaetogline, violacein, and hypomycine [3–6] (Figure 1). In this context, considerable effort has been focused in establishing such valuable frameworks, but most of these methods suffer from transition metals or harsh reaction conditions [7–12]. Therefore, developing general and effective synthetic methods for pyrrolin-2-ones and its derivatives with mild conditions has been attracting increasing attention and largely promote progress in this area [13–18]. On the other hand, the photoinduced radical cascade cyclization reaction has become a powerful tool to construct N-containing heterocycles because of its extremely high efficiency, inherently green, infinite availability, safety, and ease of operation [19–24]. However, such an efficient strategy for the synthesis of pyrrolin-2-ones has rarely been reported [25].

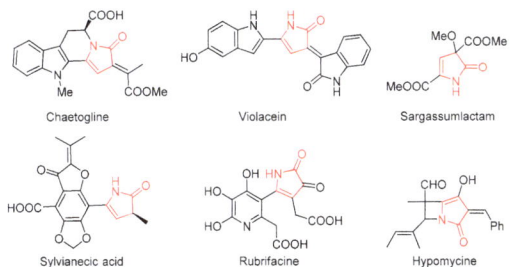

Figure 1. Examples of compounds containing pyrrolin-2-ones.

Sulfones constitute an important class of functional groups in organic synthesis that can participate in various chemical transformations [26,27] and that are found widely in the structures of natural products [28–30]. The introduction of sulfonyl functional groups can cause molecules to exhibit unique biological activity [31,32]. In this regard, a considerable amount of effort has been devoted to the development of efficient, simple, and convenient methods for synthesizing sulfonyl-containing compounds [33–38]. Among the many approaches, the difunctionalization of alkenes through a radical process has been used to prepare several sulfone-containing compounds [39–48]. Sulfonyl chloride is a readily available and easily handled source of the sulfonyl moiety and is commonly used to generate sulfonyl radicals under visible light conditions; major advances have focused on reactions with heteroaryl or aryl-tethered alkenes to produce sulfonyl-containing aromatic compounds (Scheme 1a) [49–55]. Nevertheless, the reactions of vinyl-tethered alkenes remain elusive [56,57].

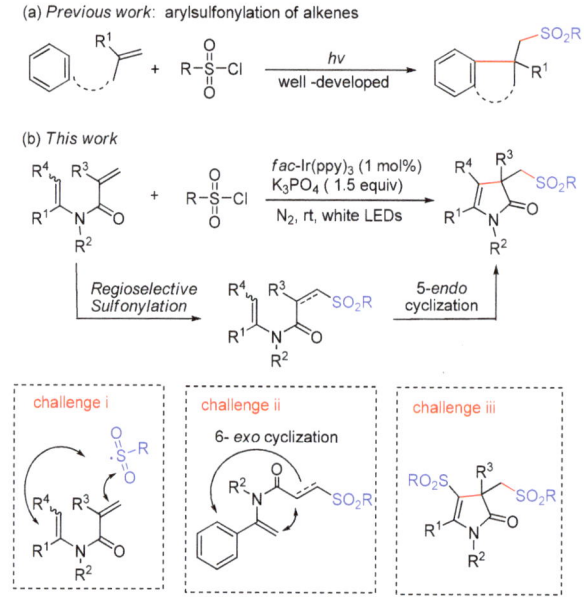

Scheme 1. Radical cyclization of tethered alkenes. Challenge i: Regioselectivity of sulfone radical addition; Challenge ii: Two pathway of cyclization; Challenge iii: 3,4-disulfonated pyrrolin-2-ones.

Considering the significance of pyrrolinones and the importance of sulfone moieties in organic synthesis. Herein, we aimed to develop an unprecedented visible-light-induced photoredox-catalyzed reaction of linear 1,5-dienes with sulfonyl chlorides via regioselective sulfonylation and 5-endo cyclization to produce important pyrrolinones (Scheme 1b). However, three challenges hinder the successful development of such a process: (i) The selective addition of the sulfone radical between two carbon-carbon double bonds is challenging. (ii) 6-Exo cyclization competes with the desired reaction and needs to be restricted. (iii) The C=C bond in the target product continues to react with the sulfonyl radical to afford 3,4-disulfonated pyrrolin-2-ones.

We then focused on the reaction of N-acetyl-N-(1-phenylvinyl)methacrylamide **1a** and p-toluenesulfonyl chloride **2a**. To our delight, when the reaction was performed in the presence of a catalytic amount of fac-Ir(ppy)$_3$ and equivalent of Na$_2$CO$_3$ in CH$_2$Cl$_2$ under irradiation with 20 W white LEDs (Light-Emitting Diodes) for 16 h, the target sulfonylated pyrrolinone **3a** could be isolated in 57% yield (Table 1, entry 1). Subsequently, other photocatalysts, such as Ru(bpy)$_3$Cl$_2$ and eosin Y, were investigated, but all failed to obtain product **3a** (entries 2, 3). After examining various bases, such as Li$_2$CO$_3$ (59%), NaHCO$_3$ (64%), K$_3$PO$_4$ (72%), and Na$_3$PO$_4$ (63%), K$_3$PO$_4$ was determined to be the best base (entries 4–8). A variety of solvents, including DCE (1,2-dichloroethane), CHCl$_3$, acetone, toluene,

THF (tetrahydrofuran), and EtOAc, were subsequently screened, but the yield of product **3a** was not promoted (entries 9–14). Next, the amounts of K_3PO_4 were evaluated (entries 15, 16). Using 1.5 equiv. of K_3PO_4 improved the yield of product **3a** by 79%. When the light source was changed to 5 W white LEDs, product **3a** was afforded in the same yield as previously obtained (entries 15 vs. 17). The results of the control experiments showed that visible light, photocatalyst [*fac*-Ir(ppy)$_3$], and base K_3PO_4 were necessary for this reaction (entries 18–20).

Table 1. Optimization of the reaction conditions [a].

Entry	Catalyst (1 mol%)	Base (Equiv.)	Solvent	Yield [b]
1	*fac*-Ir(ppy)$_3$	Na$_2$CO$_3$ (1.0)	CH$_2$Cl$_2$	57%
2	Ru(bpy)$_3$Cl$_2$	Na$_2$CO$_3$ (1.0)	CH$_2$Cl$_2$	trace
3	Eosin Y	Na$_2$CO$_3$ (1.0)	CH$_2$Cl$_2$	trace
4	*fac*-Ir(ppy)$_3$	K$_2$CO$_3$ (1.0)	CH$_2$Cl$_2$	66%
5	*fac*-Ir(ppy)$_3$	Li$_2$CO$_3$ (1.0)	CH$_2$Cl$_2$	59%
6	*fac*-Ir(ppy)$_3$	NaHCO$_3$ (1.0)	CH$_2$Cl$_2$	64%
7	*fac*-Ir(ppy)$_3$	K$_3$PO$_4$ (1.0)	CH$_2$Cl$_2$	72%
8	*fac*-Ir(ppy)$_3$	Na$_3$PO$_4$ (1.0)	CH$_2$Cl$_2$	63%
9	*fac*-Ir(ppy)$_3$	K$_3$PO$_4$ (1.0)	DCE	55%
10	*fac*-Ir(ppy)$_3$	K$_3$PO$_4$ (1.0)	CHCl$_3$	62%
11	*fac*-Ir(ppy)$_3$	K$_3$PO$_4$ (1.0)	Acetone	67%
12	*fac*-Ir(ppy)$_3$	K$_3$PO$_4$ (1.0)	Toluene	44%
13	*fac*-Ir(ppy)$_3$	K$_3$PO$_4$ (1.0)	THF	59%
14	*fac*-Ir(ppy)$_3$	K$_3$PO$_4$ (1.0)	EtOAc	32%
15	*fac*-Ir(ppy)$_3$	K$_3$PO$_4$ (1.5)	CH$_2$Cl$_2$	79%
16	*fac*-Ir(ppy)$_3$	K$_3$PO$_4$ (2.0)	CH$_2$Cl$_2$	79%
17 [c]	*fac*-Ir(ppy)$_3$	K$_3$PO$_4$ (1.5)	CH$_2$Cl$_2$	79%
18 [c]	------	K$_3$PO$_4$ (1.5)	CH$_2$Cl$_2$	0%
19 [c]	*fac*-Ir(ppy)$_3$	------	CH$_2$Cl$_2$	16%
20 [d]	*fac*-Ir(ppy)$_3$	K$_3$PO$_4$ (1.5)	CH$_2$Cl$_2$	0%

[a] Reaction conditions: **1a** (0.1 mmol), **2a** (0.2 mmol), and catalyst (1 mol%) in solvent (1 mL), which were irradiated with 20 W white LEDs at room temperature under N$_2$ for 16 h. [b] Isolated yields. [c] 5 W white LEDs was used. [d] The reaction was conducted in darkness.

2. Results and Discussion

After obtaining the optimal reaction conditions, we embarked upon exploring the substrate scope of 1,5-dienes. Different R^1, R^2, R^3 and R^4 groups of 1,5-dienes were tested with p-toluenesulfonyl chloride **2a**; the results are shown in Figure 2. Substrates with halogen atoms (F, Cl, Br, and I) and electron-donating groups (Me and MeO) at the para-positions of the benzene ring proceeded well to give target products **3b–3g** and **3g–3h** in medium to good yields. Gratifyingly, the CO$_2$Et group at the para-position of the benzene ring furnished product **3f** in an acceptable yield. The reactivity of substituents at the meta- or ortho-position was also tested, achieving yields of products **3i–3l** from 46% to 82%. Notably, substrates with an ethyl group at the β-position of the enamide moiety or an *n*-butyl group at the α-position of the acrylamide moiety smoothly converted to the corresponding product **3m** or **3n** in 85% yield or 62% yield. In addition, using propionyl or isobutyryl as the nitrogen-protecting groups was viable for this reaction to give target products **3o** and **3p** in considerable yields.

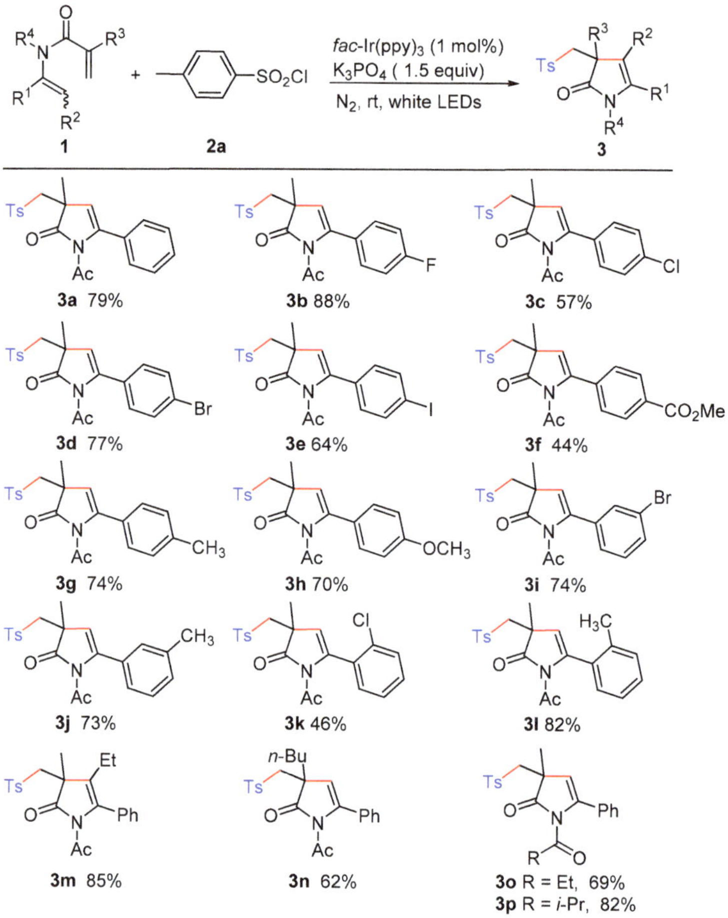

Figure 2. Substrate Scope of 1,5-dienes. Reaction conditions: **1** (0.1 mmol), **2a** (0.2 mmol), and Ir(ppy)$_3$ (1 mol%) in CH$_2$Cl$_2$ (1 mL) were irradiated with 5 W white LEDs at room temperature under N$_2$ for 16 h. The yields were isolated yields.

Next, we moved on to explore the generality of various sulfonyl chlorides (Figure 3). Arylsulfonyl chlorides bearing electron-rich (Me, McO, and *t*-Bu) groups at different positions worked well, giving corresponding sulfones **4b–4e** in 66–84% yield. Electron-poor arylsulfonyl chlorides, such as Br, I, CN, CF$_3$, and NO$_2$ groups on the benzene ring, allowed the formation of product **4f–4j** in 41% to 78% yield with the need for 20 W white LEDs as the light source. It is noteworthy that arylsulfonyl chlorides having substituents at the ortho-position were inferior to those at the para- or meta-position, mainly because of the large steric hindrance of the ortho-position (**4b** vs. **4e** and **4k** vs. **4l**). Remarkably, 2-thiophenesulfonyl chloride survived under the current conditions to achieve product **4m** in 62% yield. Moreover, alkyl-substituted sulfonyl chlorides, such as cyclopropyl and ethyl, were applicable for this reaction and transferred to **4n** and **4o** in 68% and 62% yield, respectively.

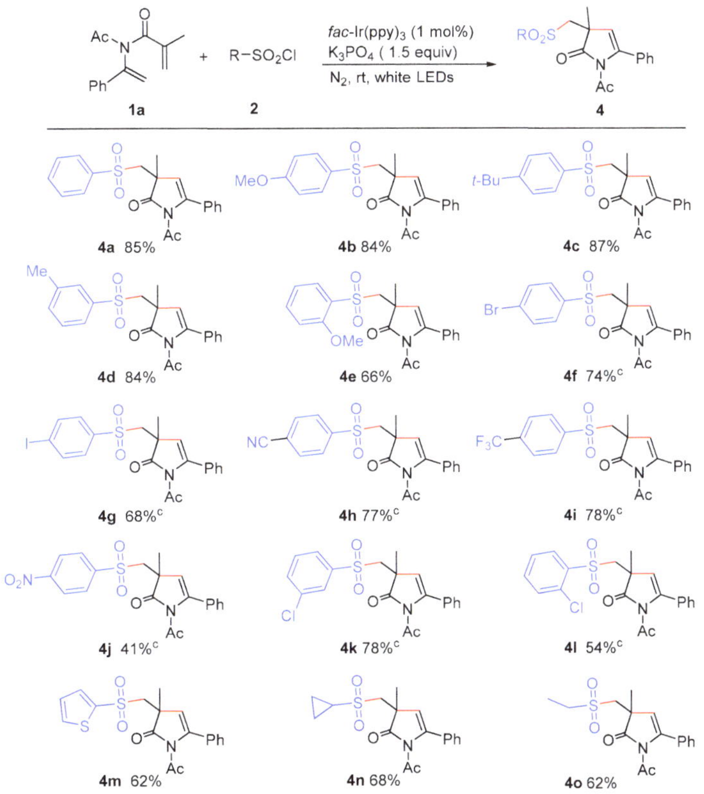

Figure 3. Substrate scope of sulfonyl chlorides. Reaction conditions: a mixture of **1a** (0.1 mmol), **2** (0.2 mmol), and Ir(ppy)$_3$ (1 mol%) in CH$_2$Cl$_2$ (1 mL), which were irradiated with 5 W white LEDs at room temperature under N$_2$ for 16 h. The yields were isolated yields. ^{c} 20 W white LEDs were used.

In order to further expand the practicality of the reaction, a gram scale reaction and removal of OAc group of compound **4a** were conducted. We were delighted to obtain the sulfonylated pyrrolinone **4a** in 78% yield with a prolonged time when the reaction was taken on 1 mmol scale (Scheme 2, (1)). Furthermore, with the addition of *n*-BuLi in THF at −78 °C, the compound **4a** could smoothly remove the OAc group, which generated the product **4aa** in 84% yield (Scheme 2, (2)).

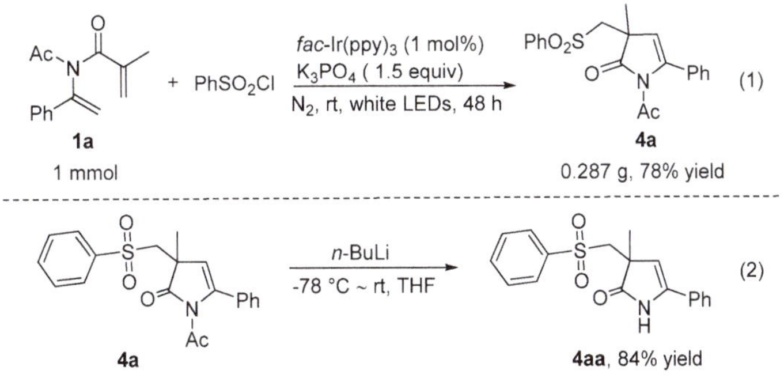

Scheme 2. Gram−scale reaction and removal of OAc group. (1): Gram-scale reaction; (2): Removal of OAc group.

To shed the possible mechanism of this visible-light-induced sulfonylation-cyclization of 1,5-dienes, some control experiments were carried out (Scheme 3). When 2.0 equivalents of TEMPO or 1,1-diphenylethylene was added to the reaction of 1,5-diene and p-toluenesulfonyl chloride under standard conditions, the transformation was completely suppressed, suggesting that a free-radical pathway may be involved in this sulfonylation-cyclization reaction. In addition, visible-light irradiation on/off experiments were performed on the model reaction, and the results show that a long-chain process was unlikely to be involved in this reaction (see Supplementary Materials).

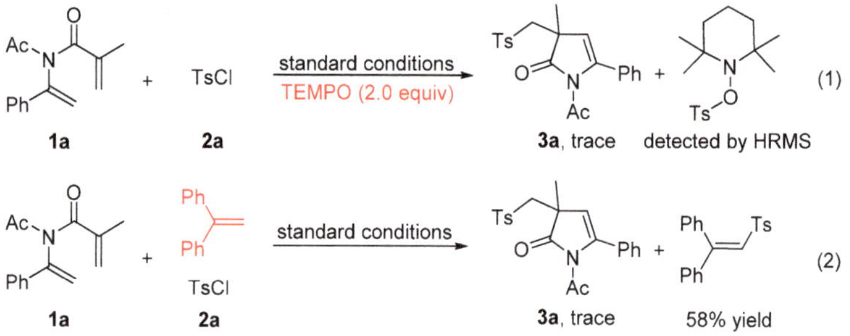

Scheme 3. Mechanistic studies. (1): TEMPO (2.0 equiv.) was added; (2): 1,1-diphenylethylene (2.0 equiv.) was added.

According to the above experimental results and previous literature reports [13–18], we propose a possible mechanism for visible-light-induced regioselective cascade sulfonylation-cyclization of 1,5-dienes (Scheme 4). First, the photocatalyst [fac-Ir(ppy)$_3$] under visible light irradiation is excited to form the strongly reducing state *[fac-Ir(ppy)$_3$]. A single electron transfer between *[fac-Ir(ppy)$_3$] and p-toluenesulfonyl chloride produces the p-toluenesulfonyl radical and oxidation state [fac-Ir(ppy)$_3$]$^+$. Second, the p-toluenesulfonyl radical was selectively added to the terminal carbon-carbon double bond of acrylamide of 1,5-diene, followed by a 5-endo cyclization to produce radical species II [58,59]. Although 5-endo cyclizations are often less favorable kinetically than their 4-exo cyclizations, the switch from 4-exo to 5-endo mode can be achieved through specific properties of the Ts radical [60,61]. The high regioselectivity can be explained by the reason that the rate of sulfonyl radical addition to the carbo–carbon double bond of acrylamide is much greater than to the enamine carbon–carbon double bond. Third, radical species II loses an electron by the oxidation of photocatalyst [fac-Ir(ppy)$_3$]$^+$ to forge tertiary cation intermediate III and to regenerate photocatalyst [fac-Ir(ppy)$_3$] for the next turnover. Last, deprotonation of cation intermediate III occurs in the presence of K$_3$PO$_4$, giving sulfonylated pyrrolinone **3a**. However, since the presence of base is important for the reaction, it cannot be ruled out that the radical II is directly deprotonated by the base to form radical anion, which is oxidized by the photocatalyst [fac-Ir (ppy)$_3$]$^+$ [62]. It is notable that arylsulfonyl radicals are prone to loss of SO$_2$ to form aryl radicals, which could induce the cyclization of 1,5-dienes in the same way as arylsulfonyl radicals, but the corresponding products have not been found in this system [63–68].

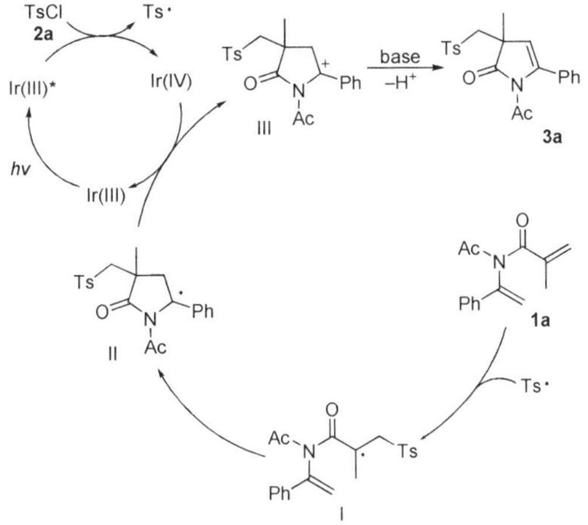

Scheme 4. Proposed reaction mechanism.

3. Materials and Methods

3.1. General Considerations

All the reagents purchased from Leyan company were directly used. ^{1}H-NMR and ^{13}C-NMR spectra of the products were recorded on a Bruker FT-NMR 400M or 600M spectrometer (Bruker Beijing Scientific Technology Co., Ltd., Beijing, China). Chemical shifts spectra are given as δ in the units of parts per million (ppm) with reference to tetramethylsilane (TMS). Multiplicities were indicated as follows: d (doublet); s (singlet); t (triplet); q (quartet); m (multiplets); etc. Coupling constants are reported as a *J* value in Hz. High-resolution mass spectral analysis (HRMS) of the products were collected on an Agilent Technologies 6540 UHD Accurate-Mass Q-TOF LC/MS (ESI) instrument (Beijing Agilent Technologies Co., Ltd, Beijing, China).

3.2. Typical Procedure for the Preparation of 3a

1,5-dienes **1a** (0.1 mmol), sulfonyl chlorides **2a** (0.2 mmol), *fac*-Ir(ppy)$_3$ (1 mol%), K$_3$PO$_4$ (1.5 equiv.), and CH$_2$Cl$_2$ (1 mL) were added into a dry 25 mL Schlenk tube containing a magnetic stirring bar under nitrogen atmosphere, Then the mixture was stirred and irradiated with 5 W white LEDs at room temperature for 16 h. After completing, the reaction mixture was directly subjected to flash column chromatography (10–40% EtOAc/Petroleum ether) to obtain the desired product **3a** as a white solid (79% yield).

3.3. Procedure for the Synthesis of the Coupling Product 4aa

n-BuLi (2.5 M, 0.24 mmol) was slowly added to the solution of compound **4a** (0.2 mmol) and THF (8 mL) at −78 °C. After 15 min, the reaction increased to room temperature. After completing, 8 mL water was added to quench the reaction and the mixture was extracted with 10 mL dichloromethane 3 times. The combined dichloromethane phases were dried over CaCl$_2$, concentrated *in vacuo* and purified by flash column chromatography (30–40% EtOAc/petroleum ether) to furnish the desired product **4aa** as a white solid (84% yield).

1-Acetyl-3-methyl-5-phenyl-3-(tosylmethyl)-1H-pyrrol-2(3H)-one (**3a**): ^{1}H NMR (600 MHz, CDCl$_3$) δ 7.71 (d, *J* = 8.3 Hz, 2H), 7.37–7.34 (m, 3H), 7.27 (d, *J* = 8.1 Hz, 2H), 7.24 (dd, *J* = 6.6, 3.0 Hz, 2H), 5.51 (s, 1H), 3.69 (d, *J* = 14.4 Hz, 1H), 3.46 (d, *J* = 14.4 Hz, 1H), 2.49 (s, 3H), 2.42 (s, 3H), 1.39 (s, 3H). δ ^{13}C NMR (151 MHz, CDCl$_3$) δ 179.60, 169.23, 145.06, 142.87, 136.57, 129.89, 128.50, 128.21, 127.88, 126.78, 115.54, 62.17, 47.76, 26.01, 24.57, 21.61.

1-Acetyl-5-(4-fluorophenyl)-3-methyl-3-(tosylmethyl)-1H-pyrrol-2(3H)-one (**3b**): ^{1}H NMR (400 MHz, CDCl$_3$) δ 7.71 (d, *J* = 8.2 Hz, 2H), 7.29 (d, *J* = 8.1 Hz, 2H), 7.26–7.20 (m, 2H), 7.05 (t, *J* = 8.7 Hz, 2H), 5.53 (s, 1H), 3.69 (d, *J* = 14.3 Hz, 1H), 3.45 (d, *J* = 14.3 Hz, 1H), 2.50 (s,

3H), 2.43 (s, 3H), 1.39 (s, 3H). ^{13}C NMR (101 MHz, CDCl$_3$) δ 179.56, 169.33, 162.72 (J = 252 Hz), 145.15, 142.02, 136.61, 129.94, 128.85, 128.77, 128.14, 115.66, 115.06, 114.85, 62.22, 47.69, 26.05, 24.53, 21.63. ^{19}F NMR (565 MHz, CDCl$_3$) δ-112.68.

1-Acetyl-5-(4-chlorophenyl)-3-methyl-3-(tosylmethyl)-1H-pyrrol-2(3H)-one (**3c**): ^{1}H NMR (600 MHz, CDCl$_3$) δ 7.70 (d, J = 8.3 Hz, 2H), 7.33 (d, J = 8.5 Hz, 2H), 7.29 (d, J = 8.0 Hz, 2H), 7.19 (d, J = 8.5 Hz, 2H), 5.56 (s, 1H), 3.68 (d, J = 14.3 Hz, 1H), 3.45 (d, J = 14.3 Hz, 1H), 2.50 (s, 3H), 2.43 (s, 3H), 1.39 (s, 3H). ^{13}C NMR (151 MHz, CDCl$_3$) δ 179.46, 169.26, 145.16, 141.90, 136.55, 134.39, 131.26, 129.94, 128.23, 128.13, 128.13, 116.05, 62.19, 47.74, 25.97, 24.48, 21.62.

1-acetyl-5-(4-bromophenyl)-3-methyl-3-(tosylmethyl)-1H-pyrrol-2(3H)-one (**3d**). ^{1}H NMR (600 MHz, CDCl$_3$) δ 7.70 (d, J = 8.2 Hz, 2H), 7.49 (d, J = 8.4 Hz, 2H), 7.29 (d, J = 8.0 Hz, 2H), 7.13 (d, J = 8.4 Hz, 2H), 5.56 (s, 1H), 3.68 (d, J = 14.3 Hz, 1H), 3.44 (d, J = 14.3 Hz, 1H), 2.50 (s, 3H), 2.43 (s, 3H), 1.39 (s, 3H). ^{13}C NMR (101 MHz, CDCl$_3$) δ 179.45, 169.27, 145.19, 141.95, 136.53, 131.74, 131.08, 129.96, 128.49, 128.14, 122.60, 116.10, 62.18, 47.77, 25.99, 24.47, 21.65.

1-Acetyl-5-(4-iodophenyl)-3-methyl-3-(tosylmethyl)-1H-pyrrol-2(3H)-one (**3e**). ^{1}H NMR (400 MHz, CDCl$_3$) δ 7.69 (dd, J = 8.0, 2.4 Hz, 4H), 7.29 (d, J = 7.9 Hz, 2H), 6.99 (d, J = 7.6 Hz, 2H), 5.56 (s, 1H), 3.69 (d, J = 14.2 Hz, 1H), 3.45 (d, J = 14.3 Hz, 1H), 2.50 (s, 3H), 2.43 (s, 3H), 1.38 (s, 3H). ^{13}C NMR (101 MHz, CDCl$_3$) δ 179.41, 169.24, 145.16, 141.99, 136.97, 136.44, 132.28, 129.93, 128.55, 128.11, 116.10, 94.28, 62.12, 47.75, 25.95, 24.44, 21.63.

Methyl-4-(1-acetyl-4-methyl-5-oxo-4-(tosylmethyl)-4,5-dihydro-1H-pyrrol-2-yl)benzoate (**3f**). ^{1}H NMR (600 MHz, CDCl$_3$) δ 8.03 (d, J = 8.3 Hz, 2H), 7.70 (d, J = 8.2 Hz, 2H), 5.61 (s, 1H), 3.93 (s, 3H), 3.70 (d, J = 14.4 Hz, 1H), 3.48 (d, J = 14.4 Hz, 1H), 2.52 (s, 3H), 2.42 (s, 3H), 1.40 (s, 3H). ^{13}C NMR (151 MHz, CDCl$_3$) δ 179.34, 169.17, 166.61, 145.19, 142.05, 137.21, 136.50, 129.95, 129.20, 128.14, 126.77, 116.93, 62.17, 52.20, 47.90, 25.85, 24.43, 21.62.

1-Acetyl-3-methyl-5-p-tolyl-3-(tosylmethyl)-1H-pyrrol-2(3H)-one (**3g**). ^{1}H NMR (400 MHz, CDCl$_3$) δ 7.71 (d, J = 8.3 Hz, 2H), 7.27 (d, J = 8.1 Hz, 2H), 7.17 (d, J = 8.1 Hz, 2H), 7.13 (d, J = 8.3 Hz, 2H), 5.49 (s, 1H), 3.69 (d, J = 14.4 Hz, 1H), 3.45 (d, J = 14.4 Hz, 1H), 2.47 (s, 3H), 2.42 (s, 3H), 2.38 (s, 3H), 1.39 (s, 3H). ^{13}C NMR (101 MHz, CDCl$_3$) δ 179.68, 169.28, 145.03, 142.88, 138.45, 136.57, 129.90, 129.76, 128.62, 128.26, 126.71, 114.96, 62.18, 47.72, 26.09, 24.61, 21.62, 21.37.

1-Acetyl-5-(4-methoxyphenyl)-3-methyl-3-(tosylmethyl)-1H-pyrrol-2(3H)-one (**3h**). ^{1}H NMR (400 MHz, CDCl$_3$) δ 7.71 (d, J = 8.3 Hz, 2H), 7.20–7.10 (m, 2H), 6.89 (d, J = 8.8 Hz, 2H), 5.45 (s, 1H), 3.84 (s, 3H), 3.69 (d, J = 14.3 Hz, 1H), 3.45 (d, J = 14.4 Hz, 1H), 2.48 (s, 3H), 2.42 (s, 3H), 1.38 (s, 3H). ^{13}C NMR (101 MHz, CDCl$_3$) δ 179.75, 169.41, 159.75, 145.04, 142.62, 136.59, 129.89, 128.25, 128.23, 125.05, 114.47, 113.35, 62.21, 55.32, 47.64, 26.17, 24.65, 21.63.

1-Acetyl-5-(3-bromophenyl)-3-methyl-3-(tosylmethyl)-1H-pyrrol-2(3H)-one (**3i**). ^{1}H NMR (600 MHz, CDCl$_3$) δ 7.70 (d, J = 8.0 Hz, 2H), 7.47 (d, J = 7.7 Hz, 1H), 7.35 (s, 1H), 7.31 (d, J = 8.0 Hz, 2H), 7.22 (t, J = 7.9 Hz, 1H), 7.16 (d, J = 7.7 Hz, 1H), 5.51 (s, 1H), 3.69 (d, J = 14.4 Hz, 1H), 3.47 (d, J = 14.4 Hz, 1H), 2.52 (s, 3H), 2.45 (s, 3H), 1.39 (s, 3H). ^{13}C NMR (151 MHz, CDCl$_3$) δ 179.33, 169.17, 145.20, 141.52, 136.52, 134.71, 131.45, 129.99, 129.66, 129.33, 128.17, 125.56, 121.91, 116.51, 62.15, 47.79, 25.89, 24.43, 21.66.

1-Acetyl-3-methyl-5-m-tolyl-3-(tosylmethyl)-1H-pyrrol-2(3H)-one (**3j**). ^{1}H NMR (400 MHz, CDCl$_3$) δ 7.74–7.66 (m, 2H), 7.28 (d, J = 7.9 Hz, 2H), 7.24 (d, J = 7.6 Hz, 1H), 7.16 (d, J = 7.6 Hz, 1H), 7.05 (s, 1H), 7.02 (d, J = 7.6 Hz, 1H), 5.49 (s, 1H), 3.69 (d, J = 14.3 Hz, 1H), 3.46 (d, J = 14.4 Hz, 1H), 2.49 (s, 3H), 2.43 (s, 3H), 2.37 (s, 3H), 1.39 (s, 3H). ^{13}C NMR (101 MHz, CDCl$_3$) δ 179.64, 169.22, 145.03, 142.97, 137.58, 136.58, 132.58, 129.92, 129.34, 128.26, 127.76, 127.32, 123.89, 115.35, 62.17, 47.76, 26.05, 24.58, 21.63, 21.46.

1-Acetyl-5-(2-chlorophenyl)-3-methyl-3-(tosylmethyl)-1H-pyrrol-2(3H)-one (**3k**). ^{1}H NMR (600 MHz, CDCl$_3$) δ 7.78 (d, J = 8.0 Hz, 2H), 7.43 (s, 1H), 7.34 (dt, J = 14.4, 4.1 Hz, 5H), 5.68 (s, 1H), 3.66 (s, 1H), 3.44 (d, J = 14.2 Hz, 1H), 2.44 (d, J = 9.1 Hz, 6H), 1.45 (s, 3H). ^{13}C NMR (151 MHz, CDCl$_3$) δ 178.67, 168.78, 145.16, 132.80, 129.98, 129.92, 129.82, 128.88, 128.11, 126.70, 116.75, 61.92, 47.61, 25.34, 24.43, 21.61. *1-Acetyl-3-methyl-5-o-tolyl-3-(tosylmethyl)-1H-pyrrol-2(3H)-one* (**3l**). ^{1}H NMR (600 MHz, CDCl$_3$) δ 7.78 (d, J = 8.0 Hz, 2H), 7.33 (d, J = 8.0 Hz, 2H), 7.28 (d, J = 7.4 Hz, 1H), 7.19 (dd, J = 15.2, 7.4 Hz, 2H), 5.58 (s, 1H), 3.67 (d, J = 14.0 Hz, 1H), 3.42 (d, J = 14.0 Hz, 1H), 2.48 (s, 3H), 2.43 (s, 3H), 2.26 (s, 3H), 1.41 (s, 3H). ^{13}C NMR

(151 MHz, CDCl$_3$) δ 179.56, 168.91, 145.09, 136.91, 133.15, 129.98, 129.57, 128.60, 128.41, 128.00, 125.37, 115.27, 62.16, 47.39, 25.73, 24.93, 21.63, 19.80.

1-Acetyl-4-ethyl-3-methyl-5-phenyl-3-(tosylmethyl)-1H-pyrrol-2(3H)-one (**3m**). ^{1}H NMR (600 MHz, CDCl$_3$) δ 7.76 (d, *J* = 7.9 Hz, 2H), 7.39 (t, *J* = 7.3 Hz, 2H), 7.36 (d, *J* = 7.2 Hz, 1H), 7.34–7.27 (m, 4H), 3.70 (d, *J* = 14.3 Hz, 1H), 3.49 (d, *J* = 14.3 Hz, 1H), 2.44 (s, 3H), 2.43 (s, 3H), 2.21 (dd, *J* = 15.2, 7.7 Hz, 1H), 1.94 (dd, *J* = 15.0, 7.5 Hz, 1H), 1.38 (s, 3H), 0.91 (t, *J* = 7.6 Hz, 3H). ^{13}C NMR (151 MHz, CDCl$_3$) δ 179.42, 169.08, 145.02, 137.67, 136.88, 132.56, 129.92, 128.32, 128.13, 128.00, 127.93, 126.10, 61.75, 50.46, 26.18, 24.64, 21.63, 18.04, 14.58.

1-Acetyl-3-butyl-5-phenyl-3-(tosylmethyl)-1H-pyrrol-2(3H)-one (**3n**). ^{1}H NMR (600 MHz, CDCl$_3$) δ 7.70 (d, *J* = 8.1 Hz, 2H), 7.38–7.34 (m, 4H), 7.26 (d, *J* = 5.4 Hz, 5H), 5.42 (s, 1H), 3.69 (d, *J* = 14.4 Hz, 1H), 3.49 (d, *J* = 14.4 Hz, 1H), 2.49 (s, 3H), 2.41 (s, 3H), 1.75–1.67 (m, 2H), 1.27 (s, 3H), 1.11 (d, *J* = 11.6 Hz, 1H), 0.85 (t, *J* = 7.0 Hz, 3H). ^{13}C NMR (151 MHz, CDCl$_3$) δ 179.40, 169.09, 145.00, 143.77, 136.68, 132.82, 129.88, 128.48, 128.22, 127.90, 126.82, 114.00, 61.79, 51.71, 38.07, 26.05, 25.64, 22.60, 21.61, 13.75.

3-Methyl-5-phenyl-1-propionyl-3-(tosylmethyl)-1H-pyrrol-2(3H)-one (**3o**). ^{1}H NMR (600 MHz, CDCl$_3$) δ 7.70 (d, *J* = 8.2 Hz, 2H), 7.38–7.33 (m, 3H), 7.27 (d, *J* = 5.6 Hz, 2H), 7.23 (dd, *J* = 6.5, 2.9 Hz, 2H), 5.51 (s, 1H), 3.70 (d, *J* = 14.4 Hz, 1H), 3.45 (d, *J* = 14.4 Hz, 1H), 2.95–2.81 (m, 2H), 2.41 (s, 3H), 1.39 (s, 3H), 1.14 (t, *J* = 7.3 Hz, 3H). ^{13}C NMR (151 MHz, CDCl$_3$) δ 179.43, 173.23, 145.03, 143.01, 136.60, 132.85, 129.87, 128.48, 128.22, 127.93, 126.70, 115.49, 62.16, 47.83, 31.58, 24.63, 21.62, 8.33.

1-Isobutyryl-3-methyl-5-phenyl-3-(tosylmethyl)-1H-pyrrol-2(3H)-one (**3p**). ^{1}H NMR (600 MHz, CDCl$_3$) δ ^{1}H NMR (600 MHz, CDCl$_3$) δ 7.69 (d, *J* = 8.3 Hz, 2H), 7.36 (dd, *J* = 5.0, 1.8 Hz, 3H), 7.24 (d, *J* = 8.0 Hz, 2H), 7.19 (dd, *J* = 6.5, 3.1 Hz, 2H), 5.49 (s, 1H), 3.70 (d, *J* = 14.4 Hz, 1H), 3.66 (s, 1H), 3.46 (d, *J* = 14.4 Hz, 1H), 2.40 (s, 3H), 1.40 (s, 3H), 1.24 (d, *J* = 6.9 Hz, 3H), 1.18 (d, *J* = 6.8 Hz, 3H). ^{13}C NMR (151 MHz, CDCl$_3$) δ 178.91, 176.67, 144.97, 143.15, 136.68, 132.81, 129.86, 128.49, 128.18, 128.05, 126.22, 115.31, 62.11, 48.11, 35.57, 24.69, 21.62, 18.60, 18.37.

1-Acetyl-3-methyl-5-phenyl-3-(phenylsulfonylmethyl)-1H-pyrrol-2(3H)-one (**4a**). ^{1}H NMR (600 MHz, CDCl$_3$) δ 7.84 (d, *J* = 7.6 Hz, 2H), 7.63 (t, *J* = 7.4 Hz, 1H), 7.49 (t, *J* = 7.8 Hz, 2H), 7.37–7.33 (m, 3H), 7.24 (dd, *J* = 6.4, 2.6 Hz, 2H), 5.50 (s, 1H), 3.71 (d, *J* = 14.4 Hz, 1H), 3.49 (d, *J* = 14.4 Hz, 1H), 2.51 (s, 3H), 1.41 (s, 3H). ^{13}C NMR (151 MHz, CDCl$_3$) δ 179.58, 169.29, 143.05, 139.60, 133.94, 132.63, 129.30, 128.54, 128.17, 127.92, 126.76, 115.37, 62.13, 47.78, 26.07, 24.53.

1-Acetyl-3-((4-methoxyphenylsulfonyl)methyl)-3-methyl-5-phenyl-1H-pyrrol-2(3H)-one (**4b**). ^{1}H NMR (600 MHz, CDCl$_3$) δ 7.74 (d, *J* = 8.8 Hz, 2H), 7.42–7.32 (m, 3H), 6.91 (d, *J* = 8.9 Hz, 2H), 5.50 (s, 1H), 3.84 (s, 3H), 3.70 (d, *J* = 14.4 Hz, 1H), 3.45 (d, *J* = 14.4 Hz, 1H), 2.50 (s, 3H), 1.39 (s, 3H).^{13}C NMR (151 MHz, CDCl$_3$) δ 179.60, 169.30, 163.90, 142.80, 132.71, 130.90, 130.46, 128.50, 127.90, 126.77, 115.66, 114.45, 62.36, 55.73, 47.80, 26.04, 24.64.

1-Acetyl-3-((4-tert-butylphenylsulfonyl)methyl)-3-methyl-5-phenyl-1H-pyrrol-2(3H)-one (**4c**). ^{1}H NMR (600 MHz, CDCl$_3$) δ 7.73 (d, *J* = 8.5 Hz, 2H), 7.47 (d, *J* = 8.5 Hz, 2H), 7.38–7.32 (m, 3H), 7.21 (dd, *J* = 3.9, 1.8 Hz, 2H), 5.45 (s, 1H), 3.71 (d, *J* = 14.4 Hz, 1H), 3.48 (d, *J* = 14.4 Hz, 1H), 2.50 (s, 3H), 1.40 (s, 3H), 1.32 (s, 9H). ^{13}C NMR (151 MHz, CDCl$_3$) δ 179.57, 169.24, 157.94, 142.81, 136.43, 132.64, 128.49, 128.04, 127.88, 126.73, 126.32, 115.56, 62.07, 47.75, 35.27, 31.02, 26.10, 24.55.

1-Acetyl-3-methyl-5-phenyl-3-((m-tolylsulfonyl)methyl)-1,3-dihydro-2H-pyrrol-2-one (**4d**). White solid; mp 136.3–138.0 °C; ^{1}H NMR (600 MHz, CDCl$_3$) δ 7.62 (d, *J* = 11.2 Hz, 2H), 7.41 (d, *J* = 7.6 Hz, 1H), 7.39–7.33 (m, 4H), 7.24 (dd, *J* = 6.6, 2.9 Hz, 2H), 5.46 (s, 1H), 3.71 (d, *J* = 14.4 Hz, 1H), 3.48 (d, *J* = 14.4 Hz, 1H), 2.53 (s, 3H), 2.32 (s, 3H), 1.40 (s, 3H). ^{13}C NMR (151 MHz, CDCl$_3$) δ 179.65, 169.31, 143.07, 139.70, 139.47, 134.73, 132.68, 129.17, 128.54, 128.48, 127.93, 126.77, 125.22, 115.33, 62.13, 47.79, 26.08, 24.51, 21.19. HRMS (ESI, *m/z*): Calcd. For C$_{21}$H$_{21}$NSO$_4$Na [M + Na]$^+$ 406.1083, found: 406.1085.

1-Acetyl-3-(((2-methoxyphenyl)sulfonyl)methyl)-3-methyl-5-phenyl-1,3-dihydro-2H-pyrrol-2-one (**4e**). White solid; mp 123.4–125.0 °C; ^{1}H NMR (600 MHz, CDCl$_3$) δ 7.76 (dd, *J* = 7.8, 1.7 Hz, 1H), 7.59–7.53 (m, 1H), 7.34–7.29 (m, 3H), 7.12 (dd, *J* = 6.5, 3.1 Hz, 2H), 7.03 (d, *J* = 8.3 Hz, 1H), 6.95 (t, *J* = 7.6 Hz, 1H), 5.37 (s, 1H), 4.02 (s, 3H), 3.95 (d, *J* = 14.5 Hz, 1H), 3.77 (d, *J* = 14.6 Hz, 1H), 2.47 (s, 3H), 1.39 (s, 3H). ^{13}C NMR (151 MHz, CDCl$_3$) δ 179.69, 169.24,

157.38, 142.70, 135.86, 132.68, 130.67, 128.39, 127.79, 127.19, 126.65, 120.87, 115.64, 112.35, 60.13, 56.47, 47.69, 26.00, 24.55. HRMS (ESI, m/z): Calcd. For $C_{21}H_{21}NO_5SNa$ [M + Na]$^+$ 422.1033, found: 422.1038.

1-Acetyl-3-((4-bromophenylsulfonyl)methyl)-3-methyl-5-phenyl-1H-pyrrol-2(3H)-one (**4f**). ^{1}H NMR (400 MHz, CDCl$_3$) δ 7.67 (d, J = 8.0 Hz, 2H), 7.61 (d, J = 7.9 Hz, 2H), 7.36 (s, 3H), 7.22 (s, 2H), 5.48 (s, 1H), 3.70 (d, J = 14.4 Hz, 1H), 3.46 (d, J = 14.3 Hz, 1H), 2.52 (s, 3H), 1.39 (s, 3H). ^{13}C NMR (101 MHz, CDCl$_3$) δ 179.45, 169.28, 143.22, 138.49, 132.66, 132.50, 129.75, 129.44, 128.67, 128.01, 126.71, 115.17, 62.20, 47.77, 26.03, 24.57. HRMS (ESI, m/z): Calcd. For $C_{20}H_{18}NO_4SBrNa$ [M + Na]$^+$ 470.0032, found: 470.0035.

1-Acetyl-3-((4-iodophenylsulfonyl)methyl)-3-methyl-5-phenyl-1H-pyrrol-2(3H)-one (**4g**). ^{1}H NMR (600 MHz, CDCl$_3$) δ 7.84 (d, J = 8.3 Hz, 2H), 7.52 (d, J = 8.4 Hz, 2H), 7.37 (d, J = 1.6 Hz, 3H), 7.22 (d, J = 3.6 Hz, 2H), 5.49 (s, 1H), 3.70 (d, J = 14.4 Hz, 1H), 3.46 (d, J = 14.4 Hz, 1H), 2.52 (s, 3H), 1.40 (s, 3H). ^{13}C NMR (151 MHz, CDCl$_3$) δ 179.41, 169.25, 143.17, 139.09, 138.63, 132.47, 129.49, 128.65, 127.99, 126.69, 115.16, 102.04, 62.12, 47.73, 26.03, 24.58.

4-(((1-Acetyl-3-methyl-2-oxo-5-phenyl-2,3-dihydro-1H-pyrrol-3-yl)methyl)sulfonyl)benzonitrile (**4h**). White solid; mp 189.4–191.5 °C; ^{1}H NMR (600 MHz, CDCl$_3$) δ 7.94 (d, J = 8.1 Hz, 2H), 7.76 (d, J = 8.1 Hz, 2H), 7.38 (s, 3H), 7.22 (d, J = 3.2 Hz, 2H), 5.43 (s, 1H), 3.72 (d, J = 14.4 Hz, 1H), 3.52 (d, J = 14.4 Hz, 1H), 2.55 (s, 3H), 1.41 (s, 3H). ^{13}C NMR (151 MHz, CDCl$_3$) δ 179.31, 169.26, 143.63, 143.57, 133.03, 132.35, 128.87, 128.79, 128.06, 126.61, 117.72, 116.90, 114.77, 62.11, 47.75, 26.05, 24.39. HRMS (ESI, m/z): Calcd. For $C_{21}H_{18}N_2O_4SNa$ [M + Na]$^+$ 417.0879, found: 417.0883.

1-Acetyl-3-methyl-5-phenyl-3-((4(trifluoromethyl)phenylsulfonyl)methyl)-1H-pyrrol-2(3H)-one (**4i**). ^{1}H NMR (400 MHz, CDCl$_3$) δ 7.96 (d, J = 7.7 Hz, 2H), 7.74 (d, J = 7.7 Hz, 2H), 7.37 (s, 3H), 7.21 (s, 2H), 5.45 (s, 1H), 3.74 (d, J = 14.4 Hz, 1H), 3.52 (d, J = 14.4 Hz, 1H), 2.52 (s, 3H), 1.41 (s, 3H). ^{13}C NMR (101 MHz, CDCl$_3$) δ 179.35, 169.30, 143.37, 142.98, 135.63 (J = 32 Hz), 132.38, 128.86, 128.74, 128.03, 126.63, 126.48 (J = 3 Hz), 125.28 (J = 250 Hz), 114.99, 76.75, 62.08, 47.74, 26.03, 24.53. ^{19}F NMR (565 MHz, CDCl$_3$) δ-63.25.

1-Acetyl-3-methyl-3-((4-nitrophenylsulfonyl)methyl)-5-phenyl-1H-pyrrol-2(3H)-one (**4j**). ^{1}H NMR (400 MHz, CDCl$_3$) δ 8.29 (d, J = 8.1 Hz, 2H), 8.01 (d, J = 8.3 Hz, 2H), 7.37 (s, 3H), 7.22 (d, J = 3.7 Hz, 2H), 5.44 (s, 1H), 3.74 (d, J = 14.3 Hz, 1H), 3.54 (d, J = 14.4 Hz, 1H), 2.55 (s, 3H), 1.41 (s, 3H). ^{13}C NMR (101 MHz, CDCl$_3$) δ 179.29, 169.27, 150.85, 145.06, 143.63, 132.28, 129.62, 128.80, 128.06, 126.57, 124.44, 114.68, 62.16, 47.75, 26.05, 24.38.

1-Acetyl-3-((3-chlorophenylsulfonyl)methyl)-3-methyl-5-phenyl-1H-pyrrol-2(3H)-one (**4k**). ^{1}H NMR (400 MHz, CDCl$_3$) δ 7.82 (s, 1H), 7.72 (d, J = 7.3 Hz, 1H), 7.60 (d, J = 7.8 Hz, 1H), 7.43 (t, J = 7.9 Hz, 1H), 7.36 (s, 2H), 7.26 (s, 2H), 5.49 (s, 1H), 3.72 (d, J = 14.4 Hz, 1H), 3.50 (d, J = 14.4 Hz, 1H), 2.55 (s, 3H), 1.41 (s, 3H). ^{13}C NMR (101 MHz, CDCl$_3$) δ 179.45, 169.26, 143.35, 141.29, 135.56, 134.13, 132.44, 130.61, 128.60, 128.13, 127.96, 126.70, 126.27, 114.91, 62.13, 47.75, 26.08, 24.45.

1-Acetyl-3-((2-chlorophenylsulfonyl)methyl)-3-methyl-5-phenyl-1H-pyrrol-2(3H)-one (**4l**). ^{1}H NMR (400 MHz, CDCl$_3$) δ 7.91 (d, J = 7.7 Hz, 1H), 7.52 (d, J = 6.7 Hz, 2H), 7.33 (s, 3H), 7.26–7.20 (m, 1H), 7.13 (d, J = 3.3 Hz, 2H), 5.29 (s, 1H), 3.92 (s, 2H), 2.53 (s, 3H), 1.40 (s, 3H). ^{13}C NMR (101 MHz, CDCl$_3$) δ 179.38, 169.33, 143.22, 137.02, 134.93, 132.62, 132.48, 131.84, 128.52, 127.86, 127.46, 126.52, 115.06, 60.08, 47.68, 26.05, 24.38.

1-Acetyl-3-methyl-5-phenyl-3-((thiophen-2ylsulfonyl)methyl)-1H-pyrrol-2(3H)-one (**4m**). ^{1}H NMR (600 MHz, CDCl$_3$) δ 7.70 (d, J = 4.4 Hz, 1H), 7.62 (d, J = 3.0 Hz, 1H), 7.40–7.33 (m, 3H), 7.26 (d, J = 4.9 Hz, 2H), 7.11–7.02 (m, 1H), 5.59 (s, 1H), 3.82 (d, J = 14.4 Hz, 1H), 3.59 (d, J = 14.4 Hz, 1H), 2.53 (s, 3H), 1.43 (s, 3H). ^{13}C NMR (151 MHz, CDCl$_3$) δ 179.45, 169.26, 143.15, 140.70, 134.67, 134.58, 132.88, 128.55, 127.92, 126.84, 115.19, 63.58, 47.89, 26.09, 24.46.

1-Acetyl-3-(cyclopropylsulfonylmethyl)-3-methyl-5-phenyl-1H-pyrrol-2(3H)-one (**4n**). ^{1}H NMR (600 MHz, CDCl$_3$) δ 7.36–7.33 (m, 3H), 7.28 (dd, J = 6.5, 2.9 Hz, 2H), 5.72 (s, 1H), 3.62 (d, J = 14.0 Hz, 1H), 3.41 (d, J = 14.0 Hz, 1H), 2.57 (s, 3H), 2.41–2.36 (m, 1H), 1.47 (s, 3H), 1.28–1.25 (m, 1H), 1.21 (dd, J = 4.8, 1.8 Hz, 1H), 1.05–1.01 (m, 2H). ^{13}C NMR (151 MHz, CDCl$_3$) δ 179.93, 169.38, 143.37, 132.73, 128.53, 127.93, 126.93, 115.39, 59.87, 47.49, 31.27, 26.11, 24.19, 5.35, 5.14.

1-Acetyl-3-((ethylsulfonyl)methyl)-3-methyl-5-phenyl-1,3-dihydro-2H-pyrrol-2-one (**4o**). Amorphous solid; ^{1}H NMR (600 MHz, CDCl$_3$) δ 7.37–7.32 (m, 3H), 7.28 (dd, *J* = 6.6, 3.0 Hz, 2H), 5.69 (s, 1H), 3.49 (d, *J* = 13.9 Hz, 1H), 3.33 (d, *J* = 13.9 Hz, 1H), 2.98 (d, *J* = 7.5 Hz, 2H), 2.57 (s, 3H), 1.46 (s, 3H), 1.38 (t, *J* = 7.5 Hz, 3H). ^{13}C NMR (151 MHz, CDCl$_3$) δ 179.90, 169.36, 143.63, 132.75, 128.55, 127.93, 126.97, 115.02, 57.84, 49.54, 47.30, 26.11, 24.15, 6.57. HRMS (ESI, *m/z*): Calcd. For C$_{16}$H$_{19}$NSO$_4$Na [M + Na]$^+$ 344.0927, found: 344.0932.

3-Methyl-5-phenyl-3-((phenylsulfonyl)methyl)-1,3-dihydro-2H-pyrrol-2-one (**4aa**). White solid; mp 186.5–188.4 °C; ^{1}H NMR (600 MHz, CDCl$_3$) δ 8.60 (s, 1H), 7.83 (d, *J* = 7.3 Hz, 2H), 7.60 (t, *J* = 7.5 Hz, 1H), 7.48–7.42 (m, 6H), 7.39 (dd, *J* = 8.2, 5.6 Hz, 1H), 5.75 (d, *J* = 1.8 Hz, 1H), 3.61 (d, *J* = 14.3 Hz, 1H), 3.50 (d, *J* = 14.3 Hz, 1H), 1.44 (s, 3H). ^{13}C NMR (151 MHz, CDCl$_3$) δ 182.28, 139.99, 139.92, 133.78, 129.49, 129.35, 129.08, 128.94, 128.18, 124.94, 107.88, 77.24, 77.03, 76.82, 61.68, 48.27, 23.52. HRMS (ESI, *m/z*): Calcd. For C$_{18}$H$_{17}$NO$_3$SNa [M + Na]$^+$ 350.0821, found: 350.0827.

(2-Tosylethene-1,1-diyl)dibenzene. ^{1}H NMR (600 MHz, CDCl$_3$) δ 7.47 (d, *J* = 8.1 Hz, 2H), 7.37 (dd, *J* = 14.0, 7.4 Hz, 2H), 7.30 (t, *J* = 7.6 Hz, 4H), 7.20 (d, *J* = 7.6 Hz, 2H), 7.15 (d, *J* = 8.1 Hz, 2H), 7.10 (d, *J* = 7.4 Hz, 2H), 6.99 (s, 1H), 2.38 (s, 3H). ^{13}C NMR (151 MHz, CDCl$_3$) δ 154.71, 143.76, 139.26, 138.63, 135.59, 130.23, 129.79, 129.34, 128.98, 128.85, 128.65, 128.58, 128.22, 127.82, 127.71, 126.05, 21.58.

4. Conclusions

In conclusion, we developed a visible-light-induced, regioselective cascade sulfonylation/cyclization of 1,5-dienes with sulfonyl chlorides. A variety of structurally significant pyrrolinones with important classes of sulfonyl group patterns were obtained in medium to high yields. This methodology features sulfonyl radical addition/cyclization of alkenes C(sp^2)-H with high regioselectivity under very mild conditions and tolerated broad functional groups.

Supplementary Materials: The following supporting information can be downloaded at: https://www.mdpi.com/article/10.3390/molecules28145473/s1. Section S1, General information. Section S2, Procedure for the synthesis of compound **3a–3p**, **4a–4o**. Section S3, Procedures for the formation of compound **4aa**. Section S4, The Transformation with the Light ON/OFF over Time. Section S5, The radical trapping reaction residue. Section S6, NMR spectra for the products.

Author Contributions: R.D. supervised the project and wrote the manuscript; B.Z. analyzed the data and discussed with R.D. and P.-L.W.; L.L., Y.-T.Y. and R.D. conducted the experiments. All authors contributed to the revision. All authors have read and agreed to the published version of the manuscript.

Funding: We gratefully acknowledge the funding support of Anhui Province Research Funding for Outstanding Young Talents in Colleges and Universities, China (No. gxyqZD2022098), Key Laboratory of Green and Precise Synthetic Chemistry and Applications, Ministry of Education (No. 2020KF02), and Anhui Grant New Material Company (No. 9341064).

Institutional Review Board Statement: Not applicable.

Informed Consent Statement: Not applicable.

Data Availability Statement: Not applicable.

Conflicts of Interest: The authors declare no conflict of interest.

Sample Availability: Samples of the compounds are available from the authors.

References

1. Drews, J. Drug Discovery: A Historical Perspective. *Science* **2000**, *287*, 1960–1964. [CrossRef] [PubMed]
2. Metzner, P.; Thuillier, A.; Katritzky, A.; MethCohn, O.; Rees, C.W. *Sulfur Reagents in Organic Synthesis*; Academic Press: London, UK, 1994.
3. Lin, S.; Yeh, T.; Kuo, C.; Song, J.; Cheng, M.; Liao, F.; Chao, M.; Huang, H.; Chen, Y.; Yang, C.; et al. Phenyl benzenesulfonylhydrazides exhibit selective indoleamine 2,3-dioxygenase inhibition with potent in vivo pharmacodynamic activity and antitumor efficacy. *J. Med. Chem.* **2016**, *59*, 419–427. [CrossRef] [PubMed]

4. Dunny, E.; Doherty, W.; Evans, P.; Malthouse, J.; Nolan, D.; Knox, A. Vinyl sulfone-based peptidomimetics as anti-trypanosomal agents: Design, synthesis, biological and computational evaluation. *J. Med. Chem.* **2013**, *56*, 6638–6647. [CrossRef]
5. Zhao, Z.; Pissarnitski, D.; Josien, H.; Wu, W.; Xu, R.; Li, H.; Clader, J.W.; Burnett, D.A.; Terracina, G.; Hyde, L.; et al. Discovery of a novel, potent spirocyclic series of γ-secretase inhibitors. *J. Med. Chem.* **2015**, *58*, 8806–8813. [CrossRef]
6. Procopiou, P.A.; Barrett, V.; Biggadike, K.; Butchers, P.R.; Craven, A.; Ford, A.J.; Guntrip, S.; Holmes, D.; Hughes, S.; Jones, A.; et al. Discovery of a rapidly metabolized, long-acting β2 adrenergic receptor agonist with a short onset time incorporating a sulfone group suitable for once-daily dosing. *J. Med. Chem.* **2014**, *57*, 159–170. [CrossRef]
7. Yang, L.; Wang, D.-X.; Huang, Z.-T.; Wang, M.-X. Cr(III)(salen)Cl catalyzed enantioselective intramolecular addition of tertiary enamides to ketones: A general access to enantioenriched 1H-pyrrol-2(3H)-one derivatives bearing a hydroxylated quaternary carbon atom. *J. Am. Chem. Soc.* **2009**, *131*, 10390–10394. [CrossRef] [PubMed]
8. Hu, R.; Tao, Y.; Zhang, X.; Su, W. 1,2-Aryl migration induced by amide C–N bond-formation: Reaction of alkyl aryl ketones with primary amines towards α, α-diaryl β, γ-unsaturated γ-lactams. *Angew. Chem. Int. Ed.* **2021**, *60*, 8425–8428. [CrossRef]
9. Liu, Y.-H.; Song, H.; Zhang, C.; Liu, Y.-J.; Shi, B.-F. Copper-catalyzed modular access to N-fused polycyclic indoles and 5-aaroyl-pyrrol-2-ones via intramolecular N–H/C–H annulation with alkynes: Scope and mechanism probes. *Chin. J. Chem.* **2020**, *38*, 1545–1552. [CrossRef]
10. Zhao, Z.; Kong, X.; Wang, W.; Hao, J.; Wang, Y. Direct use of unprotected aliphatic amines to generate N-heterocycles via β-C–H malonylation with iodonium ylide. *Org. Lett.* **2020**, *22*, 230–234. [CrossRef]
11. Kumarasamy, E.; Raghunathan, R.; Kandappa, S.K.; Sreenithya, A.; Jockusch, S.; Sunoj, R.B.; Sivaguru, J. Transposed paternò–büchi reaction. *J. Am. Chem. Soc.* **2017**, *139*, 655–659. [CrossRef]
12. Koronatov, A.N.; Rostovskii, N.V.; Khlebnikov, A.F.; Novikov, M.S. Synthesis of 3-alkoxy-4-pyrrolin-2-ones via Rhodium(II)-catalyzed denitrogenative transannulation of 1H-1,2,3-Triazoles with diazo esters. *Org. Lett.* **2020**, *22*, 7958–7963. [CrossRef] [PubMed]
13. Song, T.; Arseniyadis, S.; Cossy, J. Asymmetric synthesis of α-quaternary γ-lactams through palladium-catalyzed asymmetric allylic alkylation. *Org. Lett.* **2019**, *21*, 603–607. [CrossRef] [PubMed]
14. Ding, R.; Mao, M.-H.; Jia, W.-Z.; Fu, J.-M.; Liu, L.; Mao, Y.-Y.; Guo, Y.; Wang, P.-L. Synthesis of sulfonylated pyrrolines and pyrrolinones via Ag mediated radical cyclization of olefinic enamides with sodium sulfinates. *Asian J. Org. Chem.* **2021**, *10*, 366–370. [CrossRef]
15. He, J.-Q.; Yang, Z.-X.; Zhou, X.-L.; Li, Y.; Gao, S.; Shi, L.; Liang, D. Exploring the regioselectivity of the cyanoalkylation of 3-aza-1,5-dienes: Photoinduced synthesis of 3-cyanoalkyl-4-pyrrolin-2-ones. *Org. Chem. Front.* **2022**, *9*, 4575–4579. [CrossRef]
16. Liu, F.; Huang, J.; Wu, X.; Du, F.; Zeng, L.; Wu, J.; Chen, J. Regioselective radical-relay sulfonylation/cyclization protocol to sulfonylated pyrrolidones under transition-metal-free conditions. *J. Org. Chem.* **2022**, *87*, 6137–6145. [CrossRef]
17. Wang, X.; You, F.; Xiong, B.; Chen, L.; Zhang, X.; Lian, Z. Metal- and base-free tandem sulfonylation/cyclization of 1,5-dienes with aryldiazonium salts via the insertion of sulfur dioxide. *RSC Adv.* **2022**, *12*, 16745–16748. [CrossRef]
18. Wang, P.; Leng, Y.; Wu, Y. Copper(I)-catalyzed regioselective tandem cyanoalkylative cyclization of 1,5-dienes with Cyclobutanone Oxime Esters. *Eur. J. Org. Chem.* **2022**, *2022*, e202201091. [CrossRef]
19. Chen, B.; Wu, L.-Z.; Tung, C.-H. Photocatalytic activation of less reactive bonds and their functionalization via hydrogen-evolution cross-couplings. *Acc. Chem. Res.* **2018**, *51*, 2512–2522. [CrossRef] [PubMed]
20. Chen, Y.; Lu, L.-Q.; Yu, D.-G.; Zhu, C.-J.; Xiao, W.-J. Visible light-driven organic photochemical synthesis in China. *Sci. China Chem.* **2019**, *62*, 2462–2468. [CrossRef]
21. Liu, Q.; Wu, L.-Z. Recent Advances in Visible-light-driven organic reactions. *Natl. Sci. Rev.* **2017**, *4*, 359–363. [CrossRef]
22. Xuan, J.; Xiao, W.-J. Visible-light photoredox catalysis. *Angew. Chem. Int. Ed.* **2012**, *51*, 6828–6832. [CrossRef] [PubMed]
23. Song, H.-Y.; Jiang, J.; Wu, C.; Hou, J.-C.; Lu, Y.-H.; Wang, K.-L.; Yang, T.-B.; He, W.-M. Semi-heterogeneous g-C_3N_4/NaI dual catalytic C–C bond formation under visible light. *Green Chem.* **2023**, *25*, 3292–3296. [CrossRef]
24. Wang, Z.; Liu, Q.; Liua, R.; Ji, Z.; Li, Y.; Zhao, X.; Wei, W. Visible-light-initiated 4CzIPN catalyzed multi component tandem reactions to assemble sulfonated quinoxalin-2(1H)-ones. *Chin. Chem. Lett.* **2022**, *33*, 1479–1482. [CrossRef]
25. Hu, X.; Tao, M.; Ma, Z.; Zhang, Y.; Li, Y.; Liang, D. Regioselective photocatalytic dialkylation/cyclization sequence of 3-aza-1,5-dienes: Access to 3,4-dialkylated 4-pyrrolin-2-ones. *Adv. Synth. Catal.* **2022**, *364*, 2163–2168. [CrossRef]
26. Cassani, C.; Bernardi, L.; Fini, F.; Ricci, A. Catalytic asymmetric mannich reactions of sulfonylacetates. *Angew. Chem. Int. Ed.* **2009**, *48*, 5694–5697. [CrossRef]
27. González, P.B.; Lopez, R.; Palomo, C. Catalytic enantioselective mannich-type reaction with β-Phenyl sulfonyl acetonitrile. *J. Org. Chem.* **2010**, *75*, 3920–3922. [CrossRef]
28. Carreno, M.C. Applications of sulfoxides to asymmetric synthesis of biologically active compounds. *Chem. Rev.* **1995**, *95*, 1717–1760. [CrossRef]
29. Liu, K.-G.; Robichaud, A.J.; Bernotas, R.C.; Yan, Y.; Lo, J.R.; Zhang, M.-Y.; Hughes, Z.A.; Huselton, C.; Zhang, G.-M.; Zhang, J.-Y.; et al. 5-Piperazinyl-3-sulfonylindazoles as potent and selective 5-hydroxytryptamine-6 antagonists. *J. Med. Chem.* **2010**, *53*, 7639–7646. [CrossRef]
30. Ivachtchenko, A.V.; Golovina, E.S.; Kadieva, M.G.; Kysil, V.M.; Mitkin, O.D.; Tkachenko, S.E.; Okun, I.M. Synthesis and structure-activity relationship (SAR) of (5,7-disubstituted 3-phenylsulfonyl-pyrazolo[1,5-a]pyrimidin-2-yl) methylamines as potent serotonin 5-HT6 receptor (5-HT6R) antagonists. *J. Med. Chem.* **2011**, *54*, 8161–8173. [CrossRef]

31. Huang, Y.; Huo, L.; Zhang, S.; Guo, X.; Han, C.C.; Li, Y.; Hou, J. Sulfonyl: A new application of electron-withdrawing substituent in highly efficient photovoltaic polymer. *Chem. Commun.* **2011**, *47*, 8904–8906. [CrossRef]
32. Barbuceanu, S.-F.; Almajan, G.L.; Saramet, I.; Draghici, C.; Tarcomnicu, A.I.; Bancescu, G. Synthesis, characterization and evaluation of antibacterial activity of some thiazolo[3,2-b][1,2,4]triazole incorporating diphenylsulfone moieties. *Eur. J. Med. Chem.* **2009**, *44*, 4752–4755. [CrossRef] [PubMed]
33. Pan, X.-Q.; Zou, J.-P.; Yi, W.-B.; Zhang, W. Recent advances in sulfur- and phosphorous-centered radical reactions for the formation of S-C and P-C bonds. *Tetrahedron* **2015**, *71*, 7481–7844. [CrossRef]
34. Fang, Y.; Luo, Z.; Xu, X. Recent advances in the synthesis of vinyl sulfones. *RSC Adv.* **2016**, *6*, 59661–59676. [CrossRef]
35. Shaaban, S.; Liang, S.; Liu, N.-W.; Manolikakes, G. Manolikakes, Synthesis of sulfones via selective C–H-functionalization. *Org. Biomol. Chem.* **2017**, *15*, 1947–1955. [CrossRef]
36. Chaudhary, R.; Natarajan, P. Visible light photoredox activation of sulfonyl chlorides: Applications in organic synthesis. *ChemistrySelect* **2017**, *2*, 6458–6472. [CrossRef]
37. Zhu, J.; Yang, W.-C.; Wang, X.-D.; Wu, L. Photoredox catalysis in c-s bond construction: Recent progress in photo-catalyzed formation of sulfones and sulfoxides. *Adv. Synth. Catal.* **2018**, *360*, 386–399. [CrossRef]
38. Lv, Y.; Cui, H.; Meng, N.; Yue, H.; Wei, W. Recent advances in the application of sulfinic acids for the construction of sulfur-containing compounds. *Chin. Chem. Lett.* **2022**, *33*, 97–109. [CrossRef]
39. Rao, W.-H.; Jiang, L.-L.; Liu, X.-M.; Chen, M.-J.; Chen, F.-Y.; Jiang, X.; Zhao, J.-X.; Zou, G.-D.; Zhou, Y.-Q.; Tang, L. Copper(II)-catalyzed alkene aminosulfonylation with sodium sulfinates for the synthesis of sulfonylated pyrrolidones. *Org. Lett.* **2019**, *21*, 2890–2893. [CrossRef]
40. Wang, L.-J.; Chen, J.-M.; Dong, W.; Hou, C.-Y.; Pang, M.; Jin, W.-B.; Dong, F.-G.; Xu, Z.-D.; Li, W. Synthesis of sulfonylated lactams by copper-mediated aminosulfonylation of 2-vinylbenzamides with sodium sulfinates. *J. Org. Chem.* **2019**, *84*, 2330–2338. [CrossRef]
41. Dong, W.; Qi, L.; Song, J.-Y.; Chen, J.-M.; Guo, J.-X.; Shen, S.; Li, L.-J.; Li, W.; Wang, L.-J. Direct synthesis of sulfonylated spiro[indole-3,3′-pyrrolidines] by silver-mediated sulfonylation of acrylamides coupled with indole dearomatization. *Org. Lett.* **2020**, *22*, 1830–1835. [CrossRef]
42. Wei, W.; Liu, C.; Yang, D.; Wen, J.; You, J.; Suo, Y.; Wang, H. Copper-catalyzed direct oxysulfonylation of alkenes with dioxygen and sulfonylhydrazides leading to β-ketosulfones. *Chem. Commun.* **2013**, *49*, 10239–10241. [CrossRef]
43. Zhu, R.; Buchwald, S.J. Versatile enantioselective synthesis of functionalized lactones via copper-catalyzed radical oxyfunctionalization of alkenes. *J. Am. Chem. Soc.* **2015**, *137*, 8069–9077. [CrossRef] [PubMed]
44. Wang, L.-J.; Chen, M.; Qi, L.; Xu, Z.; Li, W. Copper-mediated oxysulfonylation of alkenyl oximes with sodium sulfinates: A facile synthesis of isoxazolines featuring a sulfone substituent. *Chem. Commun.* **2017**, *53*, 2056–2059. [CrossRef] [PubMed]
45. Li, X.-T.; Lv, L.; Wang, T.; Gu, Q.-S.; Xu, G.-X.; Li, Z.-L.; Ye, L.; Zhang, X.; Cheng, G.-J.; Liu, X.-Y. Diastereo- and enantioselective catalytic radical oxysulfonylation of alkenes in β,γ unsaturated ketoximes. *Chem* **2020**, *6*, 1692–1706. [CrossRef]
46. Gao, Y.; Tang, X.; Peng, J.; Hu, M.; Wu, W.; Jiang, H. Copper-catalyzed oxysulfenylation of enolates with sodium sulfinates: A strategy To construct sulfenylated cyclic ethers. *Org. Lett.* **2016**, *18*, 1158–1161. [CrossRef]
47. He, F.-S.; Wu, Y.; Zhang, J.; Xia, H.; Wu, J. Thiosulfonylation of alkenes with the insertion of sulfur dioxide under non-metallic conditions. *Org. Chem. Front.* **2018**, *5*, 2940–2944. [CrossRef]
48. Niu, T.-F.; Xue, L.-S.; Jiang, D.-Y.; Ni, B.-Q. Visible-Light-Induced chemoselective synthesis of α-chloro and vinyl sulfones by sulfonylation of alkenes. *Synlett* **2018**, *29*, 364–367. [CrossRef]
49. Wang, C.; Sun, G.; Huang, H.-L.; Liu, J.; Tang, H.; Li, Y.; Hu, H.; He, S.; Gao, F. Visible-light-driven sulfonylation/cyclization to Access Sulfonylated Benzo[4,5]imidazo[2,1-a]isoquinolin-6(5H)-ones. *Chem. Asian. J.* **2021**, *16*, 2618–2622. [CrossRef]
50. Sun, B.; Tian, H.-X.; Ni, Z.-G.; Huang, P.-Y.; Ding, H.; Li, B.-Q.; Jin, C.; Wu, C.-L.; Shen, R.-P. Photocatalyst-, metal- and additive-free regioselective radical cascade sulfonylation/cyclization of benzimidazole derivatives with sulfonyl chlorides induced by visible light. *Org. Chem. Front.* **2022**, *9*, 3669–3676. [CrossRef]
51. Zhou, L.; Liu, X.; Lu, H.; Deng, G.; Liang, Y.; Yang, Y.; Li, J.-H. Copper-catalyzed [3 + 2]/[3 + 2] carboannulation of dienynes and arylsulfonyl chlorides enabled by smiles rearrangement: Access to cyclopenta[a]indene-fused quinolinones. *Org. Chem. Front.* **2021**, *8*, 5092–5097. [CrossRef]
52. Liu, X.; Cong, T.; Liu, P.; Sun, P. Visible light-promoted synthesis of 4-(sulfonylmethyl)isoquinoline-1,3(2H,4H)-diones via a tandem radical cyclization and sulfonylation reaction. *Org. Biomol. Chem.* **2016**, *14*, 9416–9422. [CrossRef] [PubMed]
53. Xia, X.-F.; Zhu, S.-L.; Wang, D.; Liang, Y.-M. Sulfide and sulfonyl chloride as sulfonylating precursors for the synthesis of sulfone-containing isoquinolinonediones. *Adv. Synth. Catal.* **2017**, *359*, 859–862. [CrossRef]
54. Liu, Y.; Wang, Q.-L.; Chen, Z.; Zhou, Q.; Li, H.; Zhou, C.-S.; Xiong, B.-Q.; Zhang, P.-L.; Tang, K.-W. Visible-light-catalyzed C−C bond difunctionalization of methylenecyclopropanes with sulfonyl chlorides for the synthesis of 3-sulfonyl-1,2-dihydronaphthalenes. *J. Org. Chem.* **2019**, *84*, 2829–2839. [CrossRef] [PubMed]
55. Mao, L.-L.; Zheng, D.-G.; Zhu, X.-H.; Zhou, A.-X.; Yang, S.-D. Visible-light-induced sulfonylation/cyclization of vinyl azides: One-pot construction of 6-(sulfonylmethyl)phenanthridines. *Org. Chem. Front.* **2018**, *5*, 232–236. [CrossRef]
56. Riggi, I.D.; Gastaldi, S.; Surzur, J.-M.; Bertrand, M.P. Chemoselective ring construction from unsymmetrical 1,6-dienes via radical addition of sulfonyl halides. *J. Org. Chem.* **1992**, *57*, 6118–6125. [CrossRef]

57. Wang, C.; Russell, G.A. Chemoselective lactam formation in the addition of benzenesulfonyl bromide to N-allyl acrylamides and N-allyl 3,3-dimethylacrylamides. *J. Org. Chem.* **1999**, *64*, 2346–2352. [CrossRef]
58. Yu, Q.; Liu, Y.; Wan, J.-P. Transition metal-free synthesis of 3-trifluoromethyl chromones via tandem C-H trifluoromethylation and chromone annulation of enaminones. *Org. Chem. Front.* **2020**, *7*, 2770–2775. [CrossRef]
59. Du, K.; Zhang, Z.; Sheng, W. Copper-Catalyzed the Synthesis of 3-Trifluoromethylchromone via Trifluoromethyl Radical Addition Tandem Cyclization Reaction of 2-Hydroxyphenyl Enaminones. *Chin. J. Org. Chem.* **2021**, *41*, 3242–3248. [CrossRef]
60. Gilmore, K.; Mohamed, R.K.; Alabugin, I.V. The Baldwin rules: Revised and extended. *Comput. Mol. Sci.* **2016**, *6*, 487–514. [CrossRef]
61. Alabugin, I.V.; Timokhin, V.I.; Abrams, J.N.; Mariappan, M.; Abrams, R.; Ghiviriga, I. In Search of Efficient 5-Endo-dig Cyclization of a Carbon-Centered Radical: 40 Years from a Prediction to Another Success for the Baldwin Rules. *J. Am. Chem. Soc.* **2008**, *130*, 10984–10995. [CrossRef]
62. Studer, A.; Curran, D.P. The electron is a catalyst. *Nat. Chem.* **2014**, *6*, 765–773. [CrossRef] [PubMed]
63. Fujiwara, Y.; Dixon, J.A.; Rodriguez, R.A.; Baxter, R.D.; Dixon, D.D.; Collins, M.R.; Blackmond, D.G.; Baran, P.S. A New Reagent for Direct Difluoromethylation. *J. Am. Chem. Soc.* **2012**, *134*, 1494–1497. [CrossRef] [PubMed]
64. Zhou, Q.; Ruffoni, A.; Gianatassio, R.; Fujiwara, Y.; Sella, E.; Shabat, D.; Baran, P.S. Direct Synthesis of Fluorinated Heteroarylether Bioisosteres. *Angew. Chem. Int. Ed.* **2013**, *52*, 3949–3952. [CrossRef] [PubMed]
65. O'Hara, F.; Blackmond, D.G.; Baran, P.S. Radical-Based Regioselective C–H Functionalization of Electron-Deficient Heteroarenes: Scope, Tunability, and Predictability. *J. Am. Chem. Soc.* **2013**, *135*, 12122–12134. [CrossRef]
66. Meyer, A.U.; Straková, K.; Slanina, T.; König, B. Eosin Y (EY) Photoredox-Catalyzed Sulfonylation of Alkenes: Scope and Mechanism. *Chem. Eur. J.* **2016**, *22*, 8694–8699. [CrossRef]
67. Terent'ev, A.O.; Mulina, O.M.; Pirgach, D.A.; Demchuk, D.V.; Syroeshkin, M.A.; Nikishin, G.I. Copper(I)-mediated synthesis of β-hydroxysulfones from styrenes and sulfonylhydrazides: An electrochemical mechanistic study. *RSC Adv.* **2016**, *6*, 93476–93485. [CrossRef]
68. Gomes, G.; Wimmer, A.; Smith, J.; König, B.; Alabugin, I.V. CO_2 or SO_2: Should It Stay, or Should It Go? *J. Org. Chem.* **2019**, *84*, 6232–6243. [CrossRef]

Disclaimer/Publisher's Note: The statements, opinions and data contained in all publications are solely those of the individual author(s) and contributor(s) and not of MDPI and/or the editor(s). MDPI and/or the editor(s) disclaim responsibility for any injury to people or property resulting from any ideas, methods, instructions or products referred to in the content.

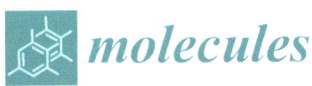

Article

First-Principles Study on Janus-Structured Sc$_2$CX$_2$/Sc$_2$CY$_2$ (X, Y = F, Cl, Br) Heterostructures for Solar Energy Conversion

Xin He [1,2], Yanan Wu [1], Jia Luo [1], Xianglin Dai [1], Jun Song [1,2] and Yong Tang [1,2,*]

[1] School of Energy Engineering, Huanghuai University, Zhumadian 463000, China; 20202086@huanghuai.edu.cn (X.H.); wuyanan@huanghuai.edu.cn (Y.W.); 10505182024@163.com (J.L.); 20202131@huanghuai.edu.cu (X.D.); songjunaa@163.com (J.S.)
[2] Henan Key Laboratory of Smart Lighting, Huanghuai University, Zhumadian 463000, China
* Correspondence: 20202127@huanghuai.edu.cn

Abstract: Two-dimensional van der Waals heterostructures have good application prospects in solar energy conversion due to their excellent optoelectronic performance. In this work, the electronic structures of Sc$_2$CF$_2$/Sc$_2$CCl$_2$, Sc$_2$CF$_2$/Sc$_2$CBr$_2$, and Sc$_2$CCl$_2$/Sc$_2$CBr$_2$ heterostructures, as well as their properties in photocatalysis and IIphotovoltaics, have been comprehensively studied using the first-principles method. Firstly, both of the three thermodynamically and dynamically stable heterostructures are found to have type-II band alignment with band gap values of 0.58 eV, 0.78 eV, and 1.35 eV. Meanwhile, the photogenerated carriers in Sc$_2$CF$_2$/Sc$_2$CCl$_2$ and Sc$_2$CF$_2$/Sc$_2$CBr$_2$ heterostructures are predicated to follow the direct Z-scheme path, enabling their abilities for water splitting. As for the Sc$_2$CCl$_2$/Sc$_2$CBr$_2$ heterostructure, its photovoltaic conversion efficiency is estimated to be 20.78%. Significantly, the light absorption coefficients of Sc$_2$CF$_2$/Sc$_2$CCl$_2$, Sc$_2$CF$_2$/Sc$_2$CBr$_2$, and Sc$_2$CCl$_2$/Sc$_2$CBr$_2$ heterostructures are enhanced more than those of the corresponding monolayers. Moreover, biaxial strains have been observed to considerably tune the aforementioned properties of heterostructures. All the theoretical results presented in this work demonstrate the application potential of Sc$_2$CX$_2$/Sc$_2$CY$_2$ (X, Y = F, Cl, Br) heterostructures in photocatalysis and photovoltaics.

Keywords: Sc$_2$CX$_2$/Sc$_2$CY$_2$ (X, Y = F, Cl, Br) heterostructures; first-principles calculations; direct Z-scheme photocatalyst; photovoltaic applications

Citation: He, X.; Wu, Y.; Luo, J.; Dai, X.; Song, J.; Tang, Y. First-Principles Study on Janus-Structured Sc$_2$CX$_2$/Sc$_2$CY$_2$ (X, Y = F, Cl, Br) Heterostructures for Solar Energy Conversion. *Molecules* **2024**, *29*, 2898. https://doi.org/10.3390/molecules29122898

Academic Editor: Sugang Meng

Received: 16 May 2024
Revised: 14 June 2024
Accepted: 17 June 2024
Published: 18 June 2024

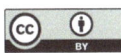

Copyright: © 2024 by the authors. Licensee MDPI, Basel, Switzerland. This article is an open access article distributed under the terms and conditions of the Creative Commons Attribution (CC BY) license (https://creativecommons.org/licenses/by/4.0/).

1. Introduction

With the depletion of traditional fossil fuels and the escalating global energy crisis, it is imperative and urgent to explore green and renewable energy sources. The use of semiconductor materials in applications such as photocatalysis or solar cells to convert abundant solar energy into clean power holds significant promise [1]. For instance, Fujishima and Honda were pioneers in demonstrating that TiO$_2$ could serve as a photocatalyst for water splitting [2]. Nevertheless, the efficiency of TiO$_2$ in converting solar energy to hydrogen is hindered by its wide band gap and high rate of carrier recombination. Chapin et al. were the first to create a solar cell using single-crystal silicon as the primary material. However, the photoelectric conversion efficiency (PCE) was disappointingly low, measuring only 6% [3]. As a result, the quest for suitable materials for photocatalysis and photovoltaics has been a prominent research area for a considerable period of time.

The discovery of graphene has sparked researchers' interest in two-dimensional (2D) materials [4,5]. The 2D materials demonstrate amazing properties, including high carrier mobility, a semiconducting band gap, prominent catalytic activities, and abundant active sites. Therefore, they can be utilized in the fields of photocatalytic water splitting and photovoltaics. At present, many 2D materials have been synthesized experimentally or theoretically, such as transition metal carbides/nitrides (MXenes) [6], transition metal dichalcogenides (TMDCs) [7], hexagonal boron nitride (h-BN) [8], black phosphorus (BP) [9], and silicene [10]. However, 2D materials have a large band gap, poor light absorption capacity, and a high carrier recombination rate, thereby leading to low efficiency. Therefore, various strategic techniques such as doping [11], metal loading [12], and constructing heterostructures have been proposed. Among these strategies, constructing van der Waals (vdW) heterostructures with type-II band alignment has promising applications in the fields of photocatalytic water splitting and solar cells due to the lower exciton binding energy and enhanced optical absorbance compared to monolayers [13]. In type-II heterostructures, the photogenerated electron–hole pairs are separated onto different monolayers, which significantly reduces the carrier recombination rate. With the deepening of research, direct Z-scheme heterostructures can be designed by selecting two appropriate monolayer materials. In the Z-scheme heterostructure, photogenerated electrons and holes accumulate on the surfaces of distinct monolayers. The Z-scheme heterostructure not only possesses a strong redox ability to drive photocatalytic reactions but also provides active sites for spatially separated oxidation and reduction processes [14]. This mechanism significantly enhances the efficiency of water splitting in the heterostructure. According to previous research, the narrow band gap of the direct Z-scheme heterostructures can achieve a broader range of solar energy harvesting [15]. The Z-scheme heterostructures show great promise in photocatalytic water splitting, photocatalytic reduction of carbon dioxide, and environmental remediation [16,17]. In recent years, more and more Z-scheme heterostructures have been discovered and studied. Indeed, examples such as the WO_3/Bi_2MoO_6 heterostructure [18], β-$SnSe/HfS_2$ heterostructure [19], $GaSe/ZrS_2$ heterostructure [20], $MoSTe/g$-GeC heterostructure [21], GeC/BSe heterostructure [22], and SnC/PtS_2 heterostructure [23] all represent direct Z-scheme heterostructures.

On the other hand, MXenes have been widely explored in applications such as photocatalysts, solar cells, heavy-metal removal, battery anodes, and electromagnetic interference shielding. MXenes are produced from their corresponding MAX phases, where M represents an early transition metal, A represents a group of IIIA or IVA elements, and X represents a C or N atom [24]. MXenes have attracted increasing attention due to their excellent stability and large specific surface area. In the field of photocatalysis, heterostructures based on MXenes, such as $Cs_2AgBiBr_6/Ti_3C_2T_x$ [25], Hf_2CO_2/WS_2 [26], AsP/Sc_2CO_2 [27], and $Sc_2CF_2/MoSSe$ [28], exhibit superior electronic properties. For the application of solar cells, Wen et al. demonstrated that the PCE of Hf_2CO_2/MoS_2 and Zr_2CO_2/MoS_2 heterostructures in solar cell applications was 19.75% and 17.13%, respectively [29]. The PCE of Ti_2CO_2/Zr_2CO_2 and Ti_2CO_2/Hf_2CO_2 heterostructures reaches 22.74% and 19.56%, respectively [30]. This indicates that MXenes have promising potential for applications as photovoltaic materials. Pure Sc_2C exhibits metallic properties; however, after functionalization by F, Cl, and Br atoms, Sc_2CF_2, Sc_2CCl_2, and Sc_2CBr_2 exhibit semiconductor characteristics with band gaps of 1.85 eV, 1.70 eV, and 1.54 eV, respectively [31]. As a member of MXenes, Sc_2CX_2 (X = F, Cl, Br) exhibits kinetic and thermal stabilities, which have potential applications in photocatalytic water splitting and solar cells [32]. However, the Sc_2CF_2 monolayer cannot facilitate the oxygen evolution reaction (OER) because its valence band maximum (VBM) is higher than that of $E_{O2/H2O}$. For Sc_2CCl_2 and Sc_2CBr_2 monolayers, the conduction band minimum (CBM) is lower than $E_{H+/H2}$, which renders them unable to meet the requirements for the HER. The construction of heterostructures using Sc_2CF_2, Sc_2CCl_2, and Sc_2CBr_2 not only addresses the mentioned deficiency of materials but also shows significant potential for photocatalytic and optoelectronic applications. Zhang et al. investigated the electrical and optical properties of $Sc_2CF_2/WSSe$ heterostructures and found that they have the potential for water splitting [33]. In addition, Sun et al. revealed that the PCE of the Sc_2CCl_2/SiS_2 heterostructure can reach 23.20%, indicating promising prospects for application in the field of solar cells [34]. It is noteworthy that the VBM and CBM of the Sc_2CF_2 monolayer are higher than those of the Sc_2CCl_2 (or Sc_2CBr_2) monolayer, and the VBM and CBM of the Sc_2CBr_2 monolayer are higher than those of the Sc_2CCl_2 monolayer. This indicates that the Sc_2CF_2/Sc_2CCl_2, Sc_2CF_2/Sc_2CBr_2, and Sc_2CCl_2/Sc_2CBr_2 heterostructures may have a type-II band alignment. In addition, the CBM in Sc_2CCl_2 (or Sc_2CBr_2) and the VBM in Sc_2CF_2 are very close. This suggests that photogenerated carrier transfer in the Sc_2CF_2/Sc_2CCl_2 and Sc_2CF_2/Sc_2CBr_2 heterostructures may follow the Z-scheme pathway. Therefore, it is worthwhile to study the Sc_2CF_2/Sc_2CCl_2, Sc_2CF_2/Sc_2CBr_2, and Sc_2CCl_2/Sc_2CBr_2 heterostructures. Their potential applications in photocatalytic water splitting and solar cells show great promise.

In this paper, three types of monolayers, namely Sc_2CF_2, Sc_2CCl_2, and Sc_2CBr_2, were successfully vertically stacked to create Sc_2CF_2/Sc_2CCl_2, Sc_2CF_2/Sc_2CBr_2, and Sc_2CCl_2/Sc_2CBr_2 heterostructures. The stacking geometries, electronic, and optical properties of the heterostructures have been systematically studied based on first-principles calculations. According to band edge alignment and charge carrier transfer processes, the Sc_2CF_2/Sc_2CCl_2 and Sc_2CF_2/Sc_2CBr_2 heterostructures were found to have a direct Z-scheme band alignment, making them promising for photocatalytic water splitting applications. On the other hand, the Sc_2CCl_2/Sc_2CBr_2 heterostructure showed potential for use in solar cells, with a notable PCE of 20.78%. The present findings indicate that Sc_2CX_2/Sc_2CY_2 (X, Y = F, Cl, Br) heterostructures have the potential for application in solar energy conversion.

2. Computation Details

In this paper, all calculations are carried out using the projection enhanced wave method based on density functional theory (DFT) [35], as implemented in the Vienna Ab initio Simulation Package (VASP5.4.4) [36]. Electron–ion interactions were explained using the projected augmented wave pseudopotential (PAW), while the exchange potential and the correlation potential were described using the generalized gradient approximation (GGA) with Perdew–Burke–Ernzerhof (PBE) functional [37]. The valence electron configurations of Sc, C, F, Cl, and Br atoms are $3p^63d^14s^2$, $2s^22p^2$, $2s^22p^5$, $3s^23p^5$, and $4s^24p^5$, respectively. The energy cutoff for obtaining the relaxed lattice vector and atomic positions was set to 500 eV. All geometrical structures were relaxed until the forces and energy on each atom converged to 0.01 eV Å^{-1} and 10^{-5} eV, respectively. For the calculation of heterostructures, we utilized the DFT-D3 method to treat the interlayer vdW interaction [38]. The K-point grid for energy convergence was set to $15 \times 15 \times 1$ for structural optimization. A vacuum layer of 20 Å was arranged along the z-axis to eliminate interactions between adjacent layers. The Heyd–Scuseria–Ernzerh (HSE06) hybrid functional was used to calculate accurate electronic and optical properties [39]. The thermal stability of the Sc_2CF_2/Sc_2CCl_2, Sc_2CF_2/Sc_2CBr_2, and Sc_2CCl_2/Sc_2CBr_2 heterostructures was further evaluated through ab initio molecular dynamics (AIMD) simulations with the NVT ensemble [40,41]. AIMD simulations were performed using a $4 \times 4 \times 1$ supercell at 300 K. In our AIMD simulation, a total simulation time of 6 ps with a time step of 1 fs was set.

3. Results and Discussion

The structural parameters and electronic properties of Sc_2CX_2 (X = F, Cl, Br) were initially studied. The atomic structures of optimized Sc_2CX_2 (X = F, Cl, Br) monolayers are displayed in Figure 1a. The lattice constant of the Sc_2CF_2 monolayer was determined to be 3.235 Å, which closely matches the theoretical value of 3.26 Å, as reported by Khang et al. [42]. The corresponding result of 3.422/3.499 Å for the Sc_2CCl_2/Sc_2CBr_2 monolayer is close to the previous theoretical value of 3.42/3.507 Å [31,43]. When the surface groups change from F to Br, the lattice parameters increase slightly due to the increase in the halogen atomic radius [31]. In addition, the band structures of the Sc_2CX_2 (X = F, Cl, Br) monolayers were calculated using the HSE06 method, as displayed in Figure 1b–d. It can be distinctly observed that the band shapes are fundamentally the same, despite the differences in band gap values. Moreover, we can observe that Sc_2CX_2 (X = F, Cl, Br) monolayers are all indirect band gap semiconductors. The CBM and VBM of the Sc_2CX_2 (X = F, Cl, Br) monolayers are located at the M point and Γ point, with corresponding band gaps of 1.80 eV, 1.70 eV, and 1.55 eV, respectively. All band gap values are in good agreement with the earlier reports, with percentage differences of less than 2% [32,44,45]. The results verify the rationality of our approach and parameterization.

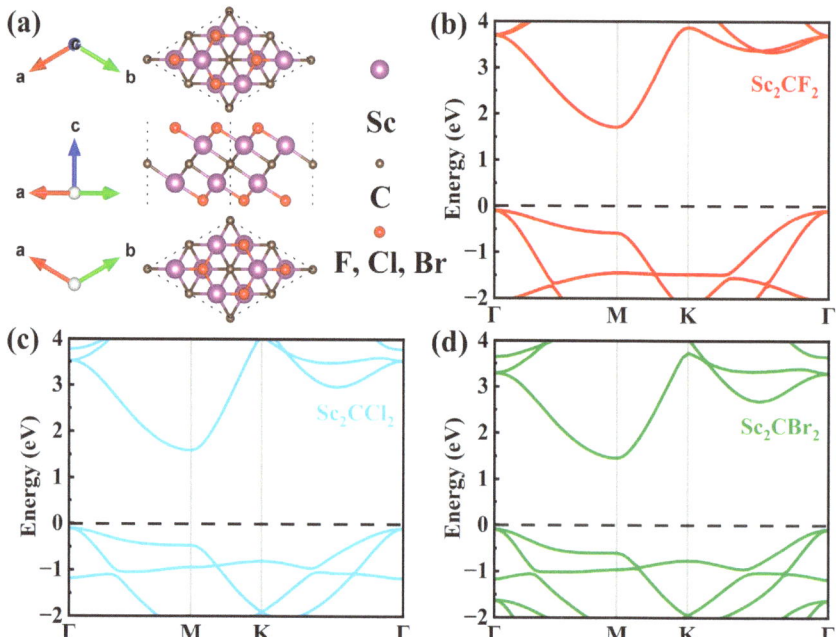

Figure 1. (a) Top view, side view, and bottom view of single-layer Sc_2CX_2 (X = F, Cl, Br). The band structures of (b) Sc_2CF_2, (c) Sc_2CCl_2, and (d) Sc_2CBr_2 monolayers.

Then, the structural properties of Sc_2CF_2/Sc_2CCl_2, Sc_2CF_2/Sc_2CBr_2, and Sc_2CCl_2/Sc_2CBr_2 heterostructures were researched in pursuit of the most stable configuration. There are three typical stacking configurations for all three heterostructures, i.e., A, B, and C, as illustrated in Figure 2. The structure coordinate information (POSCAR) is provided in Table S1. Table 1 presents various parameters associated with different stackings. For each heterostructure, the lattice constants of the three configurations closely match the lattice constants of the corresponding monolayer. In order to assess the stability of the heterostructures and determine the most stable configurations, the binding energy (E_b) values of all configurations are computed as follows:

$$E_b = \frac{E_H - E_{Sc_2CX_2} - E_{Sc_2CY_2}}{S_0}$$

where E_H represents the energy of the Sc_2CF_2/Sc_2CCl_2, Sc_2CF_2/Sc_2CBr_2, and Sc_2CCl_2/Sc_2CBr_2 heterostructures, respectively. Here, S_0 represents the interface area, while $E_{Sc_2CX_2}$ and $E_{Sc_2CY_2}$ represent the energy of the Sc_2CF_2, Sc_2CCl_2, and Sc_2CBr_2 monolayers, respectively. From Table 1, we can see that the minus E_b values for all stacking configurations manifest that the interface formation is exothermic, which is favorable for their preparation [46]. Clearly, for Sc_2CF_2/Sc_2CCl_2, Sc_2CF_2/Sc_2CBr_2, and Sc_2CCl_2/Sc_2CBr_2 heterostructures, stacking-B exhibits the smallest E_b of -35.67 meV·Å^{-2}, -28.53 meV·Å^{-2}, and -19.96 meV·Å^{-2}, indicating that stacking-B is the most stable among the three stacking configurations. In addition, this value is smaller than the previously reported $C_2N/ZnSe$ heterostructure (-12.1 meV·Å^{-2}) [47] and BiTeCl/GeSe heterostructure (-11.07 meV·Å^{-2}) [48], revealing that Sc_2CF_2/Sc_2CCl_2, Sc_2CF_2/Sc_2CBr_2, and Sc_2CCl_2/Sc_2CBr_2 are vdW heterostructures. Thus, only the stacking-B heterostructure was taken into consideration in all the following calculations. Indispensably, AIMD simulations are performed to validate the thermodynamic stability of the heterostructure. As depicted in Figure S1, the geometrical structures of the Sc_2CF_2/Sc_2CCl_2, Sc_2CF_2/Sc_2CBr_2, and Sc_2CCl_2/Sc_2CBr_2 heterostructures remained stable during the 6 ps simulation at a temperature of 300 K. No bonds were broken, and the energy fluctuation was minimal, indicating that each heterostructure is sufficiently stable at room temperature. Furthermore, to verify the dynamical stability of the Sc_2CF_2/Sc_2CCl_2, Sc_2CF_2/Sc_2CBr_2, and Sc_2CCl_2/Sc_2CBr_2 heterostructures, we calculated their phonon spectrum with a $3 \times 3 \times 1$ supercell and implemented them in the PHONOPY code with the density functional perturbation theory (DFPT), as shown in Figure S2. It can be seen that there are some insignificant imaginary frequencies near the G-point. This phenomenon also exists in the phonon spectra of some experimentally prepared 2D materials, but the imaginary frequency near the G-point can be ignored [49–51]. This phenomenon may be attributed to inadequate computational accuracy, which can be eliminated by creating a larger supercell or setting a higher parameter accuracy. Thus, the Sc_2CF_2/Sc_2CCl_2, Sc_2CF_2/Sc_2CBr_2, and Sc_2CCl_2/Sc_2CBr_2 heterostructures are dynamically stable.

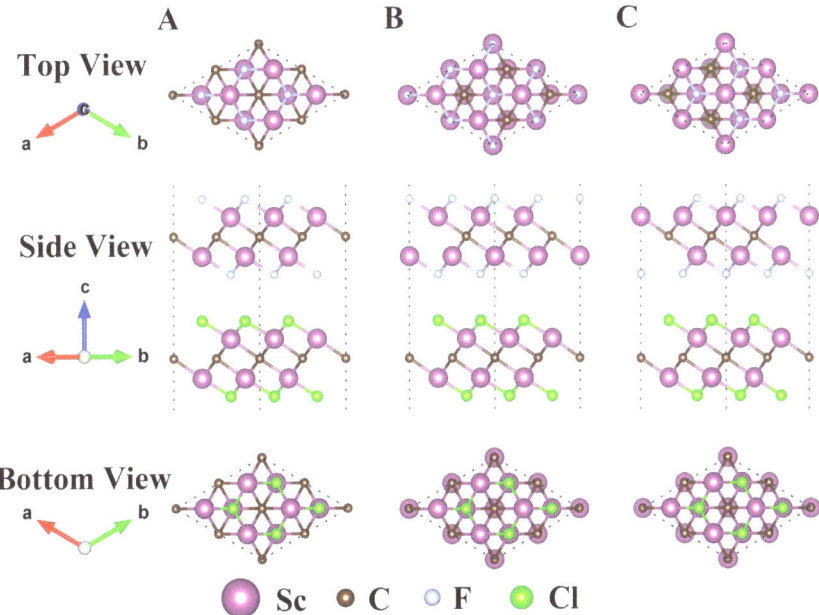

Figure 2. Top, side, and bottom views of the Sc_2CF_2/Sc_2CCl_2 heterostructure with three different stacking configurations of A, B, and C. The stacking configurations of Sc_2CF_2/Sc_2CBr_2 and Sc_2CCl_2/Sc_2CBr_2 heterostructures are similar to those of the Sc_2CF_2/Sc_2CCl_2 heterostructure.

The projected band structures of Sc_2CF_2/Sc_2CCl_2, Sc_2CF_2/Sc_2CBr_2, and Sc_2CCl_2/Sc_2CBr_2 heterostructures were calculated based on the HSE06 hybrid functional, as depicted in Figure 3a–c. It can be found that the Sc_2CF_2/Sc_2CCl_2, Sc_2CF_2/Sc_2CBr_2, and Sc_2CCl_2/Sc_2CBr_2 heterostructures all show the characteristics of semiconductors with indirect band structures. The VBM and CBM are located at the M point and Γ point, with band gaps of 0.58 eV, 0.78 eV, and 1.35 eV, respectively. Compared with the band gaps of monolayers, the significantly reduced band gaps of heterostructures are due to the interaction of vdW forces, which lead to a change in the band structure upon contact [21]. It should be noted that the smaller band gap of Sc_2CF_2/Sc_2CCl_2 and Sc_2CF_2/Sc_2CBr_2 heterostructures can lead to improved optical absorption performance during the photocatalytic reaction process. In addition, we can clearly see that the VBM and CBM of the three heterostructures are each occupied by two monolayers, demonstrating an inherent type-II heterostructure. Among them, the VBM of Sc_2CF_2/Sc_2CCl_2 and Sc_2CF_2/Sc_2CBr_2 heterostructures is mainly attributed to the Sc_2CF_2 monolayer, while the CBM mainly comes from the Sc_2CCl_2 (or Sc_2CBr_2) monolayer. Hence, electrons mainly occupy Sc_2CCl_2 (or Sc_2CBr_2), while holes mainly occupy Sc_2CF_2. Similarly, the VBM of the Sc_2CCl_2/Sc_2CBr_2 heterostructure is mainly contributed by the Sc$_2$CBr$_2$ layer, whereas the CBM is entirely dominated by the Sc$_2$CCl$_2$ layer. It is certain that the type-II band structures can separate the photoexcited electrons and holes into different monolayers, which is conducive to reducing the carrier recombination rate. This separation can improve the utilization of photogenerated carriers and extend their lifetime [44].

Table 1. The lattice constants, layer spacing (d), and binding energy (E_b) of three possible stackings in Sc$_2$CF$_2$/Sc$_2$CCl$_2$, Sc$_2$CF$_2$/Sc$_2$CBr$_2$, and Sc$_2$CCl$_2$/Sc$_2$CBr$_2$ heterostructures.

System	Configuration	Lattice Constants a (Å)	d (Å)	E_b (meV*Å^{-2})
Sc$_2$CF$_2$	-	3.235	-	-
Sc$_2$CCl$_2$	-	3.422	-	-
Sc$_2$CBr$_2$	-	3.499	-	-
Sc$_2$CF$_2$/Sc$_2$CCl$_2$	A	3.321	2.74	−35.06
	B	3.320	3.13	−35.67
	C	3.321	2.69	−34.77
Sc$_2$CF$_2$/Sc$_2$CBr$_2$	A	3.356	2.84	−27.74
	B	3.356	3.24	−28.53
	C	3.357	2.81	−27.35
Sc$_2$CCl$_2$/Sc$_2$CBr$_2$	A	3.458	3.23	−19.36
	B	3.458	3.62	−19.96
	C	3.459	3.20	−18.90

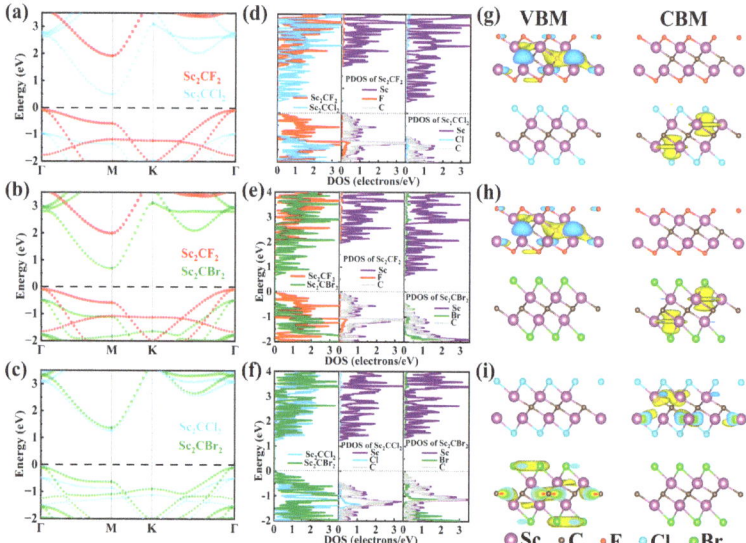

Figure 3. The projected band alignments of the (**a**) Sc$_2$CF$_2$/Sc$_2$CCl$_2$ heterostructure, (**b**) Sc$_2$CF$_2$/Sc$_2$CBr$_2$ heterostructure, and (**c**) Sc$_2$CCl$_2$/Sc$_2$CBr$_2$ heterostructures. (**d–f**) The PDOS of the Sc$_2$CF$_2$/Sc$_2$CCl$_2$, Sc$_2$CF$_2$/Sc$_2$CBr$_2$, and Sc$_2$CCl$_2$/Sc$_2$CBr$_2$ heterostructures. (**g–i**) The visualization of band decomposed charge density for Sc$_2$CF$_2$/Sc$_2$CCl$_2$, Sc$_2$CF$_2$/Sc$_2$CBr$_2$, and Sc$_2$CCl$_2$/Sc$_2$CBr$_2$ heterostructures, respectively.

In addition, Figure 3d–f shows the projected density of states (PDOS) of the Sc$_2$CF$_2$/Sc$_2$CCl$_2$, Sc$_2$CF$_2$/Sc$_2$CBr$_2$, and Sc$_2$CCl$_2$/Sc$_2$CBr$_2$ heterostructures, respectively. From Figure 3d, it can be seen that in the Sc$_2$CF$_2$/Sc$_2$CCl$_2$ heterostructure, the peak with the highest energy below the Fermi level mainly originates from the Sc and C atoms in Sc$_2$CF$_2$, while the peak with the lowest energy above the Fermi level is mainly contributed by the Sc atom in Sc$_2$CCl$_2$. This shows that the VBM of the Sc$_2$CF$_2$/Sc$_2$CCl$_2$ heterostructure is contributed by the Sc$_2$CF$_2$, while the CBM is contributed by the Sc$_2$CCl$_2$. As shown in Figure 3e, the VBM of the Sc$_2$CF$_2$/Sc$_2$CBr$_2$ heterostructure is mainly contributed by the Sc and C atoms of Sc$_2$CF$_2$, while the CBM mainly comes from the Sc atom of Sc$_2$CBr$_2$. This indicates that the VBM of the Sc$_2$CF$_2$/Sc$_2$CBr$_2$ heterostructure comes from the electronic states of Sc$_2$CF$_2$, while the CBM comes from the electronic states of Sc$_2$CBr$_2$. In Figure 3f, we can clearly observe that the CBM of the Sc$_2$CCl$_2$/Sc$_2$CBr$_2$ configuration is contributed by the Sc atom of Sc$_2$CCl$_2$. However, the VBM is not only contributed by the Sc and C atoms but also by the Br atom. This shows that the VBM of the Sc$_2$CCl$_2$/Sc$_2$CBr$_2$ heterostructure originates from the Sc$_2$CBr$_2$ monolayer, while the CBM comes from the Sc$_2$CCl$_2$ monolayer. In addition, the orbitals of the C atom and Sc atom are completely hybridized. This PDOS result further confirms that the CBM and VBM of Sc$_2$CF$_2$/Sc$_2$CCl$_2$, Sc$_2$CF$_2$/Sc$_2$CBr$_2$, and Sc$_2$CCl$_2$/Sc$_2$CBr$_2$ heterostructures are located on different monolayers.

In Figure 3g–i, we displayed the band decomposed charge densities of the VBM and CBM in Sc$_2$CF$_2$/Sc$_2$CCl$_2$, Sc$_2$CF$_2$/Sc$_2$CBr$_2$, and Sc$_2$CCl$_2$/Sc$_2$CBr$_2$ heterostructures, respectively. In Sc$_2$CF$_2$/Sc$_2$CCl$_2$ and Sc$_2$CF$_2$/Sc$_2$CBr$_2$ heterostructures, it can be observed that the VBM is located in Sc$_2$CF$_2$, while the CBM is located in Sc$_2$CCl$_2$ (or Sc$_2$CBr$_2$). Consistent with the above analysis, the VBM and CBM of the Sc$_2$CCl$_2$/Sc$_2$CBr$_2$ heterostructure are located on the lower layer (Sc$_2$CBr$_2$) and upper layer (Sc$_2$CCl$_2$), respectively. There is no charge density overlap between the VBM and CBM, indicating that heterostructures like Sc$_2$CF$_2$/Sc$_2$CCl$_2$, Sc$_2$CF$_2$/Sc$_2$CBr$_2$, and Sc$_2$CCl$_2$/Sc$_2$CBr$_2$ can effectively separate electrons and holes [52].

The above analysis shows that the Sc$_2$CF$_2$/Sc$_2$CCl$_2$, Sc$_2$CF$_2$/Sc$_2$CBr$_2$, and Sc$_2$CCl$_2$/Sc$_2$CBr$_2$ heterostructures exhibit staggered type-II band alignment. This structure can promote the effective separation of holes and electrons, reduce the carrier recombination rate, and play an important role in photocatalytic water splitting and optoelectronic devices.

The difference in work functions between two semiconductors can lead to charge redistribution and the formation of an electric field at the interface. This electric field will determine the transfer process of photogenerated charges. Thus, the work functions of the Sc$_2$CF$_2$, Sc$_2$CCl$_2$, and Sc$_2$CBr$_2$ monolayers, as well as the Sc$_2$CF$_2$/Sc$_2$CCl$_2$, Sc$_2$CF$_2$/Sc$_2$CBr$_2$, and Sc$_2$CCl$_2$/Sc$_2$CBr$_2$ heterostructures, are calculated using the following formula:

$$\Phi = E_{vac} - E_F$$

in which E_{vac} and E_F represent the vacuum level and Fermi level, respectively. As shown in Figure S3a–c, Sc$_2$CF$_2$, Sc$_2$CCl$_2$, and Sc$_2$CBr$_2$ monolayers exhibit a fixed work function of 5.02 eV, 5.86 eV, and 5.48 eV, respectively, due to their highly symmetrical crystal structure [28]. Compared to Sc$_2$CCl$_2$ and Sc$_2$CBr$_2$ monolayers, the Sc$_2$CF$_2$ monolayer exhibits a smaller work function and a higher Fermi level. Thus, in the Sc$_2$CF$_2$/Sc$_2$CCl$_2$ and Sc$_2$CF$_2$/Sc$_2$CBr$_2$ heterostructures, free electrons can migrate from Sc$_2$CF$_2$ to Sc$_2$CCl$_2$ (or Sc$_2$CBr$_2$) until their Fermi levels reach equilibrium. As shown in Figure 4a,b, the work functions of the Sc$_2$CF$_2$/Sc$_2$CCl$_2$ and Sc$_2$CF$_2$/Sc$_2$CBr$_2$ heterostructures are 5.19 eV and 4.99 eV, respectively. At the same time, there are potential drops of 5.43 eV and 3.25 eV at the Sc$_2$CF$_2$/Sc$_2$CCl$_2$ and Sc$_2$CF$_2$/Sc$_2$CBr$_2$ heterostructures, indicating the presence of a built-in electric field at the interface of the heterostructures [52]. It also indicates that electrons are inclined to flow to Sc$_2$CCl$_2$ (or Sc$_2$CBr$_2$) monolayers. The built-in electric field will create a driving force to promote the combination of photogenerated electron–hole pairs between the electrons in the CBM of Sc$_2$CCl$_2$ (or Sc$_2$CBr$_2$) and the holes in the VBM of Sc$_2$CF$_2$. As displayed in Figure 4c, the difference in monolayer work function leads to the transfer of electrons from Sc$_2$CBr$_2$ to Sc$_2$CCl$_2$, causing a decline in the Fermi level in Sc$_2$CCl$_2$ and Sc$_2$CBr$_2$. The work function of the heterostructure in the final equilibrium state is 5.34 eV. Moreover, a potential drop of 2.12 eV is found across the interface. This is proof of a built-in electric field at the interface of the Sc$_2$CCl$_2$/Sc$_2$CBr$_2$ heterostructure.

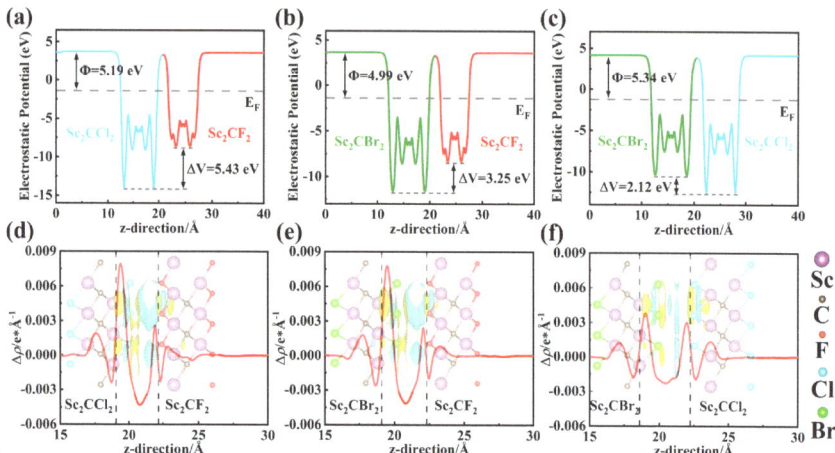

Figure 4. (**a**–**c**) The electrostatic potential along the z-axis direction of Sc_2CF_2/Sc_2CCl_2, Sc_2CF_2/Sc_2CBr_2, and Sc_2CCl_2/Sc_2CBr_2 heterostructures. (**d**–**f**) The plane-averaged charge density difference of Sc_2CF_2/Sc_2CCl_2, Sc_2CF_2/Sc_2CBr_2, and Sc_2CCl_2/Sc_2CBr_2 heterostructures. The insert is the 3D view of the charge density difference, where the yellow and blue represent the regions of electron accumulation and depletion, respectively.

During the formation of a heterostructure, the charge near the interface will be redistributed due to the presence of interlayer interactions. In order to explore the charge transfer mechanism of Sc_2CF_2/Sc_2CCl_2, Sc_2CF_2/Sc_2CBr_2, and Sc_2CCl_2/Sc_2CBr_2 heterostructures, the planar averaged charge density difference and 3D differential charge density difference were calculated using the following equation:

$$\Delta\rho = \rho_{het} - \rho_{SCX} - \rho_{SCY},$$

where the ρ_{het} stand for the density of Sc_2CF_2/Sc_2CCl_2, Sc_2CF_2/Sc_2CBr_2, and Sc_2CCl_2/Sc_2CBr_2 heterostructures, and the ρ_{SCX} and ρ_{SCY} represent the corresponding densities of Sc_2CF_2, Sc_2CCl_2, and Sc_2CBr_2 monolayers. As shown in Figure 4d,e, for Sc_2CF_2/Sc_2CCl_2 and Sc_2CF_2/Sc_2CBr_2, it can be clearly seen that a large number of negative charges are assembled in the side of Sc_2CCl_2 (or Sc_2CBr_2) monolayers, while positive charges cluster on the side of Sc_2CF_2. This leads to the formation of a built-in electric field from Sc_2CF_2 to Sc_2CCl_2 (or Sc_2CBr_2). As shown in Figure 4f, the electrons at the interface are depleted near the Sc_2CBr_2 monolayer and accumulate at the Sc_2CCl_2 monolayers, forming a built-in electric field from Sc_2CBr_2 to Sc_2CCl_2. In addition, the Bader charges obtained indicate that about 0.0072 |e| (0.0052 |e|) are transferred from the Sc_2CF_2 monolayer to the Sc_2CCl_2 (or Sc_2CBr_2) monolayers in the case of the Sc_2CF_2/Sc_2CCl_2 (Sc_2CF_2/Sc_2CBr_2) heterostructure. Furthermore, around 0.0018 |e| is transferred from Sc_2CBr_2 to Sc_2CCl_2 within the Sc_2CCl_2/Sc_2CBr_2 heterostructure.

In addition to the band gap value, the band edge alignment is also a crucial parameter for evaluating the application of the heterostructure. Therefore, we computed the band alignments of Sc_2CF_2, Sc_2CCl_2, and Sc_2CBr_2 monolayers, as well as the Sc_2CF_2/Sc_2CCl_2, Sc_2CF_2/Sc_2CBr_2, and Sc_2CCl_2/Sc_2CBr_2 heterostructures, using the method suggested by Toroker et al. [53]. Figure 5a reveals that the VBM of the Sc_2CF_2 monolayer exceeds that of $E_{O2/H2O}$. The Sc_2CCl_2 and Sc_2CBr_2 monolayers exhibit very similar characteristics in their band edge alignments, with both CBM being lower than the energy level of $E_{H+/H2}$. Based on the aforementioned analysis, the band positions of the Sc_2CF_2, Sc_2CCl_2, and Sc_2CBr_2 monolayers are unsuitable for photocatalysis. For the Sc_2CF_2/Sc_2CCl_2 and Sc_2CF_2/Sc_2CBr_2 heterostructures, the VBM and CBM of the Sc_2CF_2 layer are higher than those of the Sc_2CCl_2 (or Sc_2CBr_2) layer, further affirming that the heterostructure exhibits a type-II band alignment. For the Sc_2CCl_2/Sc_2CBr_2 heterostructure, both the VBM and CBM of Sc_2CBr_2 exceed those of the Sc_2CCl_2 layer, indicating a type-II band alignment. The CBM of Sc_2CCl_2 is lower than that of E_{H^+/H_2}, making the Sc_2CCl_2/Sc_2CBr_2 heterostructure unsuitable for photocatalytic water splitting reactions.

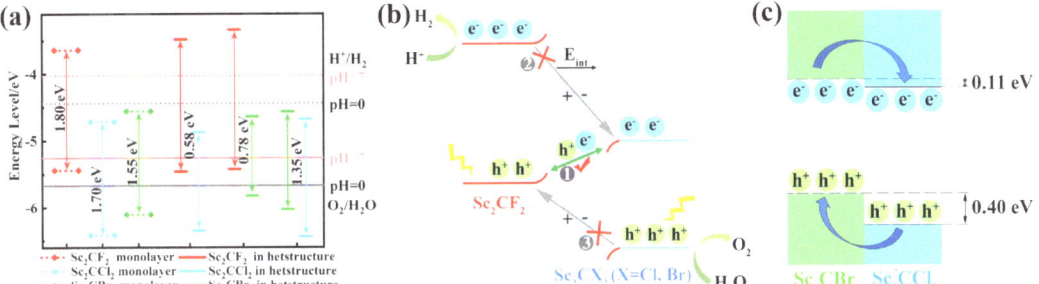

Figure 5. (**a**) The band position of monolayers and heterostructures. (**b**) Charge transfer mechanism of Sc_2CF_2/Sc_2CX_2 (X = Cl, Br). (**c**) Schematic diagram illustrating the migration of photogenerated electrons and holes at the Sc_2CCl_2/Sc_2CBr_2 heterostructure.

The photocatalytic water splitting reaction mechanism of Sc_2CF_2/Sc_2CX_2 (X = Cl, Br) is shown in Figure 5b. In general, three possible processes are considered here: ① The photoexcited holes at the VBM of Sc_2CF_2 recombine with electrons at the CBM of Sc_2CCl_2 (or Sc_2CBr_2), which represents a direct Z-scheme transfer path (indicated by the green line with double-headed arrows). ②–③ Photogenerated electrons at the CBM of Sc_2CF_2 migrate to the CBM of Sc_2CCl_2 (or Sc_2CBr_2), while photogenerated holes at the VBM of Sc_2CCl_2 (or Sc_2CBr_2) migrate to the VBM of Sc_2CF_2. This migration follows a traditional type-II path (indicated by gray lines with arrows). Electronic property analysis shows that the band alignments of the Sc_2CF_2/Sc_2CX_2 (X = Cl, Br) heterostructure are made up of the CBM of the Sc_2CCl_2 (or Sc_2CBr_2) layer and the VBM of the Sc_2CF_2 layer. Compared to the band gap of two monolayers, the heterostructure has a smaller band gap (Figure 5a), indicating a higher rate of photogenerated electron–hole pair recombination at the interface compared to the rate of intralayer recombination. Meanwhile, due to the built-in electric field from Sc_2CF_2 to Sc_2CCl_2 (or Sc_2CBr_2), the recombination of photogenerated electrons in the CBM of Sc_2CCl_2 (or Sc_2CBr_2) and photogenerated holes in the VBM of Sc_2CF_2 is accelerated, promoting the recombination of path ① carriers. In addition, electrons have varying additional potential energies at different points in the space charge region, a phenomenon known as energy band bending [54]. The positive charge on the Sc_2CCl_2 (or Sc_2CBr_2) is repelled by the holes on the Sc_2CF_2, causing the energy band to bend downward. Correspondingly, as the electrons move, the energy bands of the Sc_2CF_2 bend upward, forming a potential barrier at the interface. Due to the presence of built-in electric fields and potential barriers, the transfer of electrons from the CBM of Sc_2CF_2 to the CBM of Sc_2CCl_2 (or Sc_2CBr_2), as well as the transfer of holes from the VBM of Sc_2CCl_2 (or Sc_2CBr_2) to the VBM of Sc_2CF_2, are suppressed. Therefore, electron transfer in paths ② and ③ is repressed. After absorbing photon energy, the electrons are excited to the CBM, while the holes remain in the VBM. Due to the obstruction of path ② and path ③, photogenerated electrons gather in the CBM of Sc_2CF_2, while photogenerated holes gather in the VBM of Sc_2CCl_2 (or Sc_2CBr_2), which facilitates the efficient separation of photogenerated carriers and prolongs their lifetime [23]. Therefore, it is difficult for electrons and holes to transfer following the type-II pathway, and the Sc_2CF_2/Sc_2CX_2 heterostructure should be used as the photocatalyst for the Z-scheme. According to the above analysis, the Sc_2CF_2 layer exhibits a higher reduction ability. Photogenerated electrons and hydrogen ions undergo a reduction reaction on the CBM of the Sc_2CF_2 layer to produce hydrogen. Meanwhile, in the highly oxidizing Sc_2CCl_2

(or Sc$_2$CBr$_2$) layer, the photogenerated holes on the VBM react with hydroxyl groups to produce oxygen, thereby improving the photocatalytic performance.

Differently, the Sc$_2$CCl$_2$/Sc$_2$CBr$_2$ heterostructure is not suitable as a photocatalyst due to the fact that the CBM is lower than the energy level of E$_{H+/H2}$ (Figure 5a). However, they can function as absorption layers for solar cells. As shown in Figure 5c, the conduction band offset and valence band offset between the Sc$_2$CCl$_2$ and Sc$_2$CBr$_2$ layers are 0.11 eV and 0.40 eV, respectively. Therefore, under the influence of valence band offset, the photogenerated holes in the Sc$_2$CCl$_2$ layer tend to jump to the VBM of the Sc$_2$CBr$_2$ layer. Simultaneously, due to the lower CBM energy of Sc$_2$CCl$_2$ in the Sc$_2$CCl$_2$/Sc$_2$CBr$_2$ heterostructure, photogenerated electrons tend to move to the CBM of Sc$_2$CCl$_2$, resulting in a type-II band alignment. The very small conduction band offset can improve the energy conversion efficiency of the solar cell, while the large valence band offset limits the electrons in the Sc$_2$CCl$_2$ monolayer and the holes in the Sc$_2$CBr$_2$ monolayer [55]. Therefore, the rate of electron hole recombination will decrease, and the lifetime of photogenerated carriers will be extended. This will promote the formation of indirect excitons, which can be utilized in optoelectronic devices.

Considering that the construction of vdW heterostructures is an effective approach to enhance optical absorption and achieve excellent photovoltaic performance, therefore, to analyze the optical properties of the Sc$_2$CF$_2$/Sc$_2$CCl$_2$, Sc$_2$CF$_2$/Sc$_2$CBr$_2$, and Sc$_2$CCl$_2$/Sc$_2$CBr$_2$ heterostructures, we calculated the optical absorption of the Sc$_2$CF$_2$ monolayer, Sc$_2$CCl$_2$ monolayer, Sc$_2$CBr$_2$ monolayer, and the Sc$_2$CF$_2$/Sc$_2$CCl$_2$, Sc$_2$CF$_2$/Sc$_2$CBr$_2$, and Sc$_2$CCl$_2$/Sc$_2$CBr$_2$ heterostructures, as shown in Figure 6a–c. Among them, the optical absorption coefficient is determined by the following equation [56]:

$$\alpha(\omega) = \sqrt{2}\omega\sqrt{\sqrt{\varepsilon_1^2(\omega) + \varepsilon_2^2(\omega)} - \varepsilon_1(\omega)}$$

where $\varepsilon_1(\omega)$ and $\varepsilon_2(\omega)$ represent the real and imaginary parts of the complex dielectric function $\varepsilon(\omega)$, respectively. As illustrated in Figure 6a, we found that, compared to monolayers Sc$_2$CF$_2$ and Sc$_2$CCl$_2$, the Sc$_2$CF$_2$/Sc$_2$CCl$_2$ heterostructure has a wide absorption range from UV light to visible light due to its reduced band gap. It can be seen that the optical absorption coefficient of the Sc$_2$CF$_2$/Sc$_2$CCl$_2$ heterostructure is much larger than that of Sc$_2$CF$_2$ and Sc$_2$CCl$_2$ in both the UV and visible light ranges. More importantly, the Sc$_2$CF$_2$/Sc$_2$CCl$_2$ heterostructure shows a high absorption coefficient in the visible light region, reaching up to 2.53×10^5 cm^{-1} at a wavelength of 410 nm. The enhancement of the optical absorption coefficient is mainly due to the interlayer coupling between two monolayers of the Sc$_2$CF$_2$/Sc$_2$CCl$_2$ heterostructure [57]. Therefore, it is expected that the Sc$_2$CF$_2$/Sc$_2$CCl$_2$ heterostructure can act as an efficient visible light-harvesting photocatalyst. As can be seen from Figure 6b, compared with the Sc$_2$CF$_2$ monolayer and Sc$_2$CBr$_2$ monolayer, the significantly increased optical absorption in the UV and visible light regions of the Sc$_2$CF$_2$/Sc$_2$CBr$_2$ heterostructure is due to the interlayer coupling [58]. At the same time, compared with the Sc$_2$CF$_2$ monolayer and Sc$_2$CBr$_2$ monolayer, the increase in the optical absorption range of the Sc$_2$CF$_2$/Sc$_2$CBr$_2$ heterostructure is on account of the decrease in the band gap. Therefore, compared to the Sc$_2$CF$_2$ and Sc$_2$CBr$_2$ monolayers, the Sc$_2$CF$_2$/Sc$_2$CBr$_2$ heterostructure exhibits superior optical absorption performance, enabling efficient solar energy harvesting.

Light-absorbing materials not only need to have a suitable electronic structure but also need to have the ability to harvest solar light. Therefore, it is of great significance to study the optical properties of the Sc$_2$CCl$_2$/Sc$_2$CBr$_2$ heterostructure. The calculated absorption spectra of Sc$_2$CCl$_2$ and Sc$_2$CBr$_2$ monolayers, as well as the Sc$_2$CCl$_2$/Sc$_2$CBr$_2$ heterostructure, are shown in Figure 6c. In the UV and visible regions, the absorption intensity of Sc$_2$CCl$_2$ and Sc$_2$CBr$_2$ monolayers is weak. However, the absorption peak of the Sc$_2$CCl$_2$/Sc$_2$CBr$_2$ heterostructure in the visible region is nearly 2.33×10^5 cm^{-1}, which is 1.71 times that of the Sc$_2$CCl$_2$ monolayer. The enhancement of the optical absorption coefficient is mainly due to the interlayer coupling between two monolayers of the

Sc$_2$CCl$_2$/Sc$_2$CBr$_2$ heterostructure [58]. Compared to both monolayers, the absorption range of the Sc$_2$CCl$_2$/Sc$_2$CBr$_2$ heterostructure increases due to its reduced band gap. Therefore, it can be concluded that the Sc$_2$CCl$_2$/Sc$_2$CBr$_2$ heterostructure would be a promising material for solar cells.

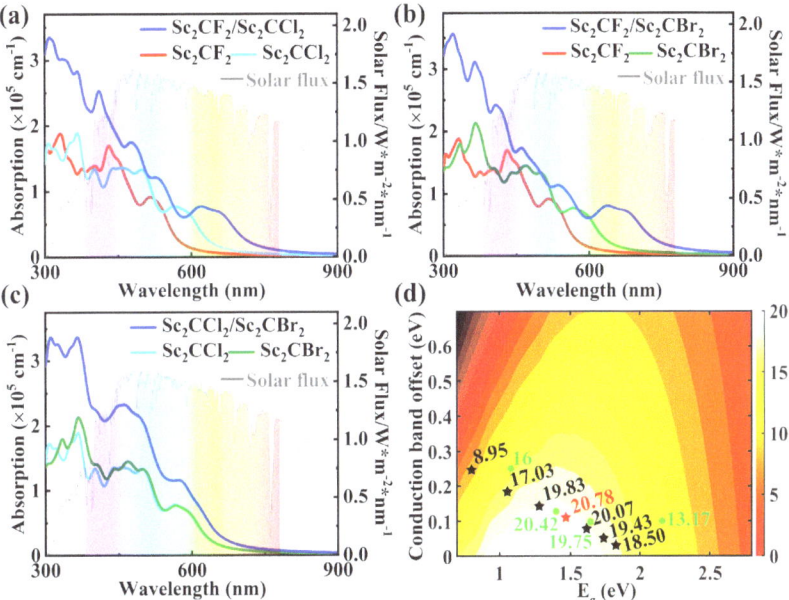

Figure 6. (a–c) Optical absorption coefficient as a function of energy for the Sc$_2$CF$_2$/Sc$_2$CCl$_2$, Sc$_2$CF$_2$/Sc$_2$CBr$_2$, and Sc$_2$CCl$_2$/Sc$_2$CBr$_2$ heterostructures, along with their respective isolated monolayers. (d) PCE as a function of donor band gap and conduction band offset of the Sc$_2$CCl$_2$/Sc$_2$CBr$_2$ heterostructure.

For device applications, in addition to the electronic and optical properties of the Sc$_2$CCl$_2$/Sc$_2$CBr$_2$ heterostructure analyzed above, such as limited band gaps, strong solar light-harvesting capabilities, and easy separation of electrons and holes with type-II band alignment, the ability to convert photon energy into electricity is also critical for solar cell applications. We use the method developed by Scharber et al. to calculate the PCE of solar cells, and its formula is as follows [59]:

$$\eta = \frac{J_{sc}V_{oc}\beta_{FF}}{P_{solar}} = \frac{0.65(E_g^d - \Delta E_c - 0.3)\int_{E_g^d}^{\infty} \frac{J_{Ph}(\hbar\omega)}{\hbar\omega}d(\hbar\omega)}{\int_0^{\infty} J_{Ph}(\hbar\omega)d(\hbar\omega)}$$

where 0.65 represents the band fill factor, E_g^d stands for the optical band gap of the donor, and ΔE_c represents the conduction band offset (CBO). The open circuit voltage is $E_g^d - \Delta E_c - 0.3$, and $J_{Ph}(\hbar\omega)$ is the 1.5 AM solar energy flux at the photon energy ($\hbar\omega$). As shown in Figure 6d, the calculated PCE of the Sc$_2$CCl$_2$/Sc$_2$CBr$_2$ heterostructure is about 20.78% (highlighted by the red star), which surpasses that of many other heterostructures, such as GeSe/AsP (16%) [13], InS/InSe (13.17%) [60], Hf$_2$CO$_2$/MoS$_2$ (19.75%) [29], and MoS$_2$/BP (20.42%) [61] heterostructures (highlighted by the green circle). Thus, we conclude that the Sc$_2$CCl$_2$/Sc$_2$CBr$_2$ heterostructure is more promising and competitive for 2D vdW heterostructure solar cells.

Strain engineering is an effective method to change the structural, electronic, and magnetic properties of 2D materials [62]. In addition, strain is unavoidable in industrial production, which comes from bending, external loads, and lattice mismatch [46]. Applying a biaxial strain will alter the band structure of the heterostructure and affect its photocatalytic and photovoltaic performance [42,45]. Then, the effects of in-plane biaxial strain on the electronic properties of Sc_2CF_2/Sc_2CCl_2, Sc_2CF_2/Sc_2CBr_2, and Sc_2CCl_2/Sc_2CBr_2 heterostructures are systematically studied. Here, the inner-layer biaxial strain (ε_{in}) is defined by $\varepsilon_{in} = [(L - L_0)/L_0] \times 100\%$, where L and L_0 are the lattice constants before and after the strain application, respectively. The applied strains η are −8%, −6%, −4%, −2%, 2%, 4%, 6%, and 8%, respectively. A negative value of η means that compressive strain is applied to the heterostructure. When η is positive, it indicates that tensile strain is applied to the heterostructure.

As shown in Figure S4, the electronic properties of the Sc_2CF_2/Sc_2CCl_2 heterostructure are significantly changed by applying biaxial strain. Compared with the Sc_2CF_2/Sc_2CCl_2 heterostructure without strain (Figure 3a), the applied strain changes the band gap of the heterostructure. From Figure 7a, it can be seen that when the compressive strain is −8%, −6%, −4%, and −2%, the band gap of the heterostructure decreases to 0.36, 0.39 eV, 0.46 eV, and 0.52 eV, respectively. Among them, the positions of the CBM and VBM have not changed and are still located at the high symmetry points M and Γ, as shown in Figure S4a–d. When the tensile strains are +2%, +4%, +6%, and +8%, respectively, the band gaps of the heterostructure increase to 0.62 eV, 0.66 eV, 0.72 eV, and 0.75 eV, respectively. The positions of the CBM and VBM are still located at the high symmetry points M and Γ, respectively (Figure S4e–h). With the increase in strain, the CBM of the Sc_2CCl_2 monolayer gradually moves away from the Fermi level, causing an increase in the band gaps. It can be seen from Figure 7b that the Sc_2CF_2/Sc_2CCl_2 heterostructure maintains a type-II band alignment throughout the strain. As for the band edge, all the heterostructures maintained photocatalytic activity under strain.

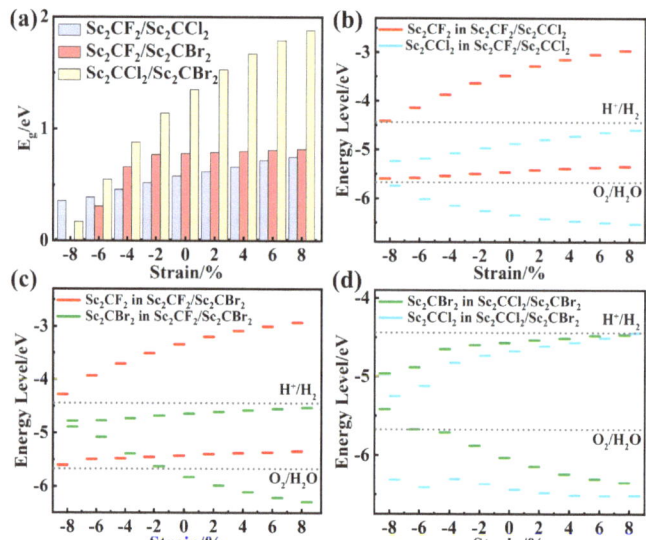

Figure 7. The (**a**) band gaps and (**b**–**d**) band alignment of strained Sc_2CF_2/Sc_2CCl_2, Sc_2CF_2/Sc_2CBr_2, and Sc_2CCl_2/Sc_2CBr_2 heterostructures.

The electronic properties of the Sc_2CF_2/Sc_2CBr_2 heterostructure changed significantly when biaxial strain was applied, as shown in Figure S5. In contrast to the strain-free Sc_2CF_2/Sc_2CBr_2 heterostructure (Figure 3b), applying strain not only alters the band gaps of the heterostructure but also changes the band alignment of the heterostructure. As can be seen from Figure 7a, the band gaps of the Sc_2CF_2/Sc_2CBr_2 heterostructure decrease to 0.31 eV, 0.66 eV, and 0.77 eV when the compression strain is −6%, −4%, and −2%, with the CBM and VBM located at highly symmetric points M and Γ (Figure S5b–d). However, when the compressive strain increases to −8%, the band gap of the Sc_2CF_2/Sc_2CBr_2 heterostructure decreases to 0 eV. This indicates that the heterostructure transitions from an indirect band gap semiconductor to a metal under −8% compressive strain because the CBM (VBM) moves below (above) the Fermi level, as shown in Figure S5a. When the tensile strain was +2%, +4%, +6%, and +8%, the CBM and VBM were located at highly symmetric points M and Γ, with band gaps increasing to 0.79 eV, 0.80 eV, 0.81 eV, and 0.82 eV, respectively, as shown in Figure S5e–h. From Figure 7c, when the compressive strain is between −6% and −4%, the VBM of the Sc_2CBr_2 layer is positioned at a higher energy level than that of the VBM of the Sc_2CF_2 layer. Consequently, the VBM of the Sc_2CF_2/Sc_2CBr_2 heterostructure shifts from the Sc_2CF_2 layer to the Sc_2CBr_2 layer, leading to a transition from type-II to type-I. In addition, when the compression strain is −2%, the VBM of Sc_2CBr_2 is higher than that of $E_{O2/H2O}$, which is unfavorable for the photocatalytic reaction. By analyzing the band structure of the Sc_2CF_2/Sc_2CBr_2 heterostructure under strain, it is considered that the strain affects the relative position of atoms as well as the bonding properties and strength of the atoms, leading to a change in the band structure. The band alignment of the Sc_2CF_2/Sc_2CBr_2 heterostructure can be changed from type-I to type-II under different strain conditions.

For the Sc_2CCl_2/Sc_2CBr_2 heterostructure, the applied biaxial strain range is still −8%~8%. As shown in Figure S6, it is noteworthy that under −8%~6% biaxial strains, the heterostructures consistently maintain type-II banding and retain indirect band gap characteristics. As displayed in Figure 7a, the band gaps of the Sc_2CCl_2/Sc_2CBr_2 heterostructure decrease to 0.17 eV, 0.55 eV, 0.88 eV, and 1.14 eV when compressive strain is applied. As the tensile strain increases, the band gap also increases, reaching 1.53 eV, 1.67 eV, 1.79 eV, and 1.88 eV, respectively. Under −8%~6% biaxial strains, the CBM and VBM are still contributed by Sc_2CCl_2 and Sc_2CBr_2, located at the M and Γ points, respectively, as depicted in Figure 7d. Unlike these changes, under the tensile strain of 8%, the CBM of the Sc_2CCl_2 layer becomes higher than the CBM of the Sc_2CBr_2 layer. Thus, the CBM of the Sc_2CCl_2/Sc_2CBr_2 heterostructure shifts from the Sc_2CCl_2 layer to the Sc_2CBr_2 layer, leading to a type-II to type-I transformation. In addition, we calculated the PCE values of the Sc_2CCl_2/Sc_2CBr_2 heterostructure under various biaxial strains, as illustrated in Figure 6d (highlighted by the black star). From Figure S7, we can see that a maximum PCE of 20.07% can be achieved under 2% tensile strain.

4. Conclusions

In summary, based on density functional theory calculations, we have systematically explored the electronic structure and optical properties towards photocatalytic water splitting as well as the photovoltaic applications for Sc_2CF_2/Sc_2CCl_2, Sc_2CF_2/Sc_2CBr_2, and Sc_2CCl_2/Sc_2CBr_2 vdW heterostructures. AIMD simulation and phonon spectrum results show that the Sc_2CF_2/Sc_2CCl_2, Sc_2CF_2/Sc_2CBr_2, and Sc_2CCl_2/Sc_2CBr_2 heterostructures are thermally and dynamically stable. Sc_2CF_2/Sc_2CCl_2, Sc_2CF_2/Sc_2CBr_2, and Sc_2CCl_2/Sc_2CBr_2 heterostructures exhibit type-II band alignments with the CBM and VBM located in different monolayers. By further analyzing the band alignment and charge carrier transfer processes, the Sc_2CF_2/Sc_2CCl_2 and Sc_2CF_2/Sc_2CBr_2 heterostructures exhibit a direct Z-scheme photocatalyst. These properties can effectively separate the photogenerated carriers, making them suitable for photocatalytic water splitting. Remarkably, a PCE of 20.78% can be achieved for the Sc_2CCl_2/Sc_2CBr_2 heterostructure, which is higher than that of many other reported heterostructures. In addition, all the heterostructures exhibit excellent optical absorption coefficients in both the visible and UV regions, reaching the order of 10^5 cm^{-1}. This theoretical work demonstrates that the Sc_2CX_2/Sc_2CY_2 (X, Y = F, Cl, Br) heterostructures are promising candidates for applications in photocatalytic and photovoltaic devices.

Supplementary Materials: The following supporting information can be downloaded at https://www.mdpi.com/article/10.3390/molecules29122898/s1, Table S1: The structure coordinate information (POSCAR) of the Sc_2CF_2/Sc_2CCl_2 heterostructure with three different stacking configurations. The POSCAR of Sc_2CF_2/Sc_2CBr_2 and Sc_2CCl_2/Sc_2CBr_2 heterostructures are the same as those of the

Sc$_2$CF$_2$/Sc$_2$CCl$_2$ heterostructure; Figure S1: (a–c) AIMD fluctuations of the total energy for the Sc$_2$CF$_2$/Sc$_2$CCl$_2$, Sc$_2$CF$_2$/Sc$_2$CBr$_2$, and Sc$_2$CCl$_2$/Sc$_2$CBr$_2$ heterostructures at 300 K with 6ps. The insets are top and side views of the final structures in the AIMD simulation; Figure S2: (a–c) Phonon dispersion structures of the Sc$_2$CF$_2$/Sc$_2$CCl$_2$, Sc$_2$CF$_2$/Sc$_2$CBr$_2$, and Sc$_2$CCl$_2$/Sc$_2$CBr$_2$ heterostructures; Figure S3: Electrostatic potential for (a) Sc$_2$CF$_2$, (b) Sc$_2$CCl$_2$, and (c) Sc$_2$CBr$_2$ monolayers; Figure S4: Relation between band gap of the Sc$_2$CF$_2$/Sc$_2$CCl$_2$ heterostructure and biaxial strain; Figure S5: The projected band structures of the Sc$_2$CF$_2$/Sc$_2$CBr$_2$ heterostructure under different vertical strains; Figure S6: Energy bands of the Sc$_2$CCl$_2$/Sc$_2$CBr$_2$ heterostructure under different strains; Figure S7: The PCE of the Sc$_2$CCl$_2$/Sc$_2$CBr$_2$ heterostructure with different strains.

Author Contributions: Conceptualization, X.H. and Y.T.; software, Y.T.; investigation, Y.W.; data curation, J.L.; writing—original draft preparation, X.H.; writing—review and editing, Y.T. and J.S.; supervision, X.D. All authors have read and agreed to the published version of the manuscript.

Funding: This research was funded by the Natural Science Foundation of Henan province (No. 232300420335) and the Scientific and Technological Breakthroughs in Henan Province (No. 232102230016, No. 242102230157, and No. 242102210164).

Institutional Review Board Statement: Not applicable.

Informed Consent Statement: Not applicable.

Data Availability Statement: Data are contained within the article and Supplementary Materials.

Conflicts of Interest: The authors declare no conflicts of interest.

References

1. Khan, K.; Tareen, A.K.; Aslam, M.; Sagar, R.U.R.; Zhang, B.; Huang, W.; Mahmood, A.; Mahmood, N.; Khan, K.; Zhang, H.; et al. Recent Progress, Challenges, and Prospects in Two-Dimensional Photo-Catalyst Materials and Environmental Remediation. *Nano-Micro Lett.* **2020**, *12*, 167. [CrossRef] [PubMed]
2. Fujishima, A.; Honda, K. Electrochemical Photolysis of Water at a Semiconductor Electrode. *Nature* **1972**, *238*, 37–38. [CrossRef] [PubMed]
3. Chapin, D.M.; Fuller, C.S.; Pearson, G.L. A New Silicon *p-n* Junction Photocell for Converting Solar Radiation into Electrical Power. *J. Appl. Phys.* **1954**, *25*, 676–677. [CrossRef]
4. Novoselov, K.S.; Geim, A.K.; Morozov, S.V.; Jiang, D.; Zhang, Y.; Dubonos, S.V.; Grigorieva, I.V.; Firsov, A.A. Electric Field Effect in Atomically Thin Carbon Films. *Science* **2004**, *306*, 666–669. [CrossRef] [PubMed]
5. Novoselov, K.S.; Geim, A.K.; Morozov, S.V.; Jiang, D.; Katsnelson, M.I.; Grigorieva, I.V.; Dubonos, S.V.; Firsov, A.A. Two-Dimensional Gas of Massless Dirac Fermions in Graphene. *Nature* **2005**, *438*, 197–200. [CrossRef] [PubMed]
6. Shakil, M.; Nazir, S.; Zafar, M.; Gillani, S.S.A.; Ali, H.E. Influence of Functional Group and Their Number of Atoms on Structural, Electronic and Optical Properties of Sc$_2$C MXenes: A DFT Study. *Comput. Condens. Matter* **2024**, *39*, e00903. [CrossRef]
7. Shen, X.; Huang, X.; Wang, H.; Zhan, H. Properties of Mo-Based TMDCs/Ti$_2$CT$_2$ (T = O, F, OH) vdWs Heterostructures for Full Spectrum Electromagnetic Absorption. *Solid State Commun.* **2022**, *346*, 114720. [CrossRef]
8. He, X.; Yu, C.; Yu, M.M.; Lin, J.; Li, Q.L.; Fang, Y.; Liu, Z.Y.; Xue, Y.M.; Huang, Y.; Tang, C.C. Synthesis of Perovskite CsPbBr$_3$ Quantum Dots/Porous Boron Nitride Nanofiber Composites with Improved Stability and Their Reversible Optical Response to Ammonia. *Inorg. Chem.* **2020**, *59*, 1234–1241. [CrossRef] [PubMed]
9. Thirugnanasambandan, T.; Karuppaiah, C.; Sankar, B.V.; Gopinath, S.C.B. Insights and Potentials of Two-Dimensional Black Phosphorous-Based Solar Cells. *Phys. Scr.* **2024**, *99*, 052002. [CrossRef]
10. Khan, U.; Saeed, M.U.; Elansary, H.O.; Moussa, I.M.; Bacha, A.-U.-R.; Saeed, Y. A DFT Study of Bandgap Tuning in Chloro-Fluoro Silicene. *RSC Adv.* **2024**, *14*, 4844–4852. [CrossRef]
11. Deng, R.; Yao, H.; Wang, Y.; Wang, C.; Zhang, S.; Guo, S.; Li, Y.; Ma, S. Interface Effect of Fe Doped NiSe/Ni$_3$Se$_2$ Heterojunction as Highly Efficient Electrocatalysts for Overall Water Splitting. *Chem. Eng. J.* **2024**, *488*, 150996. [CrossRef]
12. Zhao, H.; Jian, L.; Gong, M.; Jing, M.; Li, H.; Mao, Q.; Lu, T.; Guo, Y.; Ji, R.; Chi, W.; et al. Transition-Metal-Based Cocatalysts for Photocatalytic Water Splitting. *Small Struct.* **2022**, *3*, 2100229. [CrossRef]
13. Liu, H.-Y.; Yang, C.-L.; Wang, M.-S.; Ma, X.-G. The High Power Conversion Efficiency of a Two-Dimensional GeSe/AsP van Der Waals Heterostructure for Solar Energy Cells. *Phys. Chem. Chem. Phys.* **2021**, *23*, 6042–6050. [CrossRef]
14. Li, X.; Garlisi, C.; Guan, Q.; Anwer, S.; Al-Ali, K.; Palmisano, G.; Zheng, L. A Review of Material Aspects in Developing Direct Z-scheme Photocatalysts. *Mater. Today* **2021**, *47*, 75–107. [CrossRef]
15. Di, T.; Xu, Q.; Ho, W.; Tang, H.; Xiang, Q.; Yu, J. Review on Metal Sulphide-based Z-scheme Photocatalysts. *ChemCatChem* **2019**, *11*, 1394–1411. [CrossRef]
16. Ning, X.; Jia, D.; Li, S.; Khan, M.; Hao, A. Construction of CuS/ZnO Z-scheme Heterojunction as Highly Efficient Piezocatalyst for Degradation of Organic Pollutant and Promoting N$_2$ Fixation Properties. *Ceram. Int.* **2023**, *49*, 21658–21666. [CrossRef]

17. Liang, J.; Ren, H.; Labidi, A.; Zhu, Q.; Dong, Q.; Allam, A.; Rady, A.; Wang, C. Boosted Photocatalytic Removal of NO Using Direct Z-scheme UiO-66-NH$_2$/Bi$_2$MoO$_6$ Nanoflowers Heterojunction: Mechanism Insight and Humidity Effect. *Rare Met.* **2024**. [CrossRef]
18. Su, M.; Chen, Y.; Wang, L.; Zhao, Z.; Sun, H.; Zhou, G.; Li, P. A Z-Scheme WO$_3$/Bi$_2$MoO$_6$ Heterostructure with Improved Photocatalytic Activity: The Synergistic Effect of Heterojunction and Oxygen Vacancy Defects. *J. Phys. Chem. Solids* **2024**, *188*, 111947. [CrossRef]
19. He, L.; Long, X.; Zhang, C.; Ma, K.; She, L.; Mi, C.; Yu, M.; Xie, Z.; Wang, L. Direct Z-Scheme β-SnSe/HfS$_2$ Heterostructure for Photocatalytic Water Splitting: High Solar-to-Hydrogen Efficiency and Excellent Carrier Mobility. *Mater. Today Commun.* **2024**, *38*, 108127. [CrossRef]
20. Ge, C.; Wang, B.; Yang, H.; Feng, Q.; Huang, S.; Zu, X.; Li, L.; Deng, H. Direct Z-Scheme GaSe/ZrS$_2$ Heterojunction for Overall Water Splitting. *Int. J. Hydrogen Energy* **2023**, *48*, 13460–13469. [CrossRef]
21. Ma, D.; Li, H.; Wang, J.; Hu, J.; Yang, X.; Fu, Y.; Cui, Z.; Li, E. Direct Z-Scheme MoSTe/g-GeC Heterostructure for Photocatalytic Water Splitting: A First-Principles Study. *Int. J. Hydrogen Energy* **2024**, *51*, 1216–1224. [CrossRef]
22. Huang, X.; Cui, Z.; Shu, X.; Dong, H.; Weng, Y.; Wang, Y.; Yang, Z. First-Principles Study on the Electronic Properties of GeC/BSe van Der Waals Heterostructure: A Direct Z-Scheme Photocatalyst for Overall Water Splitting. *Phys. Rev. Mater.* **2022**, *6*, 034010. [CrossRef]
23. Liang, K.; Wang, J.; Wei, X.; Zhang, Y.; Yang, Y.; Liu, J.; Tian, Y.; Duan, L. SnC/PtS$_2$ Heterostructure: A Promising Direct Z-Scheme Photocatalyst with Tunable Electronic Optical Properties and High Solar-to-Hydrogen Efficiency. *Int. J. Hydrogen Energy* **2023**, *48*, 38296–38308. [CrossRef]
24. Singh, M.R.; Xiang, C.; Lewis, N.S. Evaluation of Flow Schemes for Near-Neutral pH Electrolytes in Solar-Fuel Generators. *Sustain. Energy Fuels* **2017**, *1*, 458–466. [CrossRef]
25. Cheng, S.; Chen, X.; Wang, M.; Li, G.; Qi, X.; Tian, Y.; Jia, M.; Han, Y.; Wu, D.; Li, X.; et al. In-Situ Growth of Cs$_2$AgBiBr$_6$ Perovskite Nanocrystals on Ti$_3$C$_2$T$_x$ MXene Nanosheets for Enhanced Photocatalytic Activity. *Appl. Surf. Sci.* **2023**, *621*, 156877. [CrossRef]
26. Zhu, B.; Zhang, F.; Qiu, J.; Chen, X.; Zheng, K.; Guo, H.; Yu, J.; Bao, J. A Novel Hf$_2$CO$_2$/WS$_2$ van Der Waals Heterostructure as a Potential Candidate for Overall Water Splitting Photocatalyst. *Mater. Sci. Semicond. Process.* **2021**, *133*, 105947. [CrossRef]
27. Guo, H.; Zhu, B.; Zhang, F.; Li, H.; Zheng, K.; Qiu, J.; Wu, L.; Yu, J.; Chen, X. Type-II AsP/Sc$_2$CO$_2$ van Der Waals Heterostructure: An Excellent Photocatalyst for Overall Water Splitting. *Int. J. Hydrogen Energy* **2021**, *46*, 32882–32892. [CrossRef]
28. Bao, J.; Zhu, B.; Zhang, F.; Chen, X.; Guo, H.; Qiu, J.; Liu, X.; Yu, J. Sc$_2$CF$_2$/Janus MoSSe Heterostructure: A Potential Z-Scheme Photocatalyst with Ultra-High Solar-to-Hydrogen Efficiency. *Int. J. Hydrogen Energy* **2021**, *46*, 39830–39843. [CrossRef]
29. Wen, J.; Cai, Q.; Xiong, R.; Cui, Z.; Zhang, Y.; He, Z.; Liu, J.; Lin, M.; Wen, C.; Wu, B.; et al. Promising M$_2$CO$_2$/MoX$_2$ (M = Hf, Zr; X = S, Se, Te) Heterostructures for Multifunctional Solar Energy Applications. *Molecules* **2023**, *28*, 3525. [CrossRef] [PubMed]
30. Zhang, Y.G.; Xiong, R.; Sa, B.; Zhou, J.; Sun, Z.M. MXenes: Promising Donor and Acceptor Materials for High-Efficiency Heterostructure Solar Cells. *Sustain. Energy Fuels* **2021**, *5*, 135–143. [CrossRef]
31. Guo, S.; Lin, H.; Hu, J.; Su, Z.; Zhang, Y. Computational Study of Novel Semiconducting Sc$_2$CT$_2$ (T = F, Cl, Br) MXenes for Visible-Light Photocatalytic Water Splitting. *Materials* **2021**, *14*, 4739. [CrossRef]
32. Modi, N.; Naik, Y.; Khengar, S.J.; Shah, D.B.; Thakor, P.B. Pressure Induced Structural, Electronic and Optical Properties of Sc$_2$CBr$_2$ MXene Monolayer: A Density Functional Approach. *Comput. Theor. Chem.* **2024**, *1232*, 114466. [CrossRef]
33. Zhang, J.; Deng, Y.; Liu, H.; Zhou, R.; Hao, G.; Zhang, R. Two-Dimensional Sc$_2$CF$_2$/WSSe van Der Waals Heterostructure for Water Splitting: A First-Principles Study. *J. Phys. Chem. Solids* **2024**, *185*, 111757. [CrossRef]
34. Sun, R.; Yang, C.-L.; Wang, M.-S.; Ma, X.-G. Two-Dimensional Sc$_2$CCl$_2$/SiS$_2$ van Der Waals Heterostructure with High Solar Power Conversion Efficiency. *Appl. Surf. Sci.* **2022**, *591*, 153232. [CrossRef]
35. Kresse, G.; Furthmüller, J. Efficiency of Ab-Initio Total Energy Calculations for Metals and Semiconductors Using a Plane-Wave Basis Set. *Comput. Mater. Sci.* **1996**, *6*, 15–50. [CrossRef]
36. Kresse, G.; Hafner, J. Ab Initio Molecular-Dynamics Simulation of the Liquid-Metal–Amorphous-Semiconductor Transition in Germanium. *Phys. Rev. B* **1994**, *49*, 14251–14269. [CrossRef] [PubMed]
37. Perdew, J.P.; Burke, K.; Ernzerhof, M. Generalized Gradient Approximation Made Simple. *Phys. Rev. Lett.* **1996**, *77*, 3865–3868. [CrossRef] [PubMed]
38. Grimme, S.; Antony, J.; Ehrlich, S.; Krieg, H. A Consistent and Accurate Ab Initio Parametrization of Density Functional Dispersion Correction (DFT-D) for the 94 Elements H-Pu. *J. Chem. Phys.* **2010**, *132*, 154104. [CrossRef] [PubMed]
39. Heyd, J.; Scuseria, G.E.; Ernzerhof, M. Hybrid Functionals Based on a Screened Coulomb Potential. *J. Chem. Phys.* **2003**, *118*, 8207–8215. [CrossRef]
40. Ramírez-Solís, A.; Maron, L. Aqueous Microsolvation of CdCl$_2$: Density Functional Theory and Born-Oppenheimer Molecular Dynamics Studies. *J. Chem. Phys.* **2014**, *141*, 094304. [CrossRef]
41. Nosé, S. A Unified Formulation of the Constant Temperature Molecular Dynamics Methods. *J. Chem. Phys.* **1984**, *81*, 511. [CrossRef]
42. Khang, N.D.; Nguyen, C.Q.; Duc, L.M.; Nguyen, C.V. First-Principles Investigation of a Type-II BP/Sc$_2$CF$_2$ van Der Waals Heterostructure for Photovoltaic Solar Cells. *Nanoscale Adv.* **2023**, *5*, 2583–2589. [CrossRef] [PubMed]

43. Meng, J.; Wang, J.; Wang, J.; Li, Q.; Yang, J. C_7N_6/Sc_2CCl_2 Weak van Der Waals Heterostructure: A Promising Visible-Light-Driven Z-Scheme Water Splitting Photocatalyst with Interface Ultrafast Carrier Recombination. *J. Phys. Chem. Lett.* **2022**, *13*, 1473–1479. [CrossRef] [PubMed]
44. Nguyen, S.T.; Nguyen, C.Q.; Hieu, N.N.; Phuc, H.V.; Nguyen, C.V. Tunable Electronic Properties, Carrier Mobility, and Contact Characteristics in Type-II BSe/Sc_2CF_2 Heterostructures toward Next Generation Optoelectronic Devices. *Langmuir* **2023**, *39*, 17251–17260. [CrossRef] [PubMed]
45. Sun, R.; Yang, C.-L.; Wang, M.-S.; Ma, X.-G. Sc_2CCl_2/WX_2 (X = Se, Te) van Der Waals Heterostructures for Photocatalytic Hydrogen and Oxygen Evolutions with Direct Z-Schemes. *Int. J. Hydrogen Energy* **2023**, *48*, 38699–38707. [CrossRef]
46. Zhang, Y.; Ding, J.; Xie, K.; Qiang, Z.; Duan, L.; Ni, L.; Fan, G. $GeC/SnSe_2$ Van Der Waals Heterostructure: A Promising Direct Z-scheme Photocatalyst for Overall Water Splitting with Strong Optical Absorption, High Solar-to-hydrogen Energy Conversion Efficiency and Superior Catalytic Activity. *Int. J. Hydrogen Energy* **2024**, *70*, 357–369. [CrossRef]
47. Rao, Y.; Zhang, F.; Zhu, B.; Li, H.; Zheng, K.; Zou, Y.; Feng, X.; Guo, H.; Qiu, J.; Chen, X.; et al. A $C_2N/ZnSe$ Heterostructure with Type-II Band Alignment and Excellent Photocatalytic Water Splitting Performance. *New J. Chem.* **2021**, *45*, 13571–13578. [CrossRef]
48. Zhu, H.; Zhang, X.; Nie, Y.; Yang, D.; Xiang, G. 2D/2D Janus BiTeCl/GeSe vdW Heterostructure as a Robust High-Performance S-Scheme Photocatalyst for Water Splitting. *Appl. Surf. Sci.* **2023**, *635*, 157694. [CrossRef]
49. Zolyomi, V.; Drummond, N.D.; Fal'ko, V.I. Electrons and Phonons in Single Layers of Hexagonal Indium Chalcogenides from Ab Initio Calculations. *Phys. Rev. B* **2014**, *89*, 205416. [CrossRef]
50. Cahangirov, S.; Topsakal, M.; Aktürk, E.; Sahin, H.; Ciraci, S. Two- and One-Dimensional Honeycomb Structures of Silicon and Germanium. *Phys. Rev. Lett.* **2009**, *102*, 236804. [CrossRef]
51. Mannix, A.J.; Zhou, X.; Kiraly, B.; Wood, J.D.; Alducin, D.; Myers, B.D.; Liu, X.; Fisher, B.L.; Santiago, U.; Guest, J.R.; et al. Synthesis of Borophenes: Anisotropic, Two-dimensional Boron Polymorphs. *Science* **2015**, *350*, 1513–1516. [CrossRef]
52. Mao, Y.; Qin, C.; Zhou, X.; Zhang, Z.; Yuan, J. First-Principles Study on GeC/β-AsP Heterostructure with Type-II Band Alignment for Photocatalytic Water Splitting. *Appl. Surf. Sci.* **2023**, *617*, 156298. [CrossRef]
53. Toroker, M.C.; Kanan, D.K.; Alidoust, N.; Isseroff, L.Y.; Liao, P.; Carter, E.A. First Principles Scheme to Evaluate Band Edge Positions in Potential Transition Metal Oxide Photocatalysts and Photoelectrodes. *Phys. Chem. Chem. Phys.* **2011**, *13*, 16644. [CrossRef]
54. Bai, S.; Li, X.; Kong, Q.; Long, R.; Wang, C.; Jiang, J.; Xiong, Y. Toward Enhanced Photocatalytic Oxygen Evolution: Synergetic Utilization of Plasmonic Effect and Schottky Junction via Interfacing Facet Selection. *Adv. Mater.* **2015**, *27*, 3444–3452. [CrossRef]
55. Guan, Y.; Li, X.; Hu, Q.; Zhao, D.; Zhang, L. Theoretical Design of BAs/WX_2 (X = S, Se) Heterostructures for High-performance Photovoltaic Applications from DFT Calculations. *Appl. Surf. Sci.* **2022**, *599*, 153865. [CrossRef]
56. Lalitha, S.; Karazhanov, S.Z.; Ravindran, P.; Senthilarasu, S.; Sathyamoorthy, R.; Janabergenov, J. Electronic Structure, Structural and Optical Properties of Thermally Evaporated CdTe Thin Films. *Phys. B* **2007**, *387*, 227–238. [CrossRef]
57. Sharma, R.; Aneesh, J.; Yadav, R.; Sanda, S.; Barik, A.R.; Mishra, A.; Maji, T.; Karmakar, D.; Adarsh, K.V. Strong Interlayer Coupling Mediated Giant two-photon Absorption in $MoSe_2$/graphene Oxide Heterostructure: Quenching of Exciton Bands. *Phys. Rev. B* **2016**, *93*, 155433. [CrossRef]
58. Wu, F.; Liu, Y.; Yu, G.; Shen, D.; Wang, Y.; Kan, E. Visible-Light-Absorption in Graphitic C_3N_4 Bilayer: Enhanced by Interlayer Coupling. *J. Phys. Chem. Lett.* **2012**, *3*, 3330–3334. [CrossRef]
59. Scharber, M.C.; Mühlbacher, D.; Koppe, M.; Denk, P.; Waldauf, C.; Heeger, A.J.; Brabec, C.J. Design Rules for Donors in Bulk-Heterojunction Solar Cells—Towards 10% Energy-Conversion Efficiency. *Adv. Mater.* **2006**, *18*, 789–794. [CrossRef]
60. Rawat, A.; Ahammed, R.; Dimple; Jena, N.; Mohanta, M.K.; De Sarkar, A. Solar Energy Harvesting in Type II van Der Waals Heterostructures of Semiconducting Group III Monochalcogenide Monolayers. *J. Phys. Chem. C* **2019**, *123*, 12666–12675. [CrossRef]
61. Mohanta, M.K.; Rawat, A.; Jena, N.; Dimple; Ahammed, R.; De Sarkar, A. Interfacing Boron Monophosphide with Molybdenum Disulfide for an Ultrahigh Performance in Thermoelectrics, Two-Dimensional Excitonic Solar Cells, and Nanopiezotronics. *ACS Appl. Mater. Interfaces* **2020**, *12*, 3114–3126. [CrossRef]
62. Kistanov, A.A.; Cai, Y.; Zhou, K.; Dmitriev, S.V.; Zhang, Y. Large Electronic Anisotropy and Enhanced Chemical Activity of Highly Rippled Phosphorene. *J. Phys. Chem. C* **2016**, *120*, 6876–6884. [CrossRef]

Disclaimer/Publisher's Note: The statements, opinions and data contained in all publications are solely those of the individual author(s) and contributor(s) and not of MDPI and/or the editor(s). MDPI and/or the editor(s) disclaim responsibility for any injury to people or property resulting from any ideas, methods, instructions or products referred to in the content.

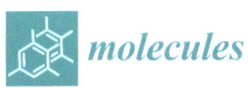

Article

First Principle Study on the Z-Type Characteristic Modulation of GaN/g-C$_3$N$_4$ Heterojunction

Meng-Yao Dai [1], Xu-Cai Zhao [1], Bo-Cheng Lei [1], Yi-Neng Huang [1,2], Li-Li Zhang [1,2,*], Hai Guo [3,*] and Hua-Gui Wang [1]

[1] Xinjiang Laboratory of Phase Transitions and Microstructures in Condensed Matter Physics, College of Physical Science and Technology, Yili Normal University, Yining 835000, China; dmy153097@sina.com (M.-Y.D.); zxc85619876@sina.com (X.-C.Z.); lbc0428@sina.com (B.-C.L.); ynhuang@nju.edu.cn (Y.-N.H.); suyi2046@sohu.com (H.-G.W.)
[2] National Laboratory of Solid State Microstructures, School of Physics, Nanjing University, Nanjing 210093, China
[3] Department of Physics, Zhejiang Normal University, Jinhua 321004, China
* Correspondence: suyi2046@sina.com (L.-L.Z.); ghh@zjnu.cn (H.G.)

Abstract: This study investigates the stability, electronic structure, and optical properties of the GaN/g-C$_3$N$_4$ heterojunction using the plane wave super-soft pseudopotential method based on first principles. Additionally, an external electric field is employed to modulate the band structure and optical properties of GaN/g-C$_3$N$_4$. The computational results demonstrate that this heterojunction possesses a direct band gap and is classified as type II heterojunction, where the intrinsic electric field formed at the interface effectively suppresses carrier recombination. When the external electric field intensity (E) falls below −0.1 V/Å and includes −0.1 V/Å, or exceeds 0.2 V/Å, the heterojunction undergoes a transition from a type II structure to the superior Z-scheme, leading to a significant enhancement in the rate of separation of photogenerated carriers and an augmentation in its redox capability. Furthermore, the introduction of a positive electric field induces a redshift in the absorption spectrum, effectively broadening the light absorption range of the heterojunction. The aforementioned findings demonstrate that the optical properties of GaN/g-C$_3$N$_4$ can be precisely tuned by applying an external electric field, thereby facilitating its highly efficient utilization in the field of photocatalysis.

Keywords: first principles; GaN/g-C$_3$N$_4$; optical properties; external electric field

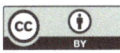

1. Introduction

Photocatalytic technology, which harnesses solar energy, has been widely applied in various domains including air purification, water splitting for hydrogen production, and self-cleaning capabilities [1–3]. The essence of photocatalytic technology lies in the development of efficient photocatalysts. However, the utilization efficiency of visible light by conventional photocatalysts such as TiO$_2$ [4], ZnO [5], and WO$_3$ [6] remains significantly low, falling below 5% [7]. Consequently, current research endeavors to enhance the light absorption range of photocatalysts in the visible spectrum while simultaneously augmenting their efficiency and stability during photocatalytic reactions [8]. Two-dimensional photocatalysts, such as g-C$_3$N$_4$ [9,10], TiS$_3$ [11], and TiS$_2$ [12], demonstrate a remarkable responsiveness to visible light and exhibit exceptional catalytic efficiency, surpassing traditional photocatalysts such as TiO$_2$ [13]. Its extensive specific surface area facilitates the formation of additional reactive sites, leading to a significant enhancement in photocatalytic performance [14,15]. However, the rapid recombination of photogenerated carriers and the limited range of light absorption continue to pose significant challenges in enhancing the photocatalytic efficiency of g-C$_3$N$_4$ [16]. Currently, the construction of heterojunctions represents a promising strategy for enhancing the efficiency of photocatalysts. The key factor of heterojunctions as excellent photocatalysts is the formation of a built-in electric field at their interface, which effectively mitigates the rapid recombination of photogenerated carriers and optimizes the optical properties of these systems [17,18]. The hydrogen production rates of the three g-C_3N_4-based heterojunctions, g-C_3N_4/SiOC, g-C_3N_4/WS_2, and g-C_3N_4/CeO_2, presented in Table 1 exhibit a significant enhancement compared to that of single-layer g-C_3N_4, with an impressive efficiency increase ranging from 46 to 93 times. This finding strongly indicates that the photocatalytic efficiency can be greatly enhanced by constructing g-C_3N_4-based heterojunctions. The band gap of these three heterojunctions is smaller than that of monolayers, indicating a significant alteration in the heterojunction structure compared to single layers. Furthermore, all three heterojunctions exhibit a type II band alignment, which is observed to significantly enhance photocatalytic efficiency compared to single-layer g-C_3N_4.

Table 1. Hydrogen production rate (H), band gap (E_g), and band structure type in g-C_3N_4-based heterojunctions.

Photocatalysts	H (μmol g^{-1} h^{-1})	E_g (eV)	Band Structure Type
Layer g-C_3N_4 [19]	2.82	2.70	/
g-C_3N_4/SiOC [20]	1020	2.64	Type II
g-C_3N_4/WS_2 [21]	599.7	2.30	Type II
g-C_3N_4/CeO_2 [22]	229.75	2.06	Type II

Data in Table 1 were determined through experimental measurements.

After analyzing the experimental results, it can be concluded that type II heterojunctions based on g-C_3N_4 exhibit superior photocatalytic efficiency compared to single-layer g-C_3N_4. Therefore, when selecting efficient photocatalysts, emphasis should be placed on g-C_3N_4-based type II heterojunctions. The band structure of the type II heterojunction is staggered, encompassing two distinct semiconductor materials, one of which must be satisfied as an oxidized type with a sufficiently low valence band position, and the other semiconductor as a reduced type with a sufficiently high conduction band position. Figure 1 illustrates the band alignment of g-C_3N_4 and confirms its adequately high conduction band position [23–25]. Accordingly, only another two-dimensional monolayer semiconductor needs to be chosen while ensuring its lower valence band position. Through screening, GaN was identified as meeting these criteria (refer to Figure 1) [26]. Based on this hypothesis, forming heterojunctions between GaN and g-C_3N_4 will lead to enhanced photocatalytic efficiency for type II heterojunctions.

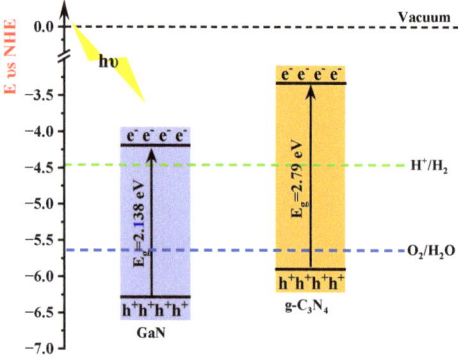

Figure 1. Schematic diagram illustrating the band alignment between a single layer of g-C_3N_4 [20] and GaN [27].

Consequently, it is plausible to anticipate the successful realization of type II GaN/g-C_3N_4. In this study, we employ first principle calculations to construct GaN/g-C_3N_4

and investigate its electronic structure and optical properties. Our findings unveil the significant potential of this heterojunction in photocatalysis, providing theoretical support for advancing efficient and stable photocatalysts. These results contribute to the application and further development of photocatalysis technology.

However, the photocatalytic efficiency of the heterojunction remains limited due to the high probability of recombination between photogenerated electron–hole pairs and the excessive loss of photogenerated carriers [28,29]. The band edge positions of the heterojunction can be precisely tuned by applying an external electric field and carefully adjusting its intensity and direction, leading to a notable enhancement in its photocatalytic performance. The proposed approach introduces novel concepts and methodologies that make a significant contribution to the advancement of photocatalytic materials, enhancing their efficiency and stability [30,31]. The influence of an external electric field on the electronic structure of the SeZrS/SeHfS heterojunction was investigated by Yang et al. [32]. Their findings demonstrate that the application of an electric field with an intensity below -0.2 V/Å or above 0.2 V/Å induces a transition from a type I to a type II heterojunction, resulting in interlaced bands. This transition significantly facilitates the efficient separation of photogenerated carriers, thereby enhancing photocatalytic efficiency. Zhao et al. [33] utilized an external electric field to modulate the electronic structure of a $PtSe_2/ZrSe_2$ heterojunction, resulting in a tunable band gap within the range of 0–0.25 eV. The bandgap initially widens and then rapidly narrows as the external electric field shifts from negative to positive values, promoting electron transitions. Moreover, under specific ranges of electric field intensity (-0.05 V/Å $< E < 0.01$ V/Å and -0.17 V/Å $< E < 0.22$ V/Å), the heterojunction type transforms from type I to type II, leading to enhanced photocatalytic performance. The aforementioned statement underscores the capacity of an external electric field to manipulate the migration pathways of photogenerated carriers, fine-tune the band alignment of the heterojunction, and optimize the photocatalytic process. Ultimately, this enhancement in heterojunction photocatalytic efficiency confers evident advantages. Consequently, the objective of this study is to construct $GaN/g-C_3N_4$ utilizing the first principle method and to manipulate its optical properties through the introduction of an external electric field. Our aim is to provide novel perspectives and theoretical models that will advance the development of highly efficient photocatalytic materials.

2. Model Structures and Stability

The present study meticulously constructed a comprehensive model $GaN/g-C_3N_4$, comprising a total of 46 atoms (as depicted in Figure 2). First, the bulk phases of $g-C_3N_4$ and GaN were cut along the (001) plane to obtain two-dimensional $g-C_3N_4$ (a = b = 4.779 Å) and GaN (a = b = 3.210 Å). Then, based on lattice matching, the single layers of both phases were expanded to form $g-C_3N_4$ (2 × 2 × 1) and GaN (3 × 3 × 1), ultimately constructing a heterojunction with $g-C_3N_4$ as the bottom layer. To effectively mitigate the impact of interlayer coupling, a substantial vacuum layer measuring 20 Å was deliberately incorporated along the c-axis direction.

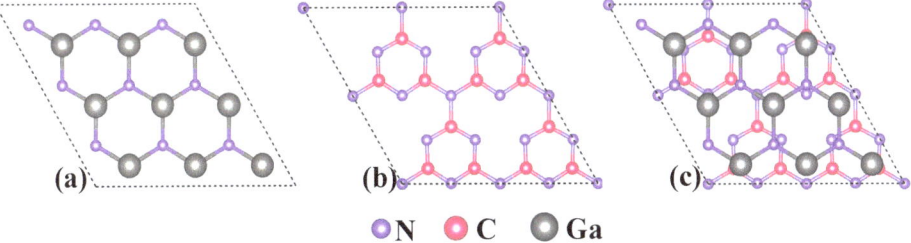

Figure 2. Structure model top views of (**a**) GaN supercell, (**b**) $g-C_3N_4$ supercell, and (**c**) $GaN/g-C_3N_4$ heterojunction.

After conducting meticulous calculations, it was conclusively determined that the lattice mismatch rate between GaN and g-C_3N_4 in the heterojunction is a mere 0.9%. This result unequivocally demonstrates the feasibility of establishing a stable heterojunction between these two materials. The three GaN/g-C_3N_4 models depicted in Figure 3 exhibit distinct stacking patterns: Model I shows precise alignment of the N-Ga ring of the GaN layer above the N-C ring of g-C_3N_4, as seen in Figure 3a; Model II features accurate positioning of the N atom of the GaN layer over that of the g-C_3N_4 layer, as shown in Figure 3b; and Model III positions the N atom of the GaN layer at the center of the N-C ring in the g-C_3N_4 layer, as illustrated in Figure 3c. Additionally, we have accurately computed the total energies by employing TS and Grimme dispersion correction methods, respectively, as summarized in Table 2. The calculation results show that the total energy value calculated by the TS method is lower, thereby showing that the TS method provided a more accurate reflection of the physical nature of intermolecular dispersion. Consequently, the calculation results are based on the TS method. Analyzing the total energy across three different modes reveals that model III exhibits the lowest calculated total energy using the TS method, which indicates its superior stability. Therefore, we chose model III as the structural model for GaN/g-C_3N_4 in this paper.

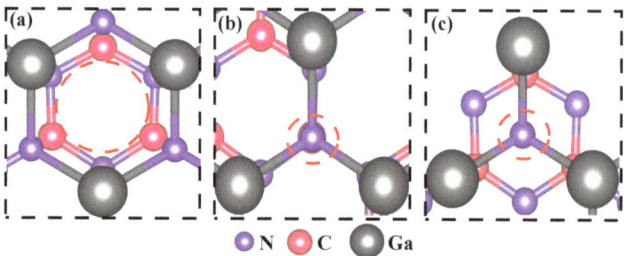

Figure 3. Three modes of GaN/g-C_3N_4 heterojunction (**a**) Model I, (**b**) Model II, (**c**) Model III. Red dashed circles represent the alignment of GaN single-layer and g-C_3N_4 single-layer stacks.

Table 2. Total energy of GaN/g-C_3N_4 heterojunctions obtained for three stacking methods using TS and Grimme dispersion correction methods.

Methods	Model I (eV)	Model II (eV)	Model III (eV)
TS	−28,134.0639	−28,134.0486	−28,134.0806
Grimme	−28,134.0480	−28,134.0237	−28,134.0534

To study the structural stability of GaN/g-C_3N_4, we calculated the binding energy at various interlayer distances. The expression for this binding energy (E_{coh}) is as follows [34]: $E_{coh} = E_T(GaN/g\text{-}C_3N_4) - E_T(GaN) - E_T(g\text{-}C_3N_4)$, where the total energies of the GaN/g-C_3N_4, the monolayer GaN, and the monolayer g-C_3N_4 are denoted as $E_T(GaN/g\text{-}C_3N_4)$, $E_T(GaN)$, and $E_T(g\text{-}C_3N_4)$, respectively. The presence of a negative binding energy signifies the inherent stability of the heterojunction structure [35]. The heterojunction structure is considered stable when the interlayer distance reaches 3.6 Å, as depicted in Figure 4a, with a corresponding minimum binding energy of −2.960 meV/Å^2.

To further validate the thermal stability of GaN/g-C_3N_4, we employed the DS-PAW (version 2023a) [36] first principle plane wave calculation software to conduct ab initio molecular dynamic (AIMD) simulations of the system at 300 K (equivalent to room temperature), as depicted in Figure 4b. After 8000 calculation steps within a timeframe of 8 ps, the system exhibits remarkable stability. The structural integrity remains intact without any chemical bond breakage, accompanied by minimal energy fluctuations. These findings underscore the exceptional thermodynamic stability of the heterojunction system at 300 K [37,38].

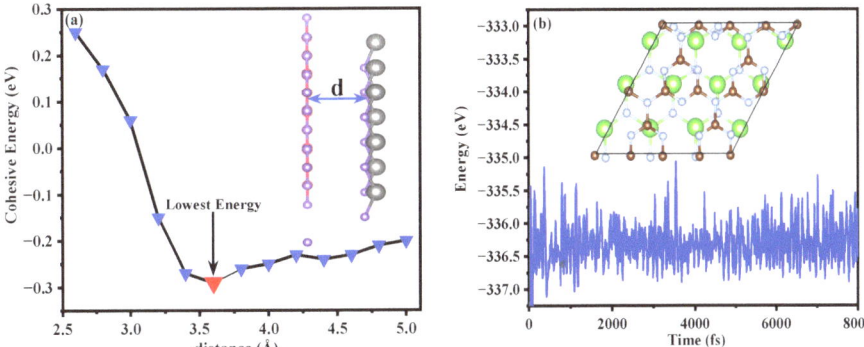

Figure 4. (a) The relationship between the binding energy of GaN/g-C$_3$N$_4$ and the interlayer spacing d; (b) The energy variation in GaN/g-C$_3$N$_4$ during the AIMD simulation lasting for 8 ps at 300 K, with the inset showing the top view of the final structure from the AIMD simulation. The illustrations shown in (a) depict gray balls representing Ga atoms, purple balls representing N atoms, and pink balls representing C atoms. The illustrations in (b) show green balls representing Ga atoms, gray balls representing N atoms, and brown balls representing C atoms.

The lattice mismatch energy (E_{miscoh}) associated with the GaN/g-C$_3$N$_4$ is expressed by the following equation [39]: $E_{miscoh} = E(g\text{-}C_3N_4)_{a1} + E(GaN)_{a2} - E(g\text{-}C_3N_4)_{a1'} - E(GaN)_{a2'}$ where the total energies of the monolayer g-C$_3$N$_4$ and GaN supercells are denoted as $E(g\text{-}C_3N_4)_{a1}$ and $E(GaN)_{a2}$, respectively, when their lattice constants are set to a. Furthermore, $E(g\text{-}C_3N_4)_{a1'}$ represents the total energy of the monolayer g-C$_3$N$_4$ with a lattice constant of $a_{1'}$, while $E(GaN)_{a2'}$ indicates the total energy of the monolayer GaN with a lattice constant of $a_{2'}$. The lattice mismatch energy of the GaN/g-C$_3$N$_4$ is calculated to be −1.230 meV/Å^2, indicating its remarkable stability. To further investigate the interaction forces at the interfaces of the heterojunction, we introduced the van der Waals energy (ΔE_{vdw}) [40] as a powerful tool for analyzing this particular heterojunction. The mathematical formulation of this energy can be expressed as follows: $\Delta E_{vdw} = |E_{coh}| + |E_{miscoh}|$, the absolute value of the binding energy for the heterojunction, denoted as $|E_{coh}|$, and the absolute value of the lattice mismatch energy within the system, denoted as $|E_{miscoh}|$, are crucial factors in this study. Notably, a van der Waals energy measurement of 4.19 meV/Å^2 indicates that the interaction force between interfaces is primarily governed by van der Waals forces.

3. Analysis and Discussion

3.1. Electronic Structure and Optical Properties

3.1.1. Energy Band Structure and Electronic Density of States

This study presents a comprehensive analysis of the band structure and electron density of states for monolayer g-C$_3$N$_4$, monolayer GaN, and the GaN/g-C$_3$N$_4$, as illustrated in Figures 5 and 6. Based on the presented data, this study focuses on the energy range spanning from −3 to 5 eV, with the Fermi level serving as the reference point at 0 eV. Moreover, the conduction band minimum and valence band maximum are both located at the identical symmetry point Γ, indicating a direct electron transition in both systems. Additionally, precise calculations demonstrate that monolayer GaN possesses a bandgap width (E_g) of 2.146 eV, which closely aligns with the calculated value of 2.138 eV by Yi et al. [27], exhibiting an error margin of only 0.37%. Conversely, monolayer g-C$_3$N$_4$ exhibits a narrower gap at 1.568 eV, deviating from the calculated result of 1.62 eV by Oreshonkov et al. [41] with a discrepancy of 3.2%. The electron density of state (DOS) diagram on the right provides evidence that N-2p states make up most of the valence band in monolayer GaN, accompanied by a minor contribution from Ga-4p states. Moreover, both the conduction band and a portion of the valence band in monolayer GaN are primarily influenced by N-2s states, consistent with observations made in its corresponding band structure diagram.

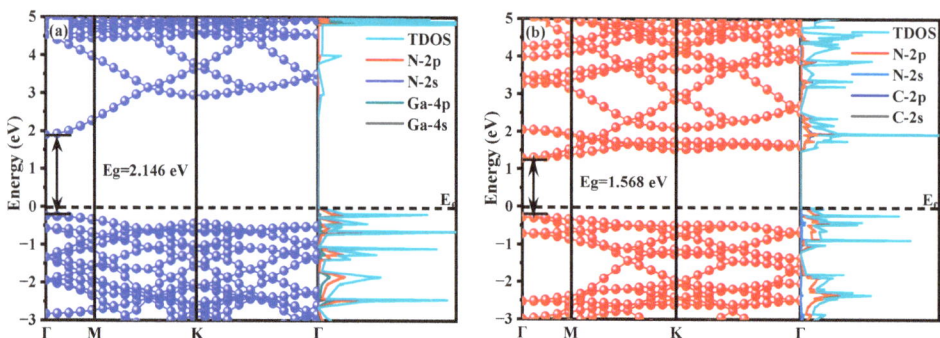

Figure 5. Energy band diagrams (left) and partial DOS diagrams (right) of monolayer GaN (**a**); monolayer g-C_3N_4 (**b**).

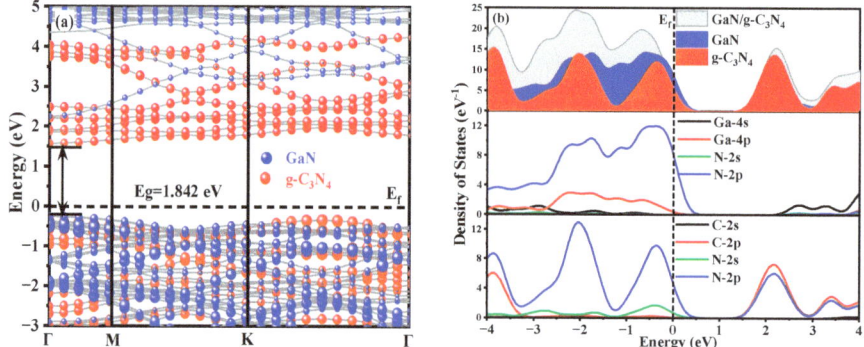

Figure 6. GaN/g-C_3N_4 heterojunction: (**a**) energy band structure diagram; (**b**) DOS diagram.

The band structure diagram of the GaN/g-C_3N_4 is depicted in Figure 6a, where the valence band maximum (VBM) and conduction band minimum (CBM) coincide at the same Γ point, indicating a direct bandgap nature with an energy value of 1.842 eV. This finding aligns consistently with previously reported literature values [42]. The CBM of GaN/g-C_3N_4 is predominantly determined by g-C_3N_4, while the VBM is primarily contributed by GaN, indicating a type-II alignment in GaN/g-C_3N_4. The present finding is in line with the experimental outcomes reported by Sarkar et al. [26]. Compared to monolayer systems, the two materials in GaN/g-C_3N_4 exhibit overlapping but maintain their respective independent electronic constructions. The combination of different materials in this process allows for the utilization of complementary advantages and the optimization of performance. Additionally, the interaction at the heterojunction interface significantly enhances the efficiency of separating photon-generated carriers.

The conduction band of the heterojunction is primarily contributed to by C-2p and N-2p states near the Fermi level, while the valence band predominantly consists of N-2p and Ga-4p states, as depicted in Figure 6b. The conduction band of the heterojunction is primarily contributed to by C-2p and N-2p states near the Fermi level, while the valence band predominantly consists of N-2p and Ga-4p states, as illustrated in Figure 6b, which can be attributed to the proximity of the valence band to the Fermi level, facilitating electron transitions from the valence band to the conduction band. Moreover, there exists an energy level overlap between the orbitals of both materials, indicating a significant hybridization of orbitals between Ga atoms and N atoms, which promotes electron transfer from Ga-4p states to N-2p states, resulting in electron accumulation at N atoms located at the heterojunction interface.

3.1.2. Work Function and Effective Mass

The work function (Φ) represents the minimum energy required for electrons to transition from the interior of a semiconductor to its surface. In this study, we conducted calculations to determine work functions for monolayer g-C_3N_4, monolayer GaN, and GaN/g-C_3N_4. The calculation formulation is outlined as follows [43]: $\Phi = E_{vac} - E_{fer}$. Here, the symbol E_{vac} denotes the vacuum energy level, while E_{fer} signifies the Fermi energy level. As depicted in Figure 7, the Φ of monolayer GaN and monolayer g-C_3N_4 are 5.956 eV and 4.097 eV, respectively, reaffirming the findings reported in the existing literature [44]. Compared to the GaN monolayer system, the Φ of the GaN/g-C_3N_4 was reduced to 5.500 eV, indicating enhanced electron excitation at the interface of this heterojunction. By comparing the minimum potential energy of GaN and g-C_3N_4, a potential difference of 1.676 eV between them is observed. It is deduced that an inherent electric field forms in the heterojunction, with its direction pointing from the g-C_3N_4 layer towards the GaN layer. Such an electric field facilitates to improve carrier mobility and efficient separation of photo-generated electron–hole pairs at the interface, ultimately resulting in a significant enhancement of photocatalytic performance for the heterojunction [45].

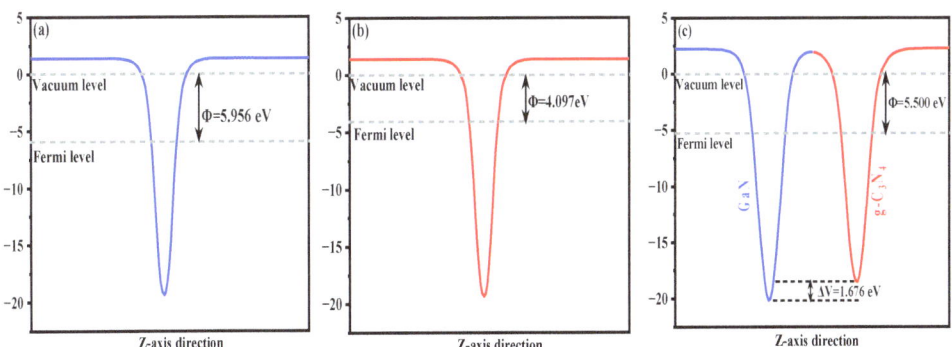

Figure 7. Work function diagrams of (a) GaN; (b) g-C_3N_4; and (c) GaN/g-C_3N_4 heterojunction (The vacuum energy level in this article is assumed to be at the reference point of 0 eV).

To gain a more comprehensive understanding of the migration behavior of electrons and holes, this study conducts an analysis by calculating the effective masses (m_e^*, m_h^*) and their ratio D = m_e^*/m_h^*, for monolayer GaN, monolayer g-C_3N_4, and GaN/g-C_3N_4. The calculation results, expressed by formulas as follows [46], are presented in Table 3:

$$m^* = \hbar^2 / (\frac{\partial^2 E}{\partial k^2})$$

Table 3. Effective masses of single-layer GaN, single-layer g-C_3N_4, and GaN/g-C_3N_4.

System	m_e^*	m_h^*	D (m_e^*/m_h^*)
GaN	0.56	0.55	0.98
g-C_3N_4	0.58	0.62	1.07
GaN/g-C_3N_4	0.67	1.29	1.93

Here, the $\partial^2 E/\partial k^2$ represents the second-order derivative of the E–K curve. The effective masses (m_e^* and m_h^*) of GaN/g-C_3N_4 are found to be 0.67 and 1.29, respectively; these values increase compared to those observed in the single-layer. The D value generally denotes the degree of separation between electrons and holes, effectively characterizing disparities between electrons and holes within a given system. A high D value indicates a significant degree of separation between electrons and holes within the system, resulting in an increased number of available electrons and holes for participation in photocatalytic water splitting reactions. In comparison to monolayer systems, GaN/g-C$_3$N$_4$ exhibits the highest D value, indicating a preference for holes and reducing the likelihood of electron–hole recombination. These findings suggest that the construction of heterojunction significantly enhances the efficiency of electron–hole separation, thus anticipating a substantial improvement in its photocatalytic performance.

3.1.3. Difference in Charge Density

In order to gain a more comprehensive understanding of the charge redistribution occurring at the heterojunction interface, this study employs formula [47] $\Delta\rho = \rho(\text{GaN/g-C}_3\text{N}_4) - \rho(\text{GaN}) - \rho(\text{g-C}_3\text{N}_4)$ to determine the planar-averaged differential charge density for GaN/g-C$_3$N$_4$. The charge densities of the GaN/g-C$_3$N$_4$, monolayer GaN, and monolayer g-C$_3$N$_4$, respectively, represent $\rho(\text{GaN/g-C}_3\text{N}_4)$, $\rho(\text{GaN})$ and $\rho(\text{g-C}_3\text{N}_4)$. As illustrated in Figure 8, a depletion of charge occurs in the GaN layer while a corresponding accumulation takes place in the g-C$_3$N$_4$ layer at the interface of GaN/g-C$_3$N$_4$. This migration of charges from the GaN layer to the g-C$_3$N$_4$ layer generates an internal electric field that is directed from the g-C$_3$N$_4$ towards the GaN region. The interface between GaN and g-C$_3$N$_4$ induces a reorganization of electron distribution. Electrons migrate from GaN towards g-C$_3$N$_4$, resulting in the establishment of a built-in electric field at the interface. The inherent electric field effectively facilitates the spatial separation of photogenerated electrons and holes, thereby significantly mitigating their recombination probability. Consequently, a higher proportion of photogenerated electrons and holes can be involved in photocatalytic reactions, thus substantially advancing the photocatalytic efficiency of the catalyst [48].

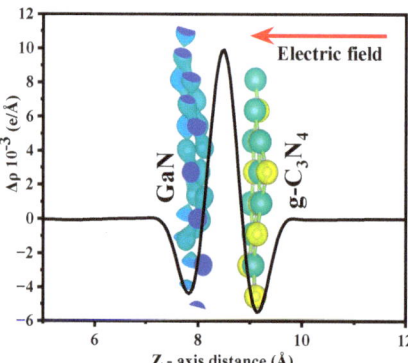

Figure 8. Plane-averaged differential charge density diagram of GaN/g-C$_3$N$_4$. The inset presents a three-dimensional diagram illustrating the differential charge density, with the yellow region indicating electron accumulation and the cyan region representing electron depletion.

3.2. Photocatalytic Performance

The optical absorption coefficient of GaN/g-C$_3$N$_4$ exhibits a remarkable enhancement within the visible light range, as illustrated in Figure 9. In comparison to monolayer g-C$_3$N$_4$, GaN/g-C$_3$N$_4$ demonstrates a significant red shift towards lower energy levels, indicating an augmented light-responsive capacity. These findings suggest that the incorporation of GaN into g-C$_3$N$_4$ can significantly enhance the optical absorption characteristics of this system.

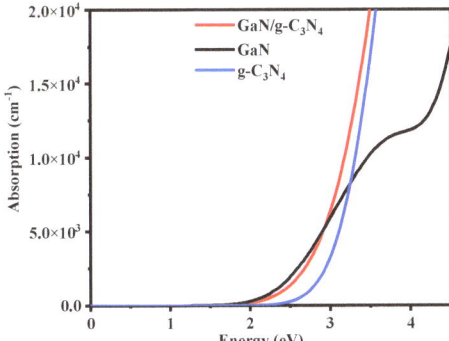

Figure 9. Absorption spectra of monolayer GaN, monolayer g-C$_3$N$_4$, and GaN/g-C$_3$N$_4$.

The CBM and VBM of single-layer GaN are −3.674 eV and −5.811 eV, respectively, as illustrated in Figure 10. Similarly, the CBM and VBM of single-layer g-C$_3$N$_4$ are −3.084 eV and −4.649 eV, respectively. The relative positions of single-layer GaN and g-C$_3$N$_4$ in the band edge alignment diagram (Figure 10) are consistent with the experimental measurements in Figure 1. During the formation of a heterojunction, electron redistribution occurs at the interface between a single-layer GaN and g-C$_3$N$_4$, resulting in downward movement of their energy bands relative to the vacuum level. However, it is important to note that the CBM and VBM of g-C$_3$N$_4$ still remain at higher energy levels compared to those of GaN, leading to the formation of a staggered band structure known as type II. Therefore, our calculation results indicate that GaN/g-C$_3$N$_4$ is a type II heterojunction.

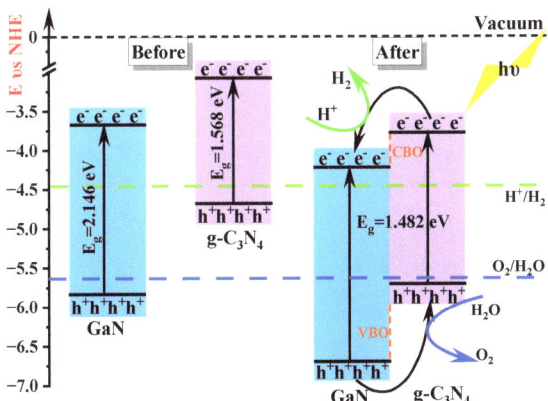

Figure 10. Band edge positions of GaN, g-C$_3$N$_4$, and GaN/g-C$_3$N$_4$ heterojunction for water oxidation and reduction. In the diagram, the green dashed line represents the energy level of H$^+$/H$_2$, while the blue dashed line corresponds to the energy level of O$_2$/H$_2$O.

3.3. External Electric Field

Extensive research has demonstrated that the bandgap and properties of heterojunction structures can be modulated by an external electric field. Therefore, in this study, we introduce an external electric field perpendicular to the planar surface of GaN/g-C$_3$N$_4$ along the c-direction. Figure 11a shows the variation in band edge positions of GaN/g-C$_3$N$_4$ under the electric field intensity range from −0.3 V/Å to 0.3 V/Å for water oxidation and reduction, wherein the valence band maximum (VBM) and conduction band minimum (CBM) of GaN and g-C$_3$N$_4$ are determined using formulae [49], which are expressed as follows: $E_{VBM} = \chi - E_{elec} + 0.5\,E_g$, $E_{CBM} = E_{VBM} - E_g$, wherein E_{elec} represents a constant value relative to the H electrode (E_{elec} = 4.5 eV), E_g denotes the bandgap of the system, and χ signifies the average electronegativity of the constituent atoms within the system [50]. According to the settlement outcome of the equations, the application of an electric field ranging from −0.1 V/Å to 0.2 V/Å sustains a higher CBM level for g-C_3N_4 compared to GaN while simultaneously maintaining a lower VBM. The aforementioned observation suggests that GaN/g-C_3N_4 possesses a staggered band structure. Furthermore, the CBM is positioned higher than the potential of H^+/H_2, while the VBM is situated lower than the potential of O_2/H_2O. The above-mentioned characteristics suggest that GaN/g-C_3N_4 can be classified as a type II heterojunction. When the electric field intensity falls below −0.1 V/Å or exceeds 0.2 V/Å, GaN/g-C_3N_4 still has a staggered band structure. However, the CBM and VBM of GaN/g-C_3N_4 are not fully straddled above and below the redox potential. Therefore, under electric field intensity, $E \leq$ −0.1 V/Å or E > 0.2 V/Å, GaN/g-C_3N_4 is not a type II heterojunction, but a Z-scheme heterojunction.

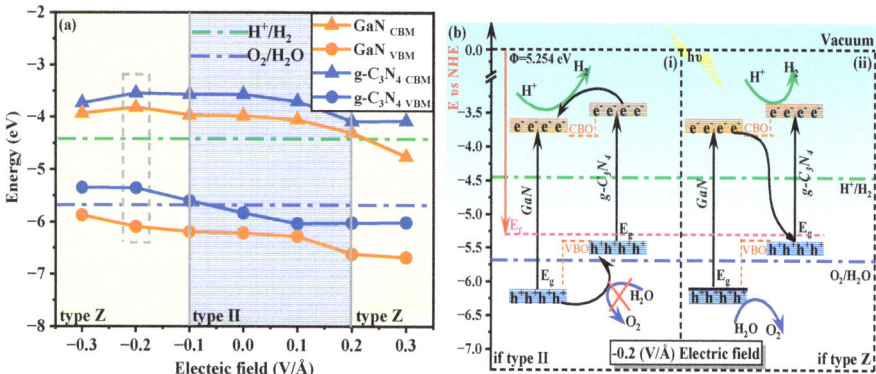

Figure 11. (**a**) Diagram illustrating the variation in band edge positions of GaN/g-C_3N_4 under the influence of sequential external electric fields for water oxidation and reduction; (**b**) Schematic representation illustrating the photocatalytic electron migration mechanism following heterojunction band edge alignment under an applied electric field intensity of −0.2 V/Å. The orange rectangle represents CB, and the blue rectangle represents VB. **b(i)** shows the assumed electron migration pathway of GaN/g-C_3N_4 as Type II, while **b(ii)** shows the assumed electron migration pathway of GaN/g-C_3N_4 as Type Z. The vacuum energy level is defined as zero eV, with the green dashed line representing oxidation potential and the blue dashed line representing reduction potential.

Subsequently, we elucidate the intrinsic mechanism of this Z-type heterojunction by considering GaN/g-C_3N_4 under a specific applied electric field strength (E = −0.2 V/A) as an illustrative example. Based on the aforementioned analysis, it is evident that the GaN/g-C_3N_4 structure exhibits a bandgap spanning characteristic, as illustrated in Figure 11b(i), suggesting its potential as a type II heterojunction [51]. However, the VBM of g-C_3N_4 is over the position of the water oxidation potential, thereby impeding hole transfer from the VBM of GaN to g-C_3N_4 and rendering it incapable of meeting the conditions required for water decomposition. This observation result negates the rationality of considering g-C_3N_4 as a type II heterojunction. Therefore, as illustrated in Figure 11b(ii), the electron transfer path occurs from the CBM of GaN with a lower reduced capacity to the VBM of g-C_3N_4 with a lower oxidized capacity, guided along a specific "Z"-type pathway, facilitating carrier recombination. Meanwhile, the electrons at the CBM of g-C_3N_4 with a higher reduced capacity and holes at the VBM of GaN with a higher oxidized capacity are selectively retained, facilitating effective spatial segregation of redox sites and improving the reactivity of the heterojunctions in the photocatalytic reaction. This new electron migration mechanism is termed as a direct Z-scheme [52]. According to this methodology, Z-scheme heterojunctions are formed in all GaN/g-C_3N_4 systems under specific electric fields (E ≤ −0.1 V/Å, E > 0.2 V/Å), as illustrated in Figure 11a.

The potential energy difference values (ΔPs) between the CBM of g-C$_3$N$_4$ and VBM of GaN were calculated based on the data presented in Figure 11a. The corresponding results are summarized in Table 4. It is observed from the table that the Z-scheme systems exhibit a higher ΔP compared to type II systems. The Z-type material exhibits a higher potential for photo-generated electrons compared to type II materials, thereby enhancing its reduction ability. Simultaneously, the Z-type material demonstrates a lower potential for holes in comparison to type II materials, leading to an augmented oxidation ability. ΔP serves as the underlying rationale for the enhanced separation of photogenerated carriers and redox capacity exhibited by Z-type heterojunctions when compared to type II heterojunctions.

Table 4. Potential difference across GaN/g-C$_3$N$_4$ under varying electric fields.

Electric Field (V/Å)	−0.3	−0.2	0.3	−0.1	0	0.1	0.2
Type	Z	Z	Z	Z	II	II	II
ΔP (eV)	2.544	2.550	2.620	2.525	2.245	2.369	2.335

The Z-type heterojunctions, as illustrated in Figure 12, exhibit significant redshifts compared to the type II heterojunctions. The redshift and absorption coefficients of Z-type heterojunction are notably enhanced at external electric field intensities of 0.2 V/Å and 0.1 V/Å, respectively. This observation aligns with the preamble comprehensive discussion on the Z-scheme GaN/g-C$_3$N$_4$, where its superior oxidation–reduction capacity has emerged as a pivotal factor in enhancing light absorption and improving photocatalytic activity.

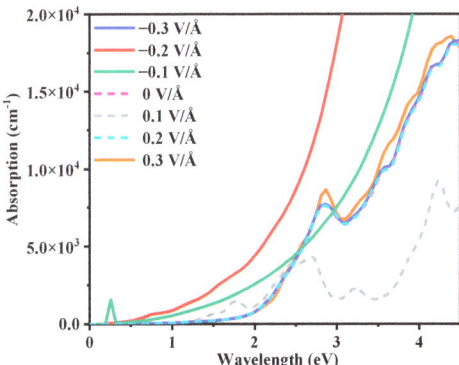

Figure 12. The absorption spectrum of GaN/g-C$_3$N$_4$ heterojunctions under the influence of different external electric field, with solid lines representing z-scheme heterojunctions and dashed lines representing type II heterojunctions.

4. Materials and Methods

The Vienna Ab initio Simulation Package (VASP 6.3) [53] based on density functional theory (DFT) [54] was employed in this study to investigate GaN/g-C$_3$N$_4$. Specifically, we selected the Perdew–Burke–Ernzerhof (PBE) exchange-correlation functional coupled with the generalized gradient approximation (GGA) [55] for our calculations. To accurately account for dispersion interactions, both the TS (Tkatchenko-Scheffler) [56] and DFT-D3 [57] methodologies were utilized. Notably, a plane wave cutoff energy of 500 eV was set, and a Monkhorst-Pack [58] scheme with a K-point grid of 3 × 3 × 1 was employed (Figure S1). Additionally, the self-consistent field (SCF) of 2 × 10^{-6} eV/atom was chosen to ensure the result precision.

5. Conclusions

First principle analysis was employed to investigate the electronic structure and optical properties of GaN/g-C_3N_4 heterojunctions under external electric fields in this study. The calculations revealed that GaN/g-C_3N_4 exhibits a lower lattice mismatch. AIMD simulations demonstrated minimal total energy fluctuations at 300 K, indicating robust thermodynamic stability and structural integrity. The GaN/g-C_3N_4 heterojunction displays a direct bandgap of 1.842 eV and exhibits a type II heterojunction configuration. The electron migration occurs from the GaN layer to the g-C_3N_4 layer, leading to the establishment of an intrinsic electric field directed towards the GaN layer. When the strength of the applied external electric field falls below 0.1 V/Å or exceeds 0.2 V/Å, the band structure of GaN/g-C_3N_4 can transition from a type II heterojunction to a Z-type heterojunction. Compared to type II materials, the Z-type material exhibits a higher potential for photo-generated electrons, which enhances its reduction ability. Additionally, it demonstrates a lower potential for holes in comparison to type II materials, resulting in an augmented oxidation ability. At external electric field intensities of 0.2 V/Å and 0.1 V/Å, respectively, the redshift and absorption coefficients of the Z-type heterojunction undergo significant enhancements. In conclusion, a precise manipulation of the external electric field can profoundly influence and optimize both band structure alignment and photocatalytic performance in these heterojunctions.

Supplementary Materials: The following supporting information can be downloaded at: https://www.mdpi.com/article/10.3390/molecules29225355/s1, Figure S1: Convergence test for supercell geometry optimization (a) Cutoff energy (b) K-point.

Author Contributions: Conceptualization, M.-Y.D., X.-C.Z., Y.-N.H., L.-L.Z. and H.G.; Data curation, L.-L.Z.; Formal analysis, M.-Y.D. and L.-L.Z.; Funding acquisition, L.-L.Z.; Investigation, M.-Y.D., X.-C.Z., B.-C.L., Y.-N.H., L.-L.Z. and H.G.; Methodology, X.-C.Z., B.-C.L., H.G. and H.-G.W.; Project administration, L.-L.Z.; Resources, L.-L.Z.; Supervision, L.-L.Z.; Validation, L.-L.Z. and H.G.; Visualization, M.-Y.D. and H.-G.W.; Writing—original draft, M.-Y.D. and B.-C.L.; Writing—review and editing, Y.-N.H., L.-L.Z. and H.G. All authors have read and agreed to the published version of the manuscript.

Funding: This research was funded by the key project at the school level of Yili Normal University (grant number 2023YSZD003), Science and Technology Plan Project of Yili Kazakh Autonomous Prefecture (grant number YZ2022B021) and Innovation and Entrepreneurship Training Project of Yili Normal University Students (grant number X2022110764022).

Data Availability Statement: The original contributions presented in this study are included in the article, and further inquiries can be directed to the corresponding authors.

Acknowledgments: We gratefully acknowledge HZWTECH for providing computation facilities.

Conflicts of Interest: The authors declare no conflicts of interest.

References

1. Dong, Y.; Zhang, Y.; Liu, S. The Impacts and Instruments of Energy Transition Regulations on Environmental Pollution. *Environ. Impact Assess. Rev.* **2024**, *105*, 107448. [CrossRef]
2. Zheng, D.; Xue, Y.; Wang, J.; Varbanov, P.S.; Klemeš, J.J.; Yin, C. Nanocatalysts in Photocatalytic Water Splitting for Green Hydrogen Generation: Challenges and Opportunities. *J. Clean. Prod.* **2023**, *414*, 137700. [CrossRef]
3. Zhou, P.; Navid, I.A.; Ma, Y.; Xiao, Y.; Wang, P.; Ye, Z.; Zhou, B.; Sun, K.; Mi, Z. Solar-to-Hydrogen Efficiency of More than 9% in Photocatalytic Water Splitting. *Nature* **2023**, *613*, 66–70. [CrossRef] [PubMed]
4. Peiris, S.; De Silva, H.B.; Ranasinghe, K.N.; Bandara, S.V.; Perera, I.R. Recent Development and Future Prospects of TiO_2 Photocatalysis. *J. Chin. Chem. Soc.* **2021**, *68*, 738–769. [CrossRef]
5. Hou, Q.; Li, W.; Xu, Z.; Liu, Y.; Sha, S. Study of the Electronic Structure and Absorption Spectrum of Co and H Doped ZnO by First-Principles. *Chem. Phys.* **2020**, *528*, 110460. [CrossRef]
6. Sun, Y.; Han, Y.; Song, X.; Huang, B.; Ma, X.; Xing, R. CdS/WO_3 S-Scheme Heterojunction with Improved Photocatalytic CO_2 Reduction Activity. *J. Photochem. Photobiol. B* **2022**, *233*, 112480. [CrossRef]
7. Yuan, J.; Wang, F.; Zhang, Z.; Song, B.; Yan, S.; Shang, M.-H.; Tong, C.; Zhou, J. Effects of Electric Field and Interlayer Coupling on Schottky Barrier of Germanene/MoSSe Vertical Heterojunction. *Phys. Rev. B* **2023**, *108*, 125404. [CrossRef]

8. Sun, X.; Huang, H.; Zhao, Q.; Ma, T.; Wang, L. Thin-Layered Photocatalysts. *Adv. Funct. Mater.* **2020**, *30*, 1910005. [CrossRef]
9. Dao, Q.D.; Nguyen, T.K.; Dang, T.T.; Kang, S.G.; Nguyen-Phu, H.; Do, L.T.; Van, V.K.; Chung, K.H.; Chung, J.S.; Shin, E.W. Anchoring Highly Distributed Pt Species over Oxidized Graphitic Carbon Nitride for Photocatalytic Hydrogen Evolution: The Effect of Reducing Agents. *Appl. Surf. Sci.* **2023**, *609*, 155305. [CrossRef]
10. Dao, D.Q.; Nguyen, T.K.A.; Kang, S.G.; Shin, E.W. Engineering Oxidation States of a Platinum Cocatalyst over Chemically Oxidized Graphitic Carbon Nitride Photocatalysts for Photocatalytic Hydrogen Evolution. *ACS Sustain. Chem. Eng.* **2021**, *43*, 14537–14549. [CrossRef]
11. Singh, J.; Sharma, P.; Tripathi, N.; Shishkina, D.; Rymzhina, A.; Boltov, E.A.; Platonov, V.; Pavelyev, V.; Volkov, V.S.; Arsenin, A.V.; et al. Synthesis of Highly Sensitive Nanomaterial for Ultra-Fast Photocatalytic Activity: A Detailed Study on Photocatalytic Capabilities of Rod-Shaped TiS_3 Nanostructures. *Catal. Commun.* **2022**, *162*, 106381. [CrossRef]
12. Telkhozhayeva, M.; Hirsch, B.; Konar, R.; Teblum, E.; Lavi, R.; Weitman, M.; Malik, B.; Moretti, E.; Nessim, G.D. 2D TiS_2 Flakes for Tetracycline Hydrochloride Photodegradation under Solar Light. *Appl. Catal. B Environ.* **2022**, *318*, 121872. [CrossRef]
13. Dai, H.; Cai, X.; Li, X.; Wang, C.; Hou, Y.; Wei, R. First-Principles Calculations on Performance of the $g-C_3N_4$/LNS-TiO_2(Cr+C) Heterojunction Photocatalyst in Water Splitting Process. *Int. J. Hydrogen Energy* **2023**, *48*, 38742–38748. [CrossRef]
14. Jiang, J.; Xiong, Z.; Wang, H.; Liao, G.; Bai, S.; Zou, J.; Wu, P.; Zhang, P.; Li, X. Sulfur-Doped $g-C_3N_4$/$g-C_3N_4$ Isotype Step-Scheme Heterojunction for Photocatalytic H_2 Evolution. *J. Mater. Sci. Technol.* **2022**, *118*, 15–24. [CrossRef]
15. Li, Y.; Zhou, M.; Cheng, B.; Shao, Y. Recent Advances in $g-C_3N_4$-Based Heterojunction Photocatalysts. *J. Mater. Sci. Technol.* **2020**, *56*, 1–17. [CrossRef]
16. Tao, J.; Huang, L.; Xiong, S.; Li, L.-X.; Wang, L.-L.; Xu, L. Two-Dimensional TMDs/MN (M = Al, Ga) van Der Waals Heterojunction Photocatalyst: A First-Principles Study. *J. Mater. Sci.* **2023**, *58*, 14080–14095. [CrossRef]
17. Ren, W.; Yang, J.; Zhang, J.; Li, W.; Sun, C.; Zhao, H.; Wen, Y.; Sha, O.; Liang, B. Recent Progress in SnO_2/$g-C_3N_4$ Heterojunction Photocatalysts: Synthesis, Modification, and Application. *J. Alloys Compd.* **2022**, *906*, 164372. [CrossRef]
18. Lin, M.; Chen, H.; Zhang, Z.; Wang, X. Engineering Interface Structures for Heterojunction Photocatalysts. *Phys. Chem. Chem. Phys.* **2023**, *25*, 4388–4407. [CrossRef]
19. Zhang, Q.; Li, Y.; Zhong, J.; Li, J. Facile Construction of CuO/$g-C_3N_4$ Heterojunctions with Promoted Photocatalytic Hydrogen Generation Behaviors. *Fuel* **2023**, *353*, 129224. [CrossRef]
20. Pan, J.; Shen, W.; Zhang, Y.; Tang, H.; Sun, H.; Zhong, W.; Yan, X. Metal-Free SiOC/$g-C_3N_4$ Heterojunction Composites with Efficient Visible-Light Photocatalytic H_2 Production. *Appl. Surf. Sci.* **2020**, *520*, 146335. [CrossRef]
21. Lin, D.; Zhou, Y.; Ye, X.; Zhu, M. Construction of Sandwich Structured Photocatalyst Using Monolayer WS_2 Embedded $g-C_3N_4$ for Highly Efficient H_2 Production. *Ceram. Int.* **2020**, *46*, 12933–12941. [CrossRef]
22. Zhang, X.; Liang, H.; Li, C.; Bai, J. 1 D CeO_2/$g-C_3N_4$ Type II Heterojunction for Visible-Light-Driven Photocatalytic Hydrogen Evolution. *Inorg. Chem. Commun.* **2022**, *144*, 109838. [CrossRef]
23. Ge, W.; Liu, K.; Deng, S.; Yang, P.; Shen, L. Z-Scheme $g-C_3N_4$/ZnO Heterojunction Decorated by Au Nanoparticles for Enhanced Photocatalytic Hydrogen Production. *Appl. Surf. Sci.* **2023**, *607*, 155036. [CrossRef]
24. Wang, H.; Liu, Z.; Wang, L.; Shou, Q.; Gao, M.; Wang, H.; Nazir, A.; Huo, P. Fabrication of $g-C_3N_4$/SnS_2 Type-II Heterojunction for Efficient Photocatalytic Conversion of CO_2. *J. Mater. Sci. Mater. Electron.* **2023**, *34*, 350. [CrossRef]
25. Wang, Y.; Zhu, X.; Zhang, H.; He, S.; Liu, Y.; Zhao, W.; Liu, H.; Qu, X. Janus MoSH/WSi_2N_4 van Der Waals Heterostructure: Two-Dimensional Metal/Semiconductor Contact. *Molecules* **2024**, *29*, 3554. [CrossRef]
26. Sarkar, K.; Kumar, P. Activated Hybrid $g-C_3N_4$/Porous GaN Heterojunction for Tunable Self-Powered and Broadband Photodetection. *Appl. Surf. Sci.* **2021**, *566*, 150695. [CrossRef]
27. Yi, Y.; Zhou, R.; Zhuang, F.; Ye, X.; Li, H.; Hao, G.; Zhang, R. First-Principles Study on the Electronic Properties and Feasibility of Photocatalytic Water Splitting on Z-Scheme GaN/MoS_2 Heterostructure. *J. Phys. Chem. Solids* **2024**, *190*, 112006. [CrossRef]
28. Zhang, Q.; Chen, P.; Liu, Q.; Sun, P.; Yi, Y.; Lei, J.; Song, T. The Electronic and Optical Properties of Type-II g-CN/GaGePS van Der Waals Heterostructure Modulated via Biaxial Strain and External Electric Field. *Mater. Sci. Semicond. Process.* **2024**, *171*, 107989. [CrossRef]
29. Xu, L.; Tao, J.; Xiao, B.; Xiong, F.; Ma, Z.; Zeng, J.; Huang, X.; Tang, S.; Wang, L.-L. Two-Dimensional AlN/g-CNs van Der Waals Type-II Heterojunction for Water Splitting. *Phys. Chem. Chem. Phys.* **2023**, *25*, 3969–3978. [CrossRef]
30. Han, S.; Wei, X.; Huang, Y.; Zhang, J.; Zhu, G.; Yang, J. Influence of Strain and External Electric Field on the Performance of PC_6/$MoSe_2$ Heterostructure. *J. Mater. Sci.* **2022**, *57*, 477–488. [CrossRef]
31. Guo, R.; Luan, L.; Cao, M.; Zhang, Y.; Wei, X.; Fan, J.; Ni, L.; Liu, C.; Yang, Y.; Liu, J.; et al. Tunable Electronic Properties of GeC/BAs van Der Waals Heterostructure under External Electric Field and Strain. *Phys. E Low-Dimens. Syst. Nanostr.* **2023**, *149*, 115628. [CrossRef]
32. Yang, G.-H.; Zhang, J.-M.; Huang, Y.-H.; Wei, X.-M. Effects of External Electric Field on the Structural and Electronic Properties of SeZrS/SeHfS van Der Waals Heterostructure: A First-Principles Study. *Thin Solid Films* **2023**, *767*, 139675. [CrossRef]
33. Zhao, X.; Niu, W.; Zhang, H.; Dai, X.; Wei, S.; Yang, L. Effects of Interlayer Coupling and Electric Field on the Electronic Properties of $PtSe_2$/$ZrSe_2$ van Der Waals Heterojunctions. *Appl. Surf. Sci.* **2020**, *510*, 145316. [CrossRef]
34. Gao, L.; Zhou, B.; Zhang, J.; Jiang, K.; Shang, L.; Hu, Z.; Chu, J. Strain and Electric Field Tunable Electronic and Optical Properties in Antimonene/C_3N van Der Waals Heterostructure. *Solid State Sci.* **2021**, *122*, 106771. [CrossRef]

35. Wang, J.; Zhang, N.; Wang, Y.; Zhao, H.; Chen, H.; Zeng, H.; Zhao, L.; Yang, Q.; Feng, B. Direct Z-Scheme Construction of $C_2N/Mg(OH)_2$ Heterojunction and First-Principles Investigation of Photocatalytic Water Splitting. *Int. J. Hydrogen Energy* **2024**, *53*, 247–255. [CrossRef]
36. Sádecký, E.; Brezina, R.; Kazár, J.; Urvölgyi, J. Immunization against Q-Fever of Naturally Infected Dairy Cows. *Acta Virol.* **1975**, *19*, 486–488.
37. Guo, X.; Gu, J.; Lin, S.; Zhang, S.; Chen, Z.; Huang, S. Tackling the Activity and Selectivity Challenges of Electrocatalysts toward the Nitrogen Reduction Reaction via Atomically Dispersed Biatom Catalysts. *J. Am. Chem. Soc.* **2020**, *142*, 5709–5721. [CrossRef]
38. Lv, L.; Shen, Y.; Liu, J.; Meng, X.; Gao, X.; Zhou, M.; Zhang, Y.; Gong, D.; Zheng, Y.; Zhou, Z. Computational Screening of High Activity and Selectivity $TM/g-C_3N_4$ Single-Atom Catalysts for Electrocatalytic Reduction of Nitrates to Ammonia. *J. Phys. Chem. Lett.* **2021**, *12*, 11143–11150. [CrossRef]
39. Liu, Y.; Jiang, Z.; Jia, J.; Robertson, J.; Guo, Y. 2D $WSe_2/MoSi_2N_4$ Type-II Heterojunction with Improved Carrier Separation and Recombination for Photocatalytic Water Splitting. *Appl. Surf. Sci.* **2023**, *611*, 155674. [CrossRef]
40. Yan, S.; Chen, W.; Xiong, W.; Yang, L.; Luo, R.; Wang, F. Dicarbon Nitride and Janus Transition Metal Chalcogenides van Der Waals Heterojunctions for Photocatalytic Water Splitting. *J. Phys. Condens. Matter* **2023**, *35*, 014003. [CrossRef]
41. Oreshonkov, A.S.; Sukhanova, E.V.; Pankin, D.V.; Popov, Z.I. Electronic Transitions and Vibrational Properties of Bulk and Monolayer $g-C_3N_4$, and a $g-C_3N_4/MoS_2$ Heterostructure from a DFT Study. *Phys. Chem. Chem. Phys.* **2024**, *26*, 23023–23031. [CrossRef] [PubMed]
42. Liu, C.-X.; Pang, G.-W.; Pan, D.-Q.; Shi, L.-Q.; Zhang, L.-L.; Lei, B.-C.; Zhao, X.-C.; Huang, Y.-N. First-principles study of influence of electric field on electronic structure and optical properties of $GaN/g-C_3N_4$ heterojunction. *Acta Phys.* **2022**, *71*, 288–296. [CrossRef]
43. Zhou, T.; Qian, G.; Huang, S.; Liang, Q.; Luo, X.; Xie, Q. The Effect of Biaxial Strain on the Electronic Structures and Optical Properties of GaS/SSnSe Heterojunction: A First-Principles Calculations. *Phys. Lett. A* **2023**, *480*, 128956. [CrossRef]
44. Lu, P.; Zhao, H.; Li, Z.; Chu, M.; Xie, G.; Xie, T.; Jiang, L. High Photocatalytic Activity of $g-C_3N_4/CdZnS/MoS_2$ Heterojunction for Hydrogen Production. *Int. J. Hydrogen Energy* **2024**, *82*, 776–785. [CrossRef]
45. Zhu, X.T.; Xu, Y.; Cao, Y.; Zhao, Y.Q.; Sheng, W.; Nie, G.-Z.; Ao, Z. Investigation of the Electronic Structure of Two-Dimensional GaN/Zr_2CO_2 Hetero-Junction: Type-II Band Alignment with Tunable Bandgap. *Appl. Surf. Sci.* **2021**, *542*, 148505. [CrossRef]
46. Hassan, A.; Nazir, M.A.; Shen, Y.; Guo, Y.; Kang, W.; Wang, Q. First-Principles Study of the Structural, Electronic, and Enhanced Optical Properties of SnS/TaS_2 Heterojunction. *ACS Appl. Mater. Interfaces* **2022**, *14*, 2177–2184. [CrossRef]
47. Qiao, F.; Liu, W.; Yang, J.; Liu, Y.; Yuan, J. Fabrication of $ZnO/CuInS_2$ Heterojunction for Boosting Photocatalytic Hydrogen Production. *Int. J. Hydrogen Energy* **2024**, *53*, 840–847. [CrossRef]
48. Liu, Y.; Yao, Y.; Liang, Z.; Gong, Z.; Li, J.; Tang, Z.; Wei, X. Two-Dimensional AlN/PtSSe Heterojunction as A Direct Z-Scheme Photocatalyst for Overall Water Splitting: A DFT Study. *J. Phys. Chem. C* **2024**, *128*, 9894–9903. [CrossRef]
49. Luan, L.; Han, L.; Zhang, D.; Bai, K.; Sun, K.; Xu, C.; Li, L.; Duan, L. $AlSb/ZrS_2$ Heterojunction: A Direct Z-Scheme Photocatalyst with High Solar to Hydrogen Conversion Efficiency and Catalytic Activity across Entire PH Range. *Int. J. Hydrogen Energy* **2024**, *51*, 1242–1255. [CrossRef]
50. Yayak, Y.O.; Topkiran, U.C.; Yagmurcukardes, M.; Sahin, H. Van Der Waals Heterostructures of AlAs and InSe: Stacking-Dependent Raman Spectra and Electric Field Dependence of Electronic Properties. *Appl. Surf. Sci.* **2024**, *654*, 159360. [CrossRef]
51. Wang, G.; Tang, W.; Xu, C.; He, J.; Zeng, Q.; Xie, W.; Gao, P.; Chang, J. Two-Dimensional CdO/PtSSe Heterojunctions Used for Z-Scheme Photocatalytic Water-Splitting. *Appl. Surf. Sci.* **2022**, *599*, 153960. [CrossRef]
52. Dai, Z.-N.; Cao, Y.; Yin, W.J.; Sheng, W.; Xu, Y. Z-Scheme SnC/HfS_2 van Der Waals Heterojunction Increases Photocatalytic Overall Water Splitting. *J. Phys. Appl. Phys.* **2022**, *55*, 315503. [CrossRef]
53. Xie, K.-X.; Zhang, Y.; Qiang, Z.-B.; Ding, J.-X.; Nouguiza, H.; Chen, H.-X.; Duan, L.; Fan, J.-B.; Ni, L. A Direct Z-Scheme GeS/GeSe van Der Waals Heterojunction as a Promising Photocatalyst with High Optical Absorption, Solar-to-Hydrogen Efficiency and Catalytic Activity for Overall Water Splitting: First-Principles Prediction. *Int. J. Hydrogen Energy* **2024**, *51*, 1381–1391. [CrossRef]
54. Zhuo, Q.; Zhang, Y.; Fu, Z.; Han, T.; Liu, X.; Ou, J.; Xu, X. First-Principles Study of Photocatalytic Mechanism and Charge Transfer of $PtS_2/MoSe_2$ S-Scheme Heterojunction. *Appl. Surf. Sci.* **2022**, *600*, 154038. [CrossRef]
55. Wang, Y.; Liu, T.; Tian, W.; Zhang, Y.; Shan, P.; Chen, Y.; Wei, W.; Yuan, H.; Cui, H. Mechanism for Hydrogen Evolution from Water Splitting Based on a MoS_2/WSe_2 Heterojunction Photocatalyst: A First-Principle Study. *RSC Adv.* **2020**, *10*, 41127–41136. [CrossRef]
56. Holmes, S.T.; Vojvodin, C.S.; Schurko, R.W. Dispersion-Corrected DFT Methods for Applications in Nuclear Magnetic Resonance Crystallography. *J. Phys. Chem. A* **2020**, *124*, 10312–10323. [CrossRef]
57. Fu, S.; Wang, D.; Ma, Z.; Liu, G.; Zhu, X.; Yan, M.; Fu, Y. The First-Principles Study on the Halogen-Doped $graphene/MoS_2$ Heterojunction. *Solid State Commun.* **2021**, *334–335*, 114366. [CrossRef]
58. Sun, Y.; Luan, L.; Zhao, J.; Zhang, Y.; Wei, X.; Fan, J.; Ni, L.; Liu, C.; Yang, Y.; Liu, J.; et al. Tunable Properties of WTe_2/GaS Heterojunction and Se-Doped WTe_2/GaS Heterojunction. *Mater. Sci. Semicond. Process.* **2023**, *166*, 107695. [CrossRef]

Disclaimer/Publisher's Note: The statements, opinions and data contained in all publications are solely those of the individual author(s) and contributor(s) and not of MDPI and/or the editor(s). MDPI and/or the editor(s) disclaim responsibility for any injury to people or property resulting from any ideas, methods, instructions or products referred to in the content.

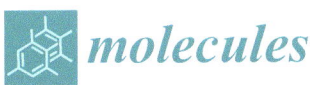

Article

Modulation of Electronic Availability in g-C$_3$N$_4$ Using Nickel (II), Manganese (II), and Copper (II) to Enhance the Disinfection and Photocatalytic Properties

Angie V. Lasso-Escobar [1], Elkin Darío C. Castrillon [1], Jorge Acosta [1], Sandra Navarro [2], Estefanía Correa-Penagos [1], John Rojas [1] and Yenny P. Ávila-Torres [1,*]

[1] Environmental Remediation and Biocatalysis Research Group (GIRAB), Institute of Chemistry, University of Antioquia UdeA, Calle 70 No. 52-21, Medellín 050014, Colombia; vanessa.lasso@udea.edu.co (A.V.L.-E.); elkindariocastellon@gmail.com (E.D.C.C.); jlacosta@utp.edu.co (J.A.); estefania.correa@udea.edu.co (E.C.-P.); jhon.rojas@udea.edu.co (J.R.)

[2] Grupo de Investigación Cecoltec, Cecoltec Services, Cra 43 A 18 sur 135, Medellín 050022, Colombia; snavarro@cecoltecservices.com

* Correspondence: yenny.avila@udea.edu.co

Abstract: Carbon nitrides can form coordination compounds or metallic oxides in the presence of transition metals, depending on the reaction conditions. By adjusting the pH to basic levels for mild synthesis with metals, composites like g-C$_3$N$_4$-M(OH)$_x$ (where M represents metals) were obtained for nickel (II) and manganese (II), while copper (II) yielded coordination compounds such as Cu-g-C$_3$N$_4$. These materials underwent spectroscopic and electrochemical characterization, revealing their photocatalytic potential to generate superoxide anion radicals—a feature consistent across all metals. Notably, the copper coordination compound also produced significant hydroxyl radicals. Leveraging this catalytic advantage, with band gap energy in the visible region, all compounds were activated to disinfect E. coli bacteria, achieving total disinfection with Cu-g-C$_3$N$_4$. The textural properties influence the catalytic performance, with copper's stabilization as a coordination compound enabling more efficient activity compared to the other metals. Additionally, the determination of radicals generated under light in the presence of dicloxacillin supported the proposed mechanism and highlighted the potential for degrading organic molecules with this new material, alongside its disinfectant properties.

Keywords: coordination compounds; disinfection; degradation; carbon nitride

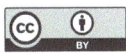

1. Introduction

Carbon nitrides have gained significant importance owing to their high physicochemical stability and low toxicity, making them suitable for applications in photocatalysis for environmental remediation and various emerging technologies [1–3]. However, certain thermodynamic properties of g-C$_3$N$_4$, such as its lipid-soluble character and the potential aggregation of its layers through hydrophobic interactions, along with considerations related to surface geometry, introduce some limitations in its electronic properties.

Notably, these compounds exhibit a high electronic recombination index, diminishing their capacity to generate electron-hole pairs. Additionally, the positioning of energy levels concerning redox potentials and the proper alignment of energy bands are critical factors influencing their efficiency and photochemical performance [4,5]. Several alternatives currently exist to enhance the optoelectronic properties of g-C$_3$N$_4$. For instance, the synthesis of heterojunctions has the potential to facilitate the efficient transfer of charge carriers between materials, mitigating undesired recombination and thereby improving the photocatalytic process [6–8].

Alternatively, the coordination of g-C$_3$N$_4$ with transition metals as composite or doping can broaden the absorption spectrum, creating active centers within the polymer mesh that facilitate light absorption, promote efficient charge transfer, and consequently increase the generation of electron-hole pairs [9–11].

Coordination with metals introduces new energy levels within the electronic structure of g-C$_3$N$_4$, influencing the position of electronic states. The stacking of graphitic carbon nitride allows coordination to metal centers through the nitrogen's lone electron pairs, in contrast to graphene. This can enhance its photocatalytic properties and charge transfer to a metal or an organic molecule. Metals such as Ni, Cu, and Mn, for example, can facilitate charge transfer in the materials, with their ions having the potential to be included in electron-rich cavities on the material's surface, providing a platform for stabilizing transition metals, even on their surface [12–16], Scheme 1a, Table S1 [13,17–27]. Previous research suggests that amino groups play a role in facilitating the transfer of photogenerated electrons. At the same time, metal ions, owing to their lower work function, can extract photogenerated electrons from semiconductors. In this scenario, coordination doping could potentially result in a synergistic effect between the amino groups and metal ions.

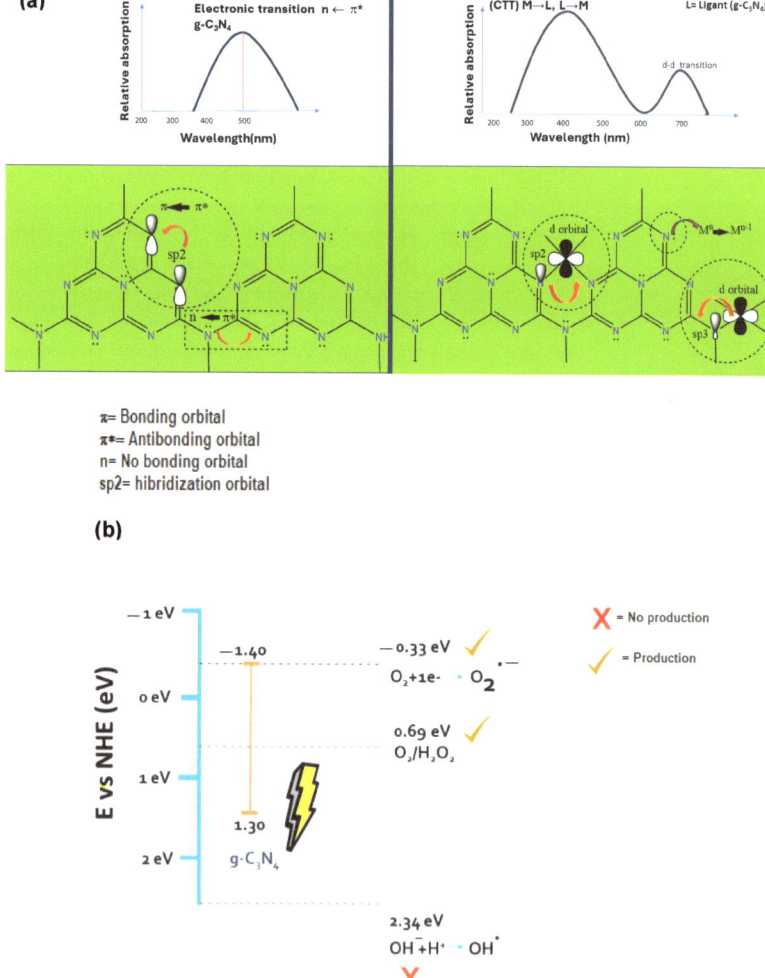

Scheme 1. (**a**) Electronic effect of metal ions on electronic properties in g-C$_3$N$_4$. (**b**) Electronic condition of g-C$_3$N$_4$ reported vs. generation of ROS.

Moreover, the generation of reactive oxygen species (ROS), such as hydroxyl radicals (•OH) and hydrogen peroxide (H_2O_2), can be achieved. For instance, Cu is effective in producing •OH, while Ni and Mn can contribute to other ROS species. Consequently, by integrating the generation of ROS with the enhanced photocatalytic properties of the coordinated material, it becomes possible for electron-hole pairs and photogenerated •OH radicals to infiltrate the bacterial cell wall. This intrusion, upon breaking the cell wall, leads to the deterioration and leakage of the cell cytoplasm, ultimately causing bacterial death [28–32]. To generate these species, the electrochemical potentials of the valence and conduction bands must energetically allow the oxidation reactions in the water molecule's hole and the reduction of oxygen in the conduction band, as shown in Scheme 1b.

Following the previous context, the present study investigated the effect of nickel (II), manganese (II), and copper (II) coordination on the g-C_3N_4 template, considering different arrangements for coordinating electron pairs of nitrogen atoms available in the structure and its co-precipitation with metallic hydroxide using soft synthesis. Subsequently, the disinfection activity against *E. coli* 25922 on the surface was evaluated for each of the characterized compounds, and finally, the best material was selected for the degradation of a recalcitrant antibiotic in hospital wastewater (dicloxacillin). Additionally, the improved photocatalytic properties of the copper modification in the presence of dicloxacillin were shown to be correlated, theoretically contributing to the adsorption equilibrium of the system versus the degradation for possible interactions of copper with the matrix and the contaminant.

2. Results

2.1. Morphology and Spectroscopic Characterization of g-C_3N_4 and Modified Materials with Copper (II), Manganese (II), and Nickel (II)

Figure S1 depicts the DRX diffraction patterns for g-C_3N_4 and modified products with divalent cations. To consider a fully polymerized tri-s-triazine-based g-C_3N_4, a structure was generated starting from the unit cell proposed by Teter and Hemley. In this study, the same reflections were also observed for the tris-triazine-based structure except for a shift towards lower angles [33].

In Figure S2a,b, the condition's reaction to basic pH evidenced different electronic spectra for each metal transition modification, finding different effects in their relationship with g-C_3N_4. Likewise, the lamp identified as adequate for the photocatalytic posterior analyses overlapped the day lamp emission spectrum (Sylvania lamps FT5T8 8500 K (40 cm length) and emitted wavelengths between 400 and 700 nm, as this range warranted the best conditions for interaction for all the materials. The function of the previous information was carried out for the optimization structures for all compounds using BIOVIA Material Studio 2017 (MS2017)—Compass II Forcefield. Energetic parameters were evaluated for structures with two coordination environments: copper (II) modification (bonding to N-aliphatic), manganese (II), and nickel (II) (bonding to N-aromatic) and high hydroxide presence, Figure S3. For hydroxide metallics, the X-ray structures that are reported and compared in Figure S1 were used. Figure S4a–d depicts the morphology and microstructure of the g-C_3N_4 samples that were revealed by SEM and TEM. The products investigated using SEM exhibited aggregated morphologies and hydroxide presence in nickel and manganese (II) modifications for layers. The TEM micrographs revealed that the g-C_3N_4 has a lamellar, sheet-like structure (Figure S4e), as has been reported previously. However, Ni-g-C_3N_4, as shown in Figure S4f, appeared to have aggregated particles, which contained many smaller crystals.

In Table 1, an elemental surface analysis was quantified from the SEM results to establish the nature of the bond to the metal ion in the function of the stoichiometric relationship. Table 2 lists the results of the leaching studies with the detection of ionic chromatography. These results investigated the stability of the compounds in aqueous solution.

Table 1. Elemental surface analysis with SEM–EDS.

Material	Theoretical Metal Amount (%)	Metal (%)	Carbon (%)	Nitrogen (%)	Oxygen (%)
g-C_3N_4	---	---	47.79	46.32	5.31
Ni-g-C_3N_4	8.23	4.89	42.36	41.42	11.1
Mn-g-C_3N_4	9.25	7.33	41.83	36.4	13.87
Cu-g-C_3N_4	12.42	15.09	31.7	39.63	13.24

Table 2. Aqueous solution stability (ionic chromatographic detection).

Sample	Concentration (ppm)
Ni-g-C_3N_4	0
Mn-g-C_3N_4	0.572
Cu-g-C_3N_4	0

Table 3 reports the PC (Potential Charge) using dynamic scattering light, which showed a residual negative charge for the graphitic nitride. After modification with metal transitions, there were significant effects on surface charge.

Table 3. Z-average (nm) particle size and PC for g-C_3N_4 and modified materials.

	g-C_3N_4	Cu-g-C_3N_4	Ni-g-C_3N_4	Mn-g-C_3N_4
z-average (nm)	2561	3714	2257	1309
PC	−27.71	−14.98	−21.94	−29.64

The microstructure of the g-C_3N_4 and modified materials was studied via nitrogen-conducting adsorption–desorption experiments, and the results are displayed in Figure S5. All materials exhibited some degree of hysteresis related to a type IV isotherm. An in-depth analysis of these hysteresis indicated that all the materials presented a distinctive, plate-shaped pore system. The pores' properties, hysteresis degree (%), and fractal dimensions were reported in Table 4.

Table 4. Pore properties in the adsorption of N_2.

Material	Pore Volume (cm^3/g)		Pore Amount (%)		Pore Width (Å)		Hysteresis Degree (%)	Fractal Dimension
	Micropore	Mesopore	Micropore	Mesopore	Micropore	Mesopore		
g-C_3N_4	0.023	0.103	13.5	86.5	10.1	51.1	1.3	2.47
Ni-g-C_3N_4	0.037	0.078	25.5	74.5	12.1	51.1	24.4	2.58
Mn-g C_3N_4	0.015	0.157	7.1	92.9	12.7	51.1	4.2	2.42
Cu-g-C_3N_4	0.013	0.120	7.8	92.2	12.1	53.4	9.8	2.48

X-ray photoelectron spectroscopy (XPS) was employed to investigate the surface chemical compositions. The full survey XPS spectrum (Figure S6a) showed the presence of Ni, Mn, and Cu at the first inflection point; it was possible to find the band gap energy values of the modified materials, which were 2.70, 2.09, and 1.50 eV for the Cu-g-C_3N_4, Mn-g-C_3N_4, and Ni-g-C_3N_4, respectively. Compared with the theoretical band gap energy of the g-C_3N_4, which is 2.65 eV, the introduction changed the band gap width because it forces the creation of new electronic transitions with the d orbitals of the transition metals and the π orbitals of the carbon nitride [34]. Figure S6b–d depicts the contributions for N1s, O1s, and Mn 2p.

2.2. Electrochemical Characterization of g-C₃N₄ and Copper (II)-, Manganese (II)-, and Nickel (II)-Modified Materials

Samples were deposited on fluorine-doped tin oxide (FTO) as a transparent substrate, and cyclic voltammetry (CV) diagrams were initially created with light, Figure 1. For the CV measurements, the scanning rate was kept at 20 mV s^{-1}. The tests were performed in three cycles between −1.5 V and +1.5 V for Cu-g-C₃N₄, Ni-g-C₃N₄, and Mn-g-C₃N₄, and between −2.2 V and 2.2 V for g-C₃N₄, as the supporting electrolyte: [Na₂SO₄] = 0.1 M. It was observed that the material exhibited an optical band gap, where the potential of the anodic and cathodic peak shifts with the interaction of light for these materials, demonstrating photoactivity or the presence of a photo response within the visible regions.

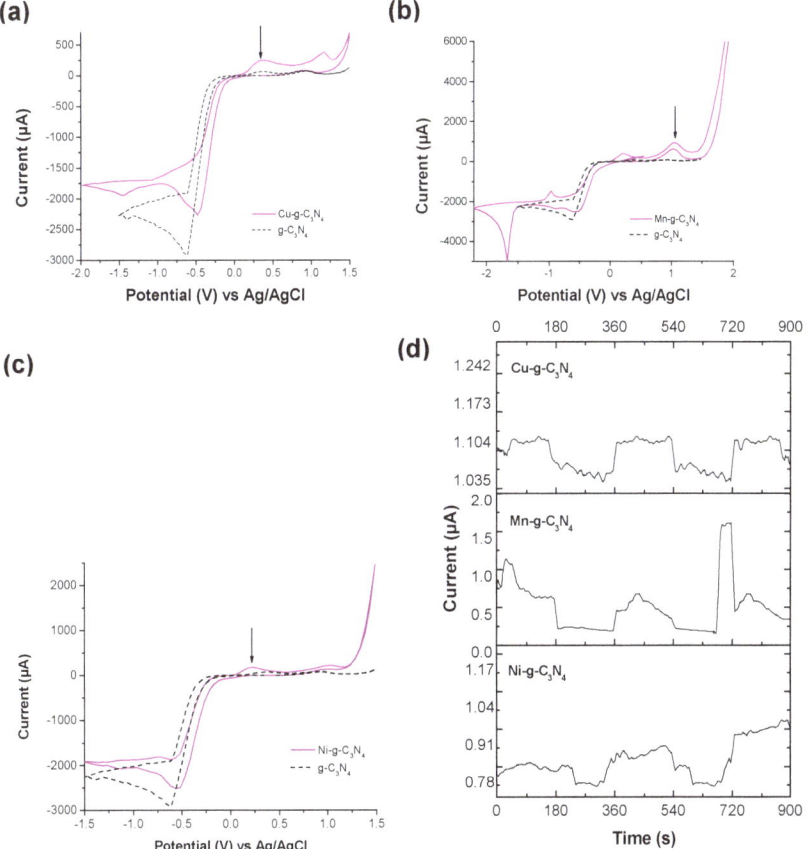

Figure 1. Cyclic voltammetry curves for (**a**) Cu-g-C₃N₄, Ni-g-C₃N₄, (**b**) Mn-g-C₃N₄, and (**c**) Ni-g-C₃N₄. Experimental conditions: sweep rate = 20 mV/s; window potential = −1.5 V and 0.0 V, supporting electrolyte: [Na₂SO₄] = 0.1 M; and [H₂O₂] = 0.01 M. (**d**) Chronoamperometry curves for Cu-g-C₃N₄, Mn-g-C₃N₄, and Ni-g-C₃N₄. Experimental conditions: V = 0.5 V; time = 15 min; supporting electrolyte: [Na₂SO₄] = 0.1 M; and [H₂O₂] = 0.01 M. The ↓ corresponds to first oxidation process.

The potential versus current plots of the carbon nitride show that the cathodic peaks shifted in metal-modified materials. It is worth noting that in the voltammogram with copper, copper (II) underwent electrochemical reduction to copper (I), demonstrating the presence of this oxidation state. However, this methodology was not entirely suitable for estimating the position of the valence and conduction bands. For this reason, Electrochemical Impedance Spectroscopy (EIS) measurements using the Mott–Schottky method were depicted to understand this mechanism.

2.3. Photocatalytic Disinfection against E. coli 25922 Using g-C_3N_4 and Modified Materials with Copper (II), Manganese (II), and Nickel (II)

To discern the contribution of the hydroxides of the respective metals independently, their antimicrobial activity against the E. coli strain was estimated simultaneously with their respective composites consisting of carbon nitrides alternated with metal hydroxides as explained previously, using the best time treatment (20 min). The hydroxide moieties showed antimicrobial activity as follows: $Cu(OH)_2$ > $Mn(OH)_2$ > $Ni(OH)_2$. With a difference between them of 3 Log units, these are not greater than the activity of each of the g-C_3N_4, Figure 2a. Figure 2b depicts the disinfection kinetic for g-C_3N_4, its modifications with metal transitions, and photolysis control in the range visible.

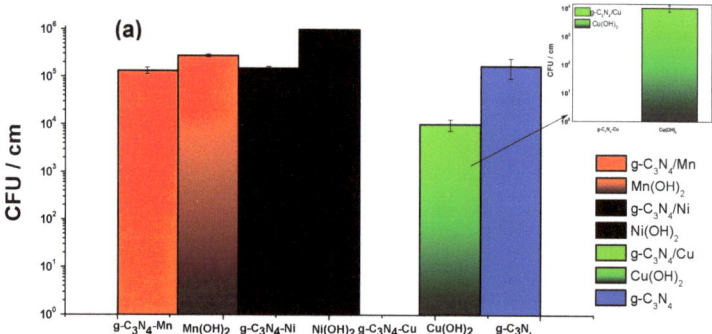

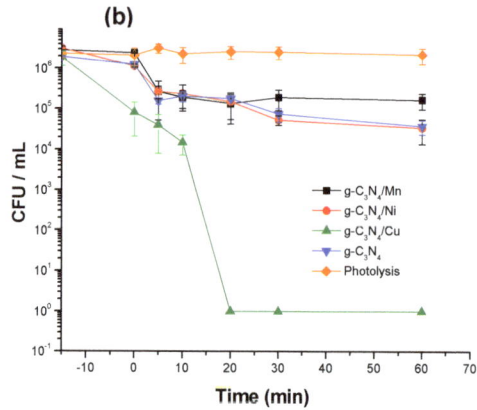

Figure 2. (**a**) Photodisinfection using hydroxides of metal ions versus materials with g-C_3N_4 after 20 min of exposure with a Xenon lamp. (**b**) Kinetic disinfection for g-C_3N_4 and modified materials with copper, manganese, and nickel against E. coli 25922 (Time = −15–60 min).

2.4. Understanding the Disinfection Mechanism of Cu-g-C_3N_4

It is particularly useful in the study of semiconducting electrodes to provide information about the charge transfer and separation process. The scans shown in Figure 3 were recorded in the potential window from −1.0 V to 0.5 V (vs. Ag/AgCl) with an increment of 0.05 V at 10 Hz frequency. The principle behind the Mott–Schottky method is based on the relationship between the capacitance of the space charge of a semiconductor electrode and the applied potential. When a positive potential is applied to the semiconductor electrode in an electrolytic solution, a space charge region is established at the semiconductor–electrolyte interface. The variation in capacitance of this region as a function of potential is known as the Mott–Schottky curve. By analyzing this curve, several key pieces of information can be extracted: (i) the position of the flat band potential or conduction band of the semiconductor within the solution, (ii) carrier density in the semiconductor, (iii) the direction of the slope of the curve, indicating whether the carriers are electrons or holes, and (iv) the conduction band and valence band. Figure 3a depicts the Nyquist diagrams and Mott–Schottky plot. The impedance curve is a semi-circular curve that shows that the process of a three-electrode system is controlled by charge transfer. A smaller semi-circular arc of impedance indicates a faster electron transfer rate on the material's surface and a more probable electrochemical redox reaction; therefore, it indicates a decrease in charge–transfer resistance [35]. Likewise, calculating for Mott–Shottky plots is commonly used to determine the flat band potential of the semiconductor catalysts, and these are shown in Figure 3b. In conclusion, regarding valence and conduction bands associated with impedance study, Figure 3c depicts these electrochemical potentials in relationship with the hydroxyl, anion superoxide formation.

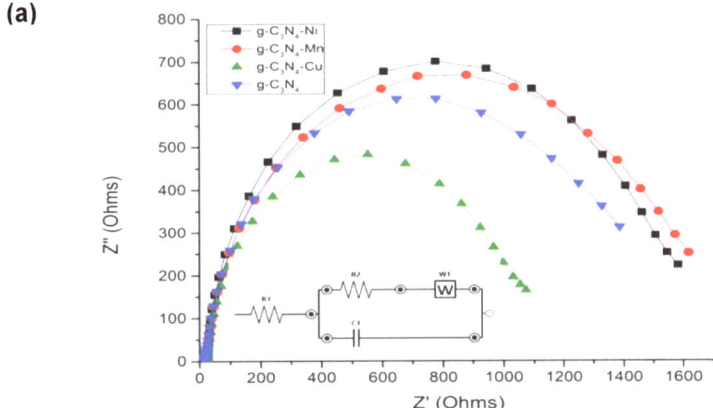

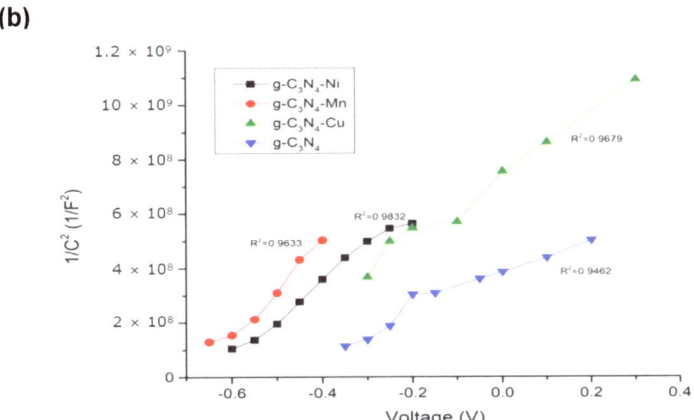

Figure 3. *Cont.*

(c)

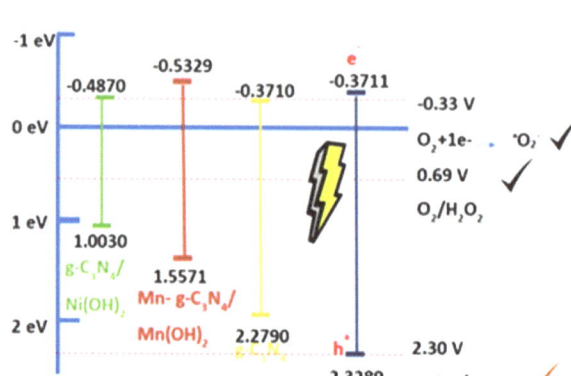

Figure 3. Electrochemical characterization of g-C_3N_4 and modified materials with copper (II), manganese (II), and nickel (II), (**a**). Nyquist diagrams, (**b**). Mott–Schottky plot, (**c**). Bands (conduction and valence) diagram construed for authors.

To confirm the presence of hydroxyl radicals in Cu-g-C_3N_4, as confirmed by electrochemical studies, scavengers like methanol (targeting hydroxyl radicals) and potassium iodide (targeting hole oxidation) were used to understand the mechanism linked to this disinfection property as compared to other materials. However, the methanol disinfection activity is well-known, complicating the interpretation of kinetic disinfection in bacterial studies. Organic molecules such as dicloxacillin are sensitive to reactive oxygen species (ROS) and, therefore, are used to examine the kinetics of degradation and to determine the evolution of ROS; the photolysis control was considered for this molecule, Figure 4a,b. Posteriorly, the scavengers (KI: holes specific; Methanol: •OH specific) were used to reveal the production of the ROS for the best material for the disinfection properties of Cu-g-C_3N_4.

This type of interaction with metal ions can modify the local electronic structure, facilitating the transfer of electrons between the orbital metals and the nitrogen atom. As described previously, copper is found around the aliphatic nitrogen located at the periphery of the carbon nitride. To understand if the interaction between the N-triazine and N-aliphatic represents lower energy in the system and low leaching, computational calculations were performed by comparing the structure of nitride with coordinated copper at the metal periphery, around the N-triazines, exerting an electrostatic adsorption interaction, Figure 5a. This resulted in the best structure of copper for interacting with dicloxacillin in the adsorption studies, Figure 5b.

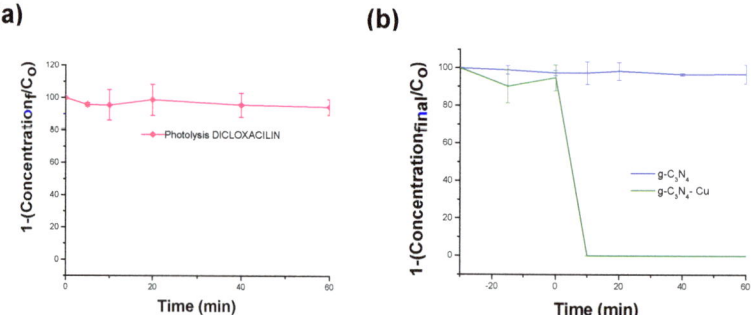

Figure 4. *Cont.*

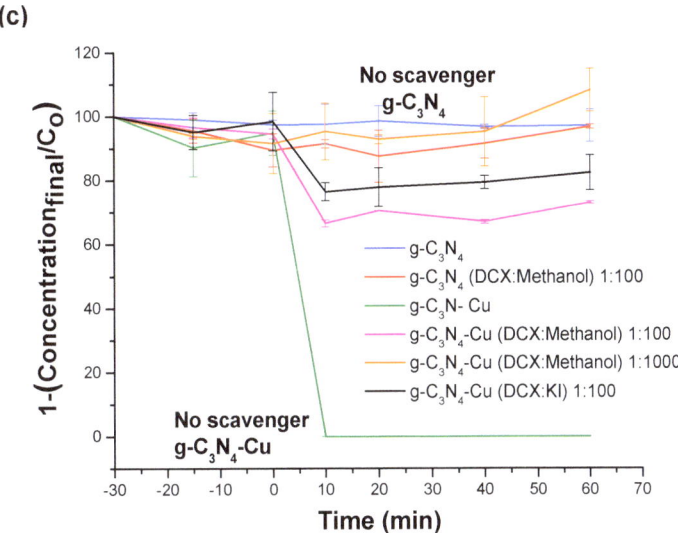

Figure 4. (**a**). Photolysis of DXC to Xenon Lamp, (**b**). Photodegradation using Cu-g-C_3-N_4 and g-C_3-N_4 with exposure to Xenon lamp, (**c**). Photodegradation using Cu-g-C_3-N_4 and g-C_3-N_4 with scavengers for •OH radical and h$^+$ activation.

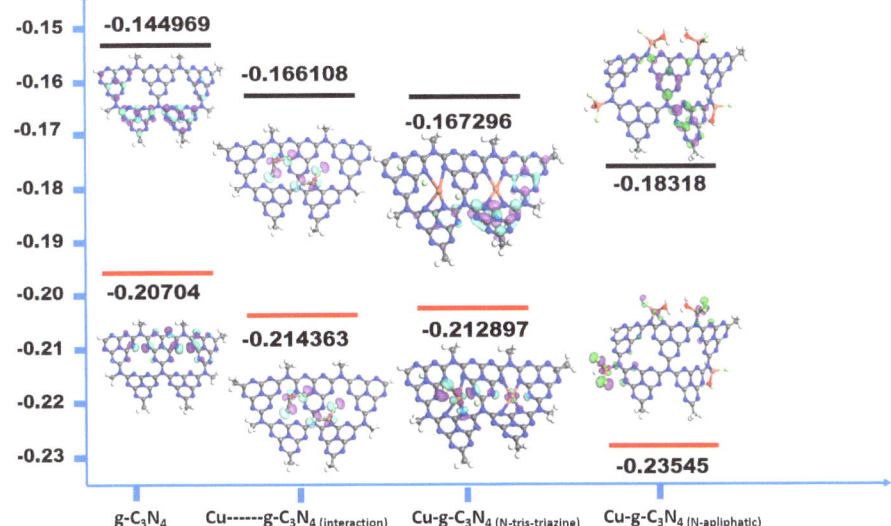

Figure 5. *Cont.*

(b)

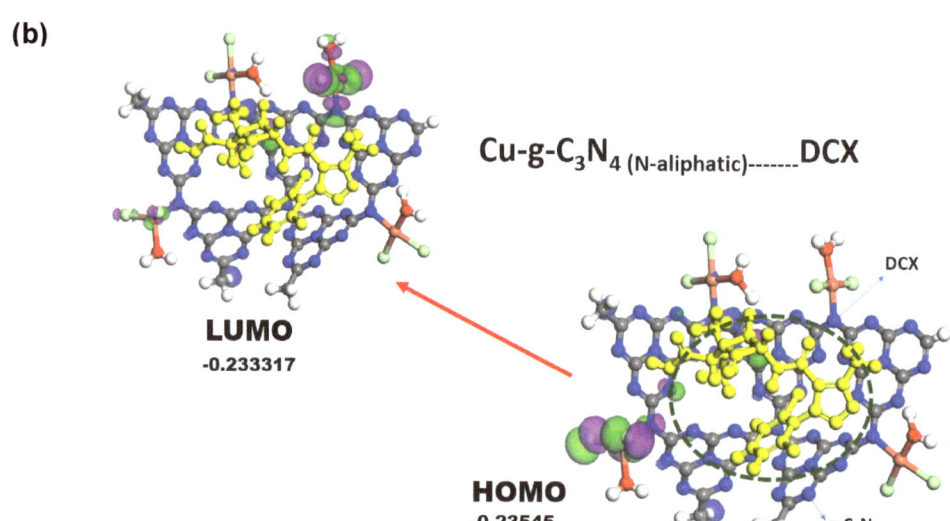

Figure 5. (**a**) Theoretical calculations for a system composed of g-C$_3$N$_4$, Cu-g-C$_3$N$_4$ (physisorption), CuN-g-C$_3$N$_4$ (Cu-coordinated N-triazine), and CuNH-g-C$_3$N$_4$ (Cu-coordinated N-aliphatic). (**b**) CuNH-g-C$_3$N$_4$ (Cu-coordinated, N-aliphatic-interacting DCX molecule). Color code structure: blue color (nitrogen atom), red (oxygen atom), grey (carbon atom), white (hydrogen atom), purple (negative density charge), green (positive density charge), and dark green (chlorine atom).

3. Discussion

Figure S1 presents, for instance, the (210) reflection observed at 2θ = 11.5°, (101) at 2θ = 17.54°, and (002) at 2θ = 27.78°, corresponding to the tris-triazine ring. The modifications related to the metal ion depend intrinsically on their ability to coexist in their hydroxylated form at the working basic pH. For example, in the case of nickel, the structure was greatly modified, having a significant contribution from the planes (001) (100) (101) corresponding to Ni(OH)$_2$ [36]. Likewise, but to a lesser extent, this phenomenon was observed for copper and manganese. Conversely, the (210) plane corresponded to the orthorhombic reflection, which was associated with the alignment of the aromatic layers. In the case of copper, the plane remains like the g-C$_3$N$_4$ material, showing a slight distortion in the conformation of the aromatic rings. This suggests that the copper ion has little effect on the planar structure and can be located on the periphery of the nitride template, located in the N-aliphatic fragment. On the other hand, nickel (II) and manganese (II) had a large contribution to the N-N-triazine structure, and, consequently, the relationship between the I_{210}/I_{002} planes distorted the aromatic rings of the triazines, which are known to have an AA stacking.

In Figure S2a,b, the Mn-g-C$_3$N$_4$ spectra presented a highly symmetric D4h coordination environment and a large planar δ electron system around 400 nm. The former gave rise to d-orbital degeneracy or near-degeneracy and the possibility of high spin multiplicity. In this case, the metal dx^2-y^2 orbital, which by convention points at the N-N-triazine, is predicted to be quite high in energy [37]. For copper (II) the electronic spectra were very different to homologs with manganese (II) and nickel (II); the band to 440 nm was related to tetrahedral environments [38]. Finally, nickel (II) presented few electronic changes; it suggested modifications in the structure due to the pH and the hydroxyl compounds in the solution. To approach this information, the lamps in the visible region were selected for the posterior analyses.

In Figure S3a–d, the structure with low energy for copper (II) is suggested for Cu-N-aliphatic. In contrast, in the manganese (II) structure, there are moderate contributions of hydroxides, but nickel stability is governed by the hydroxides nickel (II) [39,40]. This preliminary structure allows suggested different electronic properties for all modifications in relationship with carbon nitride.

In Figure S4a–d for copper micrographs, a greater distribution of the metal ion is observed, which is consistent with homogeneous coordination of the material on the periphery of the carbon nitride. Conversely, nickel- and manganese-modified materials showed a metal distribution into spots, which may be attributed to the alternation between metal hydroxides and the carbon nitride template [41]. The TEM images suggest that Ni (OH)$_2$ crystals are stacked with the g-C$_3$N$_4$, as proposed previously. The diffraction pattern shows the characteristic planes of (100), (001), and (101) attributed to nickel hydroxide in the region associated with this structure, Figure S4e,f.

In Table 1, the presence of copper in carbon nitride increases the percentage of oxygen on the surface (EDS analysis), suggesting a prevalent coordination of water molecules from the metal surface and the environment under mild reaction conditions, after the polymerization of urea. The stoichiometric relationship associated with hydroxides on the surface is few, as suggested by these results. These water molecules may complete the coordination sphere of the copper metal ion. In contrast, modification with nickel and manganese shows that the percentage of oxygen increases concerning the metal percentage in a 2:1 stoichiometry (oxygen: metal), suggesting the presence of hydroxides in the systems containing these two metals. Interestingly, for nickel, there was a slight variation in the percentage of carbon and nitrogen as compared to carbon nitride, suggesting that this graphitic structure is alternated with nickel (II) hydroxide. On the other hand, the metal leaching capability in an aqueous solution rendered the Ni-g-C$_3$N$_4$ and Cu-g-C$_3$N$_4$ materials fully stable in solution. However, the manganese compound presents moderate leaching, which is above the range put forth by the regulatory agencies (0.12 mg/L) [42], Table 2.

On the other hand, the DLS suggests deprotonation of oxygenated groups on the periphery for g-C$_3$N$_4$. However, the modification with nickel (II) and manganese (II) followed the hydroxyl group's surface. Surprisingly, the copper-modified material exhibited a more positive value in the residual potential of the system, which is explained by the metal coordination on the material's periphery compensating for the innate surface charge of carbon nitride. Likewise, the particle size increases with copper (II) modification, which is related with the disposition surface for g-C$_3$N$_4$ with a metal ion coordinated in the N-N-aliphatic, which does not limit the electronic effect of N-triazine and its availability, Table 3.

Figure S5, the g-C$_3$N$_4$, Mn-g-C$_3$N$_4$, and g-C$_3$N$_4$-Cu isotherms belonged to the H3-type isotherm, indicating a parallel and narrow plate-shaped pore conformation. Conversely, g-C$_3$N$_4$-Ni depicted an H4-type isotherm, suggesting a prevalent slit/wedge-shaped pore conformation. Particularly, Ni-g-C$_3$N$_4$, and to a lesser degree Cu-g-C$_3$N$_4$, showed a p-stacking of the g-C$_3$N$_4$ due to the tensile strength effect [43]. The specific surface areas of g-C$_3$N$_4$, Ni-g-C$_3$N$_4$, Mn-g-C$_3$N$_4$, and Cu-g-C$_3$N$_4$ were estimated to be 52.7 m^2 g^{-1}, 80.9 m^2 g^{-1}, 51.4 m^2 g^{-1}, and 47.4 m^2 g^{-1} respectively. The presence of manganese had a negligible effect on the surface area of the graphitic carbon nitride, as previously mentioned. On the contrary, the surface area of nickel carbon nitride was high due to the presence of hydroxide moieties alternated on the surface, disrupting the 3D structure of the graphitic nitride. This effect was also noticed on the surface roughness as expressed by the fractal dimension, evidencing the presence of co-structures on surfaces such as hydroxides (Table 4). Likewise, the copper-modified materials' roughness was comparable to that of carbon nitride, presuming the limited presence of surface hydroxides forming a coordination of the metallic center at the periphery of the structure. In the case of copper, the charge potential was affected by the coordination of the metal center, resulting in a large particle size. All materials were characterized as having a prevalent mesoporous system. However, the presence of nickel metal decreased the degree of mesoporosity and increased the micropore degree and width. This is explained by the presence of nickel hydroxides in the material. On the other hand, copper and manganese ions slightly increased the degree of microporosity since these metals coordinate the free electron pairs of nitrogen.

Figure S6 illustrates peaks corresponding to N1's and O1's orbitals within the 200 and 400 eV range. In the case of Cu-g-C_3N_4, the peaks observed at 400.4, 398.9, and 399.8 eV can be assigned to the bridging N atoms in $N(C)_3$ groups, and the sp^2-hybridized nitrogen triazine rings of C-N=C and the Cu-NH bond respectively, indicating that the Cu forms a coordination complex with the final amines of the carbon nitride network. Conversely, the Ni-g-C_3N_4 and g-C_3N_4 peaks at N1s at 401.1 eV suggest the presence of free amino groups (C-N-H) present in the material, suggesting that the formation of the coordination complex of these metals occurs in the triazine rings and 398.3 eV, Figure S6b [44]. From these results, we found the location of the metal in the g-C_3N_4 network. These findings are consistent with the XRD pattern, indicating a tris-triazine structure in g-C_3N_4, with metal ions interacting with its amine groups. Specifically, copper tends to interact with nitrogen aliphatic regions, as evidenced by XPS showing a greater exposure of triazine groups on the surface. In contrast, manganese ions interact with triazine groups, leading to the exposure of amine aliphatic groups. The O1's orbital demonstrates the influence of metal centers on g-C_3N_4, resulting in an energy shift from 531.16 eV to 534.07 eV for copper with water molecules and hydroxide contributions, Figure S6c. For the Mn 2p orbital, we found two contributions at 641 and 645 eV [45] corresponding to Mn-N and Mn-O, suggesting $Mn(OH)_2$ and M-N-triazine, Figure S6d.

Figure 1 shows CV results for all the modified materials and bare g-C_3N_4. All measurements were conducted at pH 5.4. According to the Pourbaix diagram for Cu, the main species at work pH is Cu(II). In Figure 1a, there is a reduction peak at 0.33 V associated with the oxidation of Cu (I) to Cu (II), and a cathodic peak at −1.44 attributed to the reduction of Cu (II) to Cu (I). Similar peaks in the CV of Mn-g-C_3N_4 (Figure 1b) and Ni-g-C_3N_4 (Figure 1c), specifically, anodic peaks at 1.03 V and 0.21 V, are linked to the oxidation of Mn (II) to Mn (IV) and Ni (II) to Ni (III), respectively, according to their Pourbaix diagram. Additionally, cathodic peaks at −0.97 V and −0.73 V are associated with the reduction of the metal species [46–49]. In Figure 1d, the Cu-gC_3N_4 photocurrent carriers were recyclable and stable under the on–off cycles, and it had the highest photocurrent. In contrast, for Mn-g-C_3N_4 and Ni-g-C_3N_4, the photocurrent changed with every on–off switch. As discussed in the previous chapter, the Cu dispersion over the g-C_3N_4 template was more homogeneous than in Mn-g-C_3N_4 and Ni-g-C_3N_4, and the presence of hydroxides affects the flow of the photocarriers over the photocatalyst surface, thereby altering the behavior of these materials.

From the spectroscopic, textural, and electrochemical characterization of new materials under soft synthesis, the disinfection against *E. coli* was determined. Figure 2 shows that the activity of the nitride structures is independent of that of the metal hydroxide, probably given that the generation of ROS in the interaction of g-C_3N_4 with the metal is more effective in oxidation processes. The Cu-g-C_3N_4 performed a complete disinfection concerning g-C_3N_4 and modified materials with manganese and nickel (II). Therefore, Cu in terms of electrical conductivity is more effective than Mn and Ni. This phenomenon is explained by the ability of a metal to participate in redox reactions and release electrons. Copper can be present in ionic forms, such as Cu (II), which can effectively participate in redox reactions and induce the formation of ROS [50]. In contrast, nickel and manganese tend to form more stable oxidation states which are not as likely to participate in redox reactions that generate ROS. Thus, when a metallic ion is integrated into a carbon nitride network, the nitrogen atoms can act as electron-pair donors to form coordination bonds with the metallic ion. This type of interaction can modify the local electronic structure, facilitating the electron transfer between the orbital metals and the nitrogen atom. The metallic ion in carbon nitride serves as a catalyst and provides active sites on the surface for oxidation reactions, these sites may have available electrons in their electronic structure. In the presence of molecular oxygen (O_2), this structure adsorbs oxygen molecules on the surface [51]. Electrons from the orbital metal can be transferred to oxygen: this electron transfer can occur due to the electrical potential difference between the metal ionic and the adsorbed species. Adsorbed oxygen captures electrons that could reduce them to superoxide species ($O_2^{\bullet -}$) [52]. The nonbonding orbitals, also called nonbonding electron pairs, can donate electrons without breaking coordination bonds. In other cases, the electronic distribution can change without breaking coordination bonds through the phenomenon of resonance. Electrons can "move" between different positions without changing the connectivity of the coordination bond [53]. On the other hand, the carbons of the triazine ring may play a significant role in donating electrons to the dopant metal. Triazine is a molecule that contains nitrogen and carbon atoms in a heterocyclic ring. Electrons from the carbon atoms in the ring can participate in the transfer of electrons through sigma bonds, stabilizing the structure, and the stability of the ring can influence the donation of electrons to the metal ion [54]. The sp^2 hybridization gives rise to an unhybridized p-orbital perpendicular to the plane of the triazine ring. This unhybridized p orbital may contain π electrons, which are more available to participate in electron donation processes. Thus, the presence of π electrons in sp^2 hybridization may allow the ring carbon atoms to participate in redox reactions, since these electrons can be more easily transferred to other chemical species including ionic metals.

Figure 3a,b is used to understand the nature and origin of ROS species with the materials that are semiconductors. Figure 3a shows that Cu- g-C_3N_4 has the lowest impedance resistance. This indicates the fastest electron transfer rate, enhancing the separation efficiency of photogenerated carriers. The transfer of charges across the interface between the semiconductor and the solution becomes easier, leading to an increase in the photocurrent and a better chemical catalytic performance [55] as compared to the other three materials [56]. The curves of g-C_3N_4, Cu-g-C_3N_4, Ni-g-C_3N_4, and Mn-g-C_3N_4-Cu are depicted in Figure 3b. The electrochemical system can be described by the Randles circuit (inset in Figure 3a), where R1 is the resistance owing to the passage of electrons between the surface of the material to the reference electrode, R2 is due to the charge transfer resistance of the redox couple, W1 is denoted as the Warburg impedance that takes into account diffusion of electroactive species towards the electrode, and C1 corresponded to the non-faradaic capacitance of the g-C_3N_4. The flat band potentials were -0.49697, -0.53287, -0.37109, and -0.37105 eV for Ni-g-C_3N_4, Mn-g-C_3N_3, Cu-g-C_3N_4, and g-C_3N_4, respectively. It can be observed that the introduction of the transition metal as a complex into the g-C_3N_4 framework modified the position of the conduction band. From the thermodynamics standpoint, a more negative conduction band position suggests a major reduction potential. This is translated into a higher production of superoxide anion radical (-0.33 eV) [57].

Knowing the band gap and the conduction band of the materials, it can be calculated the valence bands which were 1.0030, 1.5571, 2.3289, and 2.2790 eV for the Ni-g-C_3N_4, Mn-g-C_3N_4, Cu-g-C_3N_4, and g-C_3N_4, respectively. According to the previous results, it can be inferred that the oxidative potential is not enough to generate hydroxyl radicals (2.30 eV), even with the addition of the transition metal in the g-C_3N_4, manganese, and nickel systems, as is shown in Figure 3c. However, the valence band for band Cu-g-C_3N_4 was enough to produce hydroxyl radicals showing the capacity of all materials to generate superoxide anion radical, which is an ROS with a high redox potential for degrading membrane microorganisms.

In the same context, the dicloxacillin (DCX) molecule was used against scavengers to verify the ROS production. This molecule exhibited minimal degradation through photolysis within a 60 min timeframe, Figure 4a [58]. Figure 4b demonstrates that the adsorption of DCX is reduced when utilizing g-C_3N_4 and its copper-modified counterpart. DCX, when at a circumneutral pH, presents a deprotonated carboxylic group, resulting in reduced adsorption owing to the negative potential charge (PC) of the materials. Light exposure significantly influences degradation, with full degradation occurring around 10 min, possibly due to light-activated reactive oxygen species (ROS). To explore the relationship between ROS production, specifically •OH radical and h^+ activation, scavenger experiments with methanol and potassium iodide (KI) were conducted in the presence of DCX. The degradation kinetics were hindered in the presence of high concentrations of methanol, which acted as a scavenger for DCX degradation. Conversely, KI blocked approximately 15% of the degradation process, indicating direct oxidation by h^+, Figure 4c.

These findings are consistent with the positions observed in the valence and conduction bands obtained from the Mott–Schottky plot. Overall, these results suggest that •OH radicals and h⁺ play significant roles in both disinfection and degradation processes.

Finally, to comprehensively investigate the stability of the copper compound, theoretical calculations were carried out, as shown in Figure 5a. The HOMO with low energy corresponds with metal ions coordinated to nitrogen aliphatic, as was suggested in the spectroscopic characterization. The metal ion presence in the environment of carbon nitride decreased energy levels and compensated for the charge-negative surface. The geometry around copper is suggested to have a tetrahedral geometry, which is congruent with electronic spectra in the solid state [59]. Additionally, it has low stability for a structure with Cu-N-tris triazine. The interaction of the DXC with Cu-g-C_3N_4 coordinated the N- aliphatic can be explained as the DCX interacting with de sp^2-hybridization to increase the active places for the catalyst, Figure 5b.

4. Materials and Methods

4.1. Reagents

Dicloxacillin (DCX) was provided by Sinopharm Laboratories. Urea was provided by Analytical Standards M&B Laboratory Chemicals (Cape Town, South Africa). Nickel chloride hexahydrate and cupric chloride dihydrate were provided by Loba Chemie Laboratory Reagents (Colaba, India) and Fine Chemicals (Cape Town, South Africa). Manganous chloride tetrahydrate was provided by Baker (Melbourne, Australia). Reagent sodium hydroxide pellets, fluorine-doped tin oxide sheets, perchloric acid, sodium sulfate, hydrogen peroxide, formic acid, and acetonitrile were provided by Merk (Darmstadt, Germany). Nitrogen liquid was purchased from Genex (Sydney, Australia).

4.2. Modification of g-C_3N_4 Synthesis

Bulk g-C_3N_4 was prepared by pyrolyzing urea. Urea (10.0 g) was heated to 550 °C in an atmosphere-controlled oven at a heating rate of 100 °C h^{-1}. This pyrolysis was conducted for 3 h, followed by cooling until reaching room temperature. The resulting powder was purified with water and dried at 80 °C.

Modified g-C_3N_4 were prepared in a reflux system. Briefly, 0.067 g of the metal salt (copper, nickel, or manganese) was diluted in 50 mL of distilled water and was put in reflux for 0.75 h at 100 °C. Subsequently, 0.2 g of g-C_3N_4 was added to the reflux system and allowed to react for 1 h. The reaction mixture was allowed to cool down and the pH was adjusted with concentrated NaOH equimolar until reaching a pH of 10. Finally, it was filtered by gravity and allowed to dry passed through paper (75 µm).

4.3. Physicochemical and Spectroscopic Characterization

The catalyst surface morphology was observed by Transmission Electron Microscopy (TEM) using an S-4800 HITACHI at an acceleration voltage of 160 kV (Hitachi, Tokyo, Japan). The crystal structures were analyzed using an X-ray powder diffractometer (Model XPert pro-MPD, Medellín, Colombia). Copper X-ray diffraction (XRD) patterns were collected between 5° and 80° at a scan rate of 4° min^{-1} and an incident wavelength of 0.15406 nm (Cu-Kα). X-ray photoelectron spectroscopy (XPS) patterns were recorded using a PHI5300 Software ESCALAB system SID-10148252, LAXPS software with Mg Kα radiation. Pore size distribution and specific surface areas were obtained using Quantasorb equipment (Nova 1200e, Quanta chrome, Boynton Beach, FL, USA) employing nitrogen gas as adsorbate. The sorption isotherms were determined at relative pressures from 0.03 to 0.95. Dynamic Light Scattering (DLS) (ISO13321) range 0.3 nm–10 mm, humidity via. DRX AERIS High score. Scanning Electron Microscopy (ASTM E1508-12/ASTM E 766 14, 2019, M Committee E04 on Metallography, and is the direct responsibility of Subcommittee E04.11 on X-ray and Electron Metallography, USP<1181> [59]. The solid-state diffuse reflectance spectrum and the solution phase electronic spectrum were recorded on a Shimadzu UV-2401 PC spectrophotometer (Shimadzu, Tokyo, Japan) Agilent 8453 diode array spectrophotometer (Agilent, Santa Clara, CA, USA), respectively.

4.4. Electrochemical Characterization

Electrochemical Impedance Spectroscopy (EIS) and Cyclic voltammetry (CV) were performed using a PalmSens5, 2004–2022 Palm Sens BV Version 5.9.4206 Build 30281t electrochemical station coupled with a conventional three-electrode system composed of a working electrode holding the material, a counter electrode of Ir, and a reference electrode of Ag/AgCl/KCl under the Xenon lamps (60 W). Each working electrode was prepared using the impregnation method on FTO-coated glass slides (30 mm × 20 mm × 2 mm size) obtained from a commercial supplier (TechInstro, Nagpur, India). Before each experiment, the FTO sheets were soaked with $HOCl_4$ at (1×10^{-3} M) for 1 h. Approximately, 0.2 g of each material (g-C_3N_4, Ni-g-C_3N_4-, Mn-g-C_3N_4 or Cu-g-C_3N_4) was suspended in 10 mL of water, and the FTO sheet was immersed in each suspension for 30 s, followed by drying on a spin-coater. This process was repeated five times to get a complete FTO coating. The FTO-coated sheet was then calcinated in a gas control oven at 500 °C for 1 h. The latter process was repeated twice to guarantee a complete material deposition on FTO sheets. Mott–Schottky analyses were performed at a frequency of 10 Hz using an amplitude of 10 mV at several potentials. To the electrolyte (Na_2SO_4) was added H_2O_2 with a finality of oxidizing the hole.

4.5. Reaction System

The photocatalytic processes were carried out in a homemade aluminum reflective reactor containing four sunlight lamps (Sylvania FT5T8 8500 K 40 cm length, Medellín, Colombia) that emitted wavelengths between 400 and 700 nm. The photocatalytic processes were conducted at 60 W of light power. Antibiotic solutions (50 mL) were placed in beakers under constant stirring and samples were periodically taken for the analyses.

4.6. E. coli 25922 Photodisinfection

Inoculation process for the *E. coli* ATCC 25922 strain: Before each experiment, the bacterial growth culture medium was prepared by dispersing 23.5 g of HIMEDIA Plate Count Agar (PCA) in 1L of distilled millipore water. This PCA medium was dissolved, heated to boiling, and sterilized by autoclaving at 15 psi of pressure for 20 min. Subsequently, the medium was cooled to 57 ± 2 °C, and 19 ± 1 mL portions were poured into 100×15 mm sterile Petri dishes. Immediately, the culture medium underwent sterilization under UV radiation for 10 min.

The *E. coli* ATCC 25922 bacterial strain utilized in this study is part of the microbiological collection of the Research Group in *Basic and Applied Microbiology* (MICROBA). A stock suspension of 5×10^8 Forming Colony Units (FCU)/mL was prepared as follows: *E. coli* (ATCC 25922) was retrieved from glycerol at -20 °C using a loop. It was then streaked on agar contained in a petri dish, which was incubated for 18 h at 37 °C. Afterward, one colony was suspended in 5 mL of H_2O and stirred using a vortex mixer. This dispersion was analyzed at 540 nm using a Shimadzu spectrophotometer at 568 nm. A concentration of 10^8 FCU/mL was adjusted to an absorbance of 0.7.

A closed photoreaction system with temperature control composed of a 2.2 kW Xenon lamp and two vortex systems equipped with a petri dish was used. This system allows for a high interaction with light and materials. In all cases, under dark conditions, 150 mL of distilled water was mixed with 1 mL of the previously described bacterial suspension to obtain a final concentration of 5×10^6 CFU/mL, which was confirmed experimentally. Then, 150 mg/L of the chosen photocatalyst was added and stirred at 250 rpm. The lamp was turned on 15 min later, and a second sample was taken. From that time onward, sampling was conducted at various intervals (t = −15, 0, 5, 10, 20, 30, 60 min). The samples were diluted (1/10) successively in saline solution when necessary (10^5–10^2 CFU microorganisms). In all cases, the extracted bacterial suspensions were spread on plate count agar and incubated for 24 h. The number of CFUs was manually counted, and the CFU/mL was calculated. Each experiment was conducted at least in duplicate.

4.7. Dicloxacillin Degradation

Quantitative analyses of dicloxacillin were carried out using a UHPLC, Thermoscientific Dionex UltiMate 3000 instrument, equipped with an Acclaim 120 RP C18 column (5 µm, 4.6 × 150 mm) and a photodiode array detector (Thermo Fisher Scientific, Waltham, MA, USA). The wavelength of detection was 270 nm and the injection volume was 20 µL. The mobile phase was composed of a mixture of formic acid (10 mmol L^{-1}, pH 3.0) and acetonitrile at a 50:50 ratio, 0.7 mL min^{-1}).

To identify the metals' leaching, ionic chromatography was carried out with a brochure: MagIC Net and column Metro A. The injection volume was 10 µL and mixtures of nitric acid (2 mmol L^{-1})/oxalic acid (0.5 mmol L^{-1}) were used as mobile phase, conductivity detectors.

4.8. Theoretical Approximations of g-C_3N_4 and Modified Materials with Copper (II)

Computational modeling was carried out to get some information about the interaction of carbonous material with dicloxacillin and the calculations of density function theory parameters (E_{LUMO}, and E_{HUMO}). Starting from the experimental structural data within the BIOVIA Material Studio 2017 (MS2017) that was obtained using Compass II Forcefield [60], we created the Cu-g C_3N_4 for the function of spectroscopic characterization. A solid solution using water as a solvent at 100 K was considered. The module adsorption locator included within the commercial modeling software 7.0 MS2017, 2020 was used for the computational studies. BIOVIA Forcite is an advanced classical molecular mechanic tool, designed to work with a wide range of force fields, allowing for fast energy calculations and reliable geometry optimizations of molecules and periodic systems. In our study, Forcite was used to optimize the geometry of DXC and g-C_3N_4. In this sense, the BIOVIA adsorption location module was employed, which is based on simulated annealing, a metaheuristic algorithm for locating a good approximation to the global minimum of a given function of a large search space. This allows for the identification of the possible adsorption configurations by carrying out Monte Carlo searches of the configurational space of the selected surface–model molecular systems, as the temperature is slowly decreased. To identify additional local minimum energy, the process was repeated several times.

5. Conclusions

The availability of the tris-triazine template to be photoactivated and transport electrons from the valence band to the conduction band was mediated by the availability of π-unsaturation. Manganese- and nickel-modified materials contained a M-g-C_3N_4/M(OH)$_2$ composite which stabilized and blocked the active sites and prevented light from penetrating the carbon nitride template, affecting disinfection and drug degradation. However, in the copper-modified material Cu-g-C_3N_4 the stabilization of an electronic transition corresponded to a D4h environment around the metal center, with interaction in N-aliphatic. Copper-modified materials were evenly distributed due to the availability of bonds in target sections such as the periphery. This slight modification demonstrated that the copper compound can generate hydroxyl radicals and radical anion superoxide, different from other modifications. The radical hydroxyl can be generated in the h^+ as was demonstrated with the KI scavenger. The material g-C_3N_4 modified with copper (II) was an excellent photocatalyst for disinfecting *E. coli* but also was able to degrade dicloxacillin in the presence of light. It offers another opportunity for this material in the fields of degradation of organic molecules. Definitively, the hydroxides in the structures modified with the transition metals do not make important contributions to the disinfection against this microorganism; their role may be structural. It wass concluded that a transition metal coordinated in the N-aliphatic of carbon nitride allows a better electron transfer for the generation of ROS. Conversely, interaction with N-tris triazine can hinder interaction. This soft synthesis opens the opportunity to explore new transition metals by interacting with carbon nitride to degrade organic molecules and enrich disinfection processes.

Supplementary Materials: The following supporting information can be downloaded at: https://www.mdpi.com/article/10.3390/molecules29163775/s1. Figure S1. DRX patterns for g-C_3N_4 and modified materials with transition metals, the red lines (Mn(OH)$_2$ crystallographic planes reported), black lines (Ni(OH)$_2$ crystallographic planes reported), green (Cu(OH)$_2$ crystallographic planes reported), Figure S2. The absorption spectrum of (a) Cu-g-C_3N_4, g-C_3N_4, and emission spectra of the daylight lamp (red line), (b) Ni-g-C_3N_4 and Mn-g-C_3N_4 spectrum, Figure S3. Proposed structures for (a) g-C_3N_4 and modified products with (b) copper (II), (c)manganese (II), and (d) nickel (II), Figure S4. SEM images of (a) g-C_3N_4 (b) Cu-g-C_3N_4, (c) Mn-g-C_3N_4, (d)) Ni-g-C_3N_4, (e) TEM images of g-C_3N_4 and Ni-g-C_3N, and (f) diffraction pattern of Ni-g-C_3N_4, Figure S5. N_2 adsorption-desorption isotherms of g-C_3N_4 and modified materials, Table S1. Electronic properties and application in 2D-2D structures and Metal-g-C_3N_4, Figure S6. XPS spectra for modified g-C_3N_4 materials, (a) Survey XPS for g-C_3N_4 modifications, (b) High-resolution N 1s orbital contributions, (c) High-resolution O 1s orbital contributions, (d) High-resolution Mn 2p orbital contributions.

Author Contributions: Y.P.Á.-T.: conceptualization, methodology, validity tests, data curation, writing—original draft preparation, visualization, and investigation. A.V.L.-E.: visualization and investigation. E.D.C.C.: conceptualization, methodology, validity tests, data curation, writing—original draft preparation, visualization, and investigation. J.A.: visualization and investigation. E.C.-P.: validity tests, data curation, and investigation. J.R.: conceptualization, methodology, validity tests, data curation, writing—original draft preparation, visualization, and investigation. S.N.: data curation and investigation. All authors have read and agreed to the published version of the manuscript.

Funding: This work was supported by Universidad de Antioquia-financial GRANT—SGR (Sistema General de Regalías) Minciencias 2020000100587.

Institutional Review Board Statement: Not applicable.

Informed Consent Statement: Not applicable.

Data Availability Statement: The original contributions presented in the study are included in the article/Supplementary Material, further inquiries can be directed to the corresponding author/s.

Acknowledgments: This work was supported by Universidad de Antioquia—financial "Development of self-disinfecting surfaces based on materials with photochemical and magnetic activity" project.

Conflicts of Interest: The authors declare no conflict of interest.

References

1. Hong Hak, C.; Ching Sim, L.; Leong, K.H.; Chin, Y.H.; Saravanan, P. Sunlight Photodeposition of Gold nanoparticles onto Graphitic Carbon Nitride (g-C_3N_4) and Application Towards the Degradation of Bisphenol A. *IOP Conf. Ser. Mater. Sci. Eng.* **2018**, *409*, 012008. [CrossRef]
2. Alizadeh, T.; Rafiei, F. An innovative application of graphitic carbon nitride (g-C_3N_4) nano-sheets as silver ion carrier in a solid state potentiometric sensor. *Mater. Chem. Phys.* **2019**, *227*, 176–183. [CrossRef]
3. Afshari, M.; Dinari, M.; Momeni, M.M. Ultrasonic irradiation preparation of graphitic-C_3N_4/polyaniline nanocomposites as counter electrodes for dye-sensitized solar cells. *Ultrason. Sonochem.* **2018**, *42*, 631–639. [CrossRef] [PubMed]
4. Li, K.; Su, F.Y.; Zhang, W. De Modification of g-C_3N_4 nanosheets by carbon quantum dots for highly efficient photocatalytic generation of hydrogen. *Appl. Surf. Sci.* **2016**, *375*, 110–117. [CrossRef]
5. Ye, C.; Li, J.X.; Li, Z.J.; Li, X.B.; Fan, X.B.; Zhang, L.P.; Chen, B.; Tung, C.H.; Wu, L.Z. Enhanced Driving Force and Charge Separation Efficiency of Protonated g-C_3N_4 for Photocatalytic O_2 Evolution. *ACS Catal.* **2015**, *5*, 6973–6979. [CrossRef]
6. Huang, D.; Yan, X.; Yan, M.; Zeng, G.; Zhou, C.; Wan, J.; Cheng, M.; Xue, W. Graphitic Carbon Nitride-Based Heterojunction Photoactive Nanocomposites: Applications and Mechanism Insight. *ACS Appl. Mater. Interfaces* **2018**, *10*, 21035–21055. [CrossRef]
7. Wang, K.; Li, J.; Zhang, G. Ag-Bridged Z-Scheme 2D/2D $Bi_5FeTi_3O_{15}$/g-C_3N_4 Heterojunction for Enhanced Photocatalysis: Mediator-Induced Interfacial Charge Transfer and Mechanism Insights. *ACS Appl. Mater. Interfaces* **2019**, *11*, 27686–27696. [CrossRef] [PubMed]
8. Dong, F.; Zhao, Z.; Xiong, T.; Ni, Z.; Zhang, W.; Sun, Y.; Ho, W.K. In situ construction of g-C_3N_4/g-C_3N_4 metal-free heterojunction for enhanced visible-light photocatalysis. *ACS Appl. Mater. Interfaces* **2013**, *5*, 11392–11401. [CrossRef]
9. Liu, G.; Dong, G.; Zeng, Y.; Wang, C. The photocatalytic performance and active sites of g-C_3N_4 effected by the coordination doping of Fe(III). *Chin. J. Catal.* **2020**, *41*, 1564–1572. [CrossRef]

10. Shan, Q.Y.; Guo, X.L.; Dong, F.; Zhang, Y.X. Single atom (K/Na) doped graphitic carbon Nitride@MnO$_2$ as an efficient electrode Material for supercapacitor. *Mater. Lett.* **2017**, *202*, 103–106. [CrossRef]
11. Savateev, A.; Ghosh, I.; König, B.; Antonietti, M. Photoredox Catalytic Organic Transformations using Heteroge-neous Carbon Nitrides. *Angew. Chem. Int. Ed. Engl.* **2018**, *57*, 15936–15947. [CrossRef] [PubMed]
12. Ghosh, I.; Khamrai, J.; Savateev, A.; Shlapakov, N.; Antonietti, M.; König, B. Organic semiconductor photocatalyst can bifunctionalize arenes and heteroarenes. *Science* **2019**, *365*, 360–366. [CrossRef] [PubMed]
13. Wang, J.; Wang, S. A critical review on graphitic carbon nitride (g-C$_3$N$_4$)-based materials: Preparation, modification and environmental application. *Coord. Chem. Rev.* **2022**, *453*, 214338. [CrossRef]
14. Zheng, Y.; Jiao, Y.; Zhu, Y.; Cai, Q.; Vasileff, A.; Li, L.H.; Han, Y.; Chen, Y.; Qiao, S.Z. Molecule-Level g-C$_3$N$_4$ Coordinated Transition Metals as a New Class of Electrocatalysts for Oxygen Electrode Reactions. *J. Am. Chem. Soc.* **2017**, *139*, 3336–3339. [CrossRef] [PubMed]
15. Zhou, W.C.; Zhang, W. De Anchoring nickel complex to g-C$_3$N$_4$ enables an efficient photocatalytic hydrogen evolution reaction through ligand-to-metal charge transfer mechanism. *J. Colloid Interface Sci.* **2022**, *616*, 791–802. [CrossRef] [PubMed]
16. Capobianco, M.D.; Pattengale, B.; Neu, J.; Schmuttenmaer, C.A. Single Copper Atoms Enhance Photoconductivity in g-C$_3$N$_4$. *J. Phys. Chem. Lett.* **2020**, *11*, 8873–8879. [CrossRef] [PubMed]
17. Li, W.; Liu, M.; Cheng, S.; Zhang, H.; Yang, W.; Yi, Z.; Zeng, Q.; Tang, B.; Ahmad, S.; Sun, T. Polarization-independent tunable bandwidth absorber based on single-layer graphene. *Diam. Relat. Mater.* **2024**, *142*, 110793. [CrossRef]
18. Li, X.; Yu, J.; Wageh, S.; Al-Ghamdi, A.A.; Xie, J. Graphene in Photocatalysis: A Review. *Small.* **2016**, *12*, 6640–6696. [CrossRef] [PubMed]
19. Jiang, B.Q.; Hou, Y.G.; Wu, J.X.; Ma, Y.X.; Gan, X.T. In-fiber photoelectric device based on graphene-coated tilted fiber grating. *Opto-Electron. Sci.* **2023**, *2*, 230012. [CrossRef]
20. Zeng, C.; Lu, H.; Mao, D.; Du, Y.Q.; Hua, H. Graphene-empowered dynamic metasurfaces and metadevices. *Opto-Electron. Adv.* **2022**, *5*, 200098. [CrossRef]
21. Zhou, F.Y.; Mao, J.N.; Peng, X.L.; Hong, B.; Xu, J.C.; Zeng, Y.X.; Han, Y.B.; Ge, H.L.; Wang, X.Q. Magnetically separable Ni/g-C$_3$N$_4$ nanocomposites for enhanced visible-light photocatalytic degradation of methylene blue and ciprofloxacin. *Diam. Relat. Mater.* **2022**, *126*, 109070. [CrossRef]
22. Zhang, Z.; Qiu, C.; Xu, Y.; Han, Q.; Tang, J.; Loh, K.P.; Su, C. Semiconductor photocatalysis to engineering deuterated N-alkyl pharmaceuticals enabled by synergistic activation of water and alkanols. *Nat. Commun.* **2020**, *11*, 4722. [CrossRef] [PubMed]
23. Parasuraman, V.; Perumalswamy Sekar, P.; Mst Akter, S.; Ram Lee, W.; Young Park, T.; Gon Kim, C.; Kim, S. Improved photocatalytic disinfection of dual oxidation state (dos)-Ni/g-C$_3$N$_4$ under indoor daylight. *J. Photochem. Photobiol. A Chem.* **2023**, *434*, 114262. [CrossRef]
24. Kundu, A.; Pousty, D.; Kumar Vadivel, V.; Mamane, H. Cu-coated graphitic carbon nitride (Cu/CN) with ideal photocatalytic and antibacterial properties. *Carbon Trends* **2023**, *13*, 100307. [CrossRef]
25. Zhang, H.; Ren, X.; Zhang, B.; Jia, A.; Wang, Y. Size Effect of Cu Nanoparticles in Cu/g-C$_3$N$_4$ Composites on Properties for Highly Efficient Photocatalytic Reduction of CO$_2$ to Methanol. *ACS Appl. Mater. Interfaces* **2023**, *15*, 53515–53525. [CrossRef]
26. Qian, W.; Fang, Y.; Liu, H.; Deng, Y.; Li, Y.; Zhang, Y.; Diao, Z.; Li, M. Photocatalytic Degradation of Tetracycline Hydrochloride by Mn/g-C$_3$N$_4$/BiPO$_4$ and Ti/g-C$_3$N$_4$/BiPO$_4$ Composites: Reactivity and Mechanism. *Catalysts* **2023**, *13*, 1398. [CrossRef]
27. Lin, C.; Su, J.; Chen, Z. Photocatalytic oxidative degradation of methyl orange by a novel g-C$_3$N$_4$@ZnO based on graphene oxide composites with ternary heterojunction construction. *React. Kinet. Mech. Catal.* **2022**, *135*, 1651–1664. [CrossRef]
28. Xu, X.; Wang, S.; Hu, T.; Yu, X.; Wang, J.; Jia, C. Fabrication of Mn/O co-doped g-C$_3$N$_4$: Excellent charge separation and transfer for enhancing photocatalytic activity under visible light irradiation. *Dye Pigment.* **2020**, *175*, 108107. [CrossRef]
29. Murugesan, P.; Moses, J.A.; Anandharamakrishnan, C. Photocatalytic disinfection efficiency of 2D structure graphitic carbon nitride-based nanocomposites: A review. *J. Mater. Sci.* **2019**, *54*, 12206–12235. [CrossRef]
30. Yang, X.; Ye, Y.; Sun, J.; Li, Z.; Ping, J.; Sun, X. Recent Advances in g-C$_3$N$_4$-Based Photocatalysts for Pollutant Degradation and Bacterial Disinfection: Design Strategies, Mechanisms, and Applications. *Small* **2022**, *18*, 2105089. [CrossRef]
31. Liu, X.; Ma, R.; Zhuang, L.; Hu, B.; Chen, J.; Liu, X.; Wang, X. Recent developments of doped g-C$_3$N$_4$ photocatalysts for the degradation of organic pollutants. *Crit. Rev. Environ. Sci. Technol.* **2021**, *51*, 751–790. [CrossRef]
32. Cao, C.-B.; Lv, Q.; Zhu, H.-S. Carbon nitride prepared by solvothermal method. *Diam. Relat. Mater.* **2003**, *12*, 1070–1074. [CrossRef]
33. Ge, L.; Han, C.; Liu, J.; Li, Y. Enhanced visible light photocatalytic activity of novel polymeric g-C$_3$N$_4$ loaded with Ag nanoparticles. *Appl. Catal. A Gen.* **2011**, *409–410*, 215–222. [CrossRef]
34. Yang, Y.; Bian, Z. Oxygen doping through oxidation causes the main active substance in g-C$_3$N$_4$ photocatalysis to change from holes to singlet oxygen. *Sci. Total Environ.* **2021**, *753*, 141908. [CrossRef] [PubMed]
35. Muñoz-Batista, M.J.; Andrini, L.; Requejo, F.G.; Gómez-Cerezo, M.N.; Fernández-García, M.; Kubacka, A. Sunlight active g-C$_3$N$_4$-based Mn+ (M[dbnd]Cu, Ni, Zn, Mn)—Promoted catalysts: Sharing of nitrogen atoms as a door for optimizing photo-activity. *Mol. Catal.* **2020**, *484*, 110725. [CrossRef]
36. Sellers, S.P.; Korte, B.J.; Fitzgerald, J.P.; Reiff, W.M.; Yee, G.T. Canted ferromagnetism and other magnetic phenomena in square-planar, neutral manganese(II) and iron(II) octaethyltetraazaporphyrins. *J. Am. Chem. Soc.* **1998**, *120*, 4662–4670. [CrossRef]

37. Shimizu, I.; Morimoto, Y.; Faltermeier, D.; Kerscher, M.; Paria, S.; Abe, T.; Sugimoto, H.; Fujieda, N.; Asano, K.; Suzuki, T.; et al. Tetrahedral Copper(II) Complexes with a Labile Coordination Site Supported by a Tris-tetramethylguanidinato Ligand. *Inorg. Chem.* **2017**, *56*, 9634–9645. [CrossRef]
38. Fina, F.; Callear, S.K.; Carins, G.M.; Irvine, J.T.S. Structural investigation of graphitic carbon nitride via XRD and neutron diffraction. *Chem. Mater.* **2015**, *27*, 2612–2618. [CrossRef]
39. Li, F.; Zhang, L.; Evans, D.G.; Duan, X. Structure and surface chemistry of manganese-doped copper-based mixed metal oxides derived from layered double hydroxides. *Colloids Surfaces A Physicochem. Eng. Asp.* **2004**, *244*, 169–177. [CrossRef]
40. Zhao, J.; Chen, C.; Ma, W. Photocatalytic Degradation of Organic Pollutants Under Visible Light Irradiation. *Top Catal.* **2005**, *35*, 269–278. [CrossRef]
41. Spanish-Number 49g. 2023. Available online: www.HealthLinkBC.ca/more/resources/healthlink-bc-files (accessed on 19 May 2024).
42. Zhu, D.; Zhou, Q. Novel Bi_2WO_6 modified by N-doped graphitic carbon nitride photocatalyst for efficient photocatalytic degradation of phenol under visible light. *Appl. Catal. B Environ.* **2020**, *268*, 118426. [CrossRef]
43. Acosta-Vergara, J.; Torres-Palma, R.A.; Ávila-Torres, Y. Solid state pelletizing for the synthesis of new Bi-doped strontium molybdate and its development as a photocatalytic precursor for Rhodamine B degradation. *MethodsX* **2023**, *11*, 102258. [CrossRef]
44. Biesinger, M.C.; Payne, B.P.; Lau, L.W.M.; Gerson, A.; Smart, R.S.C. X-ray photoelectron spectroscopic chemical state Quantification of mixed nickel metal, oxide and hydroxide systems. *Surf. Interface Anal.* **2009**, *41*, 324–332. [CrossRef]
45. Pourbaix, M.; Zhang, H.; Pourbaix, A. Presentation of an Atlas of chemical and electrochemical equilibria in the presence of a gaseous phase. *Mater. Sci. Forum* **1997**, *251–254*, 143–148. [CrossRef]
46. Torres, L.M.; Montes-Rojas, A. Conversión de potenciales entre distintos electrodos de referencia: Una analogía para facilitar su comprensión. *Boletín Soc. Química México* **2017**, *11*, 12–14.
47. Johnstone, A.H. CRC Handbook of Chemistry and Physics—69th Edition Editor in Chief R. C. Weast, CRC Press Inc., Boca Raton, Florida, 1988, pp. 2400, price £57.50. ISBN 0-8493-0369-5. *J. Chem. Technol. Biotechnol.* **1991**, *50*, 294–295. [CrossRef]
48. Ávila-Torres, Y.; López-Sandoval, H.; Mijangos, E.; Quintanar, L.; Rodríguez, E.E.; Flores-Parra, A.; Contreras, R.; Vicente, R.; Rikken, G.L.J.A.; Barba-Behrens, N. Structure and magnetic properties of copper(II) and cobalt(II) coordination compounds derived from optically active tridentate ligands. *Polyhedron* **2013**, *51*, 298–306. [CrossRef]
49. Jiang, L.; Yuan, X.; Pan, Y.; Liang, J.; Zeng, G.; Wu, Z.; Wang, H. Doping of graphitic carbon nitride for photocatalysis: A reveiw. *Appl. Catal. B Environ.* **2017**, *217*, 388–406. [CrossRef]
50. Dong, G.; Zhang, Y.; Pan, Q.; Qiu, J. A fantastic graphitic carbon nitride (gC_3N_4) material: Electronic structure, photocatalytic and photoelectronic properties. *J. Photochem. Photobiol. C Photochem. Rev.* **2014**, *20*, 33–50. [CrossRef]
51. Yu, H.; Jiang, X.; Shao, Z.; Feng, J.; Yang, X.; Liu, Y. Metal-Free Half-Metallicity in B-Doped gh-C_3N_4 Systems. *Nanoscale Res. Lett.* **2018**, *13*, 1–7. [CrossRef]
52. Zhu, C.; Fang, Q.; Liu, R.; Dong, W.; Song, S.; Shen, Y. Insights into the Crucial Role of Electron and Spin Structures in Heteroatom-Doped Covalent Triazine Frameworks for Removing Organic Micropollutants. *Environ. Sci. Technol.* **2022**, *56*, 6699–6709. [CrossRef] [PubMed]
53. Cai, H.; Yang, Q.; Hu, Z.; Duan, Z.; You, Q.; Sun, J.; Xu, N.; Wu, J. Enhanced photoelectrochemical activity of vertically aligned ZnO-coated TiO_2 nanotubes. *Appl. Phys. Lett.* **2014**, *104*, 053114. [CrossRef]
54. Gelderman, K.; Lee, L.; Donne, S.W. Flat-band potential of a semiconductor: Using the Mott-Schottky equation. *J. Chem. Educ.* **2007**, *84*, 685–688. [CrossRef]
55. Gao, J.; Xue, J.; Jia, S.; Shen, Q.; Zhang, X.; Jia, H.; Liu, X.; Li, Q.; Wu, Y. Self-Doping Surface Oxygen Vacancy-Induced Lattice Strains for Enhancing Visible Light-Driven Photocatalytic H2Evolution over Black TiO_2. *ACS Appl. Mater. Interfaces* **2021**, *13*, 18758–18771. [CrossRef] [PubMed]
56. Torres-Palma, R.A.; Serna-Galvis, E.A.; Ávila-Torres, Y.P. Chapter 12—Photochemical and photocatalytical degradation of antibiotics in water promoted by solar irradiation. In *Nano-Materials as Photocatalysts for Degradation of Environmental Pollutants*; Elsevier: Amsterdam, The Netherlands, 2020; pp. 211–243. [CrossRef]
57. Shaban, S.Y.; Ramadan, A.E.M.M.; Ibrahim, M.M.; Elshami, F.I.; van Eldik, R. Square planar versus square pyramidal copper(II) complexes containing N_3O moiety: Synthesis, structural characterization, kinetic and catalytic mimicking activity. *Inorganica Chim. Acta* **2019**, *486*, 608–616. [CrossRef]
58. Romero-Hernandez, J.J.; Paredes-Laverde, M.; Silva-Agredo, J.; Mercado, D.F.; Ávila-Torres, Y.; Torres-Palma, R.A. Pharmaceutical adsorption on NaOH-treated rice husk-based activated carbons: Kinetics, thermodynamics, and mechanisms. *J. Clean. Prod.* **2024**, *434*, 139935. [CrossRef]
59. *Book of Standards Volume: 03.01*; Developed by Subcommittee: E04.11; ICS Code: 71.040.50; ASTM International: West Conshohocken, PA, USA, 2019; 9p. [CrossRef]
60. Suarez, M.; Caicedo, C.; Morales, J.; López, E.F.; Torres, Y. Design, theoretical study and correlation of the electronic and optical properties of diethynylphenylthiophene as photovoltaic materials. *J. Mol. Struct.* **2020**, *1201*, 127093. [CrossRef]

Disclaimer/Publisher's Note: The statements, opinions and data contained in all publications are solely those of the individual author(s) and contributor(s) and not of MDPI and/or the editor(s). MDPI and/or the editor(s) disclaim responsibility for any injury to people or property resulting from any ideas, methods, instructions or products referred to in the content.

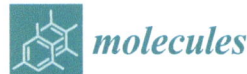 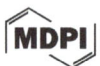

Article

Mimicking Axon Growth and Pruning by Photocatalytic Growth and Chemical Dissolution of Gold on Titanium Dioxide Patterns

Fatemeh Abshari [1,*], Moritz Paulsen [1], Salih Veziroglu [2,3], Alexander Vahl [2,3,4] and Martina Gerken [1,3,*]

[1] Chair for Integrated Systems and Photonics, Department of Electrical and Information Engineering, Faculty of Engineering, Kiel University, Kaiserstr. 2, 24143 Kiel, Germany
[2] Chair for Multicomponent Materials, Department of Materials Science, Faculty of Engineering, Kiel University, Kaiserstr. 2, 24143 Kiel, Germany
[3] Kiel Nano, Surface and Interface Science (KiNSIS), Kiel University, Christian-Albrechts-Platz 4, 24118 Kiel, Germany
[4] Leibniz Institute for Plasma Science and Technology, Felix-Hausdorff-Str. 2, 17489 Greifswald, Germany
* Correspondence: fa@tf.uni-kiel.de (F.A.); mge@tf.uni-kiel.de (M.G.); Tel.: +49-4318806255 (F.A.); +49-431886250 (M.G.)

Abstract: Biological neural circuits are based on the interplay of excitatory and inhibitory events to achieve functionality. Axons form long-range information highways in neural circuits. Axon pruning, i.e., the removal of exuberant axonal connections, is essential in network remodeling. We propose the photocatalytic growth and chemical dissolution of gold lines as a building block for neuromorphic computing mimicking axon growth and pruning. We predefine photocatalytic growth areas on a surface by structuring titanium dioxide (TiO_2) patterns. Placing the samples in a gold chloride ($HAuCl_4$) precursor solution, we achieve the controlled growth of gold microstructures along the edges of the indium tin oxide (ITO)/TiO_2 patterns under ultraviolet (UV) illumination. A potassium iodide (KI) solution is employed to dissolve the gold microstructures. We introduce a real-time monitoring setup based on an optical transmission microscope. We successfully observe both the growth and dissolution processes. Additionally, scanning electron microscopy (SEM) analysis confirms the morphological changes before and after dissolution, with dissolution rates closely aligned to the growth rates. These findings demonstrate the potential of this approach to emulate dynamic biological processes, paving the way for future applications in adaptive neuromorphic systems.

Keywords: photocatalytic deposition; chemical dissolution; gold; titanium dioxide; potassium iodide solution; indium tin oxide; neuromorphic engineering; transmission optical microscopy

1. Introduction

Neuromorphic engineering focuses on developing advanced computational systems by drawing inspiration from the structure and processes of biological neural networks, with the goal of achieving improved efficiency [1]. In neural networks, neuronal connections are dynamically and continuously reorganized. These connections evolve over different time scales: rapid synaptic plasticity results in localized adjustments at synapses between neurons, while slower processes, such as axon growth and pruning, occur throughout the broader network. Building on the dynamic reorganization of neuronal connections, axon growth represents a critical phase of neural network development, where intrinsic genetic programs and extracellular signals work in concert to extend axons toward their target regions, forming the foundational pathways for neural circuitry [2,3]. Many studies have focused on replicating rapid synaptic plasticity using memristive devices, given their unique ability to enable in-memory computing [4,5]. Ongoing research continues to investigate neuronal connections at a global scale within biological neural networks, while simultaneously developing innovative methods to integrate these mechanisms into next-generation bio-inspired systems [6].

Recent advances in neuromorphic engineering have increasingly focused on nanowire networks that exhibit memristive properties, which are being explored for their ability to emulate the dynamic and adaptable behavior of synapses in biological neural networks. These networks are gaining attention for their potential to enhance computational efficiency by replicating both short-term synaptic plasticity and long-term memory storage, paving the way for the integration of such systems into bio-inspired computing architecture [7–9]. These networks are naturally self-organizing, with nanowires forming conductive, one-dimensional (1D) pathways. The intricate topology of these networks results in collective switching behaviors, making them highly compatible with memristive architecture. In biological neural networks, the ability to dynamically regulate stimuli and control the formation and dissolution of connections is a key feature for adaptive functionality [10–12].

Axonal pruning is a critical process in the development and remodeling of neural networks, wherein excess or improperly connected axons are selectively eliminated to refine the neural circuitry, ensuring the optimal function of the nervous system [13]. This process occurs primarily during developmental stages, but also plays a role in adult neuroplasticity, where axonal pruning helps to fine-tune neural pathways based on learning, experience, and environmental stimuli [13]. Mechanistically, axonal pruning is regulated by molecular signals that induce synaptic weakening and the targeted retraction of axons, a process that parallels cellular processes, like apoptosis, ultimately contributing to the structural and functional optimization of neural circuits [14]. In the early stages, attempts to replicate the global interactions within neuronal assemblies were made by exploring global connectivity through electrolyte gating in liquid media [15].

We focus on the gradual formation of one-dimensional, long-range connections, which have the potential to enable adaptive modifications in network topology. This aspect of the research aims to mimic axonal growth through the photocatalytic deposition of conductive gold lines onto ultraviolet (UV) light-activated titanium dioxide (TiO_2) substrates. Additionally, we explore the pruning of these axonal-like structures by the chemical dissolution of the grown gold lines using a potassium iodide (KI) solution, simulating the axonal pruning process. Chemical dissolution was chosen as it allows for a gradual loss of conductivity in continuous gold lines due to the reduction in the gold line diameter. Once the gold coverage falls below the percolation threshold, conductivity is lost completely. With gold growth, the percolation threshold may be reached again, regaining conductivity. Therefore, this approach promises a reversible, stimulus-dependent growth and pruning of network connections during the learning process mimicking the situation in biological neural networks. Here, it is recognized that the density of the human dendrite network increases from birth to the age of 2 years old [16]. Subsequently, the density decreases again, which is associated with network consolidation during learning.

TiO_2 is widely utilized as a semiconductor photocatalyst due to its high photocatalytic efficiency, ease of fabrication, cost-effectiveness, non-toxic nature, and robust chemical stability [17–19]. Considering the critical role of TiO_2 as a semiconductor photocatalyst with excellent optical properties, recent studies have demonstrated its ability to facilitate photocatalytic processes under UV light, particularly for structural modifications and degradation mechanisms [20]. It was recently shown that the co-precipitation of TiO_2 with terbium and manganese effectively improves its photocatalytic performance by lowering the band gap energy and enhancing electron-hole separation, which facilitates the efficient degradation of tetracycline antibiotics under both UV- and visible-light conditions [21]. The deposition of gold onto TiO_2 thin films has been successfully achieved through the photoreduction of gold chloride ($HAuCl_4$) under UV illumination [22–24]. It has been reported that the addition of isopropanol to the $HAuCl_4$ solution can significantly accelerate the photoreduction process by acting as a hole scavenger, thereby enhancing the speed of gold nanoparticle growth under UV light [25]. In addition to the use of isopropanol, other parameters have been shown to significantly influence the morphology and coverage of the deposited gold structures. These include factors such as the crystal structure and surface morphology of the underlying TiO_2 thin film, the composition and pH of the precursor solution, as well as the intensity and duration of UV illumination [26,27].

Through UV illumination, TiO_2 facilitates the generation of electron-hole pairs, with electrons migrating to the conduction band. These electrons reduce Au^{3+} ions from the $HAuCl_4$ solution, leading to the formation of neutral gold atoms The gold atoms form solid nuclei on the TiO_2 surface, which then grow through the consecutive addition of gold atoms into gold nano- and microparticles. Simultaneously, the holes oxidize nearby molecules, completing the photocatalytic reaction [28]. The efficiency of photocatalytic processes, such as gold growth on TiO_2 surfaces, is strongly influenced by light intensity, as higher UV intensities enhance the generation of electron-hole pairs, accelerating reaction rates and structural formation [29]. These findings provide valuable insights into how UV illumination affects both the growth and morphological evolution of gold particles [30].

In this study, photocatalysis is utilized to grow gold lines on TiO_2 thin films patterned using lithography. A thin indium tin oxide (ITO) sublayer is incorporated beneath the TiO_2. Given that ITO has a higher work function compared to TiO_2, a Schottky barrier forms at the TiO_2-ITO interface, which affects the overall photocatalytic performance [31,32]. In a recent study, we demonstrated that a 6 nm ITO layer beneath TiO_2 effectively promotes localized gold growth along the edges of the TiO_2 patterns resulting in electrically conductive gold lines [33]. This study builds on these previous findings by using a consistent template with a 6 nm ITO layer beneath the TiO_2 for all experiments. Here, we investigate the sequential processes of photocatalytic gold growth followed by chemical dissolution mimicking axon growth and pruning. The schematic in Figure 1 demonstrates the abstraction process for mimicking neuronal network dynamics through a material-based approach. Figure 1a on the left presents a simplified schematic representation of a neural network, illustrating the interconnectivity between neurons in a network. This is not a true 3D neuronal network, but rather a simplified projection to communicate the idea of neuronal connectivity. Moving to the right, the neural network is translated into a 2D schematic geometry on a surface. This 2D representation simplifies the complex volumetric arrangement while retaining the essential connectivity, making it accessible for technical implementation.

Figure 1b introduces the technical methodology used to mimic axon-like connections in a proposed material system. First, a patterned template is designed to define specific regions for selective gold growth. This template mimics synapse-like nodes connected by axon-like linear pathways. Under UV illumination, the photocatalytic growth of gold structures is induced along these defined pathways, simulating the formation of axon-like connections. The resulting gold pathways provide a physical basis for mimicking neuronal connectivity in a controllable manner. Finally, the grown gold structures undergo a targeted chemical dissolution process, emulating the natural phenomenon of axonal pruning. This selective removal of gold pathways enables dynamic modifications of the network, reflecting the adaptive and self-organizing properties of biological neural circuits. This approach represents a proposed material system to mimic the formation and dissolution of axon-like connections in a simplified, reproducible framework. By combining photocatalytic growth and chemical dissolution processes, this study introduces a methodology for investigating adaptive, neuromorphic systems, laying the groundwork for further exploration in network remodeling.

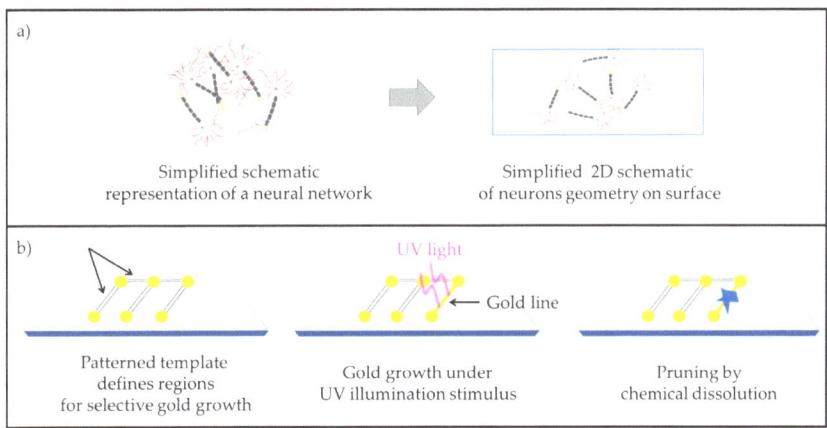

Figure 1. (**a**) Simplified schematic representation of a neural network (**left**) and its abstraction into 2D schematic geometry on a surface (**right**), retaining the essential connectivity of the network. (**b**) Process for mimicking axon-like connections: (**left**) a patterned template defines regions for selective gold growth, (**center**) UV illumination induces photocatalytic gold growth along predefined pathways, forming axon-like structures, and (**right**) chemical dissolution selectively prunes the gold connections, mimicking axonal pruning.

To further clarify this, the abstraction process depicted in Figure 1 bridges the gap between biological complexity and material implementation. The transition from a neural network to a patterned material system involves translating the functional principles of connectivity and adaptability into a simplified, physical framework. This includes using the patterned template to mimic axonal pathways, where gold deposition represents axonal growth and its selective removal represents pruning. By replicating these key features, the proposed system provides a versatile platform to study the dynamic remodeling of networks, offering insights into neuromorphic engineering and adaptive material systems.

The chemical dissolution of gold using the KI solution has proven to be an effective method for removing gold from various substrates. KI acts as a complexing agent, forming soluble gold–iodine complexes, which enable the controlled removal of gold lines grown during photocatalytic processes [34]. This dissolution process mimics the axonal pruning in neural networks, allowing for repeated cycles of growth and removal, essential for dynamic neuromorphic systems. In this paper, we aim to investigate the UV-stimulated photocatalytic growth of gold on titanium dioxide patterns, followed by chemical dissolution using KI solutions. By analyzing both real-time optical monitoring data and post-experiment scanning electron microscopy (SEM) imaging, we provide insights into the mechanisms governing these processes and their potential for precise microstructure manipulation.

2. Results

2.1. Analysis of Gold Growth Dynamics on the Edge and Surface of TiO_2

In this section, the photocatalytic growth of gold lines on TiO_2 edges is analyzed in real-time using optical transmission microscope data. As described in Section 4, a beaker was filled with 20 mL of a gold chloride precursor solution, mixed with isopropanol in a 10:1 ratio to enhance the deposition rate. The substrate was submerged in this solution and exposed to UV illumination (λ = 365 nm) for 30 min. The growth process was monitored through a transmission microscope by capturing images every 4 s over a total duration of 30 min. A certain region around the TiO$_2$ edge was selected where the gold structures predominantly grew. The selected region included the TiO$_2$ surface on the left side and the glass substrate on the right side of the TiO$_2$ edge located in the center. Figure 2a presents optical microscope images of the selected region taken at different times during the growth process: $t = 0$, $t = 10$, $t = 20$, and $t = 30$ min. A supplementary video (Video S1) is provided to offer a clearer visualization of the growth dynamics.

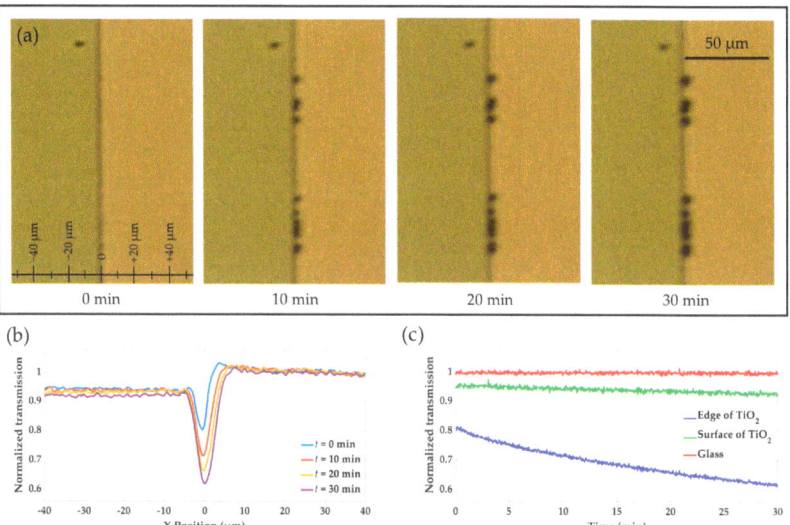

Figure 2. Real-time monitoring of gold growth (**a**) Sequential optical microscope images of a selected region around the TiO$_2$ edge, including the TiO$_2$ surface on the left side and the glass substrate on the right side, taken at various time points, $t = 0$, $t = 10$, $t = 20$, and $t = 30$ min, illustrating the gradual growth of gold structures over 30 min. (**b**) Transmission profiles across the TiO$_2$ edge at $t = 0$, $t = 10$, $t = 20$, and $t = 30$ min, normalized to the reference transmission on the glass substrate. (**c**) Time-dependent transmission curves showing dissolution progress at the TiO$_2$ edge and surface compared to the glass substrate.

For every pixel of the selected region, we measured a distinct transmitted light intensity. At each x-coordinate, we averaged the measured intensity values over all pixels with different y-coordinates to generate transmission profiles across the x-span of the selected region. These transmission curves, showing the variation in intensity as a function of x-span, are plotted in Figure 2b for four different time points: $t = 0$, $t = 10$, $t = 20$, and $t = 30$ min. All transmission values are normalized relative to the reference transmission on the bare glass substrate, located far from the TiO$_2$ edge at $x = 40$ μm.

At the beginning of the growth process ($t = 0$), the transmission at the TiO$_2$ edge ($x = 0$) was lower than those of the TiO$_2$ surface ($x < 0$) and the glass substrate ($x > 0$). This difference is attributed to light scattering at the TiO$_2$ edge, which creates a narrow dark line in the middle of the selected area, as displayed in the optical microscopy images (Figure 2a). Furthermore, the transmission on the TiO$_2$ surface ($x < 0$) was slightly lower than that of the glass substrate ($x > 0$). During the growth process, a decrease in the transmitted light intensity is observed for $x = 0$ and $x < 0$, corresponding to the growth of gold particles along the edge and on the surface of TiO$_2$ over time. At the end of the growth experiment ($t = 30$ min), the normalized transmission at the edge ($x = 0$) was significantly reduced compared to the beginning time ($t = 0$), with a total change of $\Delta T_{\text{Edge}} \approx 0.19$ over

30 min. On the surface of the TiO$_2$ ($x < 0$), the transmission was slightly reduced, with $\Delta T_{Surface} \approx 0.03$ after 30 min of growth. While a significant growth rate is achieved along the edge of TiO$_2$, little changes in transmission are observed on the left and right sides of the edge, confirming the selective formation of gold lines along the edge.

The dissolution process of gold structures on the TiO$_2$ edge and surface was analyzed by monitoring transmission changes over time. The glass substrate served as a reference, as it remained unaffected throughout the experiment. The transmission at the TiO$_2$ edge and surface increased during dissolution, indicating the gradual removal of gold structures. Figure 2 part (c) of the figure presents the time-dependent transmission curves for these regions, highlighting the sharper rise in transmission at the TiO$_2$ edge compared to the surface, reflecting the higher density of gold structures at the edge.

2.2. Analysis of Gold Dissolution Dynamics on the Edge and Surface and TiO$_2$

Following the growth process, a KI solution diluted in DI water at a ratio of 1:300 was utilized to initiate chemical dissolution of the gold structures. The dissolution process was monitored using the same method as described for the growth process. Figure 3a displays the optical microscope images of a certain area around the TiO$_2$ edge taken at different times during the dissolution process: $t = 0$, $t = 5$, $t = 10$, and $t = 30$ min. For a better visualization of the dissolution dynamics, a supplementary video (Video S2) is provided. Similar to the growth analysis, the TiO$_2$ edge is located in the center, with the TiO$_2$ surface and the glass substrate on the left and right sides, respectively. Figure 3b presents the transmission curves across the x-span of the selected region at four different time points: $t = 0$, $t = 10$, $t = 20$, and $t = 30$ min. All transmission values were normalized relative to the reference transmission on the bare glass substrate, located far from the TiO$_2$ edge at $x = 40$ μm.

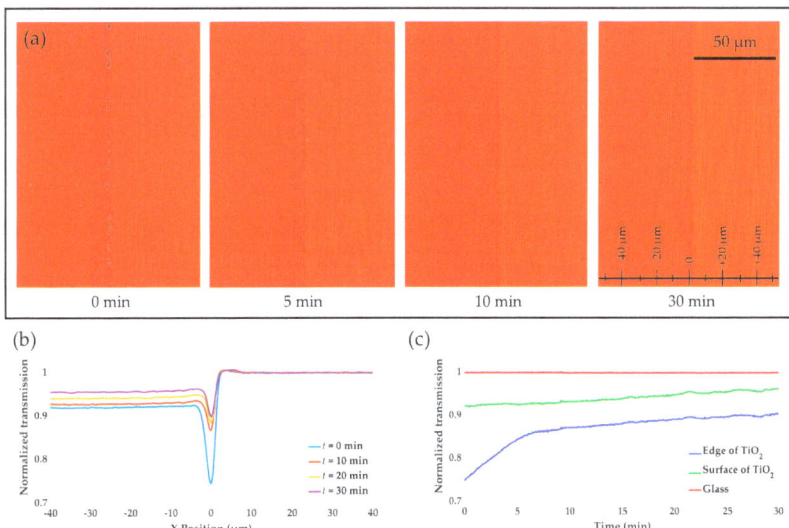

Figure 3. Real-time monitoring of gold dissolution (**a**) Sequential optical microscope images of a selected region around the TiO$_2$ edge, including the TiO$_2$ surface on the left side and the glass substrate on the right side, taken at various time points, $t = 0$, $t = 5$, $t = 10$, and $t = 30$ min, illustrating the gradual dissolution of gold structures over 30 min. (**b**) Transmission profiles across the TiO$_2$ edge at $t = 0$, $t = 10$, $t = 20$, and $t = 30$ min, normalized to the reference transmission on the glass substrate. (**c**) Time-dependent transmission curves showing dissolution progress at the TiO$_2$ edge and surface compared to the glass substrate.

At the start of the dissolution experiment ($t = 0$), the transmission at the TiO$_2$ edge ($x = 0$) was nearly 0.25 lower than that of the adjacent glass substrate ($x > 0$). This difference indicates that gold was substantially deposited along the edge of the TiO$_2$. On the surface of the TiO$_2$ ($x < 0$), the normalized transmission value was approximately 0.08 lower compared to the glass substrate, suggesting partial gold growth on the TiO$_2$ surface. As dissolution proceeded, the gold structures dissolved at varying rates on the edge and surface of TiO$_2$. While the transmission over the glass substrate remained constant throughout the experiment, a significant increase in transmission was observed on the TiO$_2$ edge and surface as the gold structures dissolved.

The dissolution process was tracked on Figure 3c by monitoring transmission changes over time, with the glass substrate as a constant reference. Figure 3c shows time-dependent transmission curves, with a sharper increase at the TiO$_2$ edge, indicating higher initial gold density, similar to the previous analysis.

2.3. Morphological Examination Using Scanning Electron Microscopy

In this section, the morphology of gold particles on a single sample was examined at different stages using SEM. The SEM imaging was performed using a Carl Zeiss Supra 55VP instrument (ZEISS AG, Oberkochen, Germany), operated at an acceleration voltage of 3 kV and a working distance of 3 mm. This technique provides high-resolution images that allow for a detailed visualization of the particles, revealing their size, shape, and distribution along the TiO$_2$ patterns. By applying SEM, the structural characteristics of the gold particles could be analyzed, both after growth and after dissolution.

SEM analysis was first conducted to observe the morphology of the gold particles formed along the edges of the titanium dioxide patterns after 30 min of UV illumination. The photocatalytic growth experiment used a precursor solution of gold chloride mixed with isopropanol in a 10:1 ratio to enhance growth. After the growth phase, SEM was also performed following the chemical dissolution of the gold particles, where the KI solution was diluted with 300 mL of deionized water to assess the effects of dissolution.

2.3.1. SEM Analysis of Grown Gold Particles on TiO$_2$ Edges

The SEM images in Figure 4 provide detailed insights into the selective growth of gold microstructures on the edge of TiO$_2$ patterns. Notably, no visible particle growth is observed on the glass substrate, confirming that the photocatalytic deposition occurred exclusively on the TiO$_2$. This result is significant, as the addition of isopropanol to the precursor solution, combined with the controlled intensity of the UV LEDs, prevented any unwanted nucleation or deposition on the glass, ensuring that growth was confined to the TiO$_2$ regions, which is consistent with the in-situ microscopy measurements where the transmission intensity on the glass substrate remained unchanged during the growth process.

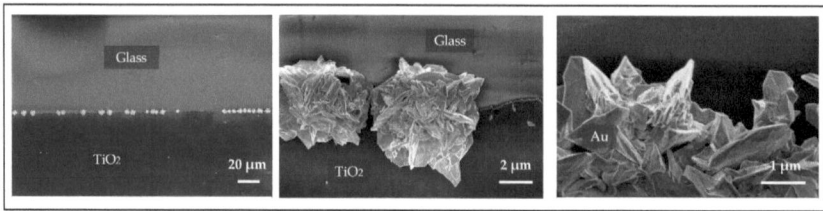

Figure 4. SEM images of the template post-growth, illustrating the formation of gold particles along the edges of the TiO$_2$ patterns.

The gold microstructures display a distinct 3D flower-like morphology, primarily concentrated along the edges of the TiO$_2$ patterns. These structures are composed of sharp, crossed plates, forming intricate flower-shaped formations. While the growth is focused along the edges, the microstructures do not form a continuous line; instead, they appear as separate clusters. This is due to the limited illumination time of 30 min in this experiment, as the focus was on studying the spontaneous growth and dissolution processes rather than forming a continuous line. With extended illumination times, a uniform and continuous gold line along the edges can be achieved [33]. In certain areas, however, the flower-shaped particles grow close together, nearly forming a connected structure along the edge. This unique morphology and spatial distribution suggest that the edges of the ITO-TiO$_2$ patterns serve as preferential nucleation sites, promoting the formation of well-defined, three-dimensional gold structures.

2.3.2. SEM Analysis After the Chemical Dissolution of Gold Structures

The SEM images in Figure 5, illustrate the morphological changes in the gold structures after the chemical dissolution process for 30 min. In some regions on the TiO$_2$ surface, clusters of flower-shaped gold particles were observed to have grown, though these areas were limited both in number and in size. Figure 5a shows one of these small regions on the surface where the characteristic flower-shaped gold particles had formed prior to the dissolution experiment.

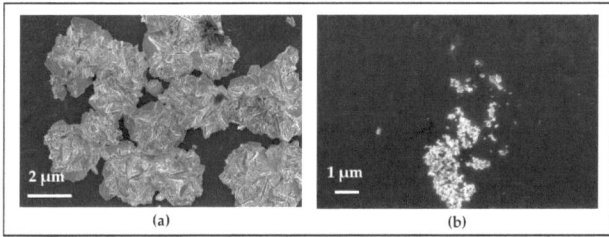

Figure 5. SEM images of gold particles on TiO$_2$: (**a**) Before dissolution, with flower-shaped particles on the surface; (**b**) After dissolution, showing reduced and irregularly shaped particles, though not fully removed.

Following chemical dissolution using the KI solution, SEM imaging of the same area in Figure 5b reveals noticeable changes. The previously well-formed, flower-like gold particles appear etched and reduced in size, suggesting the dissolution process was partially successful. The gold structures seem to have been broken down into smaller fragments, though complete dissolution was not achieved, as some remnants of gold particles are still visible. The decrease in particle size and the etched morphology indicate that the KI solution effectively initiated the dissolution, but did not fully dissolve the gold structures.

This partial etching highlights the ability of the KI solution to interact with and reduce the size of gold particles, although further refinement of the dissolution conditions may be required to achieve full removal. Additionally, the size of the gold particles noticeably decreased, and their morphology transformed from the original flower-like shapes into more irregular, amorphous spots, indicating significant structural alteration during the dissolution process.

3. Discussion

Reconfigurable long-range connections with stimulus-induced formation and stimulus-free, spontaneous dissolution over time are in high demand to implement axon-like dynamic connection schemes. Possible technical implementations range from guided wiring upon metal filament formation in liquid media upon an electrochemical redox reaction [11] toward the electrophoretic reorganization of metallic nanoparticles into anisotropic long-range nanoparticle agglomerates along electrical field gradients in nanofluids [35]. In contrast to these earlier studies, which reported on material systems for the electrically stimulated growth of long-range connections, in this study, UV illumination is applied as a stimulus. To mimic a biological neural network, growth and dissolution rates should be compatible with each other. Photocatalytic gold growth allows for UV-stimulus activated connection formation. The rate may be tailored by adjusting the chemical composition of the precursor solution or by changing the UV wavelength or intensity. We enhanced the growth rate in this experiment by using isopropanol as a hole scavenger in the precursor solution. Additionally, the implementation of two UV LEDs, positioned at an angle for even illumination, further accelerated the growth process. We decreased the gold dissolution rate by diluting the KI solution. This had the additional benefit that a higher transparency is achieved, allowing for the real-time monitoring of the dissolution with the optical transmission microscope. Based on the results of a dilution series, the 1:300 dilution was chosen. The dissolution process in this setup was slightly slower than the gold growth. This is desired as the gold lines should grow under UV stimulus and dissolve without stimulus.

The incomplete dissolution of gold structures observed in this study is attributed to the slower dissolution rate relative to the growth rate under the chosen experimental conditions. While this resulted in residual gold particles, the dissolution process can be fully completed by increasing the concentration of KI in the DI water mixture. This adjustment would accelerate the dissolution, ensuring the complete removal of gold when required. However, in the context of mimicking axon-like behaviors in neuromorphic systems, achieving a fully resolved state may not be desired. Instead, the most interesting operation point is at the percolation threshold of the gold lines. By analyzing changes in conductance during the growth and dissolution processes, the system can effectively replicate the dynamic behavior of neural connections. This conductance-based approach provides insights into dynamic behaviors without necessitating complete dissolution, highlighting the versatility of the proposed system for neuromorphic and adaptive material applications.

The SEM observations confirmed gold growth and incomplete dissolution for 30 min of each process. Small amounts of gold residue remaining after the dissolution experiment confirm the lower dissolution rate compared to the growth rate. The time scales on the minutes to hours range align well with the remodeling times of biological systems. Further tuning of the rates is possible. Regarding long-range metal connection formation and dissolution, it has to be considered that a longer gold growth is necessary to achieve a conductive gold line without gaps. On the other hand, as soon as gaps appear, the electrical conductivity is lost. In future experiments, instead of pre-grown metal lines, a photo-forming step could be utilized to initiate long-range gold connections, similar to the electroforming process in filamentary memristive devices. Once a proto-filament is formed through the photo-forming step, subsequent cycles of UV illumination and dissolution can lead to dynamic reconfigurable states, mimicking axon-like connections. This approach aligns with the foundational role of forming steps in early memristive devices, as discussed in the reviews [36].

The diameter of the gold lines in our work is comparable to the diameter of biological axons in the micrometer range [37]. In biology, the plasticity of white matter is of high importance for learning and memory [38]. The conduction time of axons is not simply regulated by the axon diameter, but myelin formation and remodeling play a key role [39]. The inhomogeneous conductivity of biological axons may be compared to the inhomogeneous nature of our grown gold lines. The dissolution mimics the reversible and localized nature of axon pruning, focusing on the functional principles of dynamic connectivity rather than the molecular complexity of biological systems. Different to biology, our two-dimensional implementation has a much lower line density and total length. In a human brain, the combined length of myelinated axons reaches approximately 160,000 km [38]. Biological network reconfiguration times are on the time scale of hours to days and longer [38]. In our study, we considered growth or pruning sequences of half-hour durations for partial growth and partial dissolution. This is comparable to biological time frames. In summary, our proposed two-dimensional approach offers a similar line diameter as well as similar reconfiguration time scales, but a much shorter overall length. While acknowledging the significant differences, stimulus-adaptive gold "axon" formation and pruning are much closer to the biological situation than the fixed conductivity of electrical connections in standard electronics.

As in biology, this neuromorphic building block only functions in a liquid environment. This is highly unusual for electronic systems and definitely poses challenges regarding system stability, leakage, etc. Nevertheless, it is an intriguing thought to mimic axonal long-range connection growth and pruning, and the system opens the possibility to study the interaction of local UV stimuli and a homeostatic environment. Different than in biology, the liquid has to be exchanged between growth and dissolution. This poses an additional challenge for further development toward applications. We envision a microfluidic realization, where the liquid is exchanged in short intervals in a flow cell. Thus, this system is in principle suitable as a building block for neuromorphic engineering, allowing for sequential growth and dissolution cycles.

The findings of this study demonstrate a controlled approach to the photocatalytic growth and chemical dissolution of gold structures on a substrate, opening potential applications in neuromorphic systems. This study represents an effort to mimic axonal dynamics on a larger scale, providing a foundation for future work aimed at achieving finer and more biologically comparable structures [7]. The ability to dynamically grow and dissolve axon-like connections reflects fundamental biological processes, such as axonal growth and pruning, which are essential for synaptic plasticity and learning [10]. This capability could eventually lead to adaptive hardware systems that reconfigure in response to stimuli, offering a pathway toward more flexible and biologically inspired artificial neural networks.

Beyond neuromorphic systems, this method holds promise for bioelectronics, particularly for the development of reconfigurable sensor arrays. Dynamically adjustable conductive pathways could enable sensors to adapt in real time to changing environmental or physiological conditions [11]. Additionally, this approach offers a platform for studying synaptic behaviors in artificial systems, enabling controlled investigations of neural processes at a larger, more accessible scale.

While there are limitations in terms of achieving the high density of three-dimensional biological systems, the versatility of the proposed system lays a foundation for adaptive and responsive material systems. By bridging biological functionality and synthetic implementation, this work represents an important step toward biologically inspired material systems that operate on scales compatible with current fabrication technologies.

4. Materials and Methods

4.1. Substrate Prepration

In this study, a single type of substrate template was used for all experiments to investigate the photocatalytic growth and dissolution processes. Soda-lime glass substrates were precisely diced into 10 mm × 10 mm squares using a Wafer Dicing System (model DAD3350, Aurotech, Santa Rosa, Philippines) to ensure uniformity and provide a consistent surface area for material deposition. The substrates were then cleaned thoroughly to remove contaminants that could interfere with the photocatalytic reactions. The cleaning process involved sequential sonication in acetone and isopropanol (both of 99% purity, Sigma-

Aldrich, St. Louis, MO, USA) in an ultrasonic bath (Martin Walter Ultraschalltechnik AG, Straubenhardt, Germany), followed by complete drying with high-purity nitrogen gas to ensure the removal of all solvent residues.

A 6 nm layer of ITO was deposited onto the cleaned glass substrates using physical vapor deposition (PVD) with an In_2O_3/SnO_2 (90/10 wt%) target (99.99% purity, Kurt J. Lesker Company GmbH, Dresden, Germany). The ITO layer, selected for its higher work function relative to TiO_2, was critical for achieving photocatalytic growth along the TiO_2 edges [33]. The deposition of this thin, uniform, ITO layer formed a heterojunction TiO_2-ITO interface, facilitating electron transfer and optimizing the conditions for gold growth during subsequent experiments.

Following ITO deposition, a 70 nm-thick layer of TiO_2 was sputtered onto the ITO-coated substrates. This was achieved using a 3-inch TiO_2 target (99.99% purity, Kurt J. Lesker Company GmbH) to ensure high-quality, uniform TiO_2 coverage across the entire substrate. The TiO_2 was deposited in its amorphous form, requiring further processing to transform it into its active photocatalytic anatase phase.

To pattern the TiO_2 layer, a standard photolithography technique was employed. The substrates were first spin-coated with AZ5214E photoresist (Microchemicals GmbH, Ulm, Germany) at 3000 rpm for 30 s to achieve a uniform resist layer. Hexamethyldisiloxane (HMDS) was used as an adhesion promoter before applying the photoresist to ensure reliable patterning. After spin coating, the substrates were prebaked at 110 °C for 50 s to solidify the resist layer.

UV exposure was performed using a mask aligner (SUSS MicroTec, Garching, Germany), with a 5-inch photomask containing reflective chromium structures for line patterns as small as 50 μm (Rose Fotomasken, Bergisch Gladbach, Germany). The exposure energy was set to 32 mJ/cm^2. Following exposure, a reversal bake at 120 °C for 2 min was performed to create the desired resist pattern, and a flood UV exposure with 320 mJ/cm^2 was applied. The unexposed areas were developed using the AZ726 developer (Microchemicals GmbH) for 1 min, after which the substrates were rinsed with deionized water and dried with nitrogen gas.

The lift-off process, used to remove the unwanted TiO_2 and ITO, involved immersing the substrates in acetone with ultrasonic agitation for 10 min, followed by a 5-min rinse in isopropanol. This process ensured that only the desired patterned regions of TiO_2 remained on the ITO layer.

Finally, to convert the sputtered TiO_2 from its amorphous state to the photocatalytically active anatase phase, the substrates were annealed in a muffle furnace at 400 °C for 90 min. This heat treatment was critical for achieving the desired crystalline structure and ensuring optimal photocatalytic properties for the TiO_2. After annealing, the substrates were rapidly cooled on a metal plate to lock in the anatase phase, preparing them for subsequent photocatalytic growth and dissolution experiments. The preparation process of the substrates, including lithographic patterning and material deposition, is schematically illustrated in Figure 6 to provide a clear overview of the procedural steps.

4.2. Photocatalytic Growth Experiment

After completing the heat treatment to convert the TiO_2 to its anatase phase, the photocatalytic growth of gold lines along the edges of the TiO_2 patterns was performed in a beaker. The precursor solution was prepared by dissolving 99.99% pure gold (III) chloride ($HAuCl_4$) powder (Sigma-Aldrich) in deionized water, with a concentration of 15 mg in 60 mL of water. This solution was thoroughly mixed to ensure the complete dissolution of the gold chloride and to create a homogeneous precursor solution, essential for consistent photocatalytic growth across the entire surface of the substrates.

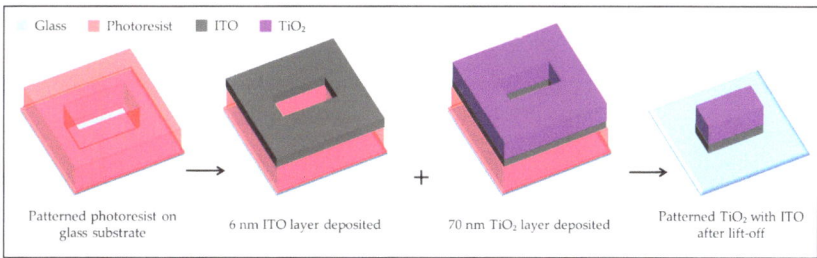

Figure 6. Schematic representation of the substrate preparation process. The glass substrate is negatively patterned with AZ5214E photoresist after lithography. A 6 nm ITO layer and a 70 nm TiO_2 layer are then deposited via sputtering. After the lift-off process, the final patterned TiO_2 structures with the underlying ITO layer are revealed.

To enhance the growth rate of the gold particles and improve the efficiency of the photocatalytic process, the precursor solution was mixed with isopropanol in a 10:1 ratio. The addition of isopropanol, which acts as a hole scavenger, plays a critical role by accelerating the reduction of Au^{3+} ions under UV illumination.

Each substrate was positioned at the bottom of a glass beaker with the TiO_2 facing upward. A total of 20 mL of the prepared precursor solution was added to the beaker, completely submerging the substrate. Two UV LEDs (Nichia, Tokushima, Japan), each emitting light at a wavelength of 365 nm, were positioned at opposite sides of the beaker with roughly 7 cm distance to the beaker, illuminating the template at an angle. The intensity of the UV light was measured using a Newport optical power meter and was found to be approximately 5 mJ/cm². The total illumination time was set to 30 min, ensuring sufficient energy input for the reduction of Au^{3+} ions and the subsequent formation of gold lines along the edges of the TiO_2 patterns. The schematic of the illumination experiment setup is shown in Figure 7. The setup is placed in a transmission microscope (DMi8 inverted microscope, Leica, Wetzlar, Germany) to allow for optical image recording of the gold growth and dissolution on the transparent substrates.

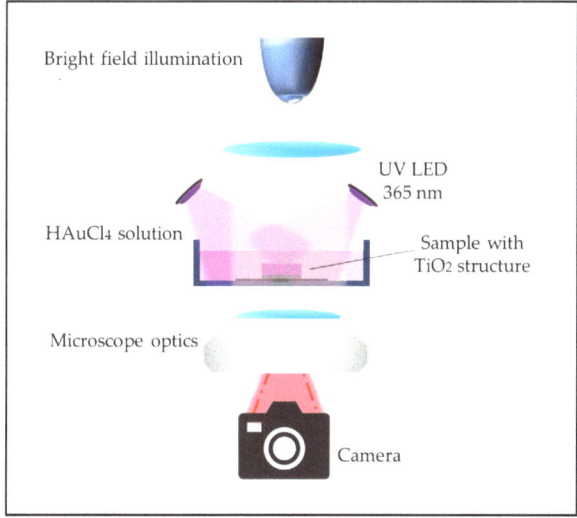

Figure 7. Schematic of the photocatalytic illumination setup. The sample with TiO_2 structures is submerged in the $HAuCl_4$ solution and illuminated by two angled UV LEDs (365 nm) under a transmission microscope connected to a camera.

4.3. Dissolution Experiment Using a KI Solution Mixed in Different Ratios with DI Water

To investigate the chemical dissolution of gold lines grown on the edge of TiO_2 patterns, a KI solution was prepared by mixing KI (Sigma-Aldrich, product number 204102) and iodine (I_2) (Sigma-Aldrich) in a ratio of 1:4:40 (DI water), which is a commonly used ratio for gold dissolution in similar chemical systems [40]. After thoroughly mixing the KI and I_2 with deionized water, the prepared solution was further diluted to different concentrations for the dissolution experiments.

Three distinct dilutions of KI solution were prepared by mixing 1 mL of the stock solution with 200 mL, 300 mL, and 400 mL of DI water. These varying concentrations were chosen to explore how different KI solution strengths impact the dissolution rate of the gold lines. The prepared solutions, exhibiting different shades of color due to varying concentrations of KI in DI, are shown in Figure 8. As the KI solution is diluted with DI water, the color transitions from dark brown to a lighter reddish hue, becoming progressively lighter with increasing amounts of DI water.

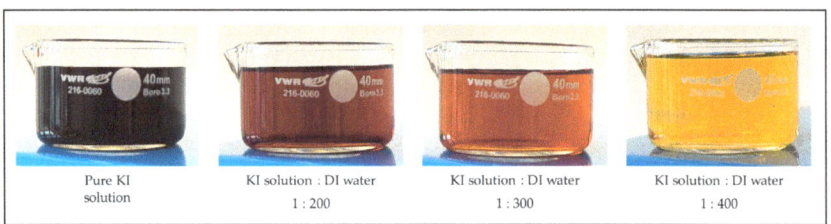

Figure 8. Visual representation of the KI solution diluted with DI water at different ratios. From left to right: pure KI solution, 1:200 KI solution to DI water, 1:300 KI solution to DI water, and 1:400 KI solution to DI water.

After preparing the KI solutions, two substrates were used for the dissolution experiments. Both substrates first underwent the photocatalytic gold growth process as described in Section 4.2. For the dissolution experiment, one of the gold-grown substrates was immersed in the KI solution diluted with 300 mL of DI water, and the other substrate was immersed in the solution mixed with 400 mL of DI water. Both samples were kept in the solution for 30 min to allow sufficient dissolution of the gold lines. The dissolution experiments were conducted under a transmission microscope connected to a camera, enabling the real-time visualization and recording of the process.

4.4. Photocatalytic Growth and Chemical Dissolution Sequence

The experiment was conducted on the substrate described in Section 4.1, using a transmission microscope for the continuous real-time observation of both the photocatalytic growth and subsequent chemical dissolution processes. The substrate was fixed in place throughout the experiment, eliminating the need for repositioning during the solution exchange steps.

In the first step, the beaker was filled with 20 mL of a $HAuCl_4$ precursor solution, which had been mixed with isopropanol in a 10:1 ratio to enhance the growth rate of the gold lines. The substrate, submerged in this solution, was then illuminated using two UV LEDs (365 nm), placed at an angle, for 30 min. This illumination initiated the photocatalytic growth of gold lines along the edges of the TiO_2 patterns on the substrate. After the growth phase, the beaker and substrate were thoroughly rinsed with deionized water to remove any residual gold precursor solution, and the substrate was dried using nitrogen gas to prepare for the next step.

In the second step, the photocatalytically grown gold Structures were subjected to chemical dissolution. The beaker was filled with 20 mL of KI solution, diluted in 30 mL of DI water. During this phase, the UV LEDs were turned off to avoid any photocatalytic effects that could interfere with the dissolution process. The substrate remained in the KI solution for 30 min, allowing the KI solution to dissolve the gold lines by forming a soluble gold–iodide complex [40]. Following the dissolution, the substrate was again rinsed with deionized water to ensure the complete removal of the KI solution, and the substrate was dried using nitrogen gas.

5. Conclusions

In this study, we demonstrated the sequential photocatalytic growth and chemical dissolution of gold structures on a patterned ITO/TiO_2 template. By optimizing the precursor solution, we achieved controlled gold growth along the edges of the ITO/TiO_2 patterns and subsequently carried out the dissolution process in an optimized KI solution. The kinetics of the growth and dissolution processes were explored through real-time monitoring using optical transmission microscopy and image processing. Although a uniform gold line was not formed within the 30 min illumination, the focus of this study was on the sequential growth and dissolution processes rather than achieving continuous lines. While the current setup did not allow simultaneous growth and dissolution, the findings suggest potential for future microfluidic systems that enable dynamic solution exchange for UV-driven growth and dissolution cycles, mimicking biological processes such as axonal growth and pruning in bio-inspired networks. This work provides a robust methodology for optimized photocatalytic growth and dissolution processes, contributing to the development of dynamic, reconfigurable material systems for neuromorphic engineering and adaptive technologies.

Supplementary Materials: The following supporting information can be downloaded at: https://www.mdpi.com/article/10.3390/molecules30010099/s1, Video S1: Gold growth dynamics in 30 min; Video S2: Gold dissolution dynamics in 30 min.

Author Contributions: Conceptualization, F.A. and M.G.; methodology, F.A. and M.G.; software, F.A., M.P. and M.G.; validation, F.A. and M.G.; formal analysis, F.A., S.V., A.V. and M.G.; investigation, F.A., S.V., A.V. and M.G.; resources, M.G.; data curation, F.A. and M.G.; writing—original draft preparation, F.A.; writing—review and editing, F.A., M.P., S.V., A.V. and M.G.; visualization, F.A.; supervision, M.G.; project administration, M.G.; funding acquisition, M.G. All authors have read and agreed to the published version of the manuscript.

Funding: This work was supported by the Deutsche Forschungsgemeinschaft (DFG, German Research Foundation)–Project-ID 434434223–SFB 1461.

Data Availability Statement: The data supporting the conclusions of this article will be made available by the corresponding authors on request.

Conflicts of Interest: The authors declare no conflict of interest.

References

1. Kendall, J.D.; Kumar, S. The Building Blocks of a Brain-Inspired Computer. *Appl. Phys. Rev.* **2020**, *7*, 011305. [CrossRef]
2. Goldberg, J.L. How Does an Axon Grow? *Genes. Dev.* **2003**, *17*, 941–958. [CrossRef]
3. Riccomagno, M.M.; Kolodkin, A.L. Sculpting Neural Circuits by Axon and Dendrite Pruning. *Annu. Rev. Cell Dev. Biol.* **2015**, *31*, 779–805. [CrossRef]
4. Strukov, D.B.; Snider, G.S.; Stewart, D.R.; Williams, R.S. The Missing Memristor Found. *Nature* **2008**, *453*, 80–83, Erratum in *Nature* **2009**, *453*, 7191. [CrossRef] [PubMed]
5. Asif, M.; Singh, Y.; Thakre, A.; Singh Ab, V.N.; Kumar, A. Synaptic Plasticity and Learning Behaviour in Multilevel Memristive Devices. *RSC Adv.* **2023**, *13*, 13292–13302. [CrossRef] [PubMed]
6. Wright, C.D. Precise Computing with Imprecise Devices. *Nat. Electron.* **2018**, *1*, 212–213. [CrossRef]

7. Vahl, A.; Milano, G.; Kuncic, Z.; Brown, S.A.; Milani, P. Brain-Inspired Computing with Self-Assembled Networks of Nano-Objects. *J. Phys. D Appl. Phys.* **2024**, *57*, 503001. [CrossRef]
8. Milano, G.; Pedretti, G.; Montano, K.; Ricci, S.; Hashemkhani, S.; Boarino, L.; Ielmini, D.; Ricciardi, C. In Materia Reservoir Computing with a Fully Memristive Architecture Based on Self-Organizing Nanowire Networks. *Nat. Mater.* **2021**, *21*, 195–202. [CrossRef] [PubMed]
9. Loeffler, A.; Diaz-Alvarez, A.; Zhu, R.; Ganesh, N.; Shine, J.M.; Nakayama, T.; Kuncic, Z. Neuromorphic Learning, Working Memory, and Metaplasticity in Nanowire Networks. *Sci. Adv.* **2023**, *9*, eadg3289. [CrossRef] [PubMed]
10. Ziegler, M.; Mussenbrock, T.; Kohlstedt, H. *Bio-Inspired Information Pathways*; Springer: Cham, Switzerland, 2023.
11. Terasa, M.I.; Birkoben, T.; Noll, M.; Adejube, B.; Madurawala, R.; Carstens, N.; Strunskus, T.; Kaps, S.; Faupel, F.; Vahl, A.; et al. Pathways towards Truly Brain-like Computing Primitives. *Mater. Today* **2023**, *69*, 41–53. [CrossRef]
12. Milano, G.; Pedretti, G.; Fretto, M.; Boarino, L.; Benfenati, F.; Ielmini, D.; Valov, I.; Ricciardi, C.; Milano, G.; Ricciardi, C.; et al. Brain-Inspired Structural Plasticity through Reweighting and Rewiring in Multi-Terminal Self-Organizing Memristive Nanowire Networks. *Adv. Intell. Syst* **2000**, *2*, 2000096. [CrossRef]
13. Cusack, C.L.; Swahari, V.; Hampton Henley, W.; Ramsey, J.M.; Deshmukh, M. Distinct Pathways Mediate Axon Degeneration during Apoptosis and Axon-Specific Pruning. *Nat. Commun.* **2013**, *4*, 1876. [CrossRef] [PubMed]
14. Mear, Y.; Enjalbert, A.; Thirion, S.; Malagón, M.M.; Kineman, R.D. GHS-R1a Constitutive Activity and Its Physiological Relevance. *Front. Neurosci.* **2013**, *7*, 87. [CrossRef]
15. Gkoupidenis, P.; Koutsouras, D.A.; Malliaras, G.G. Neuromorphic Device Architectures with Global Connectivity through Electrolyte Gating. *Nat. Commun.* **2017**, *8*, 15448. [CrossRef]
16. Seung, S. *Connectome: How the Brain's Wiring Makes Us Who We Are*; Houghton Mifflin Harcourt: New York, NY, USA, 2012.
17. Safajou, H.; Khojasteh, H.; Salavati-Niasari, M.; Mortazavi-Derazkola, S. Enhanced Photocatalytic Degradation of Dyes over Graphene/Pd/TiO$_2$ Nanocomposites: TiO$_2$ Nanowires versus TiO$_2$ Nanoparticles. *J. Colloid. Interface Sci.* **2017**, *498*, 423–432. [CrossRef]
18. Vahl, A.; Veziroglu, S.; Henkel, B.; Strunskus, T.; Polonskyi, O.; Aktas, O.C.; Faupel, F. Pathways to Tailor Photocatalytic Performance of TiO$_2$ Thin Films Deposited by Reactive Magnetron Sputtering. *Materials* **2019**, *12*, 2840. [CrossRef] [PubMed]
19. Kusmierek, E. A CeO$_2$ Semiconductor as a Photocatalytic and Photoelectrocatalytic Material for the Remediation of Pollutants in Industrial Wastewater: A Review. *Catalysts* **2020**, *10*, 1435. [CrossRef]
20. Pan, X.; Tang, S.; Chen, X.; Liu, H.; Yu, C.; Gao, Q.Z.; Zhao, X.; Yang, H.; Gao, H.; Wang, S. Temperature-Controlled Synthesis of TiO$_2$ Photocatalyst with Different Crystalline Phases and Its Photocatalytic Activity in the Degradation of Different Mixed Dyes. *Russ. J. Phys. Chem. A* **2022**, *96*, S210–S218. [CrossRef]
21. You, C.S.; Jung, S.C. Photo-Catalytic Destruction of Tetracycline Antibiotics Using Terbium and Manganese Co-Precipitated TiO$_2$ Photocatalyst. *J. Environ. Chem. Eng.* **2024**, *12*, 111666. [CrossRef]
22. Kedves, E.Z.; Pap, Z.; Hernadi, K.; Baia, L. Significance of the Surface and Bulk Features of Hierarchical TiO$_2$ in Their Photocatalytic Properties. *Ceram. Int.* **2021**, *47*, 7088–7100. [CrossRef]
23. Binas, V.; Venieri, D.; Kotzias, D.; Kiriakidis, G. Modified TiO$_2$ Based Photocatalysts for Improved Air and Health Quality. *J. Mater.* **2017**, *3*, 3–16. [CrossRef]
24. Salomatina, E.V.; Fukina, D.G.; Koryagin, A.V.; Titaev, D.N.; Suleimanov, E.V.; Smirnova, L.A. Preparation and Photocatalytic Properties of Titanium Dioxide Modified with Gold or Silver Nanoparticles. *J. Environ. Chem. Eng.* **2021**, *9*, 106078. [CrossRef]
25. Veziroglu, S.; Obermann, A.L.; Ullrich, M.; Hussain, M.; Kamp, M.; Kienle, L.; Leißner, T.; Rubahn, H.G.; Polonskyi, O.; Strunskus, T.; et al. Photodeposition of Au Nanoclusters for Enhanced Photocatalytic Dye Degradation over TiO$_2$ Thin Film. *ACS Appl. Mater. Interfaces* **2020**, *12*, 14983–14992. [CrossRef] [PubMed]
26. Guo, Y.; Siretanu, I.; Zhang, Y.; Mei, B.; Li, X.; Mugele, F.; Huang, H.; Mul, G. PH-Dependence in Facet-Selective Photo-Deposition of Metals and Metal Oxides on Semiconductor Particles. *J. Mater. Chem. A Mater.* **2018**, *6*, 7500–7508. [CrossRef]
27. Veziroglu, S.; Ghori, M.Z.; Kamp, M.; Kienle, L.; Rubahn, H.G.; Strunskus, T.; Fiutowski, J.; Adam, J.; Faupel, F.; Aktas, O.C. Photocatalytic Growth of Hierarchical Au Needle Clusters on Highly Active TiO$_2$ Thin Film. *Adv. Mater. Interfaces* **2018**, *5*, 1800465. [CrossRef]
28. Mendoza-Diaz, M.I.; Cure, J.; Rouhani, M.D.; Tan, K.; Patnaik, S.G.; Pech, D.; Quevedo-Lopez, M.; Hungria, T.; Rossi, C.; Estève, A. On the UV-Visible Light Synergetic Mechanisms in Au/TiO$_2$ Hybrid Model Nanostructures Achieving Photoreduction of Water. *J. Phys. Chem. C* **2020**, *124*, 25421–25430. [CrossRef]
29. Sari, Y.; Gareso, P.L.; Armynah, B.; Tahir, D. A Review of TiO$_2$ Photocatalyst for Organic Degradation and Sustainable Hydrogen Energy Production. *Int. J. Hydrogen Energy* **2024**, *55*, 984–996. [CrossRef]
30. Stamplecoskie, K.G.; Swint, A. Optimizing Molecule-like Gold Clusters for Light Energy Conversion. *J. Mater. Chem. A* **2015**, *4*, 2075–2081. [CrossRef]
31. Dai, W.; Wang, X.; Liu, P.; Xu, Y.; Li, G.; Fu, X. Effects of Electron Transfer between TiO$_2$ Films and Conducting Substrates on the Photocatalytic Oxidation of Organic Pollutants. *J. Phys. Chem. B* **2006**, *110*, 13470–13476. [CrossRef]

32. Irfan, F.; Tanveer, M.U.; Moiz, M.A.; Husain, S.W.; Ramzan, M. TiO$_2$ as an Effective Photocatalyst Mechanisms, Applications, and Dopants: A Review. *Eur. Phys. J. B* **2022**, *95*, 184. [CrossRef]
33. Abshari, F.; Veziroglu, S.; Adejube, B.; Vahl, A.; Gerken, M. Photocatalytic Edge Growth of Conductive Gold Lines On Microstructured TiO$_2$–ITO Substrates. *Langmuir* **2024**, *40*, 22. [CrossRef] [PubMed]
34. Tomic, P. Method for Metallization Stripping of Gold Interconnected Semiconductors Using an Aqueous Potassium Iodide Solution. *Microsc. Today* **2002**, *10*, 18–19. [CrossRef]
35. Nikitin, D.; Biliak, K.; Pleskunov, P.; Ali-Ogly, S.; Červenková, V.; Carstens, N.; Adejube, B.; Strunskus, T.; Černochová, Z.; Štěpánek, P.; et al. Resistive Switching Effect in Ag-Poly(Ethylene Glycol) Nanofluids: Novel Avenue Toward Neuromorphic Materials. *Adv. Funct. Mater.* **2024**, *34*, 2310473. [CrossRef]
36. Zhu, J.; Zhang, T.; Yang, Y.; Huang, R. A Comprehensive Review on Emerging Artificial Neuromorphic Devices. *Appl. Phys. Rev.* **2020**, *7*, 011312. [CrossRef]
37. Barazany, D.; Basser, P.J.; Assaf, Y. In Vivo Measurement of Axon Diameter Distribution in the Corpus Callosum of Rat Brain. *Brain* **2009**, *132*, 1210–1220. [CrossRef]
38. Sampaio-Baptista, C.; Johansen-Berg, H. White Matter Plasticity in the Adult Brain. *Neuron* **2017**, *96*, 1239–1251. [CrossRef] [PubMed]
39. Seidl, A.H. Regulation of Conduction Time along Axons. *Neuroscience* **2014**, *276*, 126–134. [CrossRef] [PubMed]
40. Nakao, Y.; Soneb, K. Reversible Dissolutioddeposition of Gold in Iodine-Iodide-Acetonitrile Systems. *Chem. Commun.* **1996**, *8*, 897–898. [CrossRef]

Disclaimer/Publisher's Note: The statements, opinions and data contained in all publications are solely those of the individual author(s) and contributor(s) and not of MDPI and/or the editor(s). MDPI and/or the editor(s) disclaim responsibility for any injury to people or property resulting from any ideas, methods, instructions or products referred to in the content.

MDPI AG
Grosspeteranlage 5
4052 Basel
Switzerland
Tel.: +41 61 683 77 34

Molecules Editorial Office
E-mail: molecules@mdpi.com
www.mdpi.com/journal/molecules

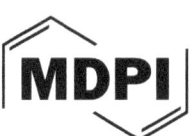

Disclaimer/Publisher's Note: The title and front matter of this reprint are at the discretion of the Guest Editor. The publisher is not responsible for their content or any associated concerns. The statements, opinions and data contained in all individual articles are solely those of the individual Editor and contributors and not of MDPI. MDPI disclaims responsibility for any injury to people or property resulting from any ideas, methods, instructions or products referred to in the content.

www.ingramcontent.com/pod-product-compliance
Lightning Source LLC
LaVergne TN
LVHW072312090526
838202LV00019B/2272